P9-AFH-220

PROGRESS IN BRAIN RESEARCH

VOLUME 87

ROLE OF THE FOREBRAIN IN SENSATION AND BEHAVIOR

Recent volumes in PROGRESS IN BRAIN RESEARCH

Volume 71: Neural Regeneration, by F.J. Seil, E. Herbert and B.M. Carlson (Eds.) – 1987
Volume 72: Neuropeptides and Brain Function, by E.R. de Kloet, V.M. Wiegant and D. de Wied (Eds.) – 1987
Volume 73: Biochemical Basis of Functional Neuroteratology, by G.J. Boer, M.G.P. Feenstra, M. Mirmiran, D.F. Swaab and F. van Haaren (Eds.) – 1988
Volume 74: Transduction and Cellular Mechanisms in Sensory Receptors, by W. Hamann and A. Iggo (Eds.) – 1988
Volume 75: Vision within Extrageniculo-striate Systems, by T.B. Hicks and G. Benedek (Eds.) – 1988
Volume 76: Vestibulospinal Control of Posture and Locomotion, by O. Pompeiano and J.H.J. Allum (Eds.) – 1988
Volume 77: Pain Modulation, by H.L. Fields and J.-M. Besson (Eds.) – 1988
Volume 78: Transplantation into the Mammalian CNS, by D.M. Gash and J.R. Sladek, Jr. (Eds.) – 1988
Volume 79: Nicotinic Receptors in the CNS, by A. Nordberg, K. Fuxe, B. Holmstedt and A. Sundwall (Eds.) – 1989
Volume 80: Afferent Control of Posture and Locomotion, by J.H.J. Allum and M. Hulliger (Eds.) – 1989
Volume 81: The Central Neural Organization of Cardiovascular Control, by J. Ciriello, M.M. Caverson and C. Polosa (Eds.) – 1989
Volume 82: Neural Transplantation: From Molecular Basis to Clinical Applications, by S. Dunnett and S.-J. Richards (Eds.) – 1990
Volume 83: Understanding the Brain through the Hippocampus, by J. Storm-Mathison, J. Zimmer and O.P. Ottersen (Eds.) – 1990
Volume 84: Cholinergic Neurotransmission: Functional and Clinical Aspects, by S.-M. Aquilonius and P.-G. Gillberg (Eds.) – 1990
Volume 85: The Prefrontal Cortex: Its Structure, Function and Pathology, by H.B.M. Uylings, C.G. van Eden, J.P.C. de Bruin, M.A. Corner and M.G.P. Feenstra (Eds.) – 1991
Volume 86: Molecular and Cellular Mechanisms of Neuronal Plasticity in Normal Aging and Alzheimer's Disease, by P.D. Coleman, G.A. Higgins and C.H. Phelps (Eds.) – 1990

PROGRESS IN BRAIN RESEARCH

VOLUME 87

ROLE OF THE FOREBRAIN IN SENSATION AND BEHAVIOR

EDITED BY

G. HOLSTEGE

Department of Anatomy, Medical School, University of Groningen, Groningen, The Netherlands

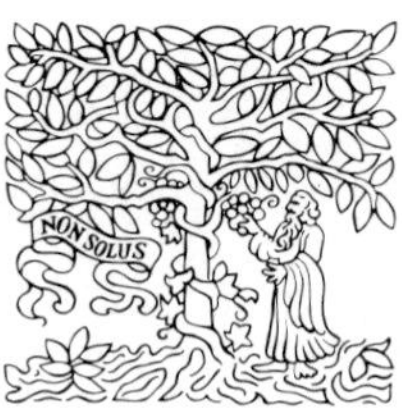

ELSEVIER
AMSTERDAM – NEW YORK – OXFORD
1991

ISBN 0-444-81181-8 (volume)
ISBN 0-444-80104-9 (series)

Published by:
Elsevier Science Publishers B.V. (Biomedical Division)
P.O. Box 211
1000 AE Amsterdam
(The Netherlands)

Sole distributors for the USA and Canada:
Elsevier Science Publishing Company, Inc.
655 Avenue of the Americas
New York, NY 10010
(U.S.A.)

This book is printed on acid-free paper
Printed in The Netherlands

List of Contributors

G.F. Alheid, University of Virginia, Department of Otolaryngology/Box 430, Charlottesville, VA 22908, U.S.A.

G. Balercia, Institute of Anatomy, Medical Faculty, Strada Le Grazie, 37134 Verona, Italy.

R. Bandler, Brain-Behavior Laboratory, Department of Anatomy, The University of Sydney, Sydney, NSW, Australia 2006.

M. Bentivoglio, Institute of Anatomy, Medical Faculty, Strada Le Grazie, 37134 Verona, Italy.

P. Carrive, Brain-Behavior Laboratory, Department of Anatomy, The University of Sydney, Sydney, NSW, Australia 2006.

P.D. Cheney, Department of Physiology and Ralph L Smith Research Center, University of Kansas Medical Center, 39th Rainbow Boulevard, Kansas City, KS 66103, U.S.A.

L. Feigenbaum Langer, Department of Brain and Cognitive Sciences, Massachusetts Institute of Technology, E25-618, 45 Carleton Street, Cambridge, MA 02139, U.S.A.

E.E. Fetz, Department of Physiology and Biophysics, University of Washington, Seattle, WA 98195, U.S.A.

J.M. Fuster, Department of Psychiatry and Brain Research Institute, School of Medicine, University of California at Los Angeles, Los Angeles, CA 90024, U.S.A.

A.M. Graybiel, Department of Brain and Cognitive Sciences, Massachusetts Institute of Technology, E25-618, 45 Carleton Street, Cambridge, MA 02139, U.S.A.

O. Hikosaka, National Institute for Physiological Sciences, Myodaiji, Okazaki 444, Japan.

L. Heimer, University of Virginia, Department of Otolaryngology/Box 430, Charlottesville, VA 22908, U.S.A.

G. Holstege, Department of Anatomy, University of California San Francisco and NASA/Ames Research Center, Moffett Field, CA 94035, U.S.A. (*Present address*): Department of Anatomy, Medical School, University of Groningen, Oostersingel 69, 9713 EZ Groningen, The Netherlands.

J. Jiménez-Castellanos, Department of Brain and Cognitive Sciences, Massachusetts Institute of Technology, E25-618, 45 Carleton Street, Cambridge, MA 02139, U.S.A.

E.G. Jones, Department of Anatomy and Neurobiology, University of California, Irvine, Irvine, CA 92717, U.S.A.

L. Kruger, Institute of Anatomy, Medical Faculty, Strada Le Grazie, 37134 Verona, Italy.

A.D. Loewy, Department of Anatomy and Neurobiology, Washington University School of Medicine, 660 South Euclid Avenue, Box 8108, St Louis, MO 63110, U.S.A.

K. Mewes, Department of Physiology and Ralph L Smith Research Center, University of Kansas Medical Center, 39th Rainbow Boulevard, Kansas City, KS 66103, U.S.A.

E.A. Murray, Laboratory of Neuropsychology, National Institute of Mental Health, Building 9, Room 1N107, Bethesda, MD 20892, U.S.A.

J. de Olmos, Instituto de Investigacion Medica, Cordoba, Argentina.

H.J. Ralston III, Department of Anatomy, University of California San Francisco, School of Medicine, San Francisco, CA 94143, U.S.A.

L.W. Swanson, Howard Hughes Medical Institute, The Salk Institute for Biological Studies, La Jolla, CA 92037, U.S.A. (*Present address*): Hedco Neurosciences Building, mc 2520, University of Southern California, Los Angeles, CA 90089, U.S.A.

Wm.D. Willis, Jr., Department of Anatomy and Neurosciences and Marine Biomedical Institute, University of Texas Medical Branch, Galveston, TX 77550, U.S.A.

L. Zaborszky, University of Virginia, Department of Otolaryngology/Box 430, Charlottesville, VA 22908, U.S.A.

S.P. Zhang, Brain-Behavior Laboratory, Department of Anatomy, The University of Sydney, Sydney, NSW, Australia 2006.

Foreword

The fourteen articles gathered in this volume constitute the Proceedings of a symposium held in honor of Dr. William R. Mehler on the occasion of his retirement from the NASA-Ames Research Center at Moffett Field, California.

Dr. Mehler's career as a neuroanatomist spanned more than three decades. Although he distinguished himself in particular by his pioneering studies on the efferent connections of the spinal cord, cerebellum, and basal ganglia, his work touched upon a multitude of other subjects within the area of Neuromorphology that recently come to be called 'Systems Neuroanatomy'. Moreover, beyond the bounds of that discipline Mehler's work inspired, and provided a beacon of light in several subsequent neurophysiological, neuropharmacological, and behavioral studies. It therefore seems most appropriate that the contents of this volume represent various research disciplines, and range over nearly all major subdivisions of the central nervous system, from spinal cord to cerebral cortex. All who are engaged in research on the brain's structure and function will find much of unique value in this volume. All who are familiar with Dr. Mehler's life's work, and especially those who, like the writer of this Foreword, have benefitted from his generosity in sharing his vast knowledge with his colleagues, will take delight in so fitting a tribute to a pioneer of Neuroscience. All will wish him well for the future.

W.J.H. Nauta

Preface

This volume of Progress in Brain Research contains the proceedings of a symposium *'Role of the forebrain in sensation and behavior'* held on May 26 and 27, 1989 in honor of William R. Mehler, who retired as senior scientist from NASA/Ames Research Center in California.

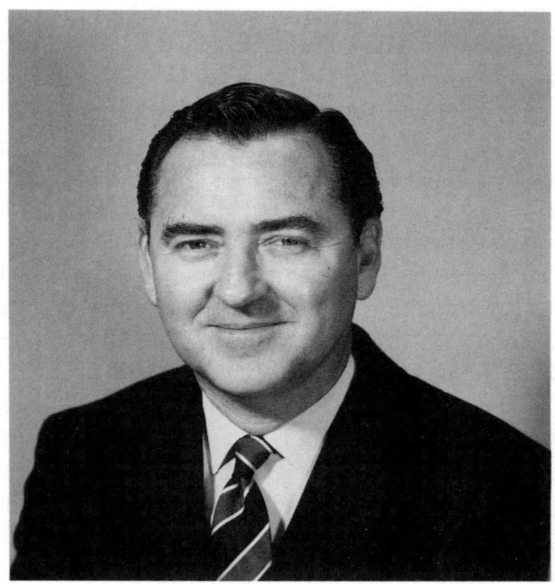

Bill Mehler was born on April 26, 1926 in Cleveland, Ohio. After highschool he served in the Hospital Corps of the United States Navy from 1944 to 1946. In 1949 he received his Bachelors degree at the John Carroll University and from 1949 to 1952 he was a graduate fellow at the Department of Anatomy, St. Louis University, St. Louis, Missouri, where he received his Masters degree in 1951. After two years in the Division of Anatomy at the University of Tennessee and one year at the Laboratory of Neuroanatomical Sciences at NIH he joined Dr. Walle Nauta (see Foreword) at the Department of Neurophysiology of the Walter Reed Army Institute of Research in Washington in 1955, where he stayed until 1962. In 1959 he received his Ph.D. in Neuroanatomy at the University of Maryland. From 1962 to 1989 Bill was research scientist at the Neurobiology Branch of NASA/Ames Research Center, a position he combined with that of lecturer in Anatomy (until 1972) and Associate Professor of Anatomy (until 1987) at the University of California, San Francisco. Nauta's influence on Mehler's scientific career is unmistakable and Bill's interest is mainly in systems or networks. Several of Bill's studies can be considered as a key to understand the function of a certain area of the brain. Perhaps best known is his work on the ascending pain pathways. He studied these pathways in monkey and man with the silver degeneration (Nauta) technique and the results can be considered as a breakthrough in our understanding of how the central nervous system processes information (see Bill Willis in the first chapter of the book). Also in the thalamic afferent system, Mehler has produced some innovative concepts. His 'idea of a new anatomy of the thalamus' was among the first in modern times to deal with the question of thalamic parcellation on the basis of afferent fiber systems, and his study served as a model for all subsequent studies of their type, according to Ted Jones in his contribution (Chapter 3) to this volume.

Bill Mehler not only has worked in the pain pathways and the thalamic afferent system, but he has studied also the basal ganglia including the dorsal and ventral striatum and substantia nigra, the amygdala as well as motor systems such as the emetic control areas in the brainstem. His interests have led us to organize a symposium in his honor, where the forebrain plays the key role, but which includes the forebrain's somatosensory afferent, and its efferent motor pathways.

Bill Willis gives an update of all the new findings on the organization of the ascending pain pathways since the first papers of Mehler (Chapter 1). Peter Ralston presents some great work on the precise terminations of the ascending pathways in the somatosensory thalamus (Chapter 2). Ted Jones brings forward the concept that the thalamus essentially has two modes of operation: the relay mode and the state dependent mode (Chapter 3). Marina Bentivoglio, Giancarlo Balercia and Lawrence Kruger review the midline thalamic nuclei, which have been encumbered with an erratic status for almost a century of experimental studies on thalamic projections (Chapter 4).

The organization of the dorsal striatum is discussed in Chaptert 5 by Laura Langer, Juan Jiménez-Castellanos and Ann Graybiel, while Okihide Hikosaka reveals how the striatum and substantia nigra influence the superior colliculus, which gives important clues for understanding the motor function of the basal ganglia (Chapter 6). The organization of the ventral striatum, including amygdala and bed nucleus of the stria terminalis (extended amygdala) is extensively reviewed by Lennart Heimer, Jose de Olmos, George Alheid and Laszlo Zaborsky (Chapter 7) and some insights in the function of the amygdala and hippocampus in memory is given by Betsy Murray (Chapter 8).

In respect to the motor output of the forebrain, Larry Swanson describes in Chapter 9 the hypothalamic circuits mediating responses to stress, and Joaquin Fuster the organization and function of the prefrontal cortex in relation to behavior (Chapter 10). How the motor cortex influences the motor output via its projections to the spinal cord is described by Paul Cheney, Eberhart Fetz and Klaus Mewes, who also include the rubrospinal tract in their review (Chapter 11). The recent findings concerning the role of the forebrain in autonomic control is discussed by Arthur Loewy in Chapter 12.

As early as 1958 Walle Nauta has published his famous paper on the limbic-midbrain circuits. Since then many other studies indicated that the midbrain periaqueductal gray with the adjacent mesencephalic tegmentum can be considered as the caudal pole of the limbic system and that the ventral forebrain uses this part of the mesencephalon as its motor output system. Richard Bandler, Pascal Carrive and Shi Ping Zhang describe the viscerotopic, somatotopic and functional organization of the periaqueductal gray in Chapter 13. In the last Chapter (14) Gert Holstege reviews the anatomy of the descending pathways of the motor system from the forebrain, including the brainstem areas which are 'used' by the forebrain motor system. His conclusion is that two different systems exist; a somatic (second) and a limbic (third) system on top of a basic (first) system consisting of the direct premotor interneurons in spinal cord and brainstem.

We are still far from a complete understanding of how the forebrain functions. However, the proceedings of this symposium show the enormous progress made since the first papers of Bill Mehler in the 1950s, a progress to which Bill himself has contributed so much.

Gert Holstege
Groningen, The Netherlands
February 1991

Acknowledgements

This volume largely represents material that was presented at a conference in honor of Dr. W.R. Mehler, held at NASA/Ames Research Center, Moffett Field, California, USA, in May 1989. The Editor acknowledges the generous financial support of the National Science Foundation (Grant BNS-8912693) and the National Aeronautics and Space Administration (NASA-grant NCC 2-491). I thank Joan Vernikos-Danellis and Cindy Bollens of the Life Science Division of NASA/Ames Research Center for their great support in organizing the symposium and Peter Room, Nel Barneveld-Schelling and Gerry Hoogenberg of the Dept. of Anatomy and Embryology of the Medical School of the Rijksuniversiteit Groningen for their editorial and administrative support.

Gert Holstege

Contents

G. Holstege (Ed.)
Progress in Brain Research, Vol. 87

CHAPTER 1

Role of the forebrain in nociception

Wm. D. Willis, Jr.

Department of Anatomy and Neurosciences and Marine Biomedical Institute, University of Texas Medical Branch, Galveston, TX 77550, U.S.A.

The experience of pain includes the sensation of pain and a number of pain reactions, including such motivational-affective responses as arousal, somatic and autonomic reflexes, and endocrine changes (Hardy et al., 1952; Melzack and Casey, 1968; Price and Dubner, 1977). The forebrain is likely to be involved in all of these, but the emphasis here will be on the role of the forebrain in the sensory aspects of pain. Evidence concerning the pathways ascending from the spinal cord that carry nociceptive information crucial to pain sensation will first be reviewed. Then experimental work on neurons in the somatosensory thalamus and cerebral cortex that respond to painful stimuli will be considered. Finally, the effects of stimulation of the somatosensory thalamus and cerebral cortex in modulating nociceptive transmission in the spinal cord will be discussed.

Ascending nociceptive pathways

Pain sensation in primates, including humans, appears to depend chiefly on information transmitted by pathways ascending in the lateral funiculus of the spinal cord. Evidence for this includes the following. A lesion of the anterolateral funiculus of the human spinal cord due to disease or to surgical intervention will result in analgesia on the contralateral side of the body below the lesion (Brown-Sequard, 1860; Gowers, 1878; Spiller, 1905; Spiller and Martin, 1912; Foerster and Gagel, 1932; White and Sweet, 1969). Similarly, an anterolateral cordotomy in the monkey reduces reactions to contralateral noxious stimulation below the level of the lesion (Yoss, 1953; Vierck and Luck, 1979). Evidently, axons from a crossed pathway that ascend in the anterolateral white matter of the spinal cord are necessary for normal pain sensation. It should be noted that months to years after an initially successful cordotomy, pain may recur (White and Sweet, 1969). The reason for this is unclear, but it is possible that there are alternative pathways that assume an important role in pain transmission some time following injury to the primary pathway(s).

A second observation concerning a role of the anterolateral quadrant in pain sensation is that pain could still be detected and localized on the contralateral side below the level of a transection of the spinal cord that spared only the anterolateral quadrant (Noordenbos and Wall, 1976). Interestingly, an unpleasant sensation without a pricking quality could also be elicited by stimulation of the ipsilateral lower extremity with a pin, suggesting that at least some aspects of pain can be mediated through uncrossed pathways. The fact that well localized pain sensation was transmitted through the contralateral anterolateral quadrant indicates that pathways in this sector of the spinal cord are sufficient for pain sensation.

A third argument favoring the idea that pain sensation depends upon transmission in the anterolateral quadrant is that stimulation within this part of the spinal cord during percutaneous cordotomy can evoke pain, provided that the appropriate parameters of electrical stimulation are used (Mayer et al., 1975).

The ascending pathways that are present within the anterolateral quadrant in the monkey and in man have been studied in detail with silver degeneration techniques by Mehler and his colleagues (Mehler et al., 1960; Mehler, 1962; 1966; 1969; 1974). Pathways that are likely to be important for nociception include the spinothalamic, spinomesencephalic and spinoreticular tracts. The most important termination sites of the spinothalamic tract include the ventral posterior lateral (VPL) nucleus and the central lateral (CL) nucleus, as shown in Fig. 1. A number of other thalamic projection targets of the spinothalamic tract have also been described, including the posterior complex, the nucleus submedius and others (Boivie, 1979; Berkley, 1980; Craig and Burton, 1981).

Based on evidence from a variety of sources, it seems reasonable to formulate a working hypothesis that the spinothalamic tract is an important pathway for mediating pain sensation. Emphasis will therefore be given here on a review of the properties of neurons belonging to this pathway. Spinomesencephalic and spinoreticular neurons are also likely to play an important role in pain. A working hypothesis is that these tracts are more important for motivational-affective pain reactions and for the activation of descending modulatory pathways than for pain sensation. Evidence for the first part of this hypothesis is that strong electrical stimulation in the central gray region of the midbrain in human subjects may

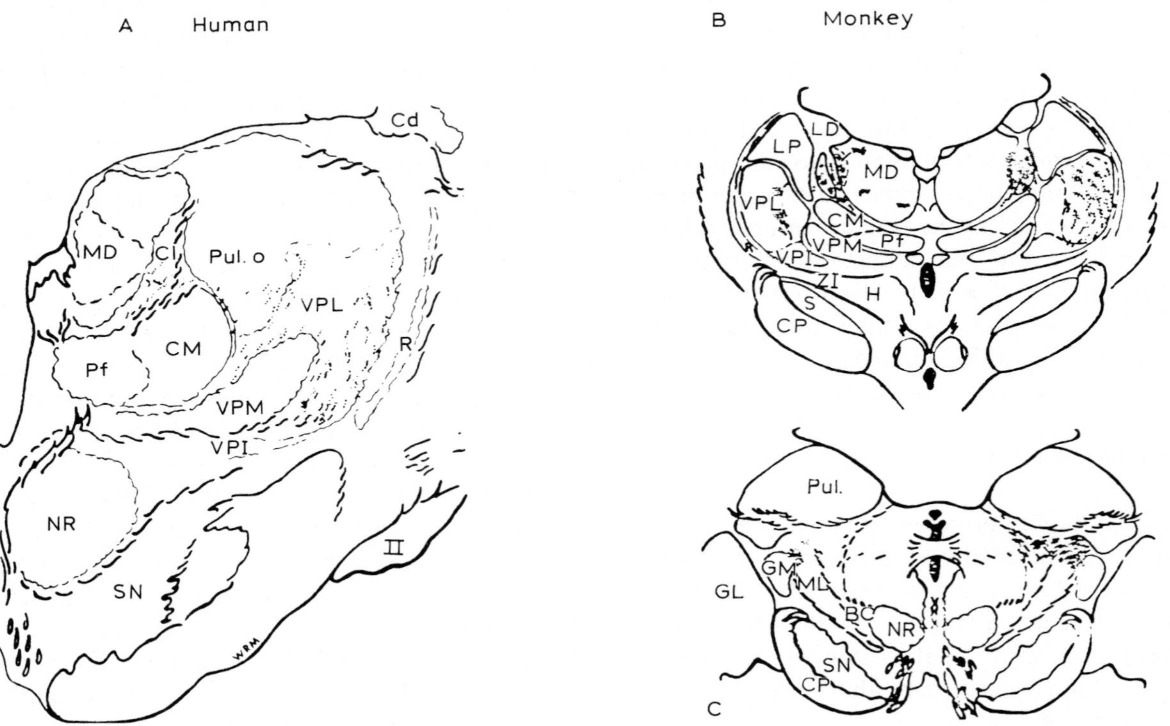

Fig. 1. Terminations of the primate spinothalamic tract as demonstrated by anterograde tracing of degeneration following anterolateral cordotomy. A shows the pattern in the human and B in the monkey. Abbreviations of thalamic nuclei: CL, central lateral; CM, centre median; DM or MD, dorsal medial; LD, lateral dorsal; LP, lateral posterior; Pul, pulvinar; VPL, ventral posterior lateral. (From Mehler, 1974; Mehler et al., 1960.)

cause emotional effects, such as fear (Nashold et al., 1969).

Spinothalamic tract neurons that project to the lateral thalamus (chiefly the VPL nucleus) have been shown by retrograde labeling with horseradish peroxidase to be concentrated in Rexed's laminae I and IV – VI of the contralateral dorsal horn (Fig. 2A; Willis et al., 1979; Apkarian and Hodge, 1989a). Neurons in similar locations project to the medial thalamus, but many of the medially projecting spinothalamic neurons are located in the ventral horn, especially in lamina VII and VIII (Fig. 2B). Recently, it has been found that most of the STT neurons in lamina I of monkeys project to the thalamus by way of the contralateral dorsal lateral funiculus, whereas most of the STT cells in laminae IV – VI and in the ventral horn project through the ventral lateral quadrant (Apkarian and Hodge, 1989b).

An electrophysiological mapping study demonstrated that many spinothalamic tract cells that can be antidromically activated from the VPL nucleus send collaterals to the CL nucleus; these are presumably the neurons that share a common location in laminae I and IV – VI with STT neurons that project only to the VPL nucleus (Giesler et al., 1981). On the other hand, STT cells that project just to the medial thalamus are located more ventrally in the spinal cord gray matter (Giesler et al., 1981). The response properties of STT cells that project to the VPL nucleus and of those that project both to the VPL and the CL nucleus are comparable, whereas the response properties of STT cells projecting just to the CL nucleus are quite different (Giesler et al., 1981), implying a different functional role for these different populations of STT cells.

STT cells that project to the VPL nucleus can be classified according to their responsiveness to cutaneous stimulation. Most of the neurons have receptive fields of a restricted size on the side of the body contralateral to the thalamic projection

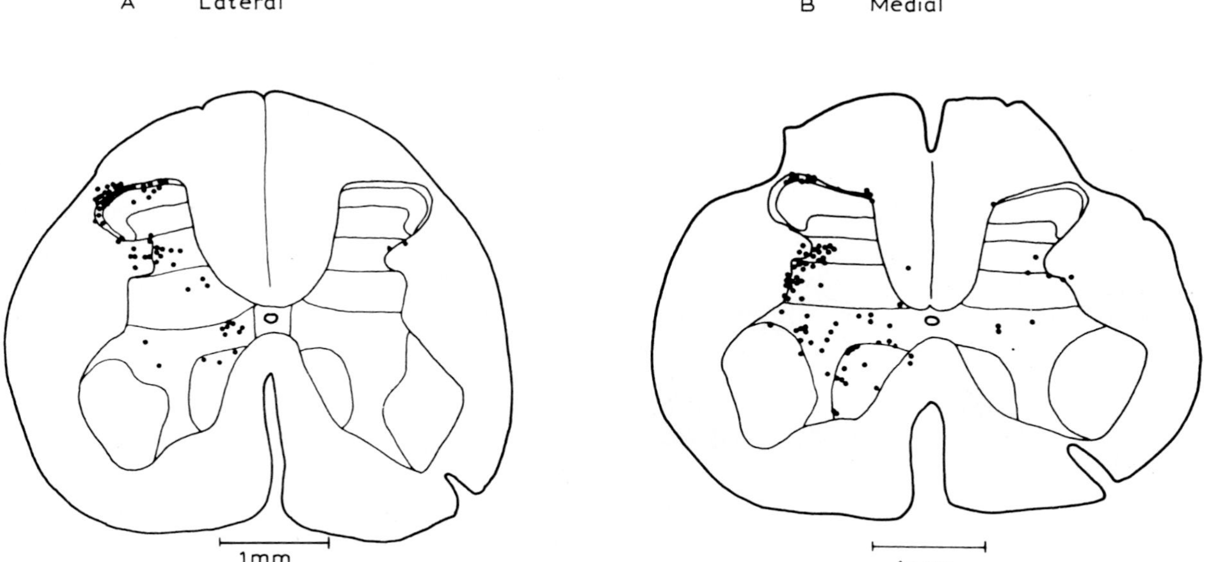

Fig. 2. Laminar distribution of spinothalamic tract cells in the monkey spinal cord. Spinothalamic tract cells were labeled retrogradely by injection of horseradish peroxidase into the thalamus. Most labeled cells were contralateral to the injection site. The locations of the labeled cells are plotted with reference to Rexed's laminae. In A are shown cells labeled from the lateral thalamus (region of the ventral posterior lateral nucleus) and in B from the medial thalamus (region of the central lateral nucleus). (From Willis et al., 1979.)

target of the neuron. STT neurons in lamina I tend to have smaller receptive fields than do STT neurons in laminae IV – VI (Fig. 3). A small proportion (about 15%) of these neurons respond best to tactile stimuli, whereas most (85 %) respond best to noxious stimuli (Fig. 4A; Chung et al., 1986a; Surmeier et al., 1988). The tactile neurons can be termed class 1 STT cells. Almost all of these are located in laminae IV – VI (Fig. 4B). At least 2 different types of nociceptive STT neurons can be distinguished. Class 2 cells have a steep stimulus-response relation throughout the noxious range, whereas class 3 cells have a stimulus-response relation that is shallow for lower intensities of noxious stimuli but steep at the higher intensities (Fig. 4A). STT cells also respond to graded noxious heat pulses (Kenshalo et al., 1979; Surmeier et al., 1986a,b). Again, neurons with steep or shallow stimulus-response functions can be recognized.

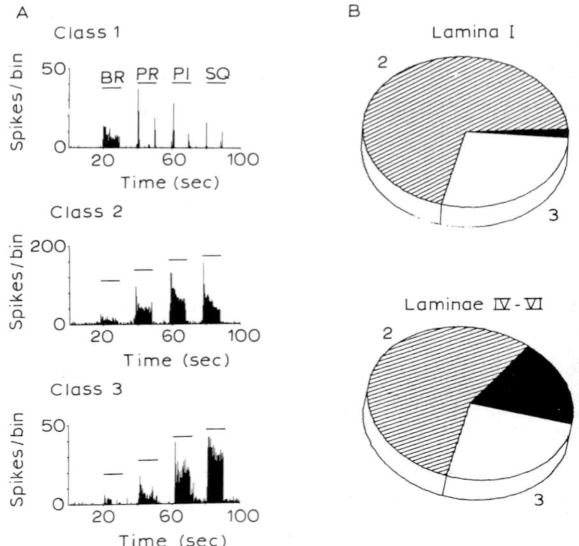

Fig. 4. Classification of primate spinothalamic tract cells. The cells were assigned to one of three types, depending upon their responses to mechanical stimulation of the skin. Typical response profiles are shown in A. Class 1 cells responded best to brushing (BR), but poorly to pressure (PR), pinch (PI) or squeeze (SQ). Class 2 cells responded about as well to PI and to SQ, but weakly to BR and PR. Class 3 cells responded best to SQ. The proportions of cells of different classes in lamina I and in laminae IV – VI are shown in B.

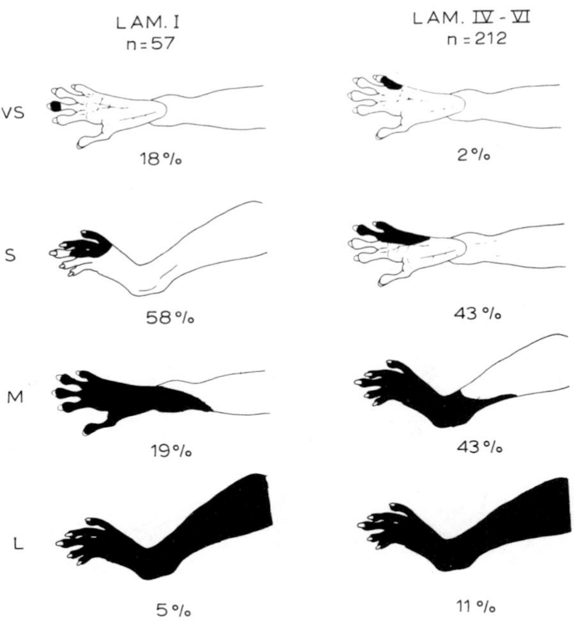

Fig. 3. Receptive fields of primate spinothalamic tract cells projecting to the ventral posterior lateral nucleus. The receptive fields were classified by size as very small (VS), small (S), medium (M) and large (L). The proportions of spinothalamic tract cells in lamina I versus laminae IV – VI having different sized receptive fields are indicated. (From Willis, 1989.)

The distinction between nociceptive neurons with steep versus shallow stimulus-response functions appears to be of importance for the role of these neurons in sensory discrimination. Similar neurons have been found in the subnucleus caudalis of the spinal nucleus of the trigeminal nerve in awake, behaving monkeys trained to discriminate between noxious heat pulses of different intensities (Maixner et al., 1989). The ability of the monkeys to make discriminations correlated well with the capacity of the nociceptive neurons with steep stimulus-response relations to discriminate between the same thermal stimuli, whereas there was no correlation of the behavioral events with the responses of the neurons with shallow stimulus-response functions.

STT cells that project only to the CL nucleus in

the medial thalamus often have very large receptive fields that encompass most or all of the surface of the body and face (Fig. 5; Giesler et al., 1981). Such neurons would be unable to provide information about stimulus location. These neurons generally responded poorly but selectively to noxious stimuli. It was suggested that they were more likely to participate in the motivational-affective component of pain than in the sensory discriminative aspects.

As mentioned earlier, pain in humans may recur months to years following an initially succesful anterolateral cordotomy. Presumably, alternative nociceptive pathways are present in areas of the spinal cord outside the anterolateral quadrant. Candidate pathways include the component of the STT that arises from lamina I (provided that this ascends in the dorsal lateral funiculus of the human, as in monkeys; this has as yet not been demonstrated), the uncrossed component of the spinothalamic tract (about 5 – 10% of the projection to the VPL nucleus from the cervical and lumbosacral enlargements is uncrossed; Willis et al., 1979; Apkarian and Hodge, 1989a), and somatosensory pathways ascending ipsilaterally in the dorsal white matter of the spinal cord. The latter include the spinocervical tract and the postsynaptic dorsal column pathway. Recently, nociceptive neurons have been demonstrated in the lateral cervical nucleus and the nucleus gracilis of the monkey that project to the contralateral VPL nucleus (Downie et al., 1988; Ferrington et al., 1988) and that may be excited by these pathways.

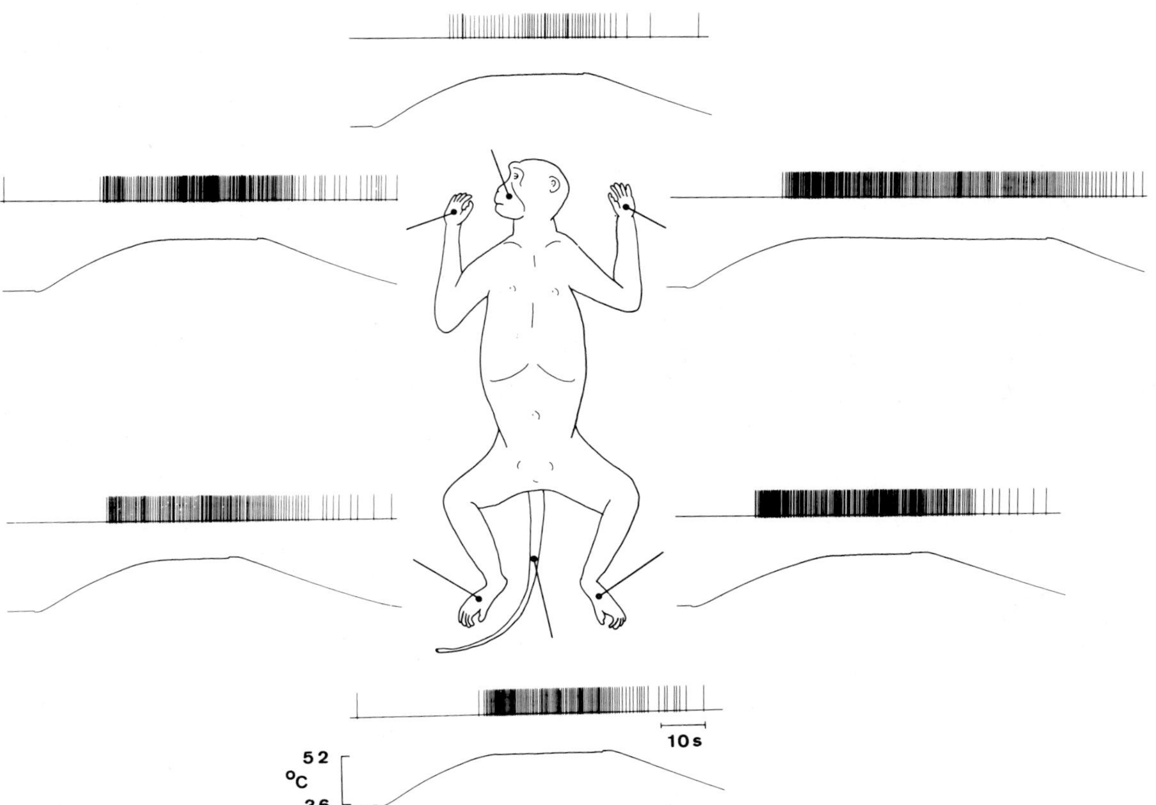

Fig. 5. Receptive field of a primate spinothalamic tract cell that projected to the medial but not to the lateral thalamus. The cell responded to the application of noxious heat pulses to all four extremities, the face and the tail. (From Giesler et al., 1981.)

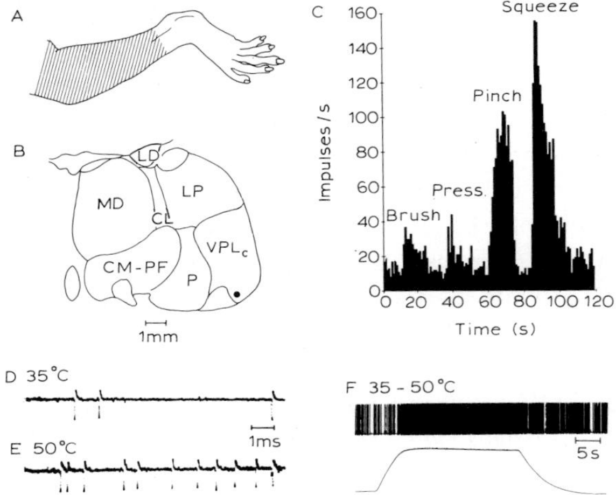

Fig. 6. Responses of a nociceptive neuron in the ventral posterior lateral nucleus of the monkey thalamus. The receptive field is shown in A and the location of the neuron in B. The cell was excited best by noxious mechanical stimulation of the skin, as shown in C. Responses to a noxious heat pulse are shown in D – F. (From Kenshalo et al., 1980.)

Nociceptive neurons of the VPL nucleus

Nociceptive responses have been observed during recordings from neurons of the VPL nucleus in the monkey (Fig. 6; Kenshalo et al., 1980; Chung et al., 1986b). In some experiments, it was possible to interfere with nociceptive transmission by placing a lesion in the spinal cord above the level of sensory input to the spinal cord. Usually, a lesion of the dorsal quadrant ipsilateral to the noxious input had little effect on the response of the VPL neuron, whereas a lesion of the contralateral lateral funiculus eliminated the response (Fig.7), indicating that the ascending pathway conveying the nociceptive information crossed at the spinal cord level and ascended in the lateral funiculus. In a few cases, however, the nociceptive input to the VPL nucleus appeared to be transmitted by way of the dorsal part of the spinal cord (Fig. 8). These observations are consistent with the view that the

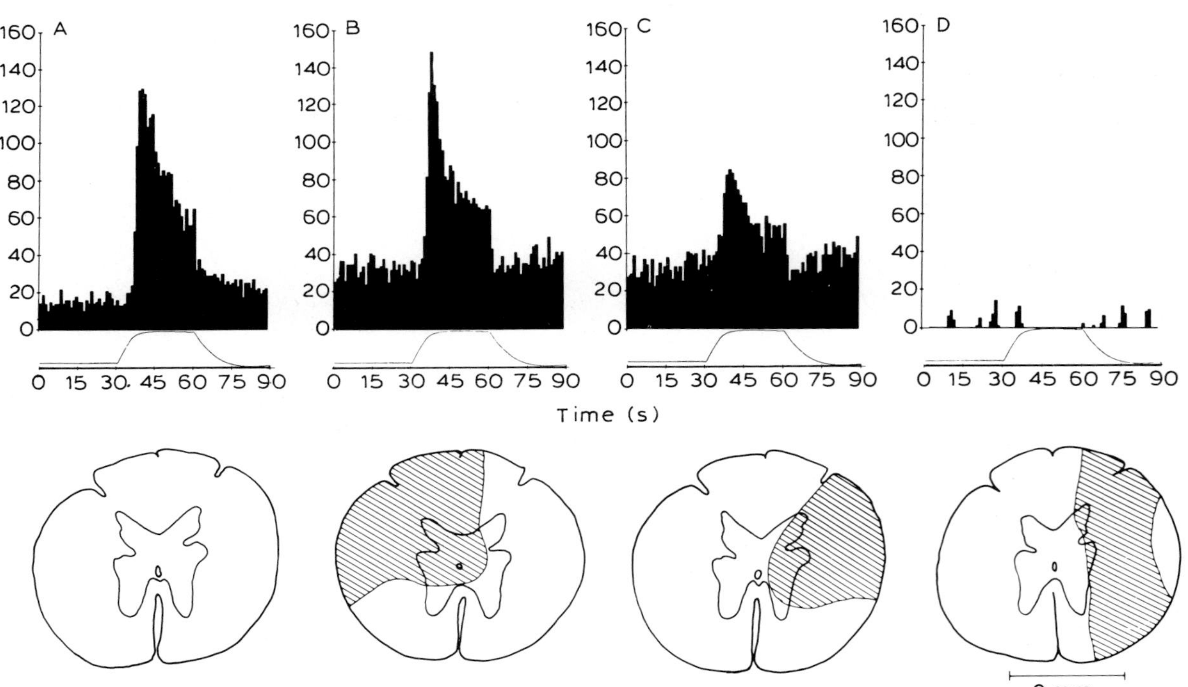

Fig. 7. Dependence of nociceptive input to a neuron of the primate ventral posterior lateral nucleus on pathways ascending in the lateral funiculus. In A is shown the response to a noxious heat pulse with the spinal cord intact. In B, the response is essentially unchanged after a lesion of the dorsal quadrant of the spinal cord ipsilateral to the noxious stimulus (contralateral to the thalamic unit). C and D show that lesioning the lateral funiculus on the opposite side eliminated the response. (From Kenshalo et al., 1980.)

STT. is the main pathway in the primate involved in transmitting nociceptive information to the VPL nucleus of the thalamus, but that other pathways, such as the spinocervical and/or postsynaptic dorsal column pathways, may play an ancillary role.

The nociceptive neurons found in the VPL nucleus were somatotopically organized (Kenshalo et al., 1980). Those having receptive fields on the contralateral lower extremity were in the lateral part of the VPL nucleus, and those with receptive fields on the upper extremity were in the medial part of the VPL nucleus. The neurons projected to the somatotopically appropriate part of the SI cortex, as shown by antidromic activation using microstimulation (Kenshalo et al., 1980). The effective stimulus sites were concentrated near the border between areas 3b and 1.

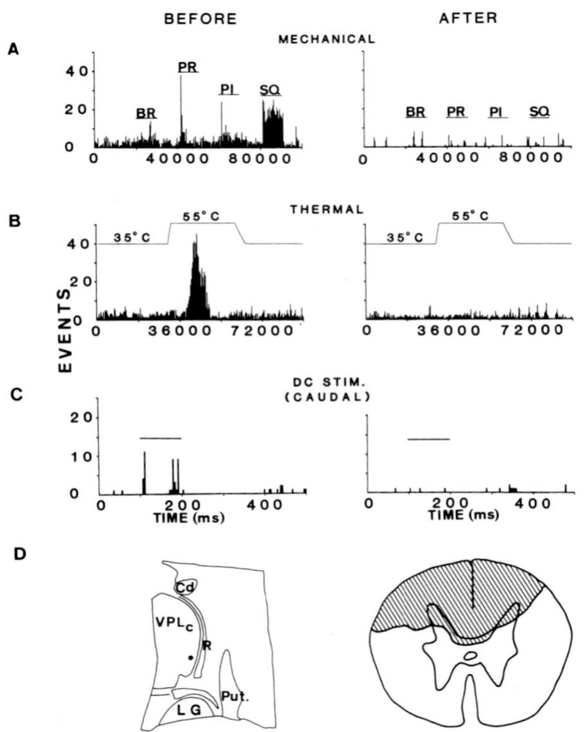

Fig. 8. Dependence of nociceptive input to a neuron of the primate ventral posterior lateral nucleus upon pathways in the dorsal part of the spinal cord. The cell responded well to squeezing the skin (SQ, A, left) and to a noxious heat pulse (B, left) before the lesion, but there was no response to these stimuli after the lesion (A, B, right). Stimulation of the dorsal column (DC) below the level of the lesion also activated the neuron before (C, left) but not after (C, right) the lesion. The location of the cell is shown to the left in D, and the maximal extent of the lesion at the right. (From Chung et al., 1986b.)

Nociceptive neurons in the SI cortex

Nociceptive responses have also been recorded from neurons in the SI cortex of both anesthetized (Kenshalo and Isensee, 1983) and awake, behaving monkeys (Kenshalo et al., 1988). Most of these cells were located in area 1. Many of the nociceptive cortical neurons had restricted contralateral receptive fields and responded best to noxious mechanical and thermal stimulation (Fig. 9). These cells appeared to be well suited for signalling the sensory discriminative aspects of pain sensation. In awake, behaving animals, the responses of such neurons correlated well with the ability of the animal to discriminate between different intensities of noxious heat stimulation (Kenshalo et al., 1988). Other neurons in the same region of the SI cortex had very large receptive fields, occupying much of the surface of the body (Kenshalo and Isensee, 1983). Such neurons may play a role in arousal or in attentional mechanisms, rather than in sensory discrimination.

Modulation of STT neurons by stimulation in the VPL nucleus

In addition to a role in the transmission of nociceptive information to the SI cortex, the ventrobasal complex appears to contribute to the modulation of the transmission of nociceptive information. Stimulation in the ventrobasal thalamus (or the adjacent internal capsule) in patients experiencing central pain is often useful in alleviating the pain (Adams et al., 1974; Hosobuchi et al., 1973; Mazars, 1975; Tsubokawa et al., 1982).

In monkeys, it has been shown that stimulation in the VPL nucleus can result in the inhibition of STT cells (Fig. 10; Gerhart et al., 1981; 1983). The inhibition can be produced by stimulating on either

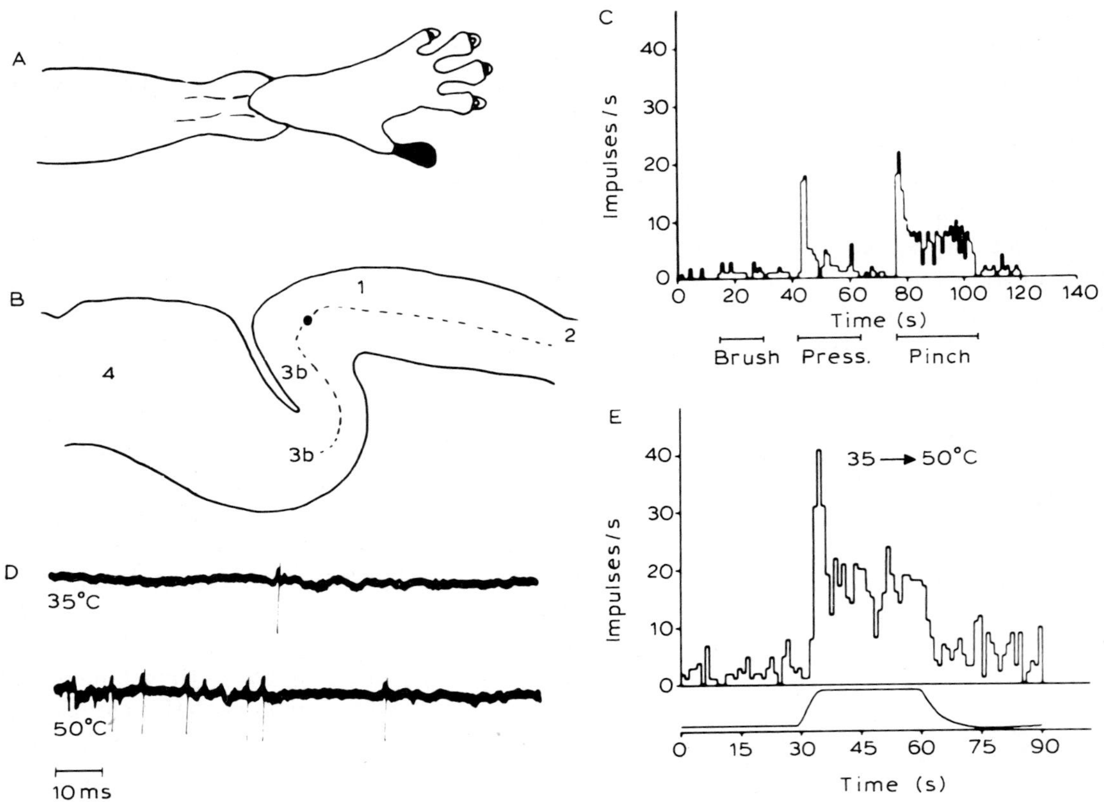

Fig. 9. Responses of a neuron in the SI cortex of a monkey to noxious stimuli. The receptive field of the cell is shown in A and its location in the middle layers of area 1 in B. The responses of the neuron to noxious mechanical and thermal stimuli are seen in C – E. (From Kenshalo and Isensee, 1980.)

side of the brain. The mechanism is uncertain. One possibility is that stimulation in the ventrobasal complex activates ascending projections from the spinal cord and brainstem antidromically, with the consequence that collaterals of the ascending axons activate neurons in modulatory structures of the brainstem, such as the periaqueductal gray (PAG) or the reticular formation, which in turn cause inhibition of spinal cord neurons. Recordings from neurons in the raphe nuclei has in fact demonstrated that such neurons can be excited following stimulation in the VPL nucleus (Tsubokawa et al., 1982; Willis et al., 1984). Another possibility is that activation of ascending projections from the ventrobasal complex (or internal capsule) engage neurons in the SI cortex that in turn modulate the activity of STT neurons (see next section).

Effects of stimulation in the sensory-motor cortex

There is clinical evidence that lesions of the SI cortex can affect pain sensation. Permanent loss of pain sensation in restricted regions of the contralateral body can be produced by cortical lesions (Russell, 1945; Marshall, 1951; Lende et al., 1971), although some clinical reports deny this (Head, 1920; Head and Holmes, 1911; Holmes, 1927). Another possible outcome of cortical lesions is the production of a central pain syndrome that resembles "thalamic pain" (see review by Cassinari and Pagni, 1969).

In monkeys, stimulation in the SI cortex or in the posterior parietal association cortex (area 5) frequently causes inhibition of STT neurons (Fig. 11; Coulter et al., 1974; Yezierski et al., 1983). The inhibition may be unselective or it may be more effective for innocuous than for noxious stimuli.

Interestingly, stimulation of the motor cortex (or the medullary pyramid) often causes excitation (or excitation followed by inhibition) of STT cells (Fig. 12; Coulter et al., 1974; Yezierski et al., 1983). The excitation appeared to depend upon the integrity of the lateral corticospinal tract, since a lesion of this pathway at an upper cervical level abolished the action. The inhibition from the parietal cortex was only partially reduced by the same lesion, suggesting that the pathway included

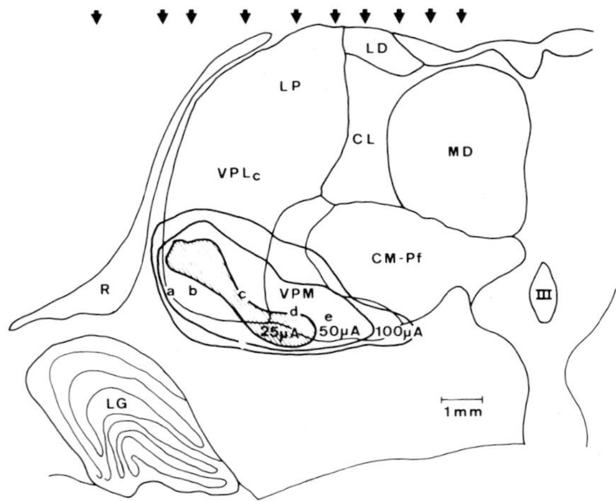

Fig. 10. Map of the sites in the ventrobasal complex of the thalamus of a monkey that when stimulated produced inhibition of a spinothalamic tract cell. The map was produced by stimulating in a grid along tracks whose trajectories are indicated by the arrows at the top of the drawing. The contours across the ventral posterior lateral (VPL) and medial (VPM) nuclei enclosed the lowest threshold regions for evoking inhibition (using 25, 50 and 100 μA stimuli). The letters a – e indicate sites at which multiunit receptive fields were recorded through the stimulating electrode to verify the location of the electrode tip. (From Gerhart et al., 1983.)

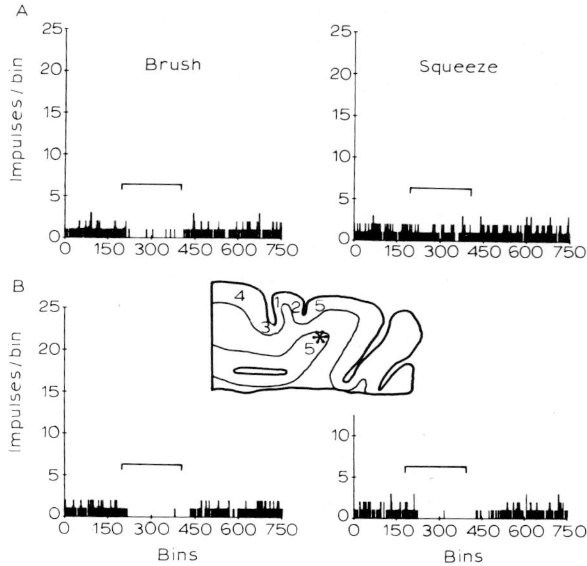

Fig. 11. Inhibition of two different primate spinothalamic neurons following stimulation in the posterior parietal cortex (area 5). The activity of the neurons was increased above background either by brushing (left column) or by squeezing (right column) the receptive field on the skin. Cortical stimulation inhibited the response of the first cell to brushing preferentially (A), but was non-selective for the second cell (B). (From Yezierski et al., 1983.)

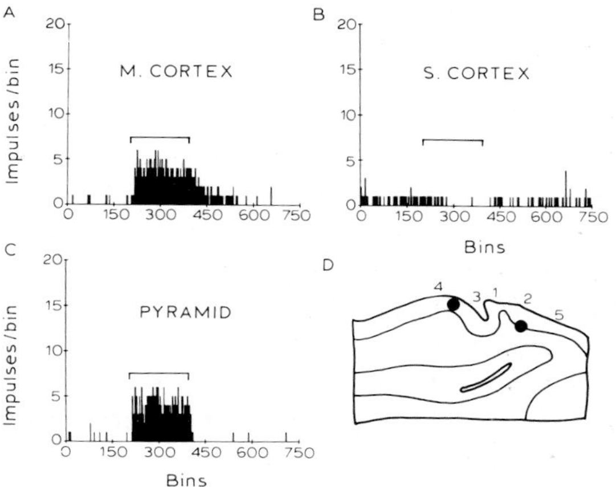

Fig. 12. Excitation of a primate spinothalamic tract cell by stimulation of the motor cortex or pyramid. The excitatory effects are shown in A and C. Stimulation of the SI cortex produced inhibition, as shown in B. The stimulus sites are indicated in D. (From Yezierski et al., 1983.)

not only the lateral corticospinal tract but axons descending in other tracts (Yezierski et al., 1983).

The excitatory effect of stimulation of the motor cortex on STT cells may be important in motor behavior. For example, there could be concomitant commands from the motor cortex to initiate exploratory activity of a hand and excitation of sensory pathways, including the spinothalamic tract, to enhance the sensitivity of such pathways to potential somatic stimuli that might be encountered during the exploratory activity.

Conclusions

Clinical and experimental evidence indicates that the forebrain plays an important role in pain sensation. Sensory discriminative processing of pain sensation appears to depend chiefly upon pathways ascending in the lateral funiculus contralateral to a painful stimulus, but ipsilateral pathways may play an ancillary role as well. Nociceptive neurons in the ventral posterior lateral nucleus transmit information about painful stimuli to neurons in the somatosensory cortex. How the nociceptive information is further processed is as yet unclear. The involvement of the somatosensory cortex in the processing of nociceptive information helps explain the transient or permanent loss of pain sensation of the contralateral side of the body that occurs in at least some cases of cortical damage. The return of pain sensation in other cases suggests that other cortical areas are also involved.

The somatosensory thalamus and sensorimotor cortex, like many structures of the brainstem, help modulate nociceptive information at a spinal cord level. Stimulation in the ventrobasal complex or in the sensory cortex or posterior parietal cortex results in the inhibition of spinothalamic tract cells, whereas stimulation in the motor cortex produces an excitation or excitation followed by inhibition of these neurons. The excitation of nociceptive tract cells by stimulation of the motor cortex may reflect an attentional mechanism. The inhibitory role of the sensory cortex may offer a partial explanation of the central pain syndrome that results in some cases of cortical damage.

In addition to these roles of the cerebral cortex in pain sensation, the forebrain is heavily involved in many other aspects of the reaction to pain. However, the analysis of these is at an early stage.

Acknowledgements

The author thanks his many collaborators for their participation in experiments that were done in his laboratory. He also thanks Griselda Gonzales for her help with the illustrations and Margie Watson for her assistance with the manuscript. The experiments were supported by NIH grants NS 09743 and NS 11255.

References

Adams, J.E., Hosobuchi, Y. and Fields, H.L. (1974) Stimulation of internal capsule for relief of chronic pain. *J. Neurosurg.*, 41: 740 – 744.

Apkarian, A.V. and Hodge, C.J. (1989a) The primate spinothalamic pathways: I. A quantitative study of the cells of origin of the spinothalamic pathway. *J. Comp. Neurol.*, 288: 447 – 473.

Apkarian, A.V. and Hodge, C.J. (1989b) The primate spinothalamic pathways: II. The cells of origin of the dorsolateral and ventral spinothalamic pathways. *J. Comp. Neurol.*, 288: 474 – 492.

Berkley, K.J. (1980) Spatial relationships between the terminations of somatic sensory and motor pathways in the rostral brainstem of cats and monkeys. I. Ascending somatic sensory inputs to lateral diencephalon. *J. Comp. Neurol.*, 193: 283 – 317.

Boivie, J. (1979) An anatomical reinvestigation of the termination of the spinothalamic tract in the monkey. *J. Comp. Neurol.*, 186: 343 – 370.

Brown-Sequard, C.E. (1860) Course of lectures on the physiology and pathology of the central nervous system. Lippincott, Philadelphia.

Cassinari, V. and Pagni, C.A. (1969) Central Pain. Harvard Univ. Press, Cambridge.

Chung, J.M., Surmeier, D.J., Lee, K.H., Sorkin, L.S., Honda, C.N., Tsong, Y. and Willis, W.D. (1986a) Classification of primate spinothalamic and somatosensory thalamic neurons based on cluster analysis. *J. Neurophysiol.*, 56: 308 – 327.

Chung, J.M., Lee, K.H., Surmeier, D.J., Sorkin, L.S., Kim, J. and Willis, W.D. (1986b) Response characteristics of neurons in the ventral posterior lateral nucleus of the monkey thalamus. *J. Neurophysiol.,* 56: 370 – 390.

Coulter, J.D., Maunz, R.A. and Willis, W.D. (1974) Effects of stimulation of sensorimotor cortex on primate spinothalamic neurons. *Brain Res.,* 351 – 356.

Craig, A.D. and Burton, H. (1981) Spinal and medullary lamina I projection to nucleus submedius in medial thalamus: a possible pain center. *J. Neurophysiol.,* 45: 443 – 466.

Downie, J.W., Ferrington, D.G., Sorkin, L.S. and Willis, W.D. (1988) The primate spinocervicothalamic pathway: responses of cells of the lateral cervical nucleus and spinocervical tract to innocuous and noxious stimuli. *J. Neurophysiol.,* 59: 861 – 885.

Ferrington, D.G., Downie, J.W. and Willis, W.D. (1988) Primate nucleus gracilis neurons: responses to innocuous and noxious stimuli. *J. Neurophysiol.,* 59: 886 – 907.

Foerster, O. and Gagel, O. (1932) Die Vorderseitenstrangdurchschneidung beim Menschen. Eine klinisch-pathophysiologisch-anatomische Studie. *Z. Ges. Neurol. Psychiat.,* 138: 1 – 92.

Gerhart, K.D., Yezierski, R.P., Fang, Z.R. and Willis, W.D. (1983) Inhibition of primate spinothalamic tract neurons by stimulation in ventral posterior lateral (VPLc) thalamic nucleus: possible mechanisms. *J. Neurophysiol.,* 49: 406 – 423.

Gerhart, K.D., Yezierski, R.P., Wilcox, T.K., Grossman, A.E. and Willis, W.D. (1981) Inhibition of primate spinothalamic tract neurons by stimulation in ipsilateral or contralateral central posterior lateral (VPLc) thalamic nucleus. *Brain Res.,* 229: 514 – 519.

Giesler, G.J., Yezierski, R.P., Gerhart, K.D. and Willis, W.D. (1981) Spinothalamic tract neurons that project to medial and/or lateral thalamic nuclei: evidence for a physiologically novel population of spinal cord neurons. *J. Neurophysiol.,* 46: 1285 – 1308.

Gowers, W.R. (1878) A case of unilateral gunshot injury to the spinal cord. *Trans. Clin. Lond.* 11: 24 – 32.

Hardy, J.D., Wolff, H.G. and Goodell, H. (1952) *Pain Sensations and Reactions.* Williams and Wilkins, New York. Reprinted by Hafner, New York, 1967.

Head, H. (1920) Studies in Neurology, vol. II. Oxford Univ. Press, London.

Head, H. and Holmes, G. (1911) Sensory disturbances from cerebral lesions. *Brain,* 34: 102 – 254.

Holmes, G. (1927) Disorders of sensation produced by cortical lesions. *Brain,* 50: 413 – 427.

Hosobuchi, Y., Adams, J.E. and Rutkin, B. (1973) Chronic thalamic stimulation for the control of facial anesthesia dolorosa. *Arch. Neurol.,* 29: 158 – 161.

Kenshalo, D.R., Jr., Chudler, E.H., Anton, F. and Dubner, R. (1988) SI nociceptive neurons participate in the encoding process by which monkeys perceive the intensity of noxious thermal stimulation. *Brain Res.,* 454: 378 – 382.

Kenshalo D.R., Jr., Giesler, G.J., Leonard, R.B. and Willis, W.D. (1980) Responses of neurons in primate ventral posterior lateral nucleus to noxious stimuli. *J. Neurophysiol.,* 43: 1594 – 1614.

Kenshalo, D.R., Jr. and Isensee, O. (1983) Responses of primate SI cortical neurons to noxious stimuli. *J. Neurophysiol.,* 50: 1479 – 1496.

Kanshalo, D.R., JR., Leonard, R.B., Chung, J.M. and Willis, W.D. (1979) Responses of primate spinothalamic neurons to graded and to repeated noxious heat stimuli. *J. Neurophysiol.,* 42: 1370 – 1389.

Lende, R.A., Kirsch, W.M. and Druckman, R. (1971) Relief of facial pain after combined removal of precentral and postcentral cortex. *J. Neurosurg.,* 34: 537 – 543.

Maixner, W., Dubner, R., Kenshalo, D.R., Jr. Bushnell, M.C. and Oliveras, J.L. (1989) Responses of monkey medullary dorsal horn neurons during the detection of noxious heat stimuli. *J. Neurophysiol.,* 62: 437 – 449.

Marshall, J. (1951) Sensory disturbances in cortical wounds with special reference to pain. *J. Neurol. Neurosurg. Psychiat.,* 14: 187 – 204.

Mayer, D.J., Price, D.D. and Becker, D.P. (1975) Neurophysiological characterization of the anterolateral spinal cord neurons contributing to pain perception in man. *Pain,* 1: 51 – 58.

Mazars, G.J. (1975) Intermittent stimulation of nucleus ventralis posterolateralis for intractable pain. *Surg. Neurol.,* 4: 93 – 95.

Mehler, W.R. (1962) The anatomy of the so-called 'pain tract' in man: an analysis of the course and distribution of the ascending fibers of the fasciculus anterolateralis. In J.D. French and R.W. Porter (Eds.) *Basic Research in Paraplegia,* Charles C Thomas, Springfield, pp. 26 – 55.

Mehler, W.R. (1966) Some observations on secondary ascending afferent systems in the central nervous system. In R.S. Knighton and P.R. Dumke (Eds.), *Pain,* Little, Brown, Boston, pp. 11 – 32.

Mehler, W.R. (1969) Some neurological species differences- a posteriori. *Ann. N.Y. Acad. Sci.* 167: 424 – 468.

Mehler, W.R. (1974) Central pain and the spinothalamic tract. *Adv. Neurol.* 4: 127 – 146.

Mehler, W.R., Feferman, M.E. and Nauta, W.J.H. (1960) Ascending axon degeneration following anterolateral cordotomy. An experimental study in the monkey. *Brain,* 83: 718 – 751.

Melzack, R. and Casey, K.L. (1968) Sensory, motivational and central control determinants of pain. In D.R. Kenshalo (Ed.), *The Skin Senses,* Charles C. Thomas, Springfield, pp. 423 – 443.

Nashold, B.S., Wilson, W.P. and Slaughter, D.G. (1969) Sensations evoked by stimulation in the midbrain of man. *J. Neurosurg.,* 30: 14 – 24.

Noordenbos, W. and Wall, P.D. (1976) Diverse sensory functions with an almost totally divided spinal cord. A case of spinal cord transection with preservation of part of one anterolateral quadrant. *Pain,* 2: 185 – 195.

Price, D.D. and Dubner, R. (1977) Neurons that subserve the sensory-discriminative aspects of pain. *Pain,* 3: 307 – 338.

Russell, W.R. (1945) Transient disturbances following gunshot wounds of the head. *Brain,* 68: 79 – 97.

Spiller, W.G. (1905) The occasional clinical resemblance between caries of the vertebrae and lumbothoracic syringomyelia, and the location within the spinal cord of the fibres for the sensations of pain and temperature. *Univ. Penn. Med. Bull.,* 18: 147 – 154.

Spiller, W.G. and Martin, E. (1912) The treatment of persistent pain of organic origin in the lower part of the body by division of the anterolateral column of the spinal cord. *J.A.M.A.,* 58: 1489 – 1490.

Surmeier, D.J., Honda, C.N. and Willis, W.D. (1986a) Responses of primate spinothalamic neurons to noxious thermal stimulation of glabrous and hairy skin. *J. Neurophysiol.,* 56: 328 – 350.

Surmeier, D.J., Honda, C.N. and Willis, W.D. (1986b) Temporal features of the responses of primate spinothalamic neurons to noxious thermal stimulation of hairy and glabrous skin. *J. Neurophysiol.,* 56: 351 – 368.

Surmeier, D.J., Honda, C.N. and Willis, W.D. (1988) Natural groupings of primate spinothalamic neurons based on cutaneous stimulation. Physiological and anatomical features. *J. Neurophysiol.,* 59: 833 – 860.

Tsubokawa, T., Yamamoto, T., Katayama, Y. and Noriyasu, N. (1982) Clinical results and physiological basis of thalamic relay nucleus stimulation for relief of intractable pain with morphine tolerance. *Appl. Neurophysiol.,* 45: 143 – 155.

Vierck, C.J. and Luck, M.M. (1979) Loss and recovery of reactivity to noxious stimuli in monkeys with primary spinothalamic cordotomies, following by secondary and tertiary lesions of other cord sectors. *Brain,* 102: 233 – 248.

White, J.C. and Sweet, W.H. (1969) *Pain, its Mechanisms and Neurosurgical Control.* Thomas, Springfield, IL.

Willis, W.D. (1989) Neural mechanisms of pain discrimination. In J.S. Lund (Ed.), *Sensory Processing in the Mammalian Brain,* Oxford University Press, New York, pp. 130 – 143.

Willis, W.D., Gerhart, K.D., Willcockson, W.S., Yezierski, R.P., Wilcox, T.K. and Cargill, C.L. (1984) Primate raphe- and reticulospinal neurons: effects of stimulation in periaqueductal gray or VPLc thalamic nucleus. *J. Neurophysiol.,* 51: 467 – 480.

Willis, W.D., Kenshalo, D.R., Jr. and Leonard, R.B. (1979) The cells or origin of the primate spinothalamic tract. *J. Comp. Neurol.* 188: 543 – 574.

Yezierski, R.P., Gerhart, K.D., Schrock, B.J. and Willis, W.D. (1983) A further examination of effects of cortical stimulation on primate spinothalamic tract cells. *J. Neurophysiol.,* 49: 424 – 441.

Yoss, R.E. (1953) Studies of the spinal cord. 3. Pathways for deep pain within the spinal cord and brain. *Neurology,* 3: 163 – 175.

G. Holstege (Ed.)
Progress in Brain Research, Vol. 87

CHAPTER 2

Local circuitry of the somatosensory thalamus in the processing of sensory information

H.J. Ralston III

Department of Anatomy, University of California, San Francisco School of Medicine, San Francisco, CA 94143, U.S.A.

Thalamic sensory nuclei that transmit information in the various sensory systems have often been termed "relay nuclei". This description is clearly a misnomer, because "relay" implies that the signal is transmitted more or less unchanged through the thalamus. It is evident from physiological studies on the visual thalamus (Burke and Sefton, 1966; Fertziger and Purpura, 1971; Sherman and Koch, 1986) that a great deal of information processing occurs during thalamic transmission. Thalamic sensory nuclei receive principal afferent fibers from their primary source of afferent information: e.g., lateral geniculate nucleus (LGN), from retina; somatosensory thalamus (VB), from spinal cord, dorsal column nuclei, lateral cervical nucleus and the trigeminal complex. In addition, LGN and VB receive GABAergic projections from the immediately adjacent thalamic reticular nucleus (TRN) (Peschanski et al., 1983; Yen et al., 1985; Yingling and Skinner, 1976) in the case of VB, or the perigeniculate nucleus in the case of LGN. There are also projections from neurons in the cerebral cortex (Ralston, 1983; Yuan et al., 1986), principally arising from cells in layers V and VI of the cortex. Recent studies have shown that thalamic nuclei also receive projections from brainstem neurons which contain various neurotransmitters, including acetylcholine, serotonin, or norepinephrine (Jones, 1985). The LGN and VB of cat and monkey contain numerous (approximately 20%) local circuit neurons (LCNs) (LeVay and Ferster, 1979) which are GABAergic (Ohara et al., 1983; Spreafico et al., 1983) and which form inhibitory synapses with thalamocortical relay cells, either by dendrodentritic (Ohara et al., 1989) or axodendritic contacts. The nature of the response properties of thalamic neurons may mimic those of the primary afferent centers which project to them, or have properties which appear to be absent in the lower centers. For instance, a recent study demonstrates a major class of LGN neurons that differs substantially in their response properties from those found in the retina (Mastronarde, 1987), suggesting that there is significant modification of the afferent input effects on thalamic neurons.

The nature of the morphological features of neurons exhibiting different physiological properties has received intensive study. More than twenty years ago Guillery, (1986) described different morphological classes of the neurons in the cat LGN. Subsequent electrophysiological studies combined with intracellular labeling (Friedlander et al., 1981) led to the hypothesis that one functional class of LGN cells (X) corresponded morphologically to Guillery's Class II cell, which exhibits numerous dendritic appendages. Further, these studies suggested that another functional class (Y) corresponded to Guillery's morphologically-described Class I cell, which had longer. aspiny dendrites than the Class II cells. Some local circuit neurons (LCNs) also have X cell physiological properties but corresponded to Guillery's Class III or Class IV cells (Friedlander et al., 1981). Recent work in the geniculate has suggested that light microscopic morphological features correlate fairly consistently with X cell physiological properties (Humphrey and Weller, 1988). Rapisardi and Miles (1984) have made the interesting observation that the number of presumed inhibitory presynaptic dendritic contacts upon LGN relay cells (Koch, 1985) are abundant on those relay cells which have numerous dendritic appendages. Because X cells in LGN exhibit numerous dendritic appendages and Y cells do not, it appears that the morphological features of these cells may predict the inhibitory mechanisms mediated by the LCN neurons upon LGN projection cells. As will be discussed in this chapter, there are similar interrelationships between dendrites of LCNs and thalamocortical relay cells in the somatosensory thalamus (VB).

The correlation between the functionally characterized properties of neurons of the somatosensory thalamus and the morphological features of these neurons is not as evident as it appears to be in the visual thalamus. For instance, Peschanski et al. (1984) examined neurons of rat VB which had been physiologically characterized and intracellularly labeled. They compared the morphology of neurons which responded to noxious stimuli with those that responded only to non-noxious stimuli, and found no obvious distinctions between them, either at the light or electron microscopic level. Similarly, a light microscopic study by Yen et al. (1985) found no correlation between the modality properties and morphological features of ventrobasal neurons in the cat.

An analysis of the issues pertaining to the structural and functional properties of thalamic somatosensory nuclei are complicated by the fact that the somatosensory thalamus receives ascending inputs from the spinal cord, the dorsal column nuclei and the lateral cervical nucleus, in the case of the region of the thalamus subserving the body, (Berkley, 1973a,b; Blomqvist et al., 1985; Boivie, 1970; Boivie, 1971; Boivie, 1979; Burton and Craig, 1983) and from different regions of the trigeminal nuclear complex for that region of VB receiving from cranial structures. In addition, there are other regions of the thalamus which receive only from the spinal cord or the nucleus caudalis of the trigeminal nuclear complex and not from the dorsal column nuclei or the principal nucleus of the trigeminal. Furthermore, there are species differences in the organization of the somatosensory thalamus. In the rat and monkey, there is extensive overlap between the terminal projection zones of the dorsal column nuclei and the spinal cord (Ma et al., 1986). In contrast, in the cat, the terminal projection fields of these two systems are largely segregated, the dorsal column nuclei projecting to the "cutaneous core" of VB and the spinal cord projecting to a "shell" region, principally lying ventral and anterior to VB (Boivie, 1971). Furthermore, there are differences in the cellular constituents of the somatosensory thalamus: the cat and monkey have numerous GABAergic LCNs, which constitute about 20–25% of the total cellular population. In contrast, the rat somatosensory thalamus lacks these GABAergic local circuit cells (Lee, 1981; Spacek and Liberman, 1974; see also Jones, this volume). The dendritic appendages of GABAergic LCNs participate in "triadic" synaptic arrays with principle afferent (e.g. medial lemniscal) axons and thalamocortical projection neurons (Ohara et al., 1989; Ralston, 1969; Ralston, 1971; Ralston 1983). These triads are organized in such a way that the afferent axon synapses directly upon the proximal dendrite of the projection neuron, the postsynaptic dendritic structure often being a dendritic spine. The afferent axon also forms a synaptic contact upon a GABAergic appendage of an LCN and the appendage in turns forms a dendrodendritic synapse (Fig. 3) upon the projection cell (Ohara et al., 1989). Thus, the initial synaptic input of the principal afferent is excitatory to the projection neuron and also depolarizes the appendage of the LCN, which then releases GABA upon the same zone of the dendrite of the thalamocortical relay cell which receives the input from the principal afferent. There is thus a monosynaptic excitatory input from principal afferent to relay cell and a disynaptic inhibitory input, via the GABAergic LCN, upon the relay cell.

Our laboratory has been concerned for several years with elucidating the nature of the synaptic circuitry of the somatosensory thalamus and much of the information described in the preceding paragraphs has been obtained by various experimental approaches which we have conducted in the analysis of this circuitry. This chapter will provide new information concerning the intrinsic circuitry of the primate thalamus and compare the findings with previously obtained findings in rat and cat.

Experimental methods

All experimental procedures were carried out in anesthetized animals, and were in accord with the guidelines of the U.S. Department of Agriculture and the UCSF Committee on Animal Research.

It is necessary to use various techniques to label elements of neural networks within the central nervous system. The principal labeling techniques which we have used are experimentally induced Wallerian degeneration following lesions in a particular neural pathway, and the orthograde transport of wheatgerm lectin conjugated to horseradish peroxidase (WGA-HRP), subsequently demonstrated by histochemical methods for light and electron microscopic analysis. Animals are first immobilized with intramuscular injections of ketamine and subsequently anesthetized with intravenous injections of pentobarbital. Using sterile neurosurgical techniques, a particular region of the nervous system (e.g. the dorsal column nuclei) is visualized and an appropriate lesion placed or a microinjection (0.01 to 0.03 μl) of WGA-HRP made into a nuclear group using pressure applied through a microsyringe. Following various survival times, the animal is reanesthetized and perfused with mixed aldehydes. The thalamus and injection site are subsequently serially sectioned on a vibratome and reacted for the presence of HRP and examined by light and electron microscopic methods. We have recently adapted the use of ammonium molybdate (Olucha, 1985) and the slow osmication technique of Henry et al. (1985) for the electron microscopic analysis of transported WGA-HRP, because these combined methods yield excellent preservation of reaction product as well as preservation of fine structure.

We have addressed the issue of convergence of the projections of the dorsal column nuclei and the spinal cord upon single thalamic neurons by utilizing degeneration of dorsal column projections combined with labelling by WGA-HRP transport of spinal cord projections. We have also compared the terminal synaptic organization of the dorsal column projections and spinal cord projections following experiments in different animals and have analyzed the axonal arbors of these two systems by making serial sections of terminal projections and reconstructing the axonal arbors with a computer-assisted program.

Results and conclusions

Electron microscopy of the primate somatosensory thalamus (VPLc) reveals the same synaptic populations that have been described in the cat (Ralston and Herman, 1969). Small synaptic profiles (< 1 μm diameter) containing round vesicles ("SR" profiles) constitute about 70% of the total synaptic population and form synapses upon the distal dendritic tree of projection neurons (Fig. 1), as well as contacting the vesicle-containing dendrites of LCNs. The majority of SR terminals arise from the cerebral cortex (Ralston, 1983), although it is possible that some may be derived from brainstem neurons that project to the thalamus.

Figure 2 shows examples of the other 3 synaptic types found in the thalamus. "F" contains a tightly packed mixture of pleomorphic vesicles, varying from round to flattened and irregular sizes. "F" profiles often exceed 2 μm in diameter, constitute about 10% of the total synaptic population of VPLc and synapse upon projection cell dendrites and cell bodies as well as the vesicle-containing dendrites of LCNs. Many, if not all, of the F pro-

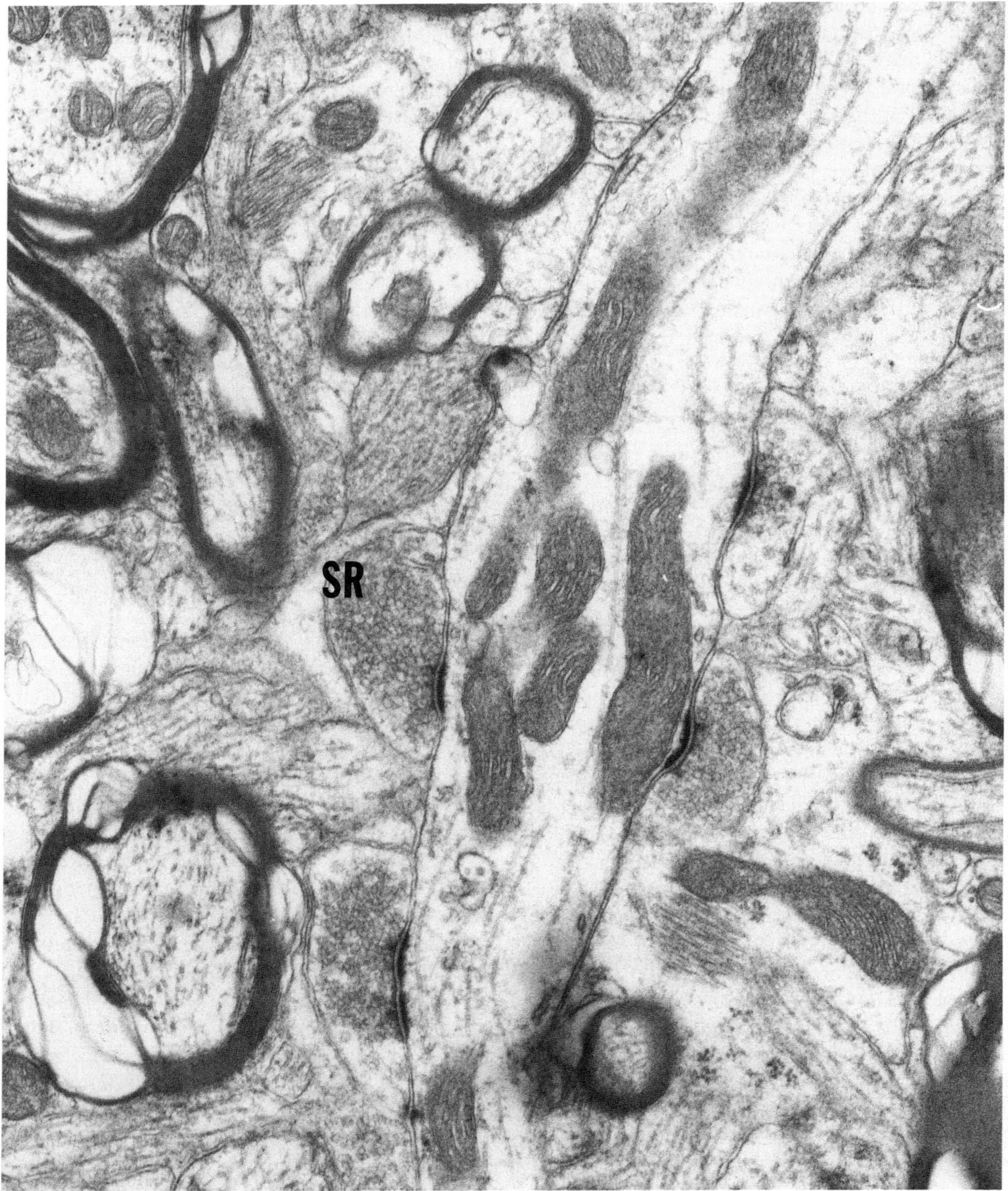

Fig. 1. A series of SR terminals (small profile, round vesicles) contacting a distal dendrite of a projection neuron in monkey VB.

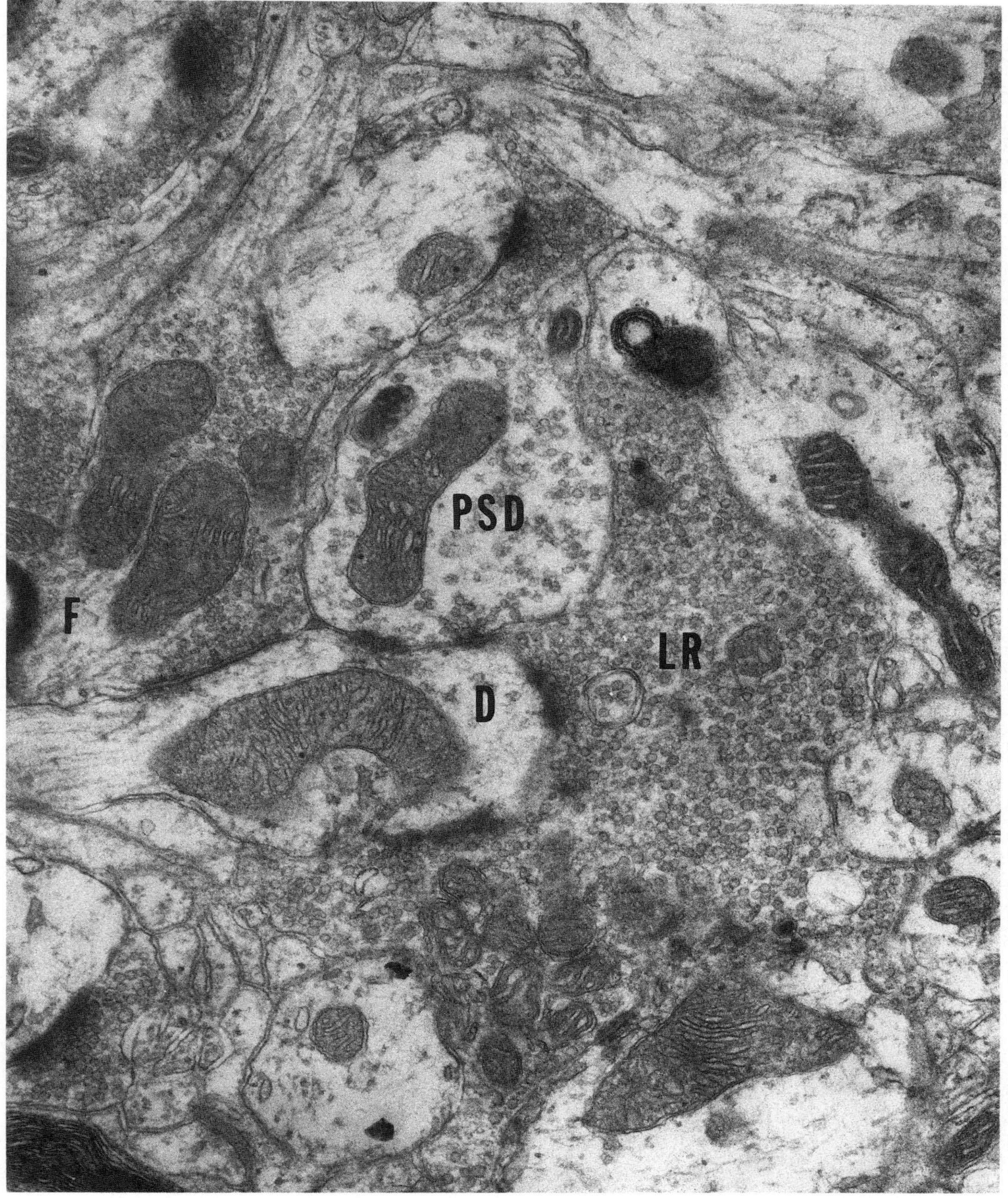

Fig. 2. An LR terminal (large profile, round vesicles) contacts a projection cell dendrite (D), which is also contacted by an F and by a PSD (presynaptic dendrite).

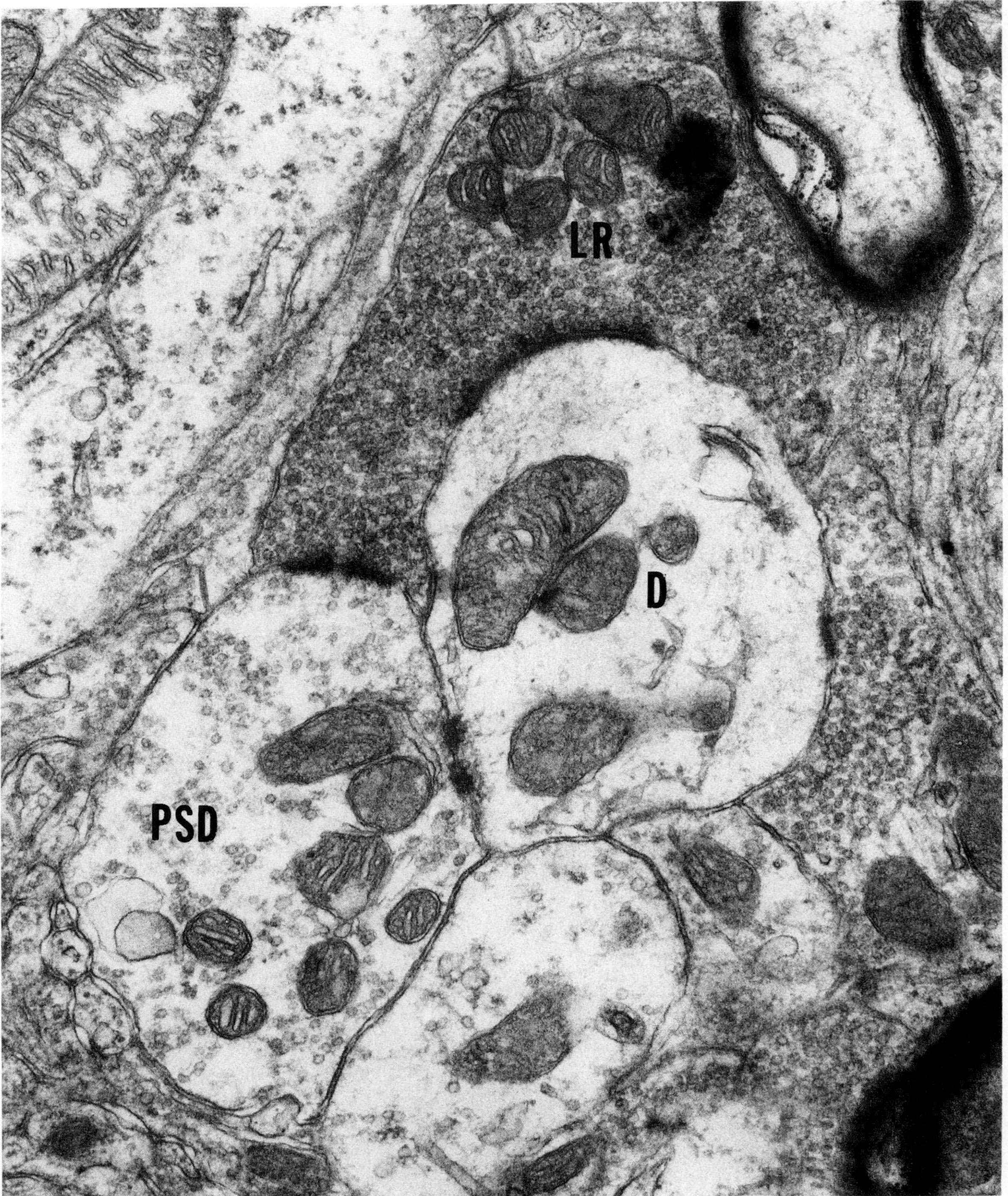

Fig. 3. A synaptic triadic complex, in which an LR profile synapses upon a projection neuron dendrite (D) and upon a PSD, which also contacts D. This synaptic array is typical of medial lemniscal terminations, and believed to mediate feed-forward, GABAergic inhibition.

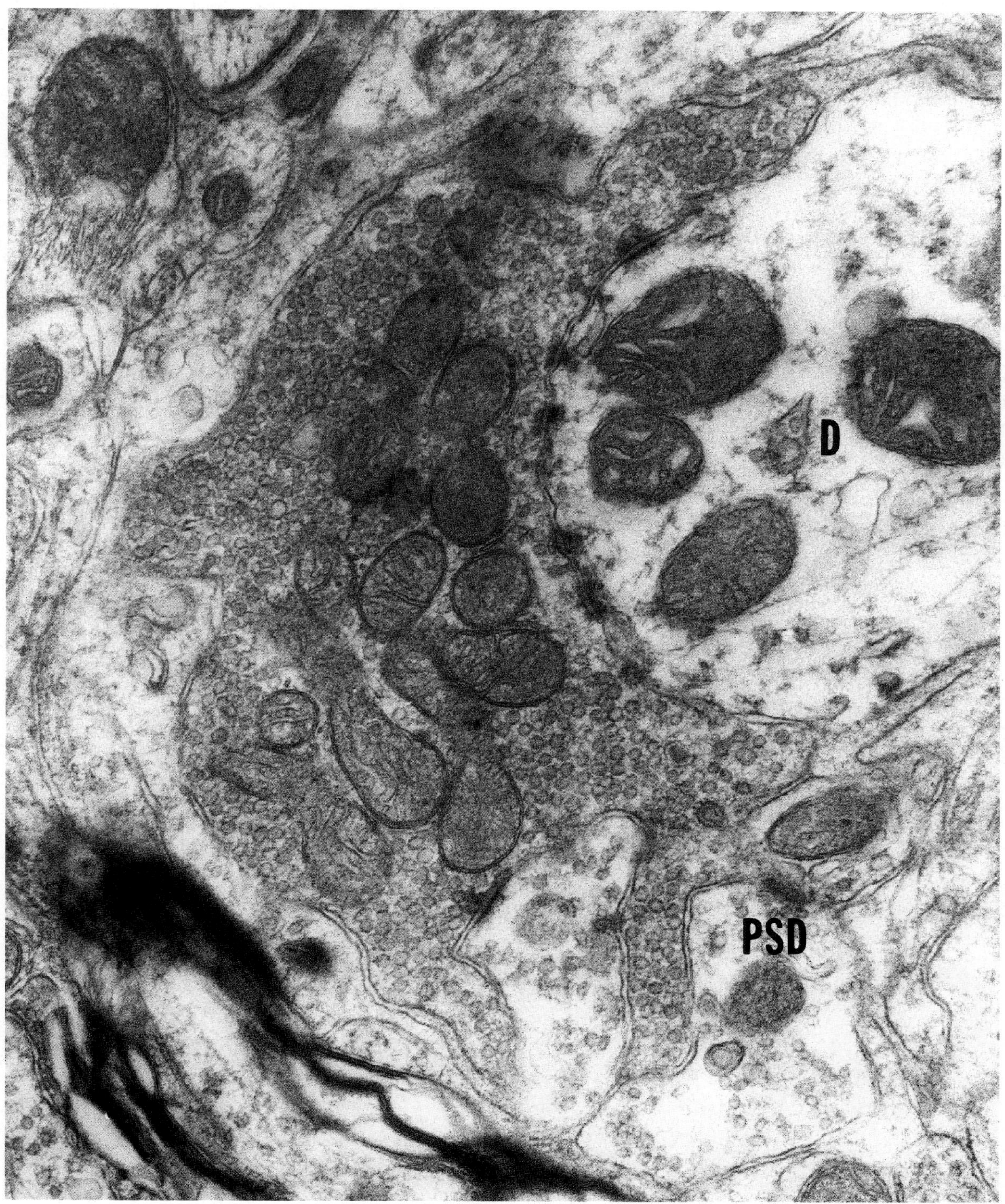

Fig. 4. An LR terminal synapsing upon a projection cell dendrite (D) and one of two PSDs.

files are GABAergic and arise from the thalamic reticular nucleus (Ohara et al., 1983; Peschanski et al., 1984). "PSD" profiles (presynaptic dendrites) have been shown in numerous studies (e.g., Ohara et al., 1989; Ralston, 1971; Ralston and Herman, 1969; Spacek and Lieberman, 1974; Spreafico et al., 1983) to be the vesicle containing shafts and appendages of GABAergic local circuit neurons. They contain scattered pleomorphic vesicles and comprise about 14% of the synaptic population of VPLc. They form synaptic contacts upon projection cell dendrites as well as upon other LCNs. They also receive synaptic contacts from the three axonal terminal types present in the thalamus (SR, F, LR) and are the only synaptic profiles which are found to be postsynaptic (Fig. 3) as well as presynaptic; there are no axoaxonal contacts in the thalamus (Ralston, 1969; Ralston and Herman, 1969) as all postsynaptic vesicle-containing profiles are the dendrites of LCNs.

The fourth synaptic type in the thalamus is a large profile with round vesicles ("LR") which measures 2 to 4 μm in diameter and constitutes about 6% of the synaptic population of VPLc. This LR profile is the axonal terminal of the principal afferent axon to the thalamus. In the case of VPLc it may be derived from the dorsal column nuclei (about 3/4 of all LR profiles), the spinal cord (about 1/4) or the lateral cervical nucleus (a very small component). LR profiles arising from the dorsal column nuclei synapse upon the proximal dendrites or dendritic appendages of projection neurons (Figs. 2, 3, 4) or the vesicle-containing dendritic appendages of LCNs (Figs.

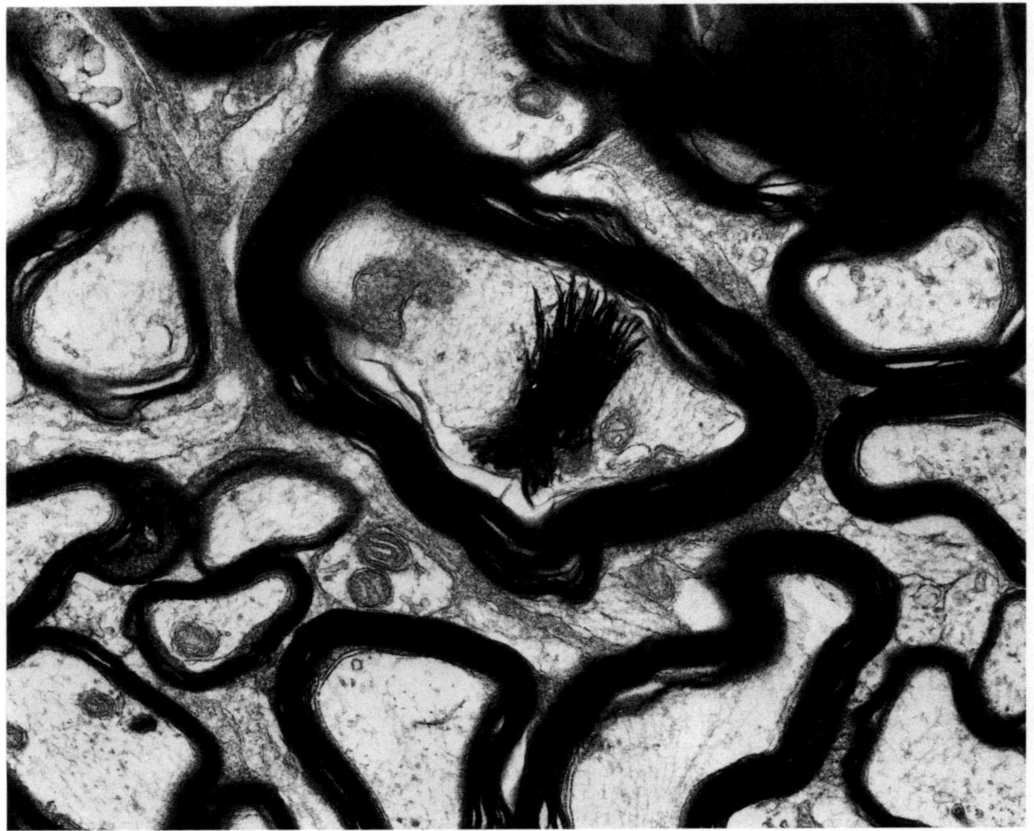

Fig. 5. Crystals of HRP reaction product inside a mylelinated axon in VPLc, following injection of WGA-HRP into the spinal cord.

3, 4). LR profiles which arise from the spinal cord (STT) as demonstrated following the axonal transport of WGA-HRP, are the terminations of small to medium-sized myelinated axons (Fig. 5). Following microinjections of WGA-HRP into the dorsal horn of the spinal cord of cervical or lumbar segments, labeled LR profiles in VPLc may be found contacting the dendrites of projection neurons (Fig. 7a, b), but only rarely are seen to synapse upon the vesicle-containing dendritic appendages of PSDs. This finding is in marked contrast to synapses formed by dorsal column projections, all of which appear to contact PSDs as well as projection neurons.

The dorsal column-medial lemniscal projections to thalamic neurons mediate nonnoxious information arising from cutaneous and deep tissues. The projections from the spinal cord, via the spinothalamic tract (STT), convey a mixture of noxious and nonnoxious information (Willis, 1987, see also Willis, this volume). In an earlier study, we have shown that the dorsal column system and the STT terminate on the same region of dendritic trees of rat VB neurons (Ma et al., 1987), being the first morphological demonstration of such convergence. Individual VB neurons of monkey have been shown to exhibit a wide range of responses when examined by the ''cluster analysis'' method of Willis and his colleagues (Chung et al., 1986). Most monkey neurons respond in varying degrees to nonnoxious or noxious peripheral input, which suggests that the cells receive varying degrees of input from the dorsal column or spinothalamic pathways. Using methods which identify dorsal column projections by causing them to degenerate following experimental ablation of the dorsal column nuclei, and the anterograde transport of WGA-HRP demonstrated by the method mentioned above, we have developed evidence that the dorsal column nuclei and STT pathways converge upon different regions of the arbors of individual thalamic neurons in the monkey, rather than ending on the same dendritic branch as they do in the rat. This raises the interesting possibility that the primate segregates the input from these two major afferent systems on seperate elements of its dendritic tree rather than having them terminate on immediately adjacent dendritic regions.

We have used computer-assisted reconstruction of serial sections through labeled medial lemniscal terminals and STT terminals to analyze the synaptic circuitry associated with these major somatosensory afferents to primate VB. The crystalline reaction product is readily visualized in medial lemniscal or STT terminals and the relationships between the labeled terminal with projection cell dendrites or the vesical-containing dendritic appendages of LCNs is easily recognized. What is not evident in single sections is the degree of complexity of the synaptic relationships of afferent terminals with projection cell dendrites and LCN appendages. Fig. 8 shows a computer generated reconstruction of the synaptic relationships of a single medial lemniscal terminal with several different GABAergic appendages of one or more

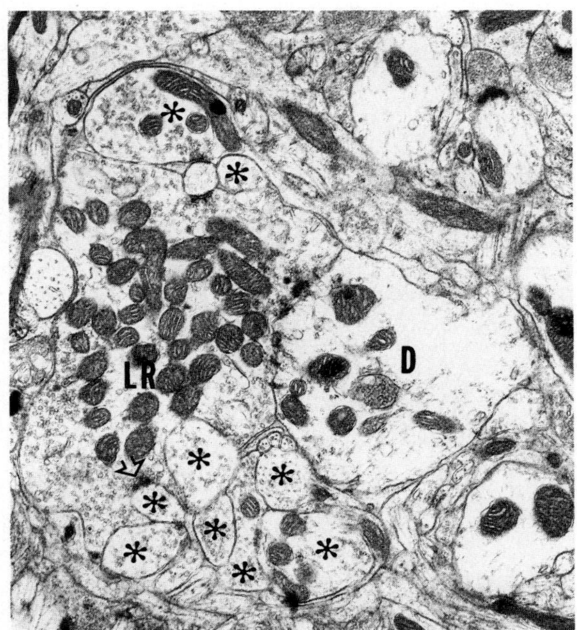

Fig. 6. An LR profile which synapses upon a projection cell dendrite (D). There are also numerous PSDs(*), one of which is contacted by an LR (arrow). Serial sections demonstrate that all the PSDs in this field are postsynaptic to LR, and presynaptic to D.

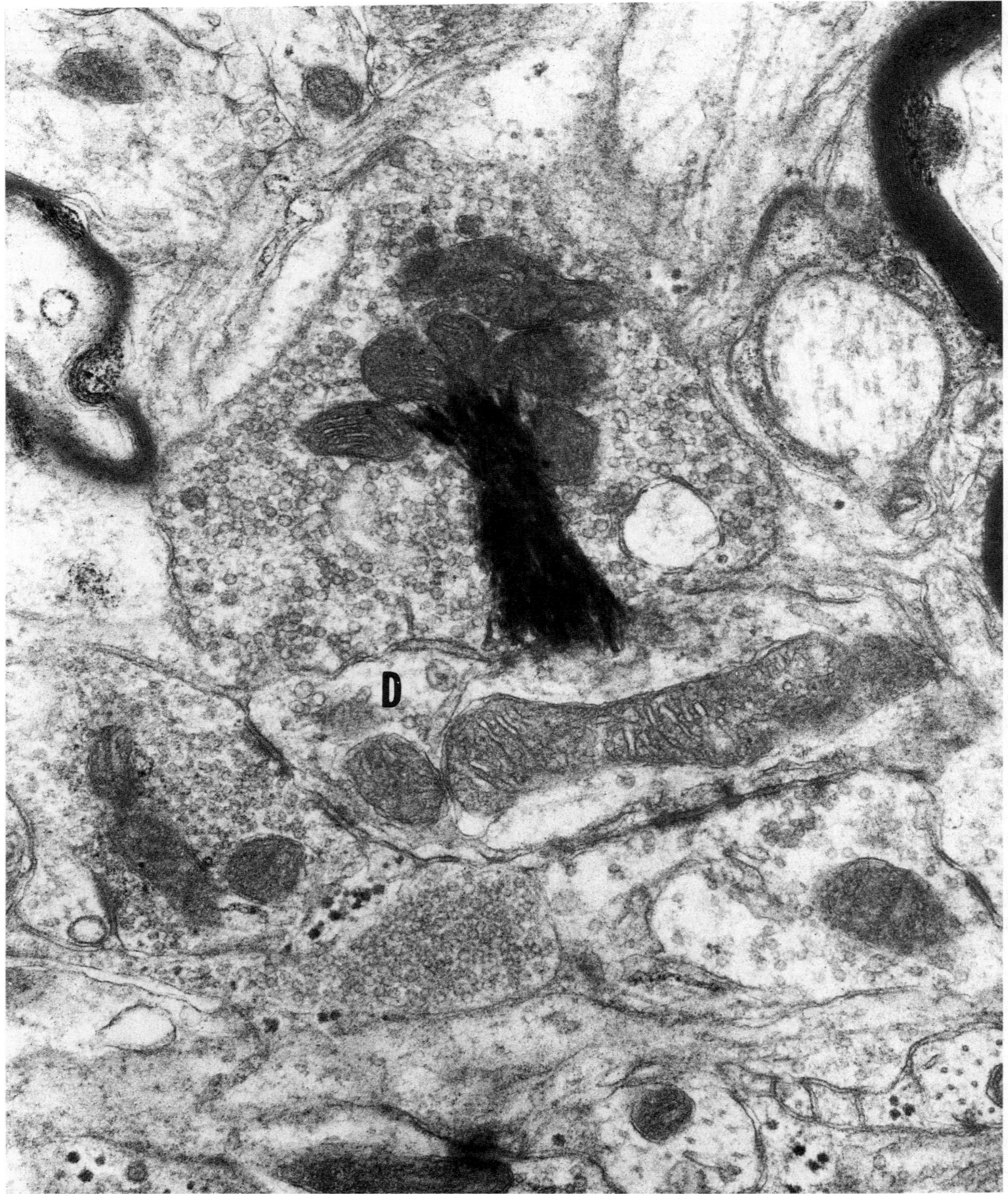

Fig. 7a, b. LR profiles containing HRP reaction product. They synapse upon projection cell dendrites, but do not contact PSDs.

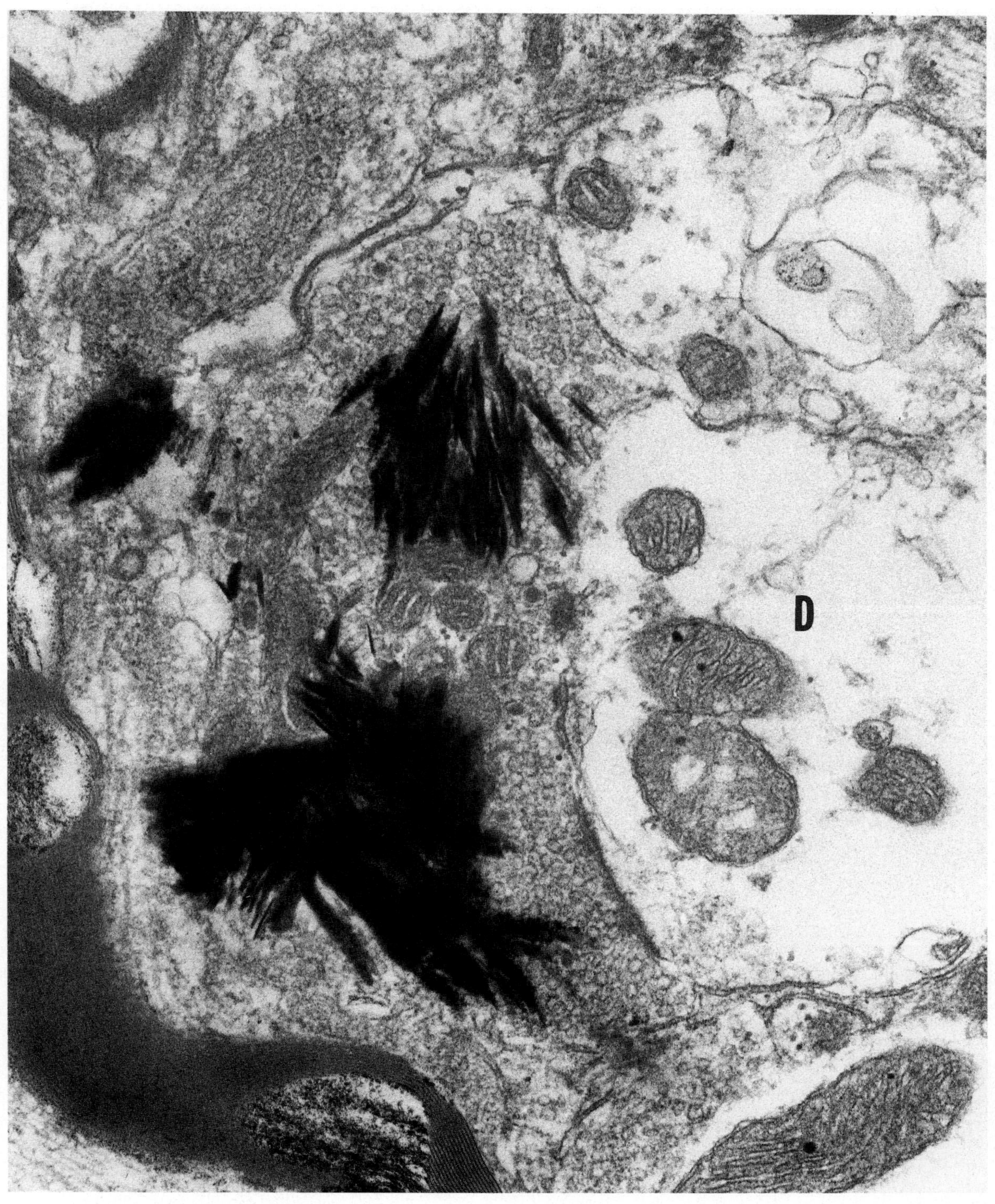
D

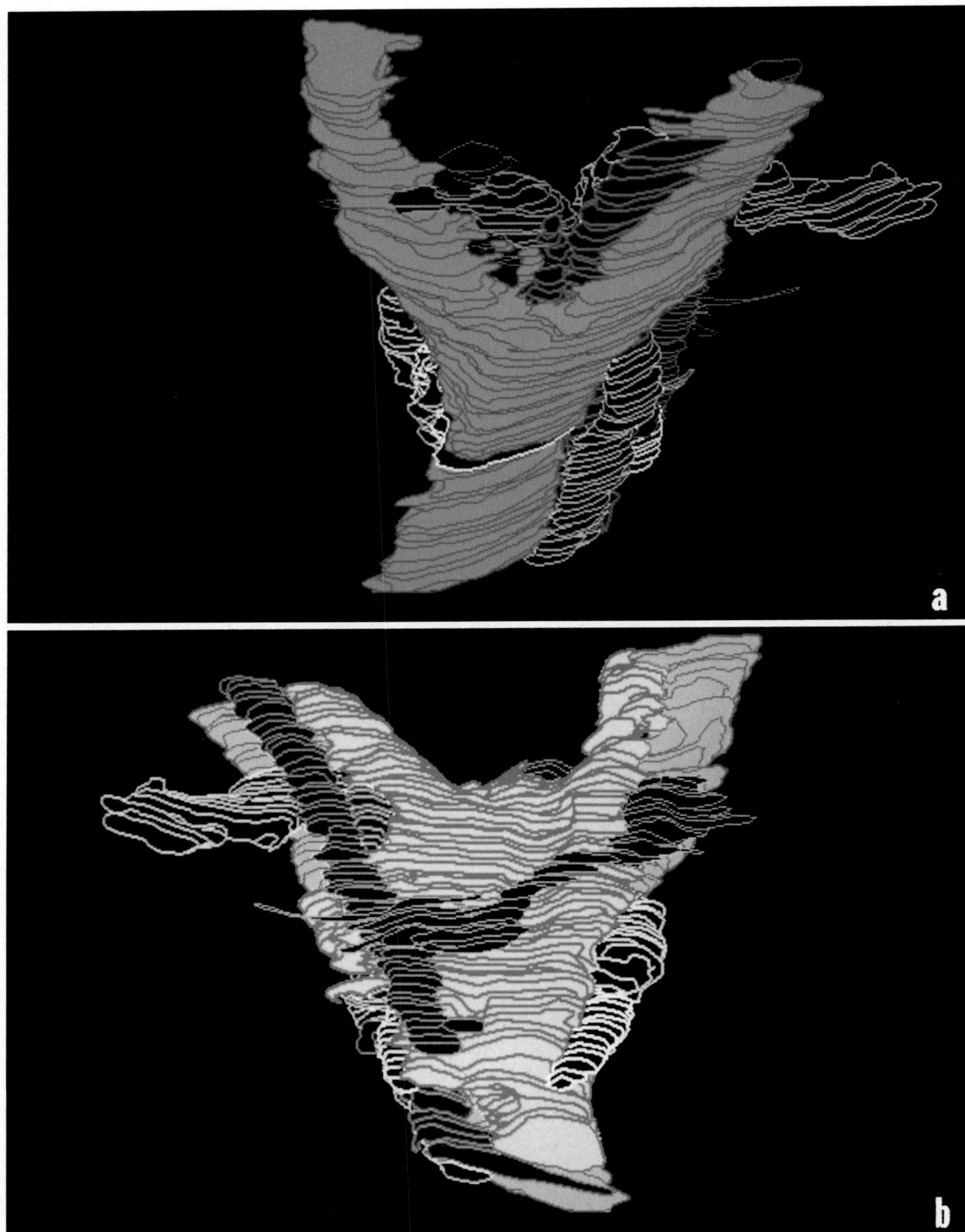

Fig. 8a, b. Computer generated reconstruction of serial sections through the LR, D and PSD profiles shown in Fig. 7. 8a and b show the images rotated 180°. The blue structure is D – the projection cell dendrite; the red structure is RL; all the other profiles are PSDs, each of which is postsynaptic to RL and presynaptic to D. (Courtesy of P.T. Ohara).

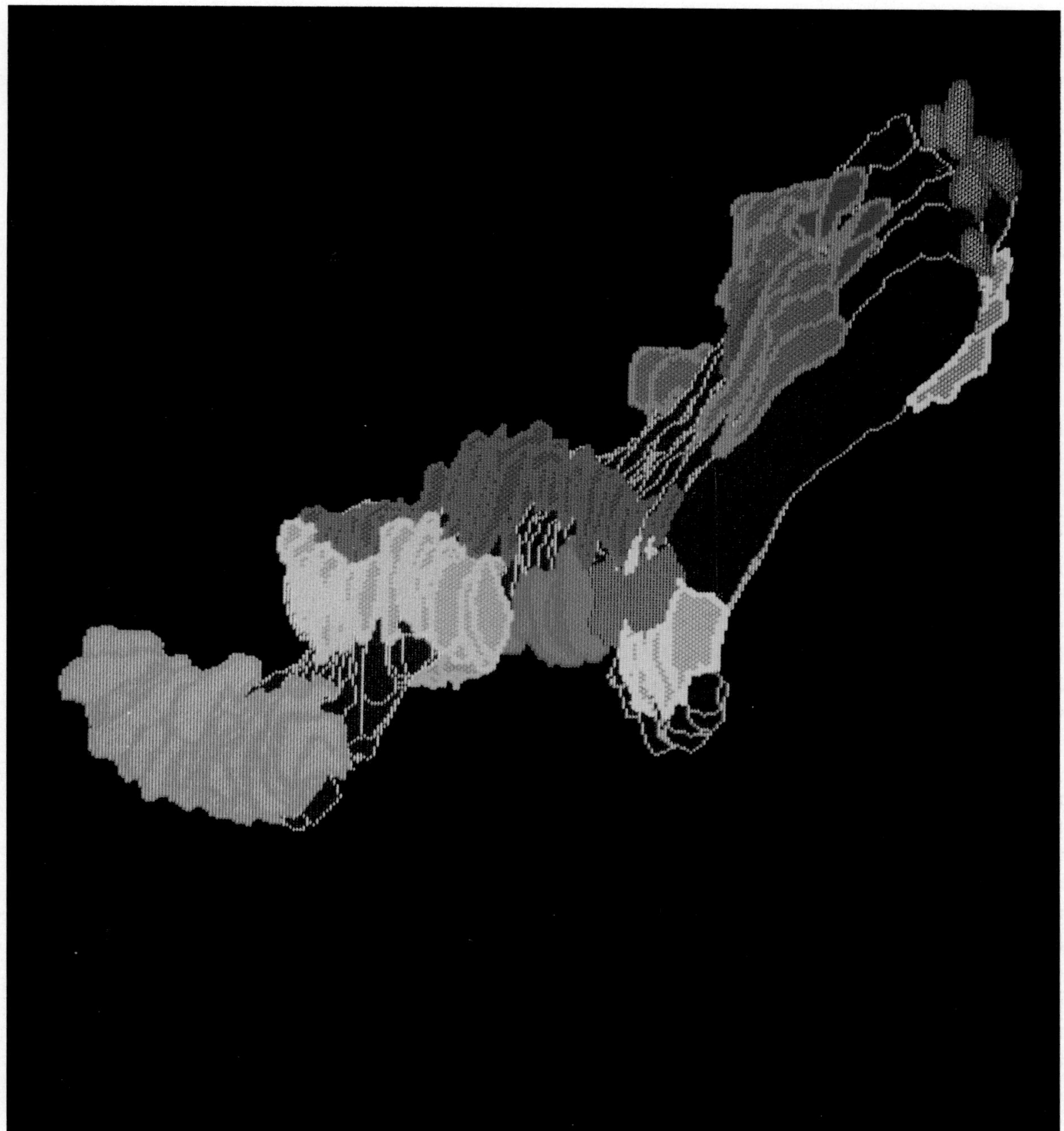

Fig. 9. Computer-generated reconstruction of synaptic profiles of labeled spinothalamic terminals, shown in various colors, all of which form axodendritic contacts with a projection cell dendrite, shown in white outline. No PSDs were found to participate in these synaptic terminations (Courtesy of D.D. Ralston).

LCNs. A single section through this complex array (Fig. 6) shows a DCN terminal forming synapses on one of the vesicle-containing LCN appendages in the field, as well as upon the dendrite of a projection neuron. Only when examined in extensive serial sections is it recognized that every one of the LCN appendages seen in Fig. 6 receives a synapse from the medial lemniscal axon and also forms synapses upon the projection cell dendrite. Thus, a single medial lemniscal axon forms multiple synaptic contacts upon a single projection cell dendrite and also forms multiple contacts upon GABAergic appendages which in turn synapse upon the projection cell dendrite. The rather simple concept of a triad between afferent axon, projection cell dendrite and dendritic appendage of an LCN is actually revealed to be a very complex series of synaptic arrays between these elements.

There is a substantial difference between the terminations of the medial lemniscal afferent to thalamic neurons and STT afferents, in that serial section reconstructions of STT terminations upon thalamic neurons reveals that most STT terminals form simple axodendritic synapses with projection cell dendrites, with no relationships with local circuit appendages (Fig. 10).

These findings suggest that the medial lemniscal projection, which conveys nonnoxious information, is subject to GABAergic modification during transmission through the thalamus on the way to the somatosensory cortex. In contrast, information conveyed by the spinothalamic system, which has a significant element of noxious information ultimately interpreted by the cerebral cortex as pain, is not subject to GABAergic modification in the thalamus and thus may have more direct, nonmodified, access to the cerebral cortex than does nonnoxious information.

In summary, it is evident that thalamocortical projection neurons that transfer information from principle afferent sources to the cerebral cortex are subject to a variety of influences: excitatory projections from the principal afferent, facilitatory influences from the cortex, GABA-mediated inhibition from the thalamic reticular nucleus and LCNs, and a mixture of excitatory and inhibitory effects from brainstem projections. We have shown that synaptic projections from two major elements of the somatosensory afferent system, the dorsal column nuclei and the spinal cord, are likely to have very different forms of information processing within the thalamus, one from the other, because of differing relationships with inhibitory LCNs. We do not yet know the nature of brainstem inputs to the thalamic neurons which may set the thalamic neurons to firing patterns which vary substantially between sleep and waking states. It is essential to understand the nature of information processing in the thalamus if we are ultimately to understand the function of the cerebral cortex, which receives information that has been processed by thalamic circuits.

Acknowledgements

Much of the work reported here has been carried out in collaboration with P.T. Ohara, Diane D. Ralston, and Joseph Wells. I thank Antonia Milroy for her expert technical assistance and Sharon Spencer for preparation of the manuscript. Supported by grants NS-21445 and NS-23347 from the NIH.

References

Berkley, K.J. (1973a) Response properties of cells in ventrobasal and posterior group nuclei of the cat. *J. Neurophysiol.*, 36: 940 – 952.

Berkley, K.J. (1973b) Afferent projections to and near the ventrobasal complex in the cat and monkey. In G. Macchi, A. Rustioni and R. Spreafico (Eds.) *Somatosensory Integration in the Thalamus,* Elsevier, Amsterdam, pp. 43 – 62.

Blomqvist, A., Flink, R., Westman, J. and Wilberg, M. (1985) Synaptic terminals in the ventroposterolateral nucleus of the thalamus from neurons in the dorsal column and lateral cervical nuclei: an electron microscopic study in the cat. *J. Neurocytol.*, 14: 869 – 886.

Boivie, J. (1970) The termination of the cervicothalamic tract in the cat: An experimental study with silver impregnation methods. *Brain Res.*, 19: 333 – 360.

Boivie, J. (1971) The termination of the spinothalamic tract in the cat: An experimental study with silver impregnation methods. *Exp. Brain Res.*, 12: 331 – 353.

Boivie, J. (1979) An anatomical reinvestigation of the termination of the spinothalamic tract in the monkey. *J. Comp. Neurol.,* 186: 343 – 370.

Burke, W. and Sefton A.J. (1966) Inhibitory mechanisms in lateral geniculate nucleus of rat. *J. Physiol. (Lond.)* 187: 231 – 246.

Burton, H. and Craig A.D. (1983) Spinothalamic neuron projections in cat, raccoon and monkey: a study based on anterograde transport of horseradish peroxidase. In G. Macchi, A. Rustioni and R. Spreafico (Eds.), *Somatosensory Integration in the Thalamus,* Elsevier, Amsterdam, pp. 17 – 42.

Chung, J.M., Lee, K.H., Surmeier, D.J., Sorkin, L.S., Kim, J. and Willis, W.D. (1986) Response characteristics of neurons in the ventral posterior lateral nucleus of the monkey thalamus. *J. Neurophysiol.,* 56: 370 – 390.

Fertziger, A.P. and Purpura D.P. (1971) Diphasic- PSPs during maintained activity of cat lateral geniculate neurons. *Brain Res.,* 33: 463 – 467.

Friedlander, M.J., Lin, C.S., Sanford, L.R. and Sherman, S.M. (1981) Morphology of functionally identified neurons in lateral geniculate nucleus of the cat. *J. Neurophysiol.,* 46: 80 – 129.

Guillery, R.W. (1966) A study of Golgi preparations from the dorsal lateral geniculate nucleus of the adult cat. *J. Comp. Neurol.,* 128: 197 – 222.

Henry, M.A., Westrum, L.E. and Johnson, L.R. (1985) Enhanced ultrastructural visualization of the horseradish peroxidase-tetramethyl benzidine reaction product. *J. Histochem. Cytochem.,* 33: 1256 – 1259.

Humphrey, A.L. and Weller, R.E. (1988) Structural correlates of functionally distinct X-cells in the lateral geniculate nucleus of the cat. *J. Comp. Neurol.,* 268: 448 – 468.

Jones, E.G. (1985) The Thalamus. Plenum Press, New York. pp. 227 – 244.

Koch, C. (1985) Understanding the instrinsic circuitry of the cat's LGN: electrical properties of the spine-triad arrangement. *Proc. R. Soc. B.,* 225: 365 – 390.

Lee, C.L. (1981) Structural and ultrastructural organization of the rat ventrobasal thalamic complex. Ph.D. thesis, University of California, San Francisco.

LeVay, S. and Ferster, D. (1979) Proportions of interneurons in the cat's lateral geniculate nucleus. *Brain Res.,* 164: 304 – 308.

Ma, W., Peschanski, M. and Besson, J.M. (1986) The overlap of spinothalamic and dorsal column nuclei projections in the ventrobasal complex of the rat thalamus: A double anterograde labeling study using light microscopic analysis. *J. Comp. Neurol.,* 245: 531 – 540.

Ma, W., Peschanski, M. and Ralston III, H.J. (1987) The differential synaptic organization of the spinal and lemniscal projections to the ventrobasal complex of the rat thalamus. Evidence for convergence of the two systems upon single thalamic neurons. *Neuroscience,* 22: 925 – 934.

Mastronarde, D.M. (1987) Two classes of single-input X-cells in cat lateral geniculate nucleus. I. Receptive-field properties and classification of cells. *J. Neurophysiol.,* 57: 357 – 380.

Ohara, P.T., Lieberman, A.R., Hunt, S.P. and Wu, J.Y. (1983) Neural elements containing glutamic acid decarboxylase (GAD) in the dorsal lateral geniculate nucleus of the rat; immunohistochemical studies by light and electron microscopy. *Neuroscience,* 8: 189 – 211.

Ohara, P.T., Chazal, G. and Ralston III, H.J. (1989) Ultrastructural analysis of GABA immunoreactive elements in the monkey thalamic ventrobasal complex. *J. Comp. Neurol.,* 283: 541 – 558.

Olucha, F., Martinez-Garcia, F. and Lopez-Garcia C. (1985) A new stablizing agent for the tetramethyl benzidine (TMD) reaction product in the histochemical detection of horseradish peroxidase (HRP). *J. Neurosci. Methods,* 13: 131 – 138.

Peschanski, M., Lee, C.L. and Ralston III, H.J. (1984) The structural organization of the ventrobasal complex of the rat revealed by the analysis of physiologically characterized neurons injected intracellularly with horseradish peroxidase. *Brain Res.,* 297: 63 – 74.

Peschanski, M., Ralston III, H.J. and Roudier, F. (1983) Reticular thalamic afferents to the ventrobasal complex of the rat thalamus: an electron microscopic study. *Brain Res.,* 270: 325 – 329.

Ralston, III H.J. (1969) The synaptic organization of lemniscal projections to the ventrobasal thalamus of the cat. *Brain Res.,* 14: 99 – 116.

Ralston, III H.J. (1971) Evidence for presynaptic dendrites and a proposal for the mechanism of action. *Nature (London)* 230: 585 – 587.

Ralston, III H.J. (1983) The synaptic organization of the ventrobasal thalamus in the rat, cat and monkey. In G. Macchi, A. Rustioni and R. Spreafico (Eds.) *Somatosensory Integration in the Thalamus,* Elsevier, Amsterdam, pp. 241 – 250.

Ralston, III H.J. and Herman, M.M. (1969) The fine structure of neurons and synapses in the ventrobasal thalamus of the cat. *Brain Res.,* 14: 77 – 98.

Rapisardi, S.C. and Miles, T.P. (1984) Synaptology of retinal terminals in the dorsal lateral geniculate nucleus of the cat. *J. Comp. Neurol.,* 223: 515 – 534.

Sherman, S.M. and Koch, C. (1986) The control of retinogeniculate transmission in the mammalian lateral geniculate nucleus. *Exp. Brain Res.,* 63: 1 – 20.

Spacek, J. and Lieberman. A.R. (1974) Ultrastructure and three-dimensional organization of synaptic glomeruli in rat somatosensory thalamus. J. Anat., 117: 487 – 516.

Spreafico, R., Schmechel, D.E., Ellis, L.C. and Rustioni, A. (1983) Cortical relay neurons and interneurons in the n. ventralis posterolateralis of cats: a horseradish peroxidase, electron microscopic, Golgi and immunocytochemical study. *Neuroscience,* 9: 491 – 509.

Willis, W.D. (1987) The spinothalamic tract in primates. In J.M. Besson, G. Guilbaud and M. Peschanski, (Eds.)

Thalamus and Pain, Exerpta Medica, Amsterdam. pp. 35 – 48.

Yen, C.T., Conley, M. and Jones, E.G. (1985) Morphological and functional types of neurons in the cat ventral posterior thalamic nucleus. *J. Neurosci.,* 5: 1315 – 1337.

Yen, C.T., Conley, M., Hendry, S.H.C. and Jones, E.G. (1985) The morphology of physiologically identified GABAergic neurons in the somatic sensory part of the thalamic reticular nucleus. *J. Neurosci.,* 5: 2254 – 2268.

Yingling, C.D. and Skinner, J.E. (1976) Selective regulation of thalamic sensory relay nuclei by nucleus reticularis thalami. *Electroenceph. Clin. Neurophysiol.,* 41: 476 – 482.

Yuan, B., Marrow, T.J. and Casey, K.L. (1986) Corticofugal influences of SI cortex on ventrobasal thalamic neurons in the awake rat. *J. Neurosci.,* 6: 3611 – 3617.

G. Holstege (Ed.)
Progress in Brain Research, Vol. 87

CHAPTER 3

The anatomy of sensory relay functions in the thalamus

Edward G. Jones

Department of Anatomy and Neurobiology, University of California, Irvine, CA 92717, U.S.A.

"...he who knows the parts the best, is most in a maze, and he who knows the least of anatomy, sees least inconsistency in the commonly received opinion."

Charles Bell (1811)

Introduction

Some years ago, Dr. William R. Mehler (1971) published his "idea of a new anatomy of the thalamus." The similarity of the title to Sir Charles Bell's (1811) "Idea of a New Anatomy of the Brain" was not coincidental. In his short, privately printed, pamphlet of 1811 Bell had set out what he saw as the dissociation of sensory and motor pathways in the brain, mentioning in an aside, the differential effects of stimulating the dorsal and ventral roots of the spinal cord and thus setting off for future generations a controversy as to his claims to priority over Magendie. Mehler was to develop the theme of sensory and motor pathway segregation in his studies of the primate thalamus in which he was able to show the separate distributions of the pallidal, cerebellar, substantia nigral, lemniscal and spinal pathways in that structure (Mehler 1966, 1969, 1971). These studies were among the first in modern times to deal with the question of thalamic parcellation on the basis of afferent fiber systems, and they serve as models for all subsequent studies of their type. The close correlation of afferent fiber distribution with cytoarchitecture and with the localized thalamocortical projections of nuclei in which afferent pathways terminate, as exemplified by Mehler's studies, is one of the keys to understanding the thalamus as the great relay center to the cerebral cortex. The thalamic nucleus with its defined set of input-output connections is the primary channel for information flow through thalamus to cortex. As work has continued on the thalamus in recent years (Jones, 1985) this time-honored organizing principle continues to hold its preeminent place. New methods of delineating thalamic nuclei and their connections, indeed, continue to reinforce it. However, the newer methods with their greater resolving power have enabled us, as it were, to peer into the nuclear relay channels and to detect within them finer and finer channels for the transfer of information to the cerebral cortex. In what follows, I shall attempt to touch on several areas of recent investigation in this field.

Histochemical delineation of thalamic nuclei: The example of the human thalamus

That certain parts of the thalamus stain more intensely than others for the enzymatic activity of, for example, cytochrome oxidase or acetylcholinesterase, has been known for some time (Olivier et al., 1970; Graybiel and Berson, 1980; Jones, 1985; Butcher and Wolf, 1986; Jones et al., 1986; Hirai and Jones, 1989). There have been some attempts to correlate differential patterns of histochemical staining with afferent and efferent connections and in some instances these patterns have been claimed as more reliable markers of the boundaries of certain fiber distributions than cytoarchitectonics. In studying the human thalamus, stained for acetylcholinesterase (Hirai and Jones, 1989), it has been possible to arrive at a more rational parcellation than previously available, since the histochemical staining patterns can be correlated closely with similar patterns in monkeys from which connectional data are already available.

The value of the histochemical approach is particularly evident in the delineation of divisions of the ventral nuclear complex. In the human it had been traditional to divide this into a large number of nuclei (Hassler, 1959) that were difficult to correlate with those of experimental primates (Olszewski, 1952; Jones, 1985) and, thus, to be confident of their inputs and outputs (Asanuma et al., 1983a,b,c). Acetylcholinesterase staining (Fig. 1) reveals five major nuclear masses in the complex: an anterior one, moderately stained, equivalent to the ventral anterior (VA) nucleus of monkeys; and anterolateral one, more densely stained, equivalent to the ventral lateral anterior (VLa) nucleus of monkeys; a very large intermediate one, very weakly stained and equivalent to the ventral lateral posterior (VLp) nucleus of monkeys; a posterior, relatively densely stained pair equivalent to the ventral posterior lateral (VPL) and ventral posterior medial (VPM) nuclei of monkeys; a moderately stained medial nucleus

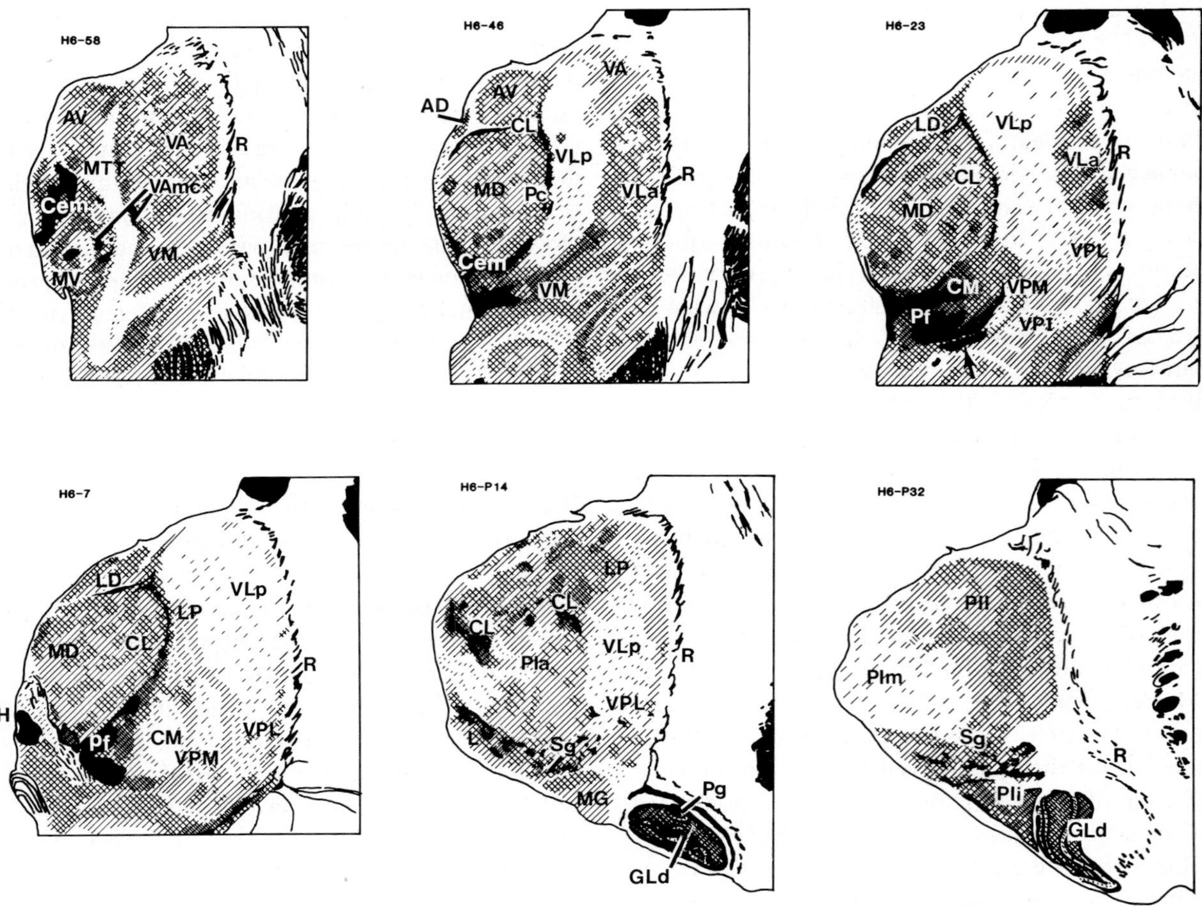

Fig. 1. Camera lucida drawings of frontal sections through a human thalamus, stained for acetylcholinesterase. Density of stain is indicated by different degrees of hatching. From Hirai and Jones (1989). Bar 1 mm.

equivalent to the principal ventral medial nucleus (VMp) of monkeys. The parcellation of these five nuclei is even more distinct in the human thalamus, presumably on account of its large size, and borders between the histochemically stained nuclei are remarkably sharp. This clear-cut delineation of the nuclei makes it extremely likely that in the human thalamus one is visualizing the separate relays of pallidal (in VLa), cerebellar (in VLp) and lemniscal (in VPL and VPM) inputs to the thalamus en route to separate regions of the cerebral cortex. Although there are still some minor controversies over details, the weight of experimental evidence in monkeys points to separate routes through the thalamus for these three great motor and sensory pathways and their projection to independent premotor, motor and sensory areas of the cerebral cortex (Kim et al., 1976; Asanuma et al., 1983a,b,c; Alexander et al., 1986). It is probable that the nigrothalamic inputs also relay separately in the VMp and VA nuclei, without overlap with the terminations of the other three pathways (Carpenter et al., 1976; Ilinsky and Kultas-Ilinsky, 1987).

The recognition of four or five major nuclear masses in the ventral group and their correlation with the major sites of termination of the above four pathways, enables the resolution of some old conflicts in the literature of the human thalamus. It is known, for example, that neuronal activity phase locked to a tremor can be recorded in regions customarily thought to correspond to Hassler's Vim nucleus (the ventral part of the current VLp) (Ohye et al., 1979; Lenz et al., 1988). In the same general region neurons also respond to proprioceptive stimuli and have customarily also been thought to occupy Vim (VLp) (Ohye et al., 1989). In monkeys, however, inputs from group I muscle afferents and other deep receptors relay in the anterior part of the VPL nucleus, (Friedman and Jones, 1981; Maendly et al., 1981; Jones and Friedman, 1982) posterior to the VLp nucleus in which inputs from the deep cerebellar nuclei terminate (Asanuma et al., 1983a,b,c). It seems clear, therefore, that proprioceptive responses in the human are recorded from the anterior part of VPL, not from Vim (VLp) (Lenz et al., 1988). It is interesting to note that the human VPL nucleus shows a cytoarchitectonic division into anterodorsal and central-posterior parts (called Vcea and Vcep by Hassler, 1959) which seem to correspond to the two physiologically definable subdivisions of the monkey VPL in which deep and cutaneous afferents relay (Jones and Friedman, 1982). These project separately to the somatic sensory cortex, the anterodorsal, "deep" relay to areas 3a and 2 and the central "cutaneous" relay to areas 3b and 1 (Fig. 2).

It is possible to make further correlations between other nuclei by matching the histochemical staining patterns in the human and monkey thalamus. The nuclei of the pulvinar and of the intralaminar system are cases in point (see Fig. 1). Four features of the intralaminar system stand out: the extension of the central lateral nucleus posterior to the mediodorsal nucleus, not always recognized in Nissl stained sections; the continuity of the intralaminar nuclei with the limitans-suprageniculate nucleus, perhaps giving credence to the old belief that the latter nucleus is part of the intralaminar system (LeGros Clark, 1936); the separation of the centre médian nucleus into two differentially stained parts that may correspond to subnuclei with different connections; the continuity of the magnocellular part of the VA nucleus with the central medial nucleus, perhaps justifying inclusion of the former in the intralaminar system (Jones, 1985).

Modular organization of a thalamic nucleus: The example of the monkey VPM nucleus

For some years now it has been evident that the relay cells of a thalamic nucleus need not all be of the same type. The original example was furnished by the dorsal lateral geniculate nucleus in which it was revealed that cells in different layers projected to different layers of the visual cortex in the cat (LeVay and Gilbert, 1976), monkey (Hubel and Livingstone, 1987) and other species (Carey et al.,

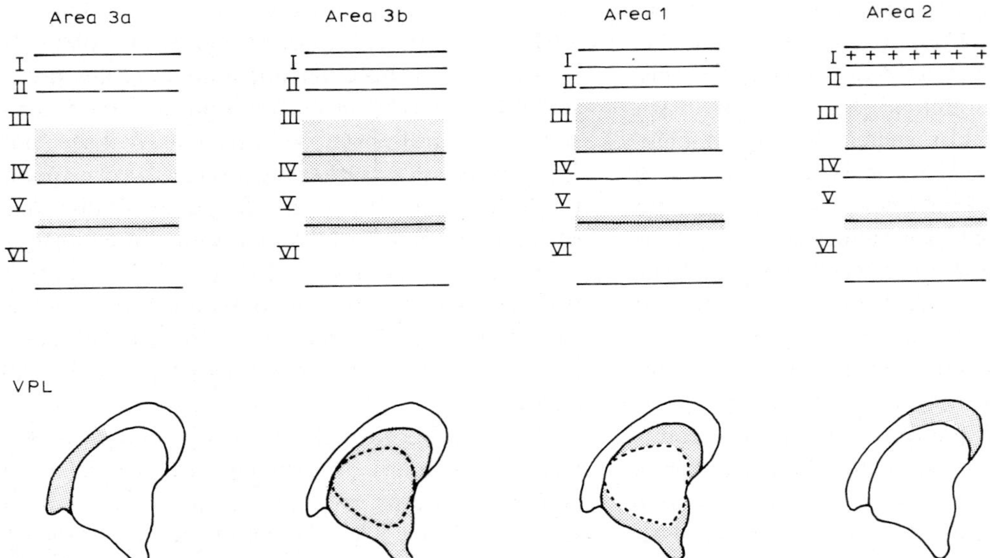

Fig. 2. Schematic diagram of the selective cortical areal and laminar distributions of axons arising from different populations of neurons in the monkey VPL nucleus (sagittal sections below). (Jones and Burton, 1976; Jones and Friedman, 1982; Jones et al., 1982).

1979). But this principle has now been extended to other nuclei as well. Different populations of cells in the monkey ventral posterior nucleus, for example (Fig.2), project upon areas 3a, 3b, 1 and 2 of the somatic sensory cortex, (Jones, 1983) and serve to transmit afferent influences from muscle, cutaneous, and deep receptors to the separate fields, (Jones and Friedman, 1982) in which their axons end selectively in layers IV and/or III (Jones, 1975; Jones and Burton, 1976). A further set of ventral posterior neurons in cats (Penny et al., 1982) and monkeys (Rausell and Jones, 1989) projects independently to layer I.

In recent studies of the monkey VPM nucleus, a very detailed modularity of organization has been revealed in which differentially projecting cells occupy different histochemically defined (Jones et al., 1986a,b; Jones and Hendry, 1989; Rausell and Jones, 1989) subcompartments of the nucleus. The monkey VPM nucleus is an L-shaped structure with a vertical limb and a horizontal limb that points medially. In it terminate both the trigeminal lemniscus and the dorsal ipsilateral trigeminal tract carrying afferent impulses from the contralateral and ipsilateral trigeminal nuclei respectively (Jones et al., 1986b; Jones and Hendry, 1989) (Fig. 3).

Single- and multi-unit mapping studies (Jones et al., 1986b) revealed that the vertical part of the nucleus contains a complete representation of the contralateral sides of the head, face and interior of the mouth while the horizontal part contains an unexpectedly large representation of the ipsilateral sides of the lips and interior of the mouth (Fig. 4). Apart from the two representations and the separate terminations of the contralateral and ipsilateral trigeminal pathways, the two parts of the nucleus are also distinguished by the fact that large numbers of tachykinin immunoreactive fibers terminate only in the vertical part of the nucleus (Molinari et al., 1987; Liu et al., 1989). These fibers make synaptic connections that suggest they are part of the trigeminal lemniscus (Liu et al., 1989) (Fig. 5).

Both parts of the VPM nucleus are divided into

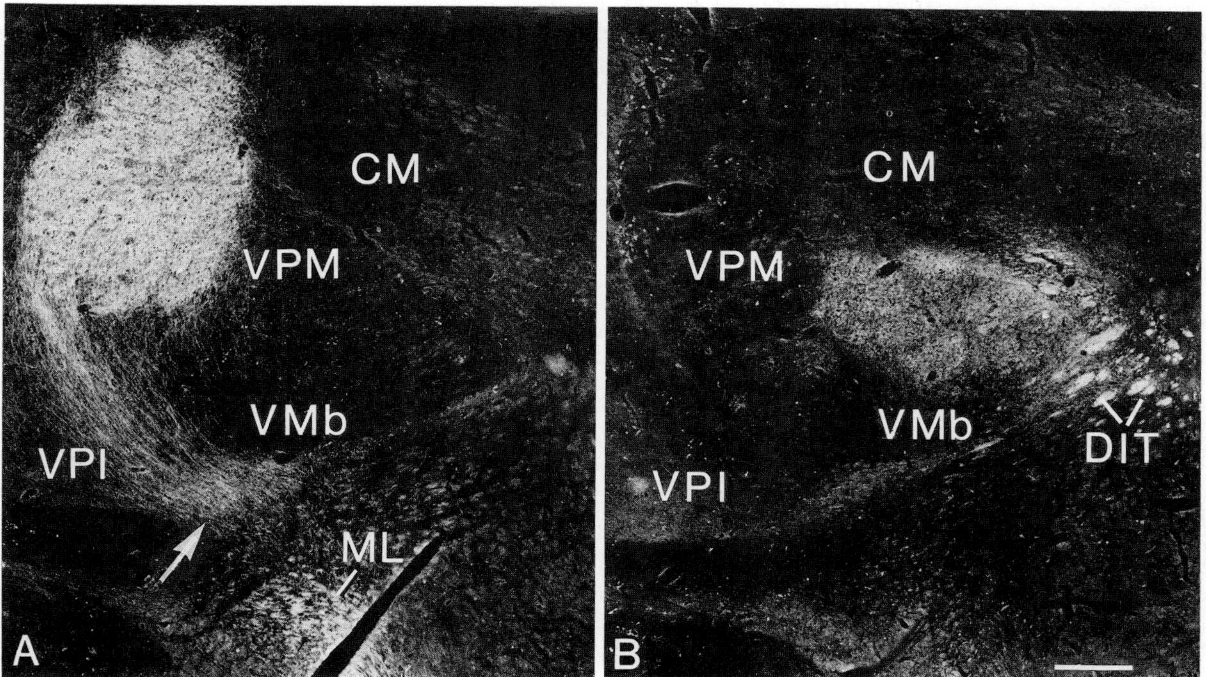

Fig. 3. Distribution of trigemino-thalamic axons, labeled by anterograde transport of horse radish peroxidase and arising in the centralateral (A) and ipsilateral (B) principal trigeminal nucleus. From Jones et al., 1986b. Bar 0.5 mm.

smaller histochemical compartments. These are detectable especially by staining for cytochrome oxidase activity (Jones et al., 1986a) but are also revealed by staining for acetylcholinesterase activity (Liu et al., 1989a) and in the vertical part of the nucleus by tachykinin immunoreactivity (Molinari et al., 1987; Liu et al., 1989b) (Fig. 6). The most conspicuous feature of the staining pattern is the presence of elongated clumps of stain that extend, rodlike, through the full anteroposterior extent of the nucleus. They have thus been named "rods." Underlying each rod of histochemical staining is a similar rod of thalamocortical relay neurons whose clumping is best revealed in the fetal thalamus (Liu et al., 1989b). What is clear from correlative anatomical and physiological studies, however, is that the cells of each rod have overlapping peripheral receptive fields, are driven by the same type of stimulus and project to one or a few narrow, column-like domains in the somatic sensory cortex (Jones et al., 1979, 1982; Jones and Friedman, 1982) (Figs. 4 and 7). This is one of the bases of the rod-to-column principle of thalamocortical organization (Jones, 1985).

The rods that show strong histochemical staining, especially for cytochrome oxidase, are embedded in a more weakly and homogenously stained background that is especially prominent in dorsomedial and ventrolateral parts of the nucleus (Rausell and Jones, 1989). This also contains thalamocortical relay neurons and a few trigeminothalamic fibers appear to terminate in it. The major zones of trigeminothalamic terminations are, however, the rods in which densely clustered fiber ramifications can be revealed by anterograde labeling (Jones et al., 1986) (Fig. 3).

The two compartments – rod and background matrix – can be demonstrated by immunocytochemical staining for the inhibitory transmitter, gamma amino butyric acid (GABA), (Hendry et al., 1979; Jones et al., 1986a; Rausell and Jones, 1989) and for two calcium binding proteins, parvalbumin and the 28Kd Vitamin D dependent calcium binding protein, calbindin (Jones and Hendry, 1989; Rausell and Jones, 1989) (Figs. 8 and 9). GABA immunostaining, which reveals the interneurons of the thalamus and their processes, is particularly dense in the rods and most GABA cells bodies are concentrated in the rods. Parvalbumin immunoreactivity is also densest in the rods and virtually all parvalbumin positive cells lie in the rods. Calbindin immunoreactivity, by contrast, is essentially confined to the background matrix, and calbindin positive cells do not intrude into the rods. A further distinction between the parvalbumin and calbindin positive cells is the fact that only the former stain with the monoclonal antibody, CAT 301, (Hendry et al., 1988) that is

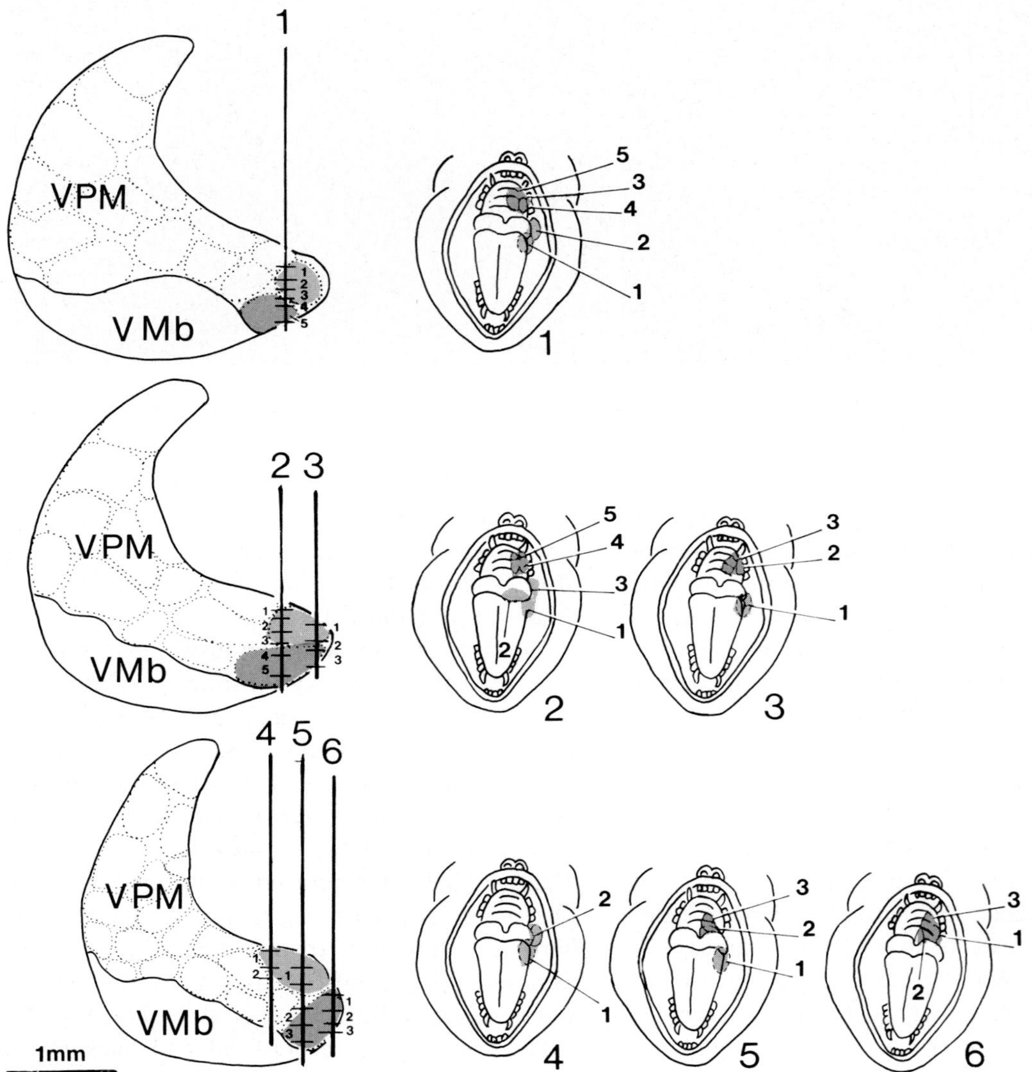

Fig. 4. Rod like distribution in VPM of neurons with receptive fields in same parts of the mouth. Sections (left) are in anteroposterior sequence and show costained rods (dotted outlines) and positions of electrode tracks (1 – 6) and of single units responding to stimulation of regions indicated on figurines (right). From Jones et al., 1986b.

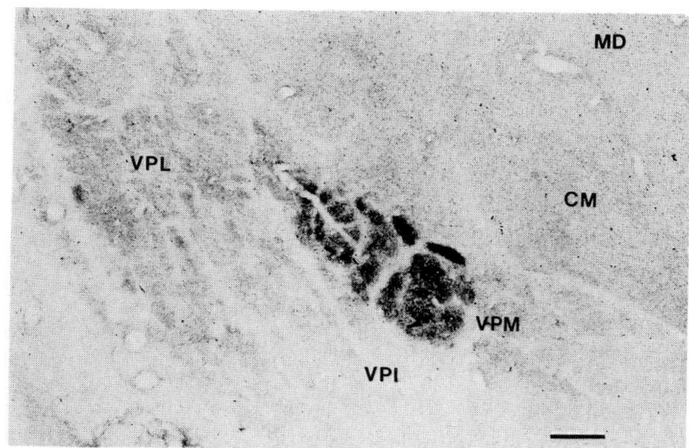

Fig. 5. Tachykinin immunoreactivity clustered in rodlike configurations and confined the dorsolateral portion of VPM in a fetal monkey. (Liu et al., 1989b) Bar 0.5 mm.

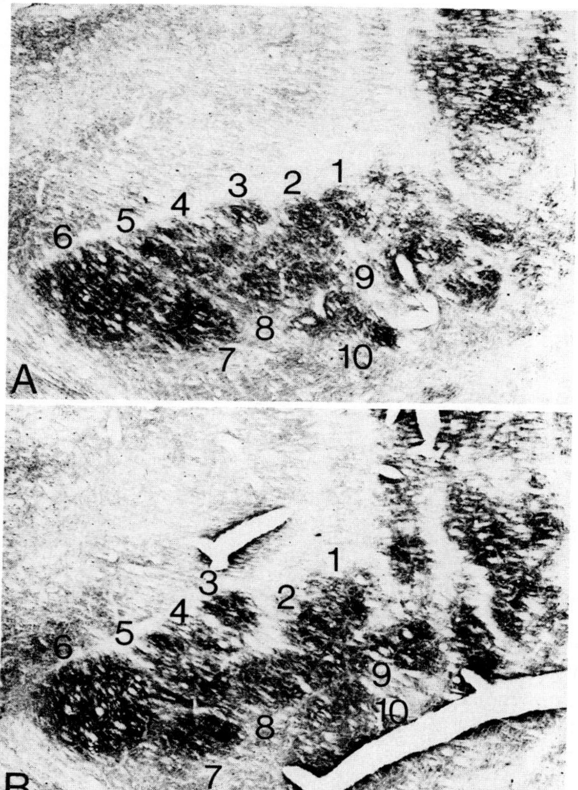

Fig. 6. Frontal sections 1mm apart through the part of monkey VPM containing the ipsilateral representation and stained for CO. The same rods are numbered in each section. From Jones et al., 1986a. Bar 0.5 mm.

directed against a surface proteoglycan (Zaremba et al., 1989) (Fig. 10). Neither cell type co-stains for GABA (Jones and Hendry, 1989). This is suggestive of their relay character and is confirmed by retrograde tracing studies which reveal that the parvalbumin/CAT 301 positive cells project to middle layers of the somatic sensory cortex while the calbindin positive cells project to superficial layers (Rausell and Jones, 1989).

These studies have revealed a very highly structured organization of the VPM nucleus that may be indicative of one of the underlying principles of organization of all thalamic nuclei. That is, the presence of subpopulations of relay neurons whose axons project to different layers of the cerebral cortex. In the dorsal lateral geniculate nucleus these are largely segregated by layers; in the VPM

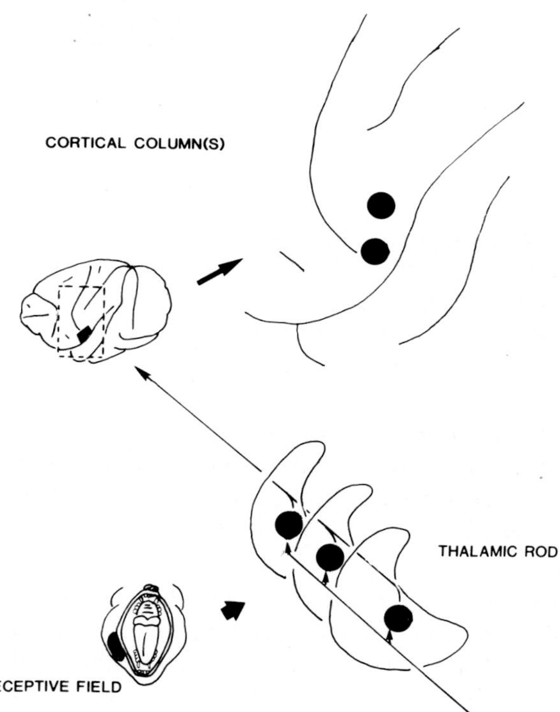

Fig. 7. Schematic representation of the rod-to-column principal of thalamo-cortical connectivity. The same receptive fields are represented along an anteroposterior sequence of thalamic cells whose axons project collectively to one of a few focal cortical domains.

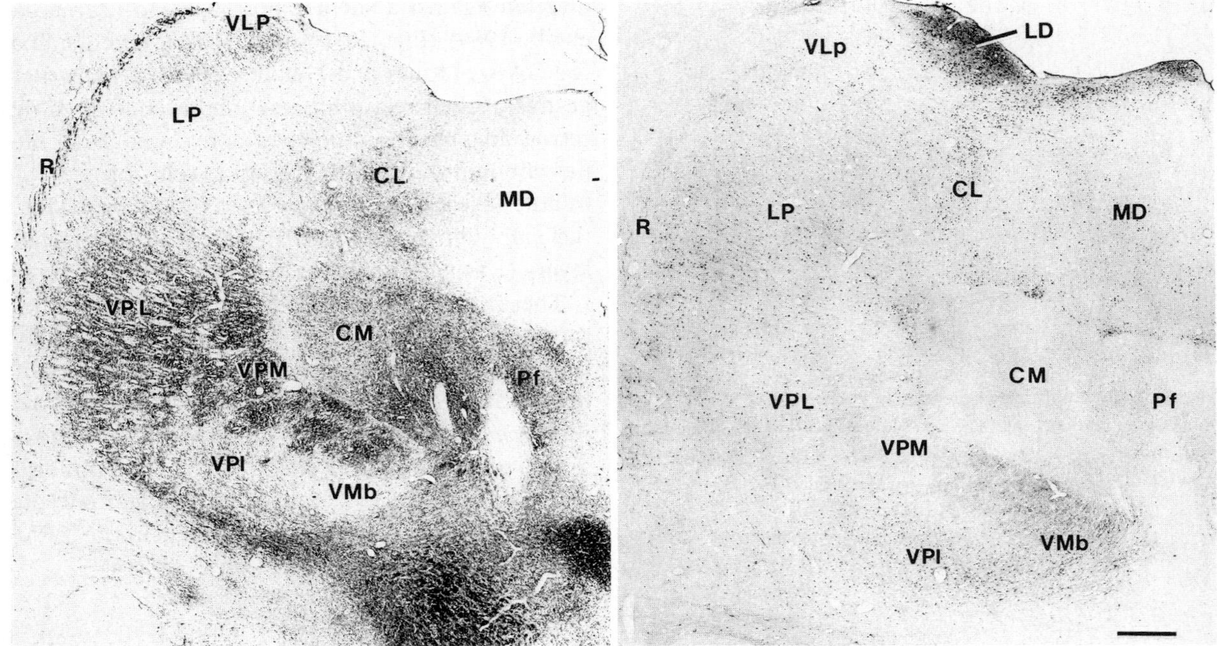

Fig. 8. Alternating frontal sections through the thalamus of a monkey stained immunocytochemically for parvalbumin (left) or calbindin (right) and showing the virtually complementary nature of cell and fiber staining. From Jones and Hendry, 1989. Bar 1 mm.

nucleus they are equally compartmentalized but along lines that reflect the particular topography of the nucleus. Other patterns of segregation of differentially projecting relay neurons may be found in other nuclei.

Specification of classes of thalamic relay neurons by differential calcium binding protein immunoreactivity: The example of the monkey thalamus

Extension of the studies on the VPM nucleus to the thalamus in general, revealed patterns of immunoreactivity for parvalbumin and calbindin that distinguish thalamic nuclei from one another and that serve to differentiate cell types in many nuclei (Jones and Hendry, 1989). A partial map of the distribution patterns is shown in Fig. 9. There it can be seen that many dorsal thalamic nuclei, e.g. the centre médian nucleus, show immunoreactivity

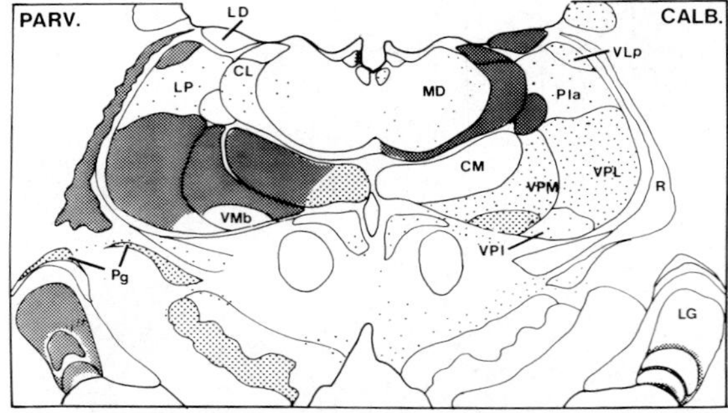

Fig. 9. Camera lucida drawings transferred to left and right sides of the same monkey thalamus showing the differential distribution of parvalbumin (Parv.) and calbindin (Calb.) immunoreactive neurons. From Jones and Hendry, 1989. Bar 1 mm.

for parvalbumin alone; others, e.g. the lateral dorsal nucleus, show immunoreactivity for calbindin alone; others show immunoreactivity for both. Where immunoreactive staining is demonstrable, it includes neuronal somata, afferent fibers entering the nucleus and efferent fibers leaving the nucleus to join the internal capsule. Parvalbumin positive afferent fibers can be traced back into the medial lemniscus, optic tract and brachium of the inferior colliculus. Calbindin positive fibers can be traced back into the midbrain tegmental pathways and into the optic tract. Both types of efferent fibers can be traced to the cerebral cortex and both parvalbumin- and calbindin-positive cells can be retrogradely labeled from injections of fluorescent dyes into the cortex (Jones and Hendry, 1989; Rausell and Jones, 1989).

Where nuclei contain both parvalbumin and calbindin positive relay cells, the patterns of distribution are extremely varied. That in the VPM nucleus has already been mentioned. In some nuclei, islands of cells immunoreactive for one calcium binding protein are completely segregated from those immunoreactive for the other. A good example is the rostral group (Rh, CL, Pc, CeM) of intralaminar nuclei where most cells are positive for calbindin but a few islands are positive for parvalbumin. In the caudal group (CM, Pf) of intralaminar nuclei virtually all cells are parvalbumin positive. Another example of segregation is furnished by the dorsal lateral geniculate nucleus in which parvalbumin positive cells are confined to the main laminae and calbindin positive cells are restricted to the S-layers and interlaminar zones. In nuclei where the two populations are mixed, e.g. VPL, most cells are either parvalbumin or calbindin positive but a few cells stain for both (Jones and Hendry, 1989).

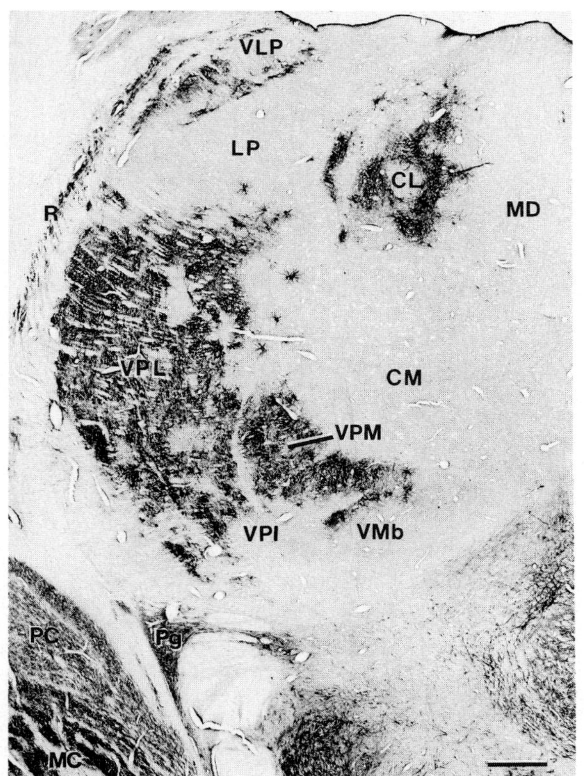

Fig. 10. Immunoreactive staining of selected populations of neurons in the monkey thalamus by the monoclonal antibody. CAT 301. From Hendry et al., 1988. Bar 0.5 mm.

It had been reported in earlier studies on the dorsal lateral geniculate nucleus of the cat (Stichel et al., 1987) that parvalbumin immunoreactivity characterized the GABAergic interneurons of that nucleus, not the relay neurons. In the studies on the monkey, the vast majority of cells staining positively for the calcium binding proteins in the dorsal thalamus were GABA negative (Jones and Hendry, 1989). A few GABA cells, however, costained for parvalbumin in the dorsal lateral geniculate nucleus and in the magnocellular medial geniculate nucleus. In the ventral thalamus, the situation is quite different with all cells in the reticular nucleus and many in the zona incerta staining for both GABA and parvalbumin.

The significance of the differential distributions of the two calcium binding proteins among thalamic relay neurons is not clear at present. When originally reported in other parts of the nervous system, these calcium binding proteins were thought to correlate closely with the presence of fast spiking behavior (Celio, 1986), that is in neurons whose action potentials are rapidly cut down by the appearance of a sudden, large conductance change (McCormick et al., 1985). In the cerebral cortex, in particular, this was thought to be especially characteristic of the nonspiny intrinsic neurons (McCormick et al., 1985) which are both GABA- and calbindin- or parvalbumin-positive (Celio, 1986; Hendry et al., 1989). In the monkey thalamus, however, while the GABAergic interneurons can be expected to display fast spiking behavior (Andersen et al., 1964), it is the relay neurons that are the predominant population displaying immunoreactivity for the calcium binding proteins and the vast majority of GABA neurons, except in the ventral thalamus, are negative (Jones and Hendry, 1989). Although one may feel disappointed at the lack of a functional correlate, the capacity to stain individual populations of thalamic relay neurons opens up many possibilities for anatomical studies of thalamic organization.

Other neuronal markers in the thalamus

Most work involving the specification of cell types in the thalamus has been of a physiological kind in which cells are characterized by their receptive fields and discharge properties. Molecular and chemical markers of cell individuality are now however, starting to appear. The calcium binding proteins, mentioned above, are a case in point. Other markers include the CAT 301 antibody, also mentioned above, which specifically stains certain populations of relay neurons in the dorsal thalamus and the GABAergic neurons of the reticular nucleus (Hendry et al., 1988) (Fig. 10). Dorsal thalamic nuclei containing CAT 301 positive cells in the monkey are the anterodorsal nucleus of the anterior group, central lateral, cen-

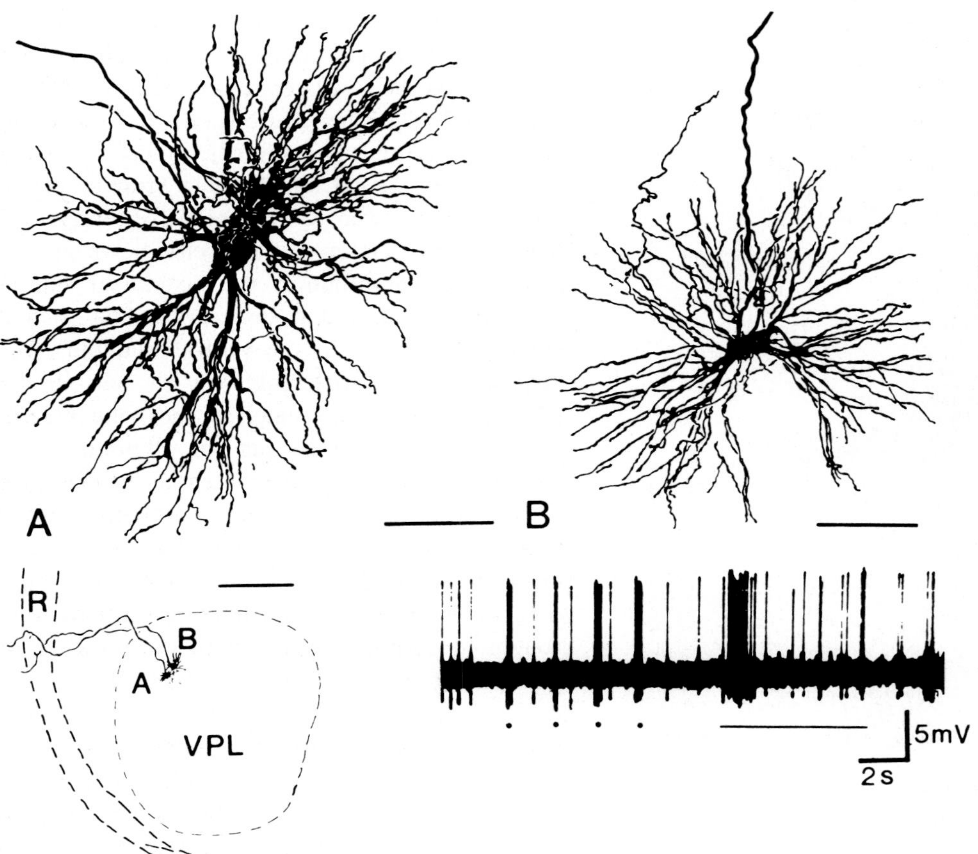

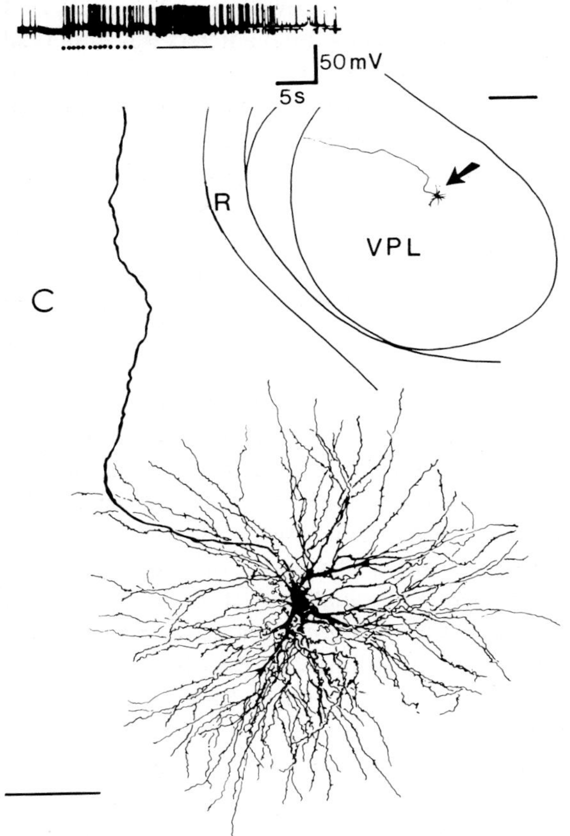

Fig. 11. Intracellularly injected type I (A,B) and type II (C) relay neurons in the cat VPL nucleus. Type I cells respond with transient discharges to a stimulus (dots, bar) while most type II cells respond with a sustained discharge. From Yen et al., 1985b. Bars 1 mm, 100 μm.

tral medial and para-central of the intralaminar group, the suprageniculate-limitans nucleus of the posterior group, the VPL, VPM, VLp and VLa nuclei of the ventral group, the magnocellular medial geniculate nucleus and the dorsal lateral geniculate nucleus. All other dorsal thalamic nuclei contain no or virtually no stained cells. The distribution of CAT-301 positive cells in the dorsal lateral geniculate nucleus is not uniform. 70% of the neurons in the magnocellular layers are CAT-301 positive but less than 40% in the parvocellular layers and none in the S layers and intercalated layers.

An interesting complementarity appears when the monkey dorsal lateral geniculate nucleus is stained immunocytochemically for a neuronal phosphoprotein, the calcium-calmodulin dependent protein kinase, CAM II kinase (S.H.C. Hendry, M.B. Kennedy and E.G. Jones, unpublished). Then, only the S and intercalated layer relay cells are stained. These are the same cells that stain for calbindin. In other parts of the dorsal thalamus, virtually all relay cells appear to stain for CAM II kinase. The differential staining for CAM II kinase in the dorsal lateral geniculate nucleus is especially interesting given the fact that this enzyme, once activated is capable of self-phosphorylation (Miller and Kennedy, 1986) and thus should be able to hold the "memory" of a calcium transient in the cell. In this there may be a determining influence on the temporal characteristics of a cell's discharges. With the discovery of additional neuronal markers of this kind it may become possible to specify different classes of thalamic relay cells with greater fidelity than in the past and from a perspective that transcends both the anatomical and the physiological.

Relay neurons and interneurons: the example of the cat VPL nucleus

The security and fidelity with which the sensory nuclei of the thalamus relay information from the periphery to the cerebral cortex is a well known fact, although it is becoming recognized again after a period of neglect that the relay capacities of the sensory nuclei are very much state dependent and influenced by brainstem mechanisms (Steriade and Deschênes, 1984; Hobson and Steriade, 1987; Steriade and Llinás, 1988). The faithfulness of the relay mode of thalamic function is dependent upon the presence of specific sets of relay neurons with secure input synapses and a focussed projection upon the cerebral cortex (Jones, 1985). Studies in the visual system have revealed at least three sets of relay cells in the dorsal lateral geniculate nucleus and which are selectively innervated by different classes of retinal ganglion cells. These have been traditionally referred to as X, Y and W cells, the distinction among them being primarily based upon their capacity for the summation of discharges resulting from stimulation by grating stimuli of different spatial frequencies (Enroth-Cugell and Robson, 1966; Sherman and Koch, 1986). Other criteria, at least in monkeys (Hubel and Livingstone, 1987; Livingstone and Hubel, 1987) are now also being used to classify these various cell types. In the dorsal lateral geniculate nucleus of the cat there seem to be very clear morphological differences between most members of the X, Y and W cell classes (Friedlander et al., 1981; Stanford et al., 1983; Wilson et al., 1984; Raczowski et al., 1988) and in the terminal distributions of the ganglion cell axons that appear selectively to innervate them (Sur and Sherman, 1982; Bowling and Michael, 1984; Garraghty et al., 1986).

In searching for analogous correlations in the somatic sensory system, the focus has been largely on analyzing cells and lemniscal axons in terms of their submodality properties (Yen et al., 1985b; Hirai et al., 1988). In making morphological correlations in the cat VPL, however, this has proven less fruitful than the analysis of the cells in terms of tonicity or transiency of discharge in response to a peripheral stimulus. Two major classes of relay cells were identified by intracellular injection. One, by far the majority, was characterized by tufted dendrites, lacking appendages, and a thick axon. It included cells with both cutaneous and deep receptive fields and which responded in a transient manner to peripheral stimulation (Fig. 11). The other, characterized by more slender, dichotomously branching dendrites covered in thin appendages and a thin axon, also included cells with both cutaneous and deep receptive fields that usually discharged in a sustained manner to peripheral stimulation. The key to cell differences as reflected in morphology, appears, therefore, to lie in discharge patterns rather than in receptive field type (Yen et al., 1985b).

The study was extended to the arriving lemniscal axons to determine the extent to which their morphologies reflected functional differences (Hirai et al., 1988). The distribution of conduction velocities and parent axon diameters was unimodal and broadly extended. Differences were revealed, however, when the patterns of axonal distribution, as determined by intra-axonal injection of horseradish peroxidase, were examined (Fig. 12). Medial lemniscal fibers activated by joint movement terminated mainly in anterodorsal parts of the nucleus while those activated by cutaneous stimulation terminated in the central core of the nucleus, a differential distribution reflecting the segregation of deep and cutaneous modalities in the nucleus of cats and monkeys (Friedman and Jones, 1981; Jones and Friedman, 1982; Hirai et al., 1988). All axons irrespective of their zone of termination and the submodality represented ended in localized terminal fields that were extended anteroposteriorly. The major differences were in the number of terminal boutons on each axon and the extent of termination. Joint axons had the least extensive terminations and the fewest boutons. Pressure, sustained axons had the most extensive terminations and largest number of boutons. Hair, sustained axons had small terminations and few boutons. Hair, transient axons had medium-sized terminations and many boutons. It would appear, therefore, that the principal central correlate of submodality specificity at the anatomical level may be the number of relay cells contacted by individual axon types.

The exact nature of the synaptic relationships between afferent fibers and relay cells probably plays a substantial role in determining the character of the relay cells' discharge patterns. This and the influence of local interneurons may be especially important in determining that cells whose membrane properties, as revealed by in vitro studies (Jahnsen and Llinás, 1983a,b) and in intact preparations (Roy et al., 1984), are fundamentally similar, can consistently relay different information in the intact animal. Where it has been examined in the dorsal lateral geniculate nucleus of cats, the synaptic relationships between optic tract axons and X and Y neurons are quite different. Retinal afferents end on X cells mainly on den-

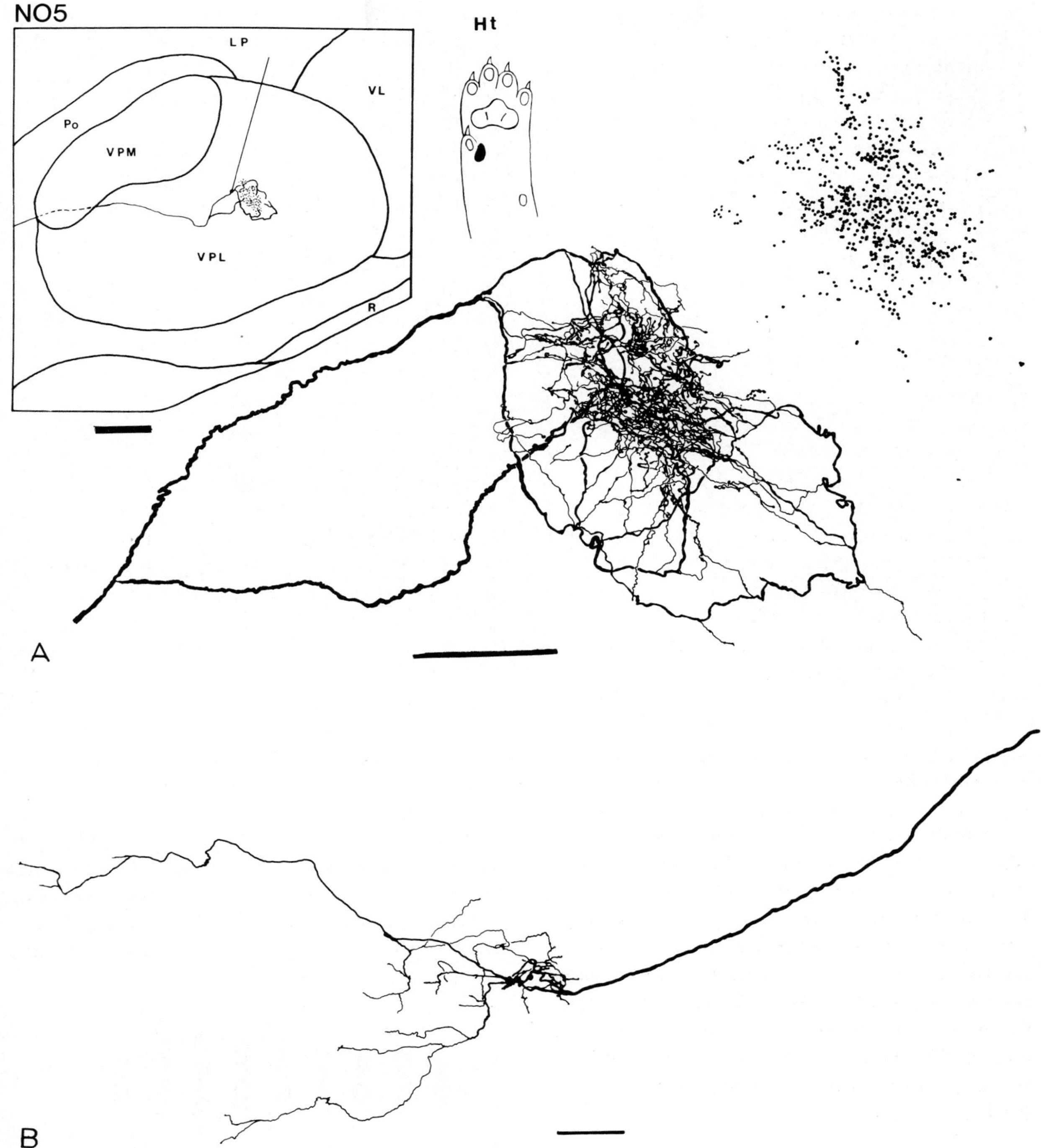

Fig. 12. Intra-axonally injected medial lemniscal (12A) and spinothalamic tract (12B) axons in the cat VPL nucleus. Dots in A indicate terminal boutons extracted form main camera lucida drawing. From Hirai et al., 1988; Yen, Honda and Jones (unpublished). Bar 1 mm, 100 μm.

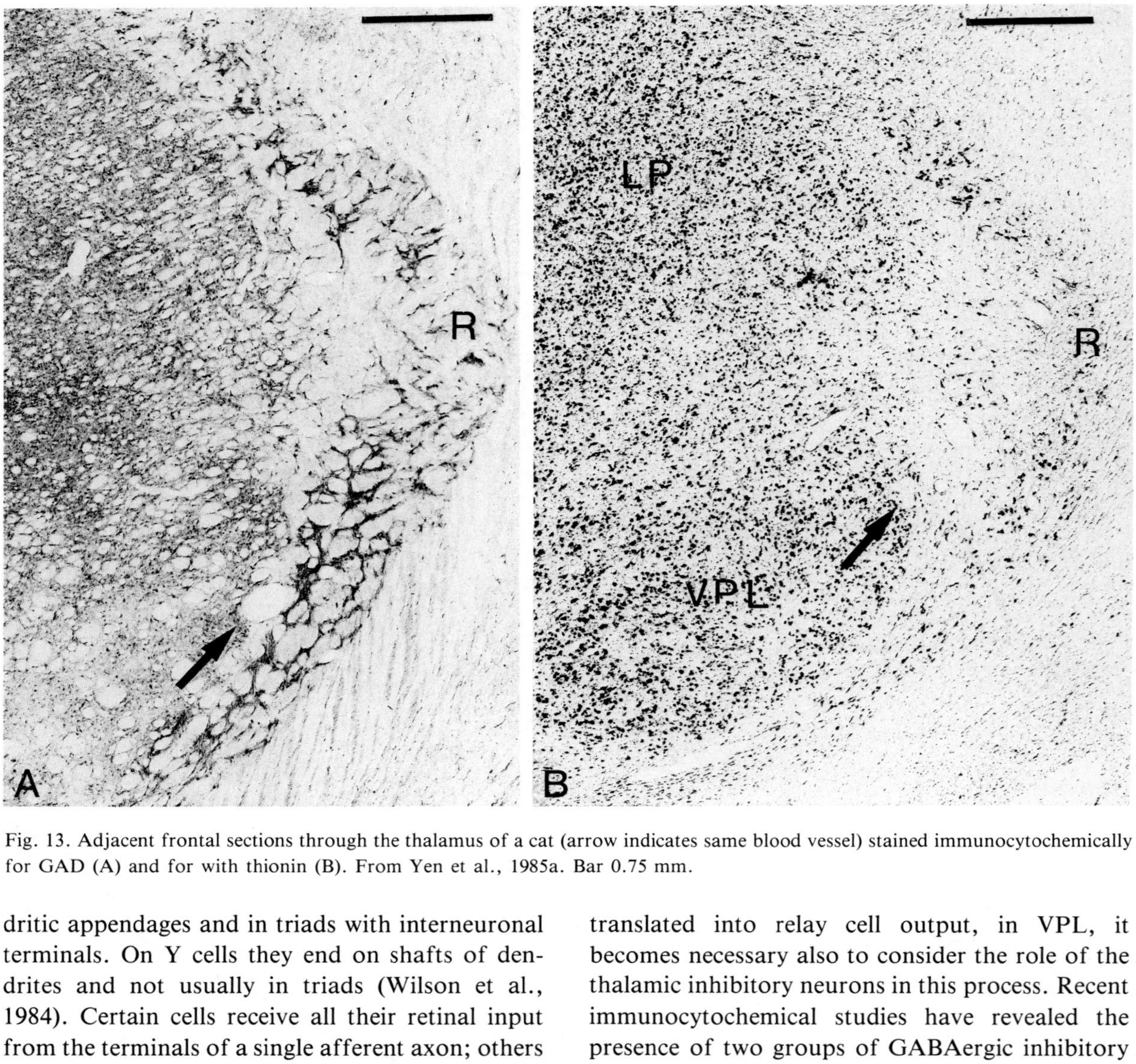

Fig. 13. Adjacent frontal sections through the thalamus of a cat (arrow indicates same blood vessel) stained immunocytochemically for GAD (A) and for with thionin (B). From Yen et al., 1985a. Bar 0.75 mm.

dritic appendages and in triads with interneuronal terminals. On Y cells they end on shafts of dendrites and not usually in triads (Wilson et al., 1984). Certain cells receive all their retinal input from the terminals of a single afferent axon; others receive terminals from several afferent axons (Hamos et al., 1987). The geography of synapses on the surfaces of the relay neurons, thus, varies and in this there may be clues to the different responsivity of the two relay cell classes to afferent driving.

Inhibitory neurons in the thalamus: instrinsic and reticular nucleus

On enquiring into how lemniscal input is translated into relay cell output, in VPL, it becomes necessary also to consider the role of the thalamic inhibitory neurons in this process. Recent immunocytochemical studies have revealed the presence of two groups of GABAergic inhibitory

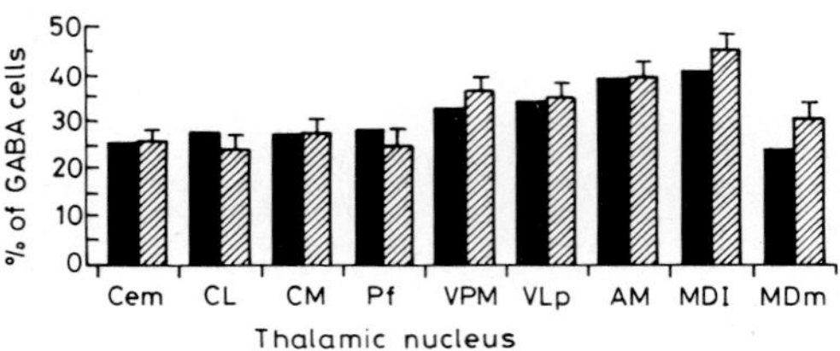

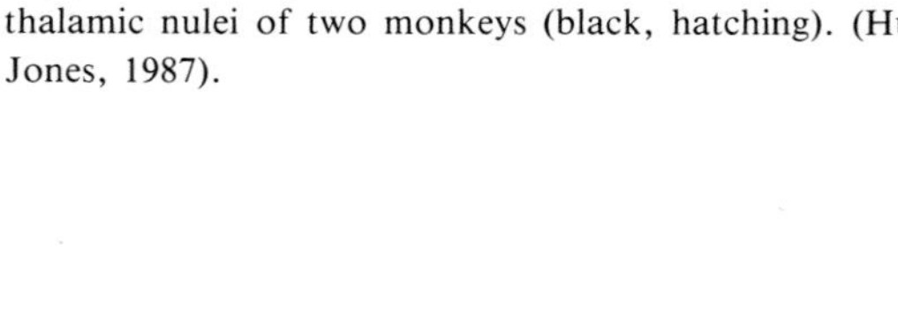

Fig. 14. Percentages of GABA immunoreactive cells in selected thalamic nulei of two monkeys (black, hatching). (Hunt and Jones, 1987).

neuron innervating dorsal thalamic relay nuclei such as the ventral posterior (Jones, 1985). One of these groups is formed by the intrinsic neurons of the dorsal thalamus, the other by the cells of the reticular nucleus (Fig. 13).

In the ventral posterior nucleus of cats and monkeys, GABA or GAD immunoreactive neurons form approximately 20% of the total neuronal population (Penny et al., 1983; Hunt and Jones, 1987) (Fig. 14). A similar percentage of GABAergic neurons is found in the dorsal lateral geniculate nucleus of the two species (Penny et al., 1984; Montero and Zempel, 1985; Montero, 1986). These and other dorsal thalamic nuclei are also innervated by GABA neurons whose cell bodies occupy a sector of the reticular nucleus that is specified for a particular dorsal thalamic nucleus (Jones, 1975; Pollin and Rokyta, 1982; Montero and Singer, 1984; Jones, 1985; Sherman and Koch, 1986; Sumitomo et al., 1988). All the reticular nucleus cells are GABA or GAD immunoreactive (Oertel et al., 1983; Montero and Singer, 1984; Yen et al., 1985a) (Fig. 13).

The general structure of these two groups of

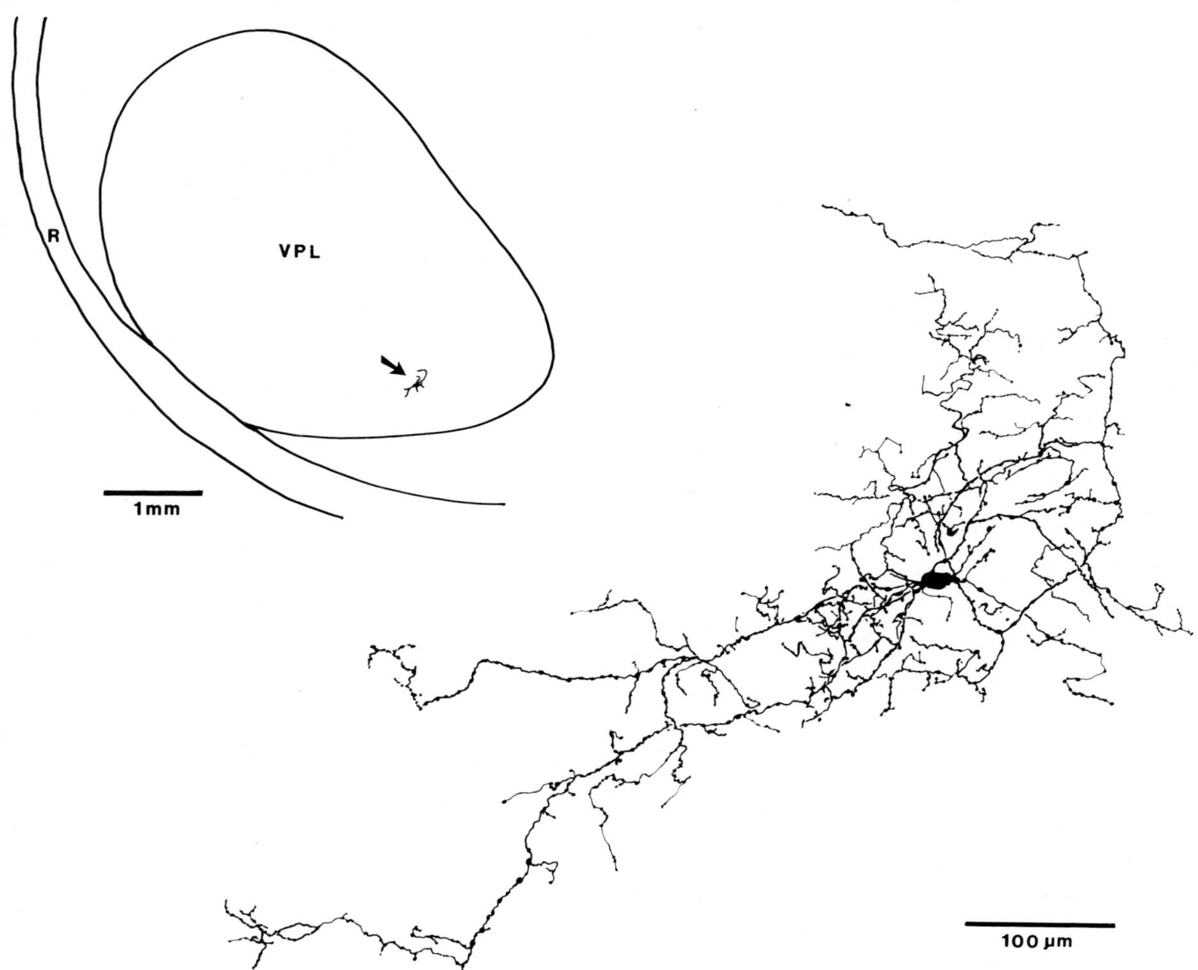

Fig. 15. Intracellularly injected interneuron in VPL nucleus of a cat. From Yen et al., 1985a.

thalamic inhibitory neurons has been known for some time from Golgi studies (Jones, 1985) and these have been confirmed and extended by recent intracellular staining studies (Yen et al., 1985b; Sherman and Friedlander, 1988). In both the ventral posterior and dorsal lateral geniculate nuclei, the intrinsic neurons are revealed as having very small somata and a series of angular dendrites covered in bulbous protrusions and dilatations (Fig. 15) which prove on electron microscopic analysis to be the presynaptic dendritic terminals of earlier electron microscopic studies (Ralston and Herman, 1969; Ralston, 1971) and which prove also to be GABA and GAD immunoreactive (Fitzpatrick et al., 1984; Montero and Singer, 1984; Jones, 1985).

The reticular nucleus cells in a sector of the nucleus connected with a particular dorsal thalamic nucleus (Jones, 1975) have receptive fields that reflect inputs from and convergence of the collateral branches of thalamocortical axons emanating from that nucleus. When intracellularly injected and recovered histologically, reticular nucleus cells prove to have a very extensively rami-

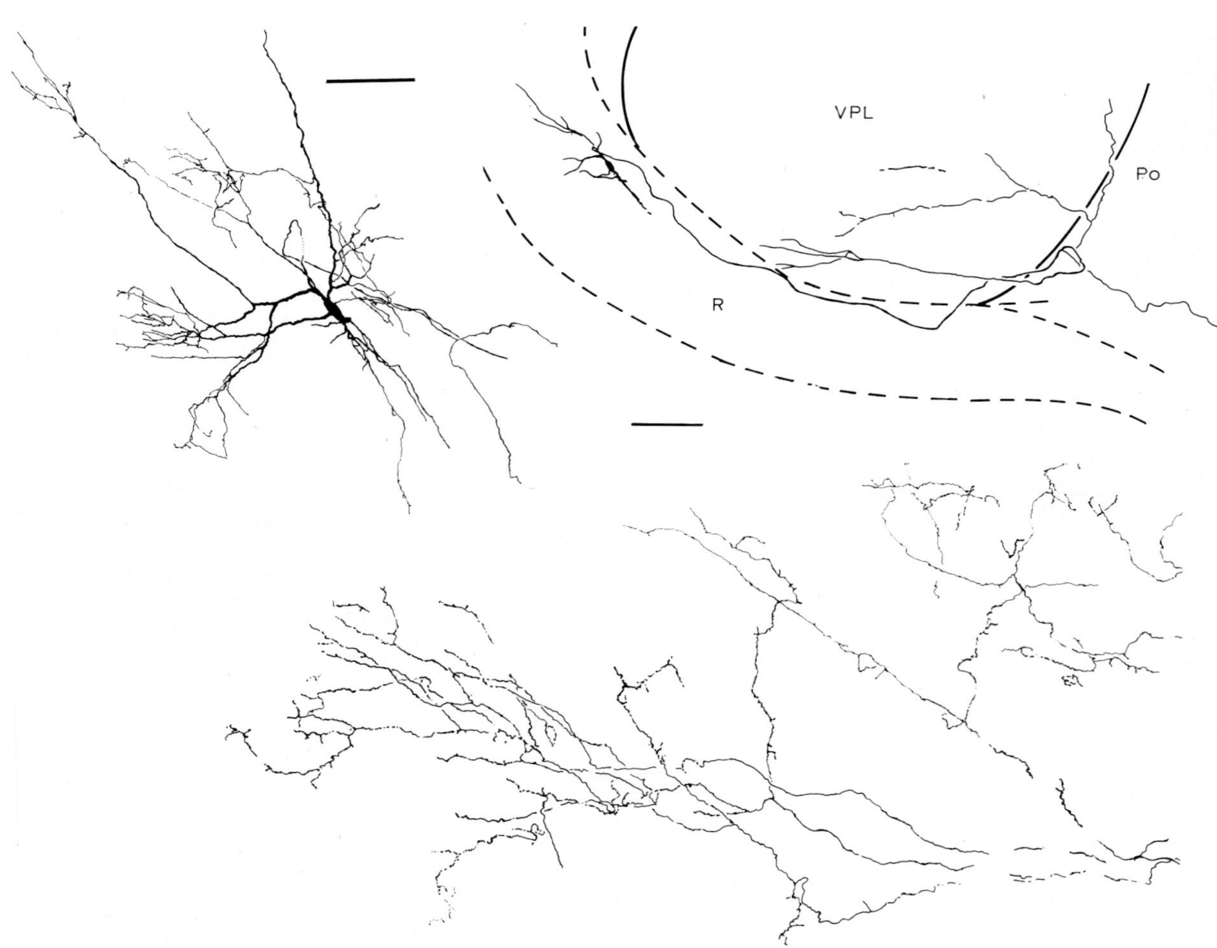

Fig. 16. Intracellularly injected neuron of the reticular nucleus of a cat (Yen et al., 1985a) with its axon ramifying widely in VPL. Part of the axonal ramification is enlarged in lower figure. Bars 100 μm (left, lower) 0.5 mm (right).

fying axon distributing in the dorsal thalamus (Yen et al., 1985a) (Fig. 16) and local collaterals in the reticular nucleus itself. The dendrites of the reticular nucleus cells also show evidence of protrusions that prove on thin sectioning to be presynaptic dendritic terminals that are also GABA immunoreactive (Yen et al., 1985a; see also Ralston, this volume). These apparently serve to couple together adjacent cells of the reticular nucleus.

The effects of GABA synapses in the dorsal thalamus have been variously reported. In the ventral posterior nucleus blockade of GABA receptors by bicuculline, is said to enlarge the cutaneous receptive fields of many neurons (Hicks et al., 1986) and to block the process whereby tonic lemniscal inputs to certain cells are converted by the cell into a transient output (Gottschaldt et al., 1983). In the dorsal lateral geniculate nucleus, the center-surround antagonism of relay neurons appears to be maintained by GABA mechamisms (Sillito and Kemp, 1983). The relative contributions of intrinsic and reticular nucleus GABA neurons to these functions are not known. There are some data to suggest, however, that the two types of GABA synapse may be concentrated on different parts of the dendritic trees of the relay neurons. Reticular nucleus axons are reported to end on the soma and proximal dendrites while the presynaptic dendrites of the intrinsic neurons appear to terminate closer to the first branchings of the dendrites and beyond (Ohara et al.,1980; Montero and Scott, 1981; Peschanski and Besson, 1984; Liu et al., 1989). GABA immunoreactive presynaptic dendrites also terminate distal to GABA immunoreactive axon terminals in electron microscopic immunocytochemical studies (Liu et al., 1989a). The selective activities of these two separately targeted sets of inhibitory synapses on relay cell function await physiological and pharmacological exploration.

Other transmitters and related compounds in the thalamus: the importance of the brainstem

The neurochemical transmitters of the thalamic relay neurons and of the great afferent pathways terminating in the thalamus still elude detection. Repeated hints, however, point to the possibility of an acidic amino acid or combination of amino acids. More is known of the transmitters expressed by the diffuse pathways of brainstem and basal forebrain region that permeate the thalamus (Mesulam et al., 1983; Cropper et al., 1984; De Lima et al., 1985; Butcher and Woolf, 1986; De Lima and Singer, 1987) and which seem to be involved in the state dependent activities of the thalamus (Hobson and Steriade, 1987) (Fig. 17). Noradrenergic fibers emanating from the locus coeruleus, serotoninergic fibers emanating from the dorsal raphe of the midbrain and cholinergic fibers emanating from the peribrachial region of the pons and the basal forebrain, are distributed widely in the dorsal thalamus and are especially concentrated in the reticular nucleus. The effects of stimulating these systems, especially the cholinergic, (McCormick and Prince, 1986; Prince and McCormick, 1987) are becoming better known. Acetyl choline, for example, suppresses reticular cell excitability but causes the cells to discharge in a burst pattern (McCormick and Prince, 1986). The anatomy of their synapses is far less well known. Recent studies on the dorsal lateral geniculate nucleus (De Lima et al., 1985) indicate that cholinergic terminals end in symmetrical contacts on dendrites of relay neurons and on presynaptic dendrites of putative GABAergic neurons. Serotonin immunoreactive fibers have relatively few synapses and many may end without synaptic specialization (De Lima and Singer, 1987).

Immunocytochemistry is also revealing the likely presence of certain neuropeptides in afferent fiber systems innervating the thalamus and in certain thalamic cells (Graybiel and Elde, 1983). The presence of tachykinin immunoreactivity in trigeminal fibers innervating the VPM nucleus in monkeys was mentioned above (Fig. 5). Cholecystokinin immunoreactivity has also been reported in fibers of dorsal column nuclear origin innervating the rat VPL (Hunt and Jones, 1987) and cholecystokinin, tachykinin and enkephalin immunoreactivity has been reported in fibers of spinal origin that innervate more medial parts of the thalamus in rats, monkeys and humans (Gall et al., 1987; Molinari et al., 1987; Hirai and Jones, 1989). Also entering the thalamus from brainstem, basal forebrain, hypothalamic and/or prethalamic sites are fibers immunoreactive for neuropeptide

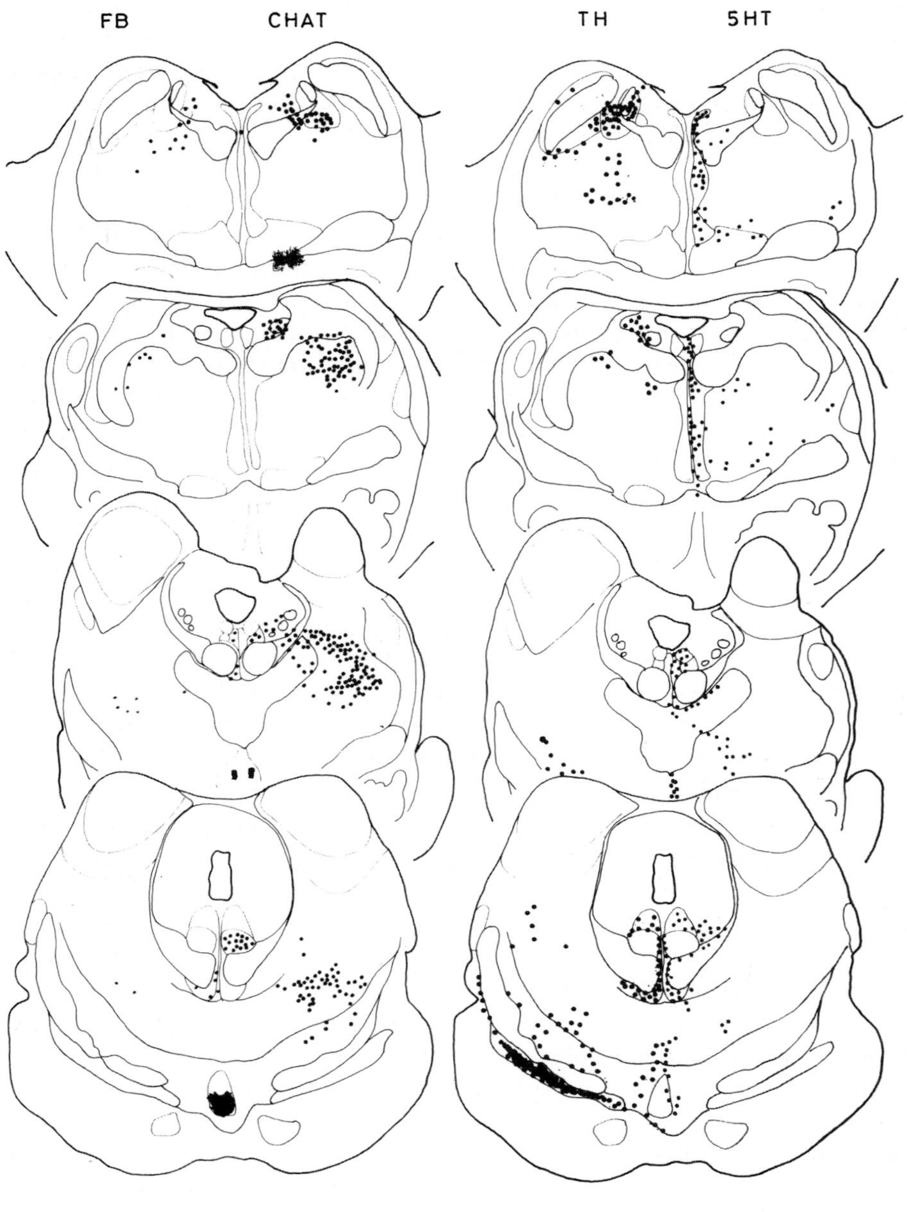

Fig. 17. Distribution of neurons retrogradely labeled with Fast Blue (FB) following an injection of the tracer in the ipsilateral VPL nucleus of a monkey, correlated with the distribution of choline acetyl transferase (ChAT) and serotonin (5HT) immunoreactive cells in the same animal. Unpublished work from the author's laboratory.

Y, somatostatin, cholecystokinin, tachykinins and neurotensin (Swanson and Hartman, 1975; Cuello and Kanazawa, 1978; Finlay et al., 1981; Inagaki et al., 1983; Johannson et al., 1983; Fallon and Leslie, 1986; Molinari et al., 1987). Most of these have relatively selective zones of termination involving one or a few nuclei. Apart from the tachykinin positive fibers in the VPM nucleus, however, the synapses formed by these various peptide positive fibers have not been identified and their functions have not been explored.

Conclusion

This brief review of some recently discovered aspects of thalamic organization has ranged over a variety of topics that involve examination of the thalamus as a sensory relay center at different levels of resolution. Sensitive histochemical methods reveal that the nuclear parcellation of the thalamus is still valid and that the gross nuclei represent the macrochannels for the relay of sensory and motor related pathways to the cerebral cortex. Charles Bell's idea and William Mehler's reformulation of it are, thus, still with us. Within each of these macrochannels, however, are a series of finer channels that can be revealed as constellations of relay cells with preferential staining properties and differential cortical projections. At an even finer level are the individual cells themselves whose dendritic structure and the synaptic geography of whose inputs seem to be directly correlated with the cells' capacities to relay different patterns of afferent activity. These functional properties appear to be under the influence of both local GABA neurons and GABA neurons of the reticular nucleus whose effects seem to be to maintain the security and faithfulness of the relay of sensory information through thalamus to cortex. Imposed on all of these channels, however, and apparently serving to regulate the level of excitability of the thalamus and through that the state of arousal of the cerebral cortex, are the diffuse brainstem pathways whose transmitters are now known. In all of these topics there is much opportunity for further productive work and for further development of a field to which William Mehler contributed so much.

Acknowledgements

Personal work was supported by grant numbers NS21377 and NS22317 from the National Institutes of Health, United States Public Health Science.

Abbreviations

AD	Anterodorsal nucleus
AM	Anteromedial nucleus
AV	Anteroventral nucleus
CALB	Calbindin
CeM	Central medial nucleus
ChAT	Choline acetyltransferase
CL	Central lateral nucleus
CM	Centre médian nucleus
DIT	Dorsal ipsilateral trigeminal tract
FB	Fast Blue
GLD, LG	Dorsal lateral geniculate nucleus
H	Habenular nuclei
Ht	Hair transient response
L	Limitans nucleus
LD	Lateral dorsal nucleus
MC	Magnocellular layers, dorsal lateral geniculate nucleus
MD	Mediodorsal nucleus
MDl	Mediodorsal nucleus, lateral division
MDm	Mediodorsal nucleus, medial division
ML	Medial lemniscus
MV	Medioventral nucleus
PARV	Parvalbumin
PC	Parvocellular layers, dorsal lateral geniculate nucleus
Pc	Paracentral nucleus
Pf	Parafascicular nucleus
Pg	Pregeniculate nucleus
Pla	Anterior pulvinar nucleus
Pli	Inferior pulvinar nucleus
Pll	Lateral pulvinar nucleus
Plm	Medial pulvinar nucleus
Po	Posterior nucleus
R	Reticular nucleus
Sg	Suprageniculate nucleus
TH	Tyrosine hydroxylase
VA	Ventral anterior nucleus
VAmc	Ventral anterior nucleus, magnocellular division

VL	Ventral lateral nucleus
VLa	Ventral lateral anterior nucleus
VLp	Ventral lateral posterior nucleus
VMb	Basal ventral medial nucleus
VPI	Ventral posterior inferior nucleus
VPL	Ventral posterior lateral nucleus
VPM	Ventral posterior medial nucleus
5HT	Serotonin.

References

Alexander, G.E., DeLong, M.R. and Strick, P.L. (1986) Parallel organization of functionally integrated circuits linking basal ganglia and cortex. *Ann. Rev. Neurosci.,* 9: 357 – 382.

Andersen, P., Eccles, J.C. and Sears, T.A. (1964) The ventrobasal nucleus of the thalamus: types of cells, their responses and their functional organization. *J. Physiol. Lond.,* 174: 307 – 399.

Asanuma, C., Thach, W.T. and Jones, E.G. (1983a) Cytoarchitectonic delineation of the ventral lateral thalamic region in monkeys. *Brain Res. Rev.,* 5: 219 – 235.

Asanuma, C., Thach, W.T. and Jones, E.G. (1983b) Distribution of cerebellar terminations and their relation to other afferent terminations in the ventral lateral thalamic region of the monkey. *Brain Res. Rev.,* 5: 237 – 265.

Asanuma, C., Thach, W.T. and Jones, E.G. (1983c) Anatomical evidence for segregated focal groupings of efferent cells and their terminal ramifications in the cerebellothalamic pathways. *Brain Res. Rev.,* 5: 267 – 297.

Bell, C. (1811) Idea of a New Anatomy of the Brain, Privately printed.

Bowling, D.B. and Michael, C.R. (1984) Terminal patterns of single, physiologically characterized optic tract fibers in the cat's lateral geniculate nucleus. *J. Neurosci.,* 4: 198 – 216.

Butcher, L.L. and Woolf, N.J. (1986) Central cholinergic systems: a synopsis of anatomy and overview of physiology and pathology. In A.B. Scheibel and A.F. Wechsler (Eds.), *The Biological Substrates of Alzheimer's Disease,* Academic Press, New York, pp. 73 – 86.

Carey, R.G., Fitzpatrick, D. and Diamond, I.T. (1979) Layer I of striate of *Tupaia glis* and *Galago senegalensis:* Projections from thalamus and claustrum revealed by retrograde transport of horseradish peroxidase. *J. Comp. Neurol.,* 186: 393 – 438.

Carpenter, M.B., Nakano, K. and Kim, R. (1976) Nigrothalamic projections in the monkey demonstrated by autoradiographic technics. *J. Comp. Neurol.,* 165: 401 – 415.

Celio, M.R. (1986) Parvalbumin in most y-aminobutyric acid-containing neurons of the rat cerebral cortex. *Science,* 231: 995 – 997.

Clark, W.E., LeGros (1936) The thalamic connections of the temporal lobe of the brain in the monkey. *J. Anat.,* 70: 447 – 464.

Conrath, M., Covenas, R., Romo, R., Cheramy, A., Bourgoin, S. and Hamon, M. (1986) Distribution of Met-enkephalin immunoreactive fibres in the thalamus of the cat. *Neurosci Lett.,* 65: 299 – 303.

Cropper, E.C., Eisenman, J.S. and Azmitia, E.C. (1984) An immunocytochemical study of the serotonergic innervation of the thalamus of the rat. *J. Comp. Neurol.,* 224: 38 – 50.

Cuello, A.C. and Kanazawa, I. (1978) The distribution of substance P immunoreactive fibers in the rat central nervous system. *J. Comp. Neurol.,* 178: 129 – 156.

DeFelipe, J., Hendry, S.H.C. and Jones, E.G. (1989) Visualization of chandelier cell axons by parvalbumin immunoreactivity in monkey cerebral cortex. *Proc. Natl. Acad. Sci. USA,* 86: 2093 – 2097.

De Lima, A.D. and Singer, W. (1987) The serotoninergic fibers in the dorsal lateral geniculate nucleus of the cat: distribution and synaptic connections demonstrated with immunocytochemistry. *J. Comp. Neurol.,* 258: 339 – 351.

De Lima, A.D., Montero, V.M. and Singer, W. (1985) The cholinergic innervation of the visual thalamus: an EM immunocytochemical study. *Exp. Brain Res.,* 59: 206 – 212.

Enroth-Cugell, C.C. and Robson, J.G. (1966) The contrast sensitivity of retinal ganglion cells of the cat. *J. Physiol. Lond.,* 187: 517 – 534.

Fallon, J.H. and Leslie, F.M. (1986) Distribution of dynorphin and enkephalin peptides in the rat brain. *J. Comp. Neurol.,* 249: 293 – 336.

Finlay, J.C.W., Maderdrut, J.L., Roger, L.J. and Petrusz, P. (1981) The immunocytochemical localization of somatostatin-containing neurons in rat central nervous system. *Neuroscience,* 6: 2173 – 2192.

Fitzpatrick, D., Penny, G.R. and Schmechel, D.E. (1984) Glutamic acid decarboxylase-immunoreactive neurons and terminals in the lateral geniculate nucleus of the cat. *J. Neurosci.,* 4: 1809 – 1829.

Friedlander, M.J., Lin, C.-S., Stanford, L.R. and Sherman, S.M. (1981) Morphology of functionally identified neurons in lateral geniculate nucleus of cat. *J. Neurophysiol.,* 46: 80 – 129.

Friedman, D.P. and Jones, E.G. (1981) Thalamic input to areas 3a and 2 in monkey, *J. Neurophysiol.,* 45: 59 – 85.

Gall, C., Lauterborn, J., Burks, D. and Seroogy, K. (1987) Colocalization of enkephalin and cholecystokinin in discrete areas of rat brain. *Brain Res.,* 403: 403 – 408.

Garraghty, P.E., Sur, M. and Sherman, S.M. (1986) Morphology of retinogeniculate X and Y axon arbors in monocularly enucleated cats. *J. Comp. Neurol.,* 251: 198 – 215.

Gottschaldt, K.-M., Vahle-Hinz, C. and Hicks, T.P. (1983) Electrophysiological and micropharmacological studies on mechanisms of input-output transformation in single neurones of the somato-sensory thalamus. In G. Macchi, A. Rustioni and R. Spreafico (Eds.), *Somatosensory Integration in the Thalamus,* Elsevier, Amsterdam, pp. 199 – 216.

Graybiel, A.M. and Berson, D.M. (1980) Histochemical identification and afferent connections of subdivisions in the lateralis posterior-pulvinar complex and related thalamic nuclei in the cat. *Neuroscience,* 5: 1175 – 1238.

Graybiel, A.M. and Elde, R.P. (1983) Somatostatin-like immunoreactivity characterizes neurons of the nucleus reticularis thalami in the cat and monkey. *J. Neurosci.,* 3: 1308 – 1321.

Hamos, J.E., Van Horn, S.C., Raczkowski, D. and Sherman, S.M. (1987) Synaptic circuits involving an individual retinogeniculate axon in the cat. *J. Comp. Neurol.,* 259: 165 – 192.

Hassler, R. (1959) Anatomy of the Thalamus. In G. Schaltenbrand and P. Bailey (Eds.), *Introduction to Stereotaxis with an Atlas of the Human Brain,* Thieme, Stuttgart, pp. 230 – 290.

Hendry, S.H.C., Jones, E.G., Emson, P.C., Lawson, D.E.M., Heizmann, C.W. and Streit, P. (1989) Two classes of cortical GABA neurons defined by differential calcium binding protein immunoreactivities. *Exp. Brain Res.* 76: 467 – 472.

Hendry, S.H.C., Jones, E.G. and Graham, J. (1979) Thalamic relay nuclei for cerebellar and certain related fiber system in the cat. *J. Comp. Neurol.,* 185: 679 – 714.

Hendry, S.H.C., Jones, E.G., Hockfield, S. and McKay, R.D.G. (1988) Neuronal populations stained with the monoclonal antibody Cat-301 in the mammalian cerebral cortex and thalamus. *J. Neurosci.,* 8: 518 – 542.

Hicks, T.P., Metherate, R., Landry, P. and Dykes, R.W. (1986) Bicuculline-induced alterations of response properties in functionally identified ventroposterior thalamic neurones. *Exp. Brain Res.,* 63: 248 – 264.

Hirai, T. and Jones, E.G. (1988) Segregation of lemniscal inputs and motor cortex outputs in cat ventral thalamic nuclei: application of a novel technique. *Exp. Brain Res.,* 71: 329 – 344.

Hirai, T. and Jones, E.G. (1989a) A new parcellation of the human thalamus on the basis of histochemical staining. *Brain Res. Rev.,* 14: 1 – 34.

Hirai, T. and Jones, E.G. (1989b) Distribution of tachykinin- and enkephalin-immunoreactive fibers in the human thalamus. *Brain Res. Rev.,* 14: 35 – 52.

Hirai, T., Schwark, H.D., Yen, C.-T., Honda, C.N. and Jones, E.G. (1988) Morphology of physiologically characterized medial lemniscal axons terminating in cat ventral posterior thalamic nucleus. *J. Neurophysiol.* 60: 1439 – 1459.

Hobson, J.A. and Steriade, M. (1987) Neuronal basis of behavioral state control. In J.M. Brookhart et al. (Eds.), *Handbook of Physiology - The nervous system* Volume IV, Amer. Physiol. Soc., Washington D.C., pp. 701 – 823.

Hubel, D.H. and Livingstone, M.S. (1987) Segregation of form, color and stereopsis in primate area 18. *J. Neurosci.,* 7: 3378 – 3415.

Hubel, D.H. and Wiesel, T.N. (1969) Anatomical demonstration of columns in the monkey striate cortex. *Nature,* 221: 747 – 750.

Hunt, C.A. and Jones, E.G. (1987) Distribution of Gamma-aminobutyric acid-positive neurons and acetylcholinesterase in the monkey thalamus. *Neurosci. Abstr.,* 13: 953.

Hunt, C.A., Seroogy, K.B., Gall, C.M. and Jones, E.G. (1987) Cholecystokinin innervation of rat thalamus, including fibers to ventroposterolateral nucleus from dorsal column nuclei. *Brain Res.,* 426: 257 – 269.

Ilinsky, I.A. and Kultas-Ilinsky, K. (1987) Sagittal cytoarchitectonic maps of the *Macaca mulatta* thalamus with a revised nomenclature of the motor-related nuclei validated by observations on their connectivity. *J. Comp. Neurol.,* 262: 331 – 364.

Inagaki, S., Kubota, Y., Shinoda, K., Kawai, Y. and Tohyama, M. (1983) Neurotensin-containing pathway from the endopiriform nucleus and the adjacent prepiriform cortex to the dorsomedial thalamic nucleus in the rat. *Brain Res.,* 260: 143 – 146.

Jahnsen, H. and Llinás, R. (1983a) Electrophysiological properties of guinea-pig thalamic neurons: an in vitro study. *J. Physiol. Lond.,* 349: 205 – 226.

Jahnsen, H. and Llinás, R. (1983b) Ionic basis for the electroresponsiveness and oscillatory properties of guinea-pig thalamic neurones in vitro. *J. Physiol. Lond.,* 349: 227 – 248.

Johannson, O., Hökfelt, T. and Elde, R.P. (1984) Immunohistochemical distribution of somatostatin-like immunoreactivity in the central nervous system of the adult rat. *Neuroscience,* 13: 265 – 239.

Jones, E.G. (1975) Lamination and differential distribution of thalamic afferents in the sensory-motor cortex of the squirrel monkey. *J. Comp. Neurol.,* 160: 167 – 204.

Jones, E.G. (1975) Some aspects of the organization of the thalamic reticular complex, *J. Comp. Neurol.,* 162: 285 – 307.

Jones, E.G. (1983a) Lack of collateral thalamocortical projections to fields of the first somatic sensory cortex in monkeys. *Exp. Brain Res.,* 52: 375 – 384.

Jones, E.G. (1983b) The Thalamus. In P.C. Emson (Ed.), *Chemical Neuroanatomy,* Raven Press, New York, pp. 257 – 293.

Jones, E.G. (1985) *The Thalamus,* Plenum, New York.

Jones, E.G. (1988) GABA neurons and their cotransmitters in the primate cerebral cortex. In M. Avoli, T.A. Reader, R.W. Dykes, P. Gloor (Eds.), *Neurotransmitters and Cortical function: From Molecules to Mind,* Plenum, New York, pp. 125 – 152.

Jones, E.G. and Burton, H. (1976) Areal differences in the laminar distribution of thalamic afferents in cortical fields of the insular, parietal and temporal regions of primates. *J. Comp. Neurol.,* 168: 197 – 248.

Jones, E.G. and Friedman, D.P., Projection pattern of functional components of thalamic ventrobasal complex on monkey somatosensory cortex. *J. Neurophysiol.,* 48: 521 – 544.

Jones, E.G., Friedman, D.P. and Hendry, S.H.C. (1982) Thalamic basis of place and modality-specific columns in monkey somatosensory cortex: a correlative anatomical and physiological study. *J. Neurophysiol.,* 48: 545 – 568.

Jones, E.G. and Hendry, S.H.C. (1989) Differential calcium binding protein immunoreactivity distinguishes two classes of relay neurons in monkey thalamic nuclei. *Eur. J. Neurosci.* 1: 222 – 246.

Jones, E.G., Hendry, S.H.C. and Brandon, C. (1986a) Cytochrome oxidase staining reveals functional organization of monkey somatosensory thalamus. *Exp. Brain Res.,* 62: 438 – 442.

Jones, E.G., Schwark, H.D. and Callahan, P.J. (1986b) Extent of the ipsilateral representation in the ventral posterior medial nucleus of the monkey thalamus. *Exp. Brain Res.,* 63: 310 – 320.

Jones, E.G., Wise, S.P. and Coulter, J.D. (1979) Differential thalamic relationships of sensory motor and parietal cortical fields in monkeys. *J. Comp. Neurol.,* 183: 833 – 882.

Kim, R., Nakano, K., Carpenter, M.B. and Jayaraman, A. (1976) Projections of the globus pallidus and adjacent structures: an autoradiographic study in the monkey. *J. Comp. Neurol.,* 169: 263 – 290.

Lenz, F.A., Dostrovsky, J.O., Tasker, R.R., Yamashiro, K., Kwan, H.C. and Murphy, J.T. (1988) Single-unit analysis of the human ventral thalamic nuclear group: somatosensory responses. *J. Neurophysiol.,* 59: 299 – 316.

Lenz, F.A., Tasker, R.R., Kwan, H.C., Schnider, S., Kwong, R., Murayama, Y., Dostrovsky, J.O. and Murphy, J.T. (1988) Single unit analysis of the human ventral thalamic nuclear group: correlation of thalamic "tremor" cells with the 3-6Hz component of Parkinsonian tremor. *J. Neurosci.,* 8: 754 – 764.

LeVay, S. and Gilbert, C.D. (1976) Laminar patterns of geniculocortical projection in the cat. *Brain Res.,* 113: 1 – 20.

Liu, X.-B., Honda, C.N. and Jones, E.G. (1989a) Distribution of GABA terminals on identified thalamocortical neurons in the VPL nucleus of the cat. *Neurosci. Abstr.,* 15: 383.

Liu, X.-B., Jones, E.G., Huntley, G.W. and Molinari, M. (1989b) Tachykinin immunoreactivity in terminals of trigeminal afferent fibers in adult and fetal monkey thalamus. *Exp. Brain Res.* (in press).

Livingstone, M.S. and Hubel, D.H. (1987) Psychophysical evidence for separate channels for the perception of form, color, movement, and depth. *J. Neurosci.,* 7: 3416 – 3468.

Maendly, R., Rüegg, D.G., Wiesendanger, M., Wiesendanger, R., Lagowska, J. and Hess, B. (1981) Thalamic relay for group I muscle afferents of forelimb nerves in the monkey. *J. Neurophysiol.,* 46: 901 – 917.

McCormick, D.A., Connors, B.W., Lighthall, J.N. and Prince, D.A. (1985) Comparative electrophysiology of pyramidal and sparsely spiny stellate neurons of the neocortex. *J. Neurophysiol.,* 54: 782 – 806.

McCormick, D.A. and Prince, D.A. (1986) Acetylcholine induces burst firing in thalamic reticular neurones by activating a potassium conductance. *Nature,* 319: 402 – 405.

Mehler, W.R. (1966) Some observations on secondary ascending afferent systems in the central nervous system. In R.S. Knighton and P. Dumke (Eds.), *Pain,* Little, Brown and Co., Boston, pp. 11 – 32.

Mehler, W.R. (1969) Some neurological species differences – *a posteriori. Ann. NY Acad. Sci.,* 167: 424 – 468.

Mehler, W.R. (1971) Idea of a new anatomy of the thalamus. *J. Psychiatr.,* 8: 203 – 217.

Mesulam, M.-M., Mufson, E.J., Wainer, B.H. and Levey, A.I. (1983) Central cholinergic pathways in the rat: an overview based on an alternative nomenclature (Ch1-Ch6). *Neuroscience,* 10: 1185 – 1202.

Miller, S.G. and Kennedy, M.B. (1986) Regulation of brain type II Ca^{+}/calmodulin-dependent protein kinase by autophosphorylation: a Ca^{2+}-triggered molecular switch, *Cell,* 44: 861 – 870.

Molinari, M., Hendry, S.H.C. and Jones, E.G. (1987) Distribution of certain neuropeptides in the primate thalamus. *Brain Res.,* 426: 270 – 289.

Montero, V.M. (1986) The interneuronal nature of GABAergic neurons in the lateral geniculate nucleus of the rhesus monkey: a combined HRP and GABA-immunocytochemical study. *Exp. Brain Res.,* 64: 615 – 622.

Montero, V.M. and Scott, G.L. (1981) Synaptic terminals in the dorsal lateral geniculate nucleus from neurons of the thalamic reticular nucleus: a light and electron microscopic autoradiographic study. *Neuroscience,* 6: 2561 – 2578.

Montero, V.M. and Singer, W. (1984) Ultrastructure and synaptic relations of neural elements containing glutamic acid decarboxylase (GAD) in the perigeniculate nucleus of the cat: A light and electron microscopic immunocytochemical study. *Exp. Brain Res.,* 56: 115 – 125.

Montero, V.M. and Zempel, J. (1985) Evidence for two types of GABA-containing interneurons in the A-laminae of the cat lateral geniculate nucleus: a double-label HRP and GABA-immunocytochemical study. *Exp. Brain Res.,* 60: 603 – 609.

Oertel, W.H., Graybiel, A.M., Mugnaini, E., Elde, R.P., Schmechel, D.E. and Kopin, I.J. (1983) Coexistence of glutamic acid decarboxylase and somatostatin-like immunoreactivity in neurons of the feline nucleus reticularis thalami. *J. Neurosci.,* 3: 1322 – 1332.

Ohara, P.T., Sefton, A.J. and Lieberman, A.R. (1980) Mode of termination of afferents from the thalamic reticular nucleus in the dorsal lateral geniculate nucleus of the rat. *Brain Res.,* 197: 503 – 506.

Ohye, C., Imai, S., Nakajima, H., Shibazaki, T. and Hirai, T. (1979) Experimental study of spontaneous postural tremor induced by a more successful tremor-producing procedure in the monkey. *Adv. Neurol.*, 24: 83 – 91.

Ohye, C., Shibazaki, T., Hirai, T., Wada, H., Hirato, M. and Kawashima, Y. (1989) Further physiological observation on the ventralis intermedius neurons in the human thalamus. *J. Neurophysiol.*, 61: 488 – 500.

Olivier, A., Parent, A. and Poirier, L.J. (1970) Identification of the thalamic nuclei on the basis of their cholinesterase content in the monkey. *J. Anat. Lond.*, 106: 37 – 50.

Olszewski, J. (1952) *The thalamus of the* Macaca mulatta. *An atlas for use with the stereotaxic instrument.* S. Karger, New York.

Parent, A. and Butcher, L.L. (1976) Organization and morphologies of acetylcholinesterase containing neurons in the thalamus and hypothalamus of the rat. *J. Comp. Neurol.*, 170: 205 – 225.

Penny, G.R., Conley, M., Schmechel, D.E. and Diamond, I.T. (1984) The distribution of glutamic acid decarboxylase immunoreactivity in the diencephalon of the opossum and rabbit. *J. Comp. Neurol.*, 228: 38 – 56.

Penny, G.R., Itoh, K. and Diamond I.T. (1982) Cells of different sizes in the ventral nuclei project to different layers of the somatic cortex in the cat. *Brain* 242: 55 – 65.

Penny, G.R., Fitzpatrick, D., Schmechel, D.E. and Diamond, I.T. (1983) Glutamic acid decarboxylase immunoreactive neurons and horseradish peroxidase labeled projection neurons in the ventral posterior nucleus of the cat and *Galago senegalensis. J. Neurosci.*, 3: 1868 – 1887.

Peschanski, M. and Besson, J.M. (1984) Diencephalic connections of the raphe nuclei of the rat brain-stem: an anatomical study with reference to the somatosensory system. *J. Comp. Neurol.*, 224: 503 – 534.

Peschanski, M., Ralston, H.J. and Roudier, F. (1983) Reticularis thalami afferents to the ventrobasal complex of the rat thalamus: an electron microscopic study. *Brain Res.*, 270: 325 – 329.

Pollin, B. and Rokyta, R. (1982) Somatotopic organization of nucleus reticularis thalami in chronic awake cats and monkeys. *Brain Res.*, 250: 211 – 222.

Prince, D.A. and McCormick, D.A. (1987) Actions of acetylcholine in the guinea-pig and cat medial and lateral geniculate nuclei, in vitro. *J. Physiol.*, 392: 147 – 165.

Raczowski, D., Hamos, J.E. and Sherman, S.M. (1988) Synaptic circuitry of physiologically identified W-cells in the cat's dorsal lateral geniculate nucleus. *J. Neurosci.*, 8: 31 – 48.

Ralston, H.J. (1971) Evidence for presynaptic dendrites and a proposal for their mechanism of action. *Nature*, 230: 585 – 587.

Ralston, H.J. and Herman, M.M. (1969) The fine structure of neurons and synapses in the ventrobasal thalamus of the cat. *Brain Res.*, 14: 77 – 97.

Rausell, E. and Jones, E.G. (1989) Modular organization of the thalamic VPM nucleus in monkeys. *Neurosci. Abstr.*, 15: 311.

Roy, J.P., Clercq, M., Steriade, M. and Deschênes, M. (1984) Electrophysiology of neurons of lateral thalamic nuclei in cat: mechanisms of long-lasting hyperpolarizations. *J. Neurophysiol.*, 51: 1220 – 1235.

Sherman, S.M. and Friedlander, M.J. (1988) Identification of X versus Y properties for interneurons in the A-laminae of the cat's lateral geniculate nucleus. *Exp. Brain Res.*, 73: 384 – 392.

Sherman, S.M. and Koch, C. (1986) The control of retinogeniculate transmission in the mammalian lateral geniculate nucleus. *Exp. Brain Res.*, 63: 1 – 20.

Shosaku, A. and Sumitomo, I. (1983) Auditory neurons in the rat thalamic reticular nucleus. *Exp. Brain Res.*, 49: 432 – 442.

Sillito, A.M. and Kemp, J.A. (1983) The influence of GABAergic inhibitory processes on the receptive field structure of X and Y cells in cat dorsal lateral geniculate nucleus (dLGN). *Brain Res.*, 277: 55 – 62.

Stanford, L.R., Friedlander, M.J. and Sherman, M.S. (1983) Morphological and physiological properties of geniculate W-cells of the cat: a comparison with X- and Y- cells. *J. Neurophysiol.*, 50: 582 – 608.

Steriade, M. and Deschênes, M. (1984) The thalamus as a neuronal oscillator. *Brain Res. Rev.*, 8: 1 – 63.

Steriade, M. and Llinás, R.R. (1988) The functional states of the thalamus and the associated neuronal interplay. *Physiol. Reviews*, 68: 649 – 742.

Stichel, C.C., Singer, W., Heizmann, C.W. and Norman, A.W. (1987) Immunohistochemical localization of calcium-binding proteins, parvalbumin and calbindin-D 28k, in the adult and developing visual cortex of cats: a light and electron microscopic study. *J. Comp. Neurol.*, 262: 563 – 577.

Sumitomo, I., Hsiao, C.-F. and Fukuda, Y. (1988) Two types of thalamic reticular cells in relation to the two visual thalamocortical systems in the rat. *Brain Res.*, 446: 354 – 362.

Sur, M. and Sherman, S.M. (1982) Retinogeniculate terminations in cats: morphological differences between X and Y cell axons. *Science*, 218: 389 – 391.

Swanson, L.W. and Hartman, B.K. (1975) The central adrenergic system: an immunofluorescence study of the location of cell bodies and their efferent connections in the rat utilizing dopamine-B-hydroxylase as a marker. *J. Comp. Neurol.*, 163: 467 – 506.

Wilson, J.R., Friedlander, M.J. and Sherman, S.M. (1984) Fine structural morphology of identified X- and Y-cells in the cat's lateral geniculate nucleus. *Proc. R. Soc. London, B.*, 221: 411 – 436.

Wong-Riley, M. (1979) Changes in the visual system of monocularly sutured or enucleated cats demonstrable with cytochrome oxidase histochemistry. *Brain Res.*, 171: 11 – 28.

Yen, C.-T., Conley, M., Hendry, S.H.C. and Jones, E.G. (1985a) The morphology of physiologically identified GABAergic neurons in the somatic sensory part of the thalamic reticular nucleus in the cat. *J. Neurosci.*, 5:

2254 – 2268.

Yen, C.-T., Conley, M. and Jones, E.G. (1985b) Morphological and functional types of neurons in cat ventral posterior thalamic nucleus. *J. Neurosci.,* 5: 1316 – 1338.

Zaremba, S., Guimaraes, A., Kalb, R.G. and Hockfield, S. (1989) Characterization of an activity-dependent, neuronal surface proteoglycan identified with monoclonal antibody Cat-301. *Neuron,* 2: 1207 – 1219.

G. Holstege (Ed.)
Progress in Brain Research, Vol. 87

CHAPTER 4

The specificity of the nonspecific thalamus: The midline nuclei

Marina Bentivoglio, Giancarlo Balercia and Lawrence Kruger[1]

Institute of Anatomy, University of Verona, Strada Le Grazie, 37134 Verona, Italy

Introduction

Historical background

The concept of a dual origin of thalamic innervation of the cerebral cortex stems from the observation, summarized by Lorente de Nó in 1938 on the basis of Golgi impregnation, of two modes of laminar organization of thalamocortical projections: "specific" fibers which arborize densely in layer IV of a restricted cortical target, and "nonspecific" fibers, reaching layer I with sparse termination and a multiareal distribution. Subsequently, a dichotomy was also found in the electrophysiological properties of thalamic nuclei. Repetitive low-frequency stimulation of the nonspecific thalamic structures elicited "recruiting" responses over a wide cortical territory, whereas stimulation of specific structures (such as the main sensory relay nuclei) elicited augmenting responses in the respective cortical target (Morison and Dempsey, 1942; Dempsey and Morison, 1942). In the latter type of response, a biphasic positive-negative primary response was augmented by repetition of the stimulus. In the recruiting phenomenon, the response increased to maximum amplitude during repetitive stimulation, and appeared over widespread cortical areas. The recruiting type of response could be elicited from a wide region of the thalamus, located medially within the internal medullary lamina or adjacent to it, as well as at the rostral thalamic pole. This region in the cat included the thalamic reticular nucleus, and structures located at the midline (central medial, reuniens and rhomboid nuclei), the anterior and posterior intralaminar nuclei (central lateral, paracentral, parafascicular and centre median), the medial and rostral sectors of the ventral complex (ventromedial and ventral anterior nuclei), and a posterior thalamic region interposed between the ventrobasal complex, medial geniculate body and pulvinar.

On the basis of these electrophysiological data, the origin of the nonspecific diffuse innervation of cortical superficial layers observed by Lorente de Nó was ascribed to the structures from which recruiting responses had been evoked. A decade after Lorente de Nó's description, Jasper (1949) stated: "It seems well established now that there exists a diffuse thalamocortical system with independent projection to the cortex overlapping that of the better known specific projection system." Thus, the definition of thalamic "nonspecificity" was grounded on structural and electrophysiological correlates, and the principle was introduced that the cortical activity and the en-

[1] On leave from the Department of Anatomy and Cell Biology, UCLA, Los Angeles, CA, USA.

coding of cortical information could be differentially regulated by multiple sets of thalamic afferents. Forty years later the ''specific'' projection systems are still ''better known'' than the others.

The concept of a nonspecific thalamus has been substantially revised in the last forty years, so that we now know that it is composed of a heterogeneous collection of individually signatured cell groups. The term nonspecific has been dismissed, but it has left behind a great deal of confusion and the embarrassing impression that the nonspecific thalamus has not found a satisfactory anatomical identity. The midline thalamic region reviewed in this chapter is part of this complex territory. This brief overview is aimed at a definition of the midline thalamus as a collection of cell groups whose structural features and circuits differ greatly from those of adjacent structures and from all other portions of the ''nonspecific'' thalamus. The midline will be discussed in relation to the intralaminar thalamus since these two regions have been unified historically in the same entity, and they are still often considered as a single group. This is due to the common belief that midline and intralaminar nuclei share functional features, based on their preferential innervation from the brain stem core and their robust connections with the basal ganglia (see later).

The ambiguous status of the midline thalamus

The midline thalamic nuclei have been encumbered with an erratic status for almost a century of experimental studies on thalamic projections. It was known from the original studies of Franz Nissl (1913) and later elaborated by Rose and Woolsey (1943) that some portions of the thalamic midline undergo retrograde atrophy following large telencephalic ablations. The latter authors grouped these structures in the ''central commissural system'', but separated some nuclei which they believed deserved distinct status on a variety of grounds. Thus, they excluded the parafascicular-centre median complex, which they called the ''postmedial group'', largely because of its pronounced phyletic expansion in some mammals. The paraventricular complex was relegated to the epithalamus, together with the habenula and pretectal nuclei, based on developmental findings (Rose, 1942) as well as the apparent absence of ''endbrain-dependency'' of these nuclei (Rose and Woolsey, 1943, 1949). Early electrophysiological studies of cortical activation from midline regions as part of the recruiting structures (Morison and Dempsey, 1942; Dempsey and Morison, 1942) resulted in obfuscation of the complexity of this thalamic domain. This was compounded by discrepant nomenclature employed by various authors and the findings in macaque monkeys that these nuclei did not degenerate after massive cortical ablations (Walker, 1938; Powell and Cowan, 1956; Peacock and Combs, 1965a,b) and therefore required an extensive difficult analysis based on subcortical lesions. Early studies with the retrograde axonal transport of horseradish peroxidase (HRP) as a tracer led Jones and Leavitt (1974) to separate the paraventricular nuclei as the singular midline group that apparently lacked a projection to the cerebral cortex or striatum. Uncertainties concerning thalamo-amygdala connections via fibers traversing the hypothalamus accounted for a separate indeterminate classification of some nuclei, notably for the paraventricular and subparafascicular neurons (e.g. Ajmone Marsan, 1965), until a seminal and provocative summary article by Mehler (1980) on connections of the amygdala, based on retrograde HRP labeling, attempted to bring a sense of order and consistent nomenclature to this subject.

The significance of midline fusion of symmetrical nuclei with unilateral projections to form a ''massa intermedia'' of varying extent in individual specimens of human brain and of the dense fiber bundles crossing the midline and extending into the internal medullary lamina remains obscure, but the past decade has yielded some new and relevant information for re-evaluation of this subject. The findings suggest that previous constructs applied to the midline nuclei, designating these thalamic cell groups as part of ''diffuse'', "nonspecific", "generalized" or "commissural" systems, constitute misleading simplifications. A consideration of some recent observations may lead to new insights concerning these structures.

Oversimplification by introducing neologisms for vaguely related and poorly understood relations abound in descriptions of neuroanatomical systems; such popular terms as "limbic" and "reticular formation" are often resorted to evading and thereby subverting rigorous definition. It may thus be a valuable exercise to examine to what extent subsuming the diverse thalamic nuclei in or near the midline into a unitary "system" warrants legitimacy on grounds other than location. Attempts to develop broad general principles risks ignoring significant details. Differences which are addressed here, without pretension of comprehensive review, are for the purpose of examining the difficulties inherent in applying multiple, and often unrelated criteria to systematization of the "midline" nuclei. Cellular and fiber architecture, development, afferent and efferent connections, peptide and enzyme distribution and selective localization of exotic proteins and poorly understood receptor molecules may all be relevant to this task, but the findings most frequently lack congruency.

Components of the thalamic midline

Cell groups and development

The neurons that fuse to form a central (i.e. midline) condensation in early postnatal life are paired structures in fetal stages, each projecting to the ipsilateral forebrain: although some cells appear to cross the midline following fusion, these nuclei retain their essential laterality of projection and bilateral symmetry (see below). This feature is applicable to all of the components of the thalamic midline. These are represented by the dorsally placed paraventricular (Pv) nuclei, a centromedial group, sometimes divided on the basis of the surrounding structures into interanteromedial (IAM) and intermediodorsal (IMD) nuclei (or designated on the basis of cytoarchitectural features as centralis densocellularis), a rhomboid (Rh) complex and a ventral reuniens (Re) or medioventral nucleus (Fig. 1). Some authors (e.g. Mehler, 1980) give separate status to the ventrolateral wings of

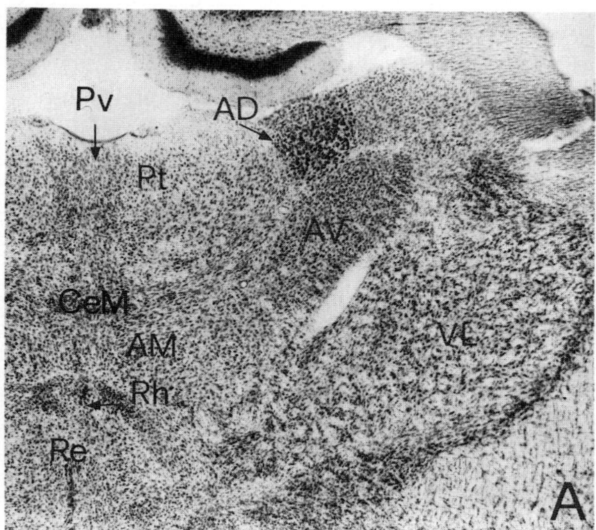

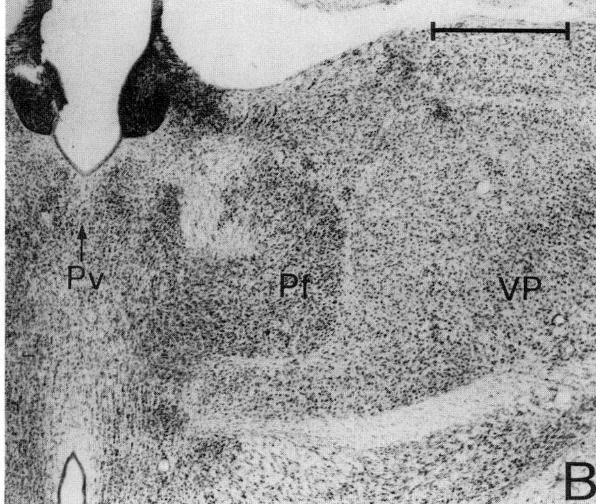

Fig. 1. Cresyl-violet stained transverse sections through the thalamus of the rat, showing the nuclear structures of the midline and the adjacent nuclei. Scale bar: 500 μm.

the Re nucleus, although they do not fuse medially. The paired paratenial (Pt) nuclei (Fig. 1A) are also generally included in the midline group, although these also do not fuse medially, but, lacking association with the internal medullary lamina, they are assigned to the midline by default rather than rigorous definition.

Nearly a century of description in a vast array of mammalian species has yielded some agreement on the boundaries, if not the names of several midline structures; certainly, this applies to the Pv, Pt and Re nuclei. But what about the range of opinions concerning the central medial grouping, including the status of "interanteromedial" and "intermediodorsal" nuclei and the discrepant accounts for the limits and arrangement of Rh? It is also interesting to note that fiber and Nissl-stained patterns are less readily matched here than for most thalamic structures. Without elaborating the issue excessively, it is not unusual to find disagreement concerning the limits of these nuclei, and even individual authors have proven inconsistent with their own previous accounts using the same material. The "wings" of the midline Re and Rh nuclei serve as an example; they are often described as medioventral, ventromedial, submedial, gelatinosus and even a "gustatory" nucleus is sometimes named, although its limits are but vaguely established in any species (see Kruger and Mantyh, 1989 for review).

The neurons of the Pv nuclear complex extend along the dorsal midline position, lining the third ventricle from the anterior end of the thalamus to the habenular nuclei, and appear to be among the most stable structures in terms of position and relative size throughout mammalian evolution (Kruger, 1959). They are often architecturally subdivided into anterior and posterior subnuclei, but share projections consonant with a single functional nuclear complex (see below). The Pv nuclei differentiate earlier in development than the other midline structures which derive from the middle thalamic plate of the embryo called "dorsal thalamus", consistent with the interpretation of the Pv complex as a derivative of the embryonic dorsal "epithalamic" plate (Rose, 1942). More recent studies based on [^{3}H]-thymidine dating of developing Pv neurons (Altman and Bayer, 1988) may render such distinctions less certain if the range of neuron "birthdates" constitutes the most suitable criterion for determining the sequence of formation of thalamic nuclei.

The central medial (CeM) nucleus subdivides the midline into a dorsal and a ventral sector. CeM cells are embedded in fibers of the internal medullary lamina, so that CeM could be considered part of the rostral intralaminar group, although it is topographically located at the midline: the relationships of CeM efferents with the cortex share many features of the anterior intralaminar projections (Macchi and Bentivoglio, 1986).

Developmental remodeling

Recent studies based on double retrograde tracing with fluorescent dyes in the rat (Takada et al., 1987; Minciacchi and Granato, 1988, 1989) have provided evidence of a considerable rearrangement in the thalamic midline during late embryonic and early postnatal stages. Cells retrogradely labeled from the forebrain, situated bilaterally, fuse into the thalamic midline, with intermingling of neurons which cross the midline and maintain unilateral projections regardless of the laterality of their perikarya. In the medial thalamus, the overlap zone between the neurons which project to either the ipsi- or the contralateral frontal cortex (which includes the midline structures, the medial part of the mediodorsal, MD, nucleus, and the ventromedial, VM, nucleus) is three times wider in neonates than in adults (Minciacchi and Granato, 1988, 1989; Fig. 2). Thus, a massive developmental reduction of the cell population projecting to the contralateral cortex occurs at the midline, which could be ascribed to phenomena of cell death or to other strategies of developmental rearrangement.

Input to midline thalamus

General organization

The limited data available on the cortical and subcortical afferents to the thalamic midline provide evidence of a substantial difference among the inputs to adjacent nuclear structures. According to studies in the rat (Swanson, 1976; Saper et al., 1979; Cornwall and Phillipson, 1988b), the main subcortical projections to the midline thalamus derive from a variety of hypothalamic nuclei (anterior, ventromedial arcuate, lateral hypothalamic areas and dorsomedial hypothalamus), and in particular from the entire extent of the periventricular nucleus. Central periaqueductal grey cells also project to the midline thalamus (Eberhart et al., 1985), such that the latter receives a robust input from a ''periventricular system'' surrounding the third ventricle and the cerebral aqueduct (Cornwall and Phillipson, 1988b). The rostral and dorsal portion of the thalamic midline is innervated by efferents of the septal nuclei and the bed nucleus of stria terminalis (Meibach and Siegel, 1977a; Swanson and Cowan, 1979; Cornwall and Phillipson, 1988b), which terminate preferentially in Pv and Pt (Swanson and Cowan, 1979). Brainstem input to the thalamic midline derives from the reticular core and monoaminergic cell groups (see below), as well as from the nucleus of the solitary tract and the parabrachial nuclei (Ricardo and Koh, 1978; Herkenham, 1978; Saper and Loewy, 1980; Cornwall and Phillipson, 1988b; Groenewegen, 1988). Altogether, the pattern of subcortical inputs indicates that the thalamic midline receives dense innervation by cell groups involved in visceral, autonomic and gustatory functions.

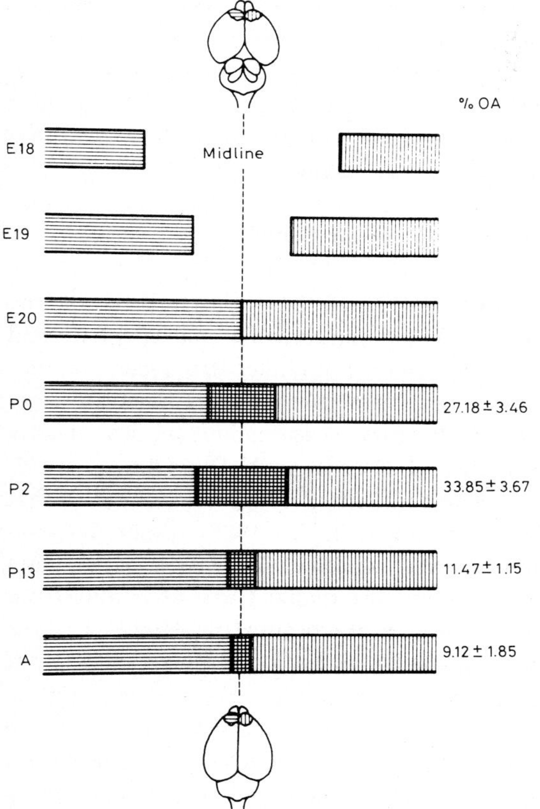

Fig. 2. Schematic representation of the time course of thalamic labeling observed at prenatal (E), postnatal (P) and adult (A) ages in the rat after bilateral injections of different tracers in the frontal cortex. Horizontally and vertically striped ares indicate the thalamic regions which contain tightly packed cells labeled from each cortical injection; squared areas represent the areas of overlap (OA) of the two cell populations in the medial thalamus. Mean values and standard deviations for the percent value of the overlap area (%OA) are indicated on the right side. Note that the overlap of the neurons labeled from each cortical injection is restricted in adulthood to a limited portion of the thalamic midline, and it is at birth about three times wider than in adults, indicating that a developmental remodeling of the midline projection cells occurs after fusion of the two hemithalami. (Reproduced with permission from Minciacchi and Granato, 1988).

The cortical afferents to the midline, as described in the rat by means of retrograde tracing (Cornwall and Phillipson, 1988b), derive largely from the ventral subiculum and perirhinal cortex (and reciprocate the midline output to these structures: see below). Data on perirhinal efferents to the medial thalamus, obtained in the cat with anterograde tracing, indicate that they are concentrated in Re and spare all the rest of the midline and the intralaminar nuclei (Witter and Groenewegen, 1986). Thus, hippocampal and parahippocampal corticothalamic projections sharply differentiate the midline, where they are concentrated, from the adjacent thalamic structures and in particular from MD. The differences in the areal origin of other corticothalamic inputs to MD and the midline are less clear-cut, since a dense innervation of the midline has been traced anterogradely in the rat from the rostral and ventral prelimbic and medial "prefrontal" fields (Sesack et al., 1989), and bilaterally in the monkey from the prefrontal cortex (Preuss and Goldman-Rakic, 1987), which also project to MD (rat: Groenewegen 1988; Cornwall and Phillipson, 1988a; cat: Velayos and Reinoso-Suárez, 1985; monkey: Preuss and Goldman-Rakic, 1987). As for the subcortical input, the forebrain projections to the midline and MD seem to delineate two different systems: the afferents to the midline derive from sectors of the hypothalamus and basal forebrain situated more medially than those projecting to MD (Cornwall and Phillipson, 1988a,b). Furthermore, amygdaloid efferents are concentrated in the more medial sectors of MD in the rat (Krettek and Price, 1977b) and in the medial magnocellular part of MD in the monkey (Porrino et al., 1981; Aggleton and Mishkin, 1984; Russchen et al., 1987), whereas only a light amygdaloid innervation of the midline region, and in particular of Re, has been reported in the rat (Herkenham, 1978) and monkey (Aggleton and Mishkin, 1984). Therefore, as emphasized by Cornwall and Phillipson (1988b), information from the amygdala is conveyed to the midline thalamus mostly via an indirect route through the bed nucleus of the stria terminalis.

The midline also receives input from the spinal cord: spinothalamic tract fibers in the cat are distributed not only to paramedian regions (e.g. the nucleus submedius) but also penetrate into the midline (Burton and Craig, 1983; Mantyh, 1983), terminating throughout Pv and extending dorsolaterally to Pt (Burton and Craig, 1983). A low density of spinothalamic innervation was detected in midline structures in the monkey (Burton and Craig, 1983; Apkarian and Hodge, 1989).

The extrinsic innervation of the intralaminar nuclei is largely different from that of the midline: spinothalamic fibers terminate much more densely in the anterior intralaminar structures than in the midline; moreover, the anterior intralaminar nuclei are densely innervated by cerebellothalamic fibers and the posterior intralaminar group by efferents of the globus pallidus (see Macchi and Bentivoglio, 1986, and Bentivoglio et al., 1988b for review) which do not innervate the midline. Therefore, the major inputs to the intralaminar nuclei appear strongly related to sensory-motor information processing, indicating that intralaminar and midline regions may belong to different functional systems (see below).

Inputs from the brain stem

Besides the afferents from the nucleus of the solitary tract and parabrachial nuclei mentioned above, the thalamic midline also receives input from the brain stem core. Studies based on tract tracing in different mammalian species, mostly subprimates (Edwards and De Olmos, 1976; Robertson and Feiner, 1982; Jones and Yang, 1985; Vertes and Martin, 1988), pointed to intralaminar and midline regions as the main thalamic targets of reticular fibers ascending from medial portions of the brain stem. However, these studies consistently showed that the reticular input is denser in the intralaminar than in the midline region. Within the latter, fibers deriving from the medullary and pontine medial reticular formation display a ventral predominance, innervating preferentially Rh and Re (Jones and Yang, 1985).

Moruzzi and Magoun (1949) introduced the concept of a rostrally directed brain stem reticular system which influences the basic pattern of cortical activity contributing to EEG activation. Recent electrophysiological data support the concept that the ascending brain stem reticular projections contribute to tonic activation of the thalamocortical system (see Steriade and Deschênes, 1984, for review). The anatomical data mentioned above indicate that the midline thalamus would play a minor role compared to the intralaminar thalamus in tonic cortical activation.

The thalamic innervation deriving from

chemically-signatured brain stem structures, such as the noradrenergic locus coeruleus and the serotonergic raphe nuclei, is concentrated in the midline (see below). Efferents of the mesopontine cholinergic cell groups (i.e. the pedunculopontine and laterodorsal tegmental nuclei) terminate in medial thalamic regions (Hallänger and Wainer, 1988), as well as in the other thalamic relay nuclei (see Jones' chapter in this volume). However, the midline does not appear as a preferential site of cholinergic innervation (see below). This is also supported by the finding obtained with *Phaseolus* leucoagglutinin (PHA-L) anterograde tracing in the rat (Groenewegen, 1988) that Pv is only lightly innervated by the laterodorsal tegmental nucleus, which, instead, projects heavily upon the medial portion of MD adjacent to Pv.

The input from the thalamic reticular nucleus

The midline nuclei receive afferents from the rostral pole of the reticular nucleus (rat: Herkenham, 1978; Cornwall and Phillipson, 1988b, Wouterlood et al., 1990; Cornwall et al., 1990; cat: Velayos et al., 1989). Through its inhibitory projections to the dorsal thalamus, the reticular nucleus plays a pacemaker role in the regulation of spindle activity of thalamocortical cells (see Spreafico et al., 1987, and Steriade and Deschênes, 1984 for review; see also chapters of Jones and Ralston in this volume). The intrathalamic distribution of reticular nucleus efferents is uneven: in the cat it spares the anterior nuclei, and is more densely distributed in some territories, such as the intralaminar thalamus, than in others (Steriade et al., 1984). The retrograde study by Velayos et al (1989) on the reticular nucleus innervation of medial and paramedian sectors of the cat thalamus, reported that the reticular nucleus cells projecting to the midline are much less numerous than those projecting to MD or the intralaminar nuclei. The sharp contrast between the heavy concentration of anterogradely labeled terminals in the intralaminar thalamus and the paucity of anterograde labeling in the midline after tritiated amino acid injection in the rostral pole of the reticular nucleus in the rat (see Fig. 12 in Herkenham, 1986) further substantiates this differential distribution. Therefore, the intrathalamic circuitry regulating midline cells is different, at least from the quantitative point of view, from that of adjacent cell groups, and in particular from the intralaminar thalamus.

The relationships of the midline with the reticular nucleus are reciprocal: Re efferents, labeled with PHA-L, distribute terminals within the reticular nucleus in their course through the inferior thalamic peduncle (Wouterlood et al., 1990), similarly in this respect to the other thalamic efferents, which emit a collateral to the reticular nucleus in their thalamofugal pathway (see Harris, 1987).

Midline output channels

As for most structures which are known to project upon several targets, a comprehensive overview on the efferent connections of the thalamic midline is difficult to assemble. Data scattered throughout studies on a variety of circuits indicate that the thalamic midline innervates limbic structures, neocortical areas and the striatum.

Midline-amygdala connection

Studies on the afferents to the amygdala based on the HRP retrograde transport in the rat (Veening, 1978; Ottersen and Ben-Ari, 1979), cat (Ottersen and Ben-Ari, 1979; Russchen, 1982) and monkey (Aggleton et al., 1980; Mehler, 1980) have consistently reported that the midline provides the main source of thalamic input to the amygdala (Fig. 3) and, conversely, that thalamic midline efferents are widely distributed within the amygdaloid complex. Recent data based on multiple retrograde tracing in the rat (Su and Bentivoglio, 1990) have confirmed previous findings on the large number of midline cells projecting to the amygdala, and have provided a detailed topographical analysis of this cell population.

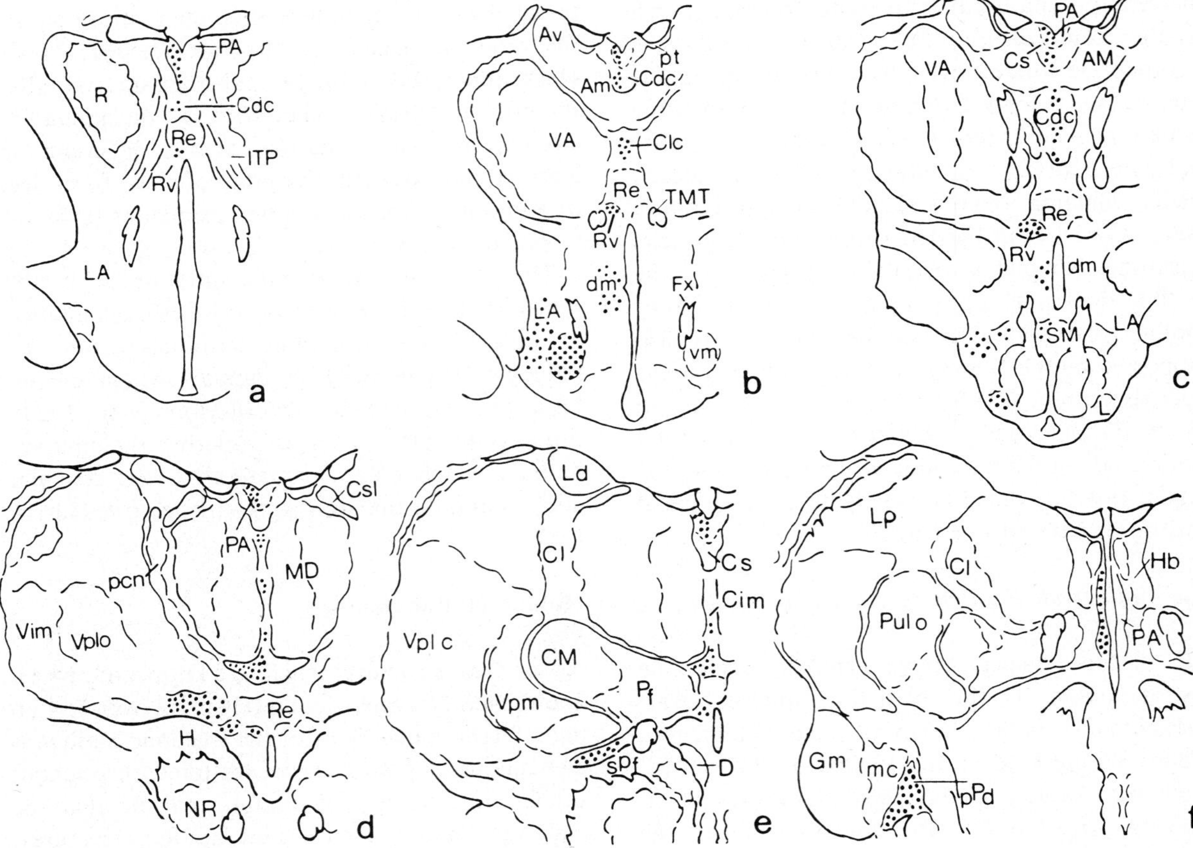

Fig. 3. Schematic representation of rostrocaudal (a – f) coronal sections through the monkey diencephalon summarizing the distribution of cells (indicated by black dots) retrogradely labeled following various injections of horseradish peroxidase in the amygdala. Note that in the thalamus the labeled neurons are concentrated in midline nuclear structures. (Modified from Mehler, 1980).

Neurons projecting to the amygdaloid complex are distributed in the rat throughout the rostrocaudal extent of the midline, with an anterior prevalence and a consistent regional concentration: dorsally, throughout the anteroposterior extent of Pv, and ventrally, in the medial and ventral portion of Re (Fig. 4); amygdala-projecting cells are also located in CeM and Rh, as well as in the medial part of Pt. In the dorsal part of Pv, many of the neurons projecting to the amygdala are concentrated closer to the ependymal lining than the cell populations projecting to the hippocampal formation and nucleus accumbens (Figs. 4 and 5A). The dendrites of thalamo-amygdaloid neurons extend towards the ependyma, arborizing profusely in the subependymal portion of Pv (Su and Bentivoglio, 1990) (Fig. 5B).

Midline efferents to the hippocampus, entorhinal and perirhinal cortices: the reuniens-cortical connection

The thalamic innervation of the hippocampal formation (here defined as dentate gyrus, Ammon's horn and subicular complex) has been "discovered" with the introduction of the sensitive tracing axonal transport methods, which showed afferents from many thalamic nuclei, and in particular from the midline. Anterograde and retrograde tracing studies have consistently reported that the Re nucleus is a major source of thalamic projections to the hippocampus in several mammalian species (rat: Herkenham, 1978, 1986; Wyss et al., 1979; Baisden et al., 1979; Riley and Moore, 1981; Wouterlood et al., 1990; cat: Yanagihara et al., 1987; monkey: Amaral and Cowan, 1980). Multiple retrograde tracing data in the rat (Su and Bentivoglio, 1990) have confirmed that Re is the main midline relay to the hippocampal formation, whereas the other midline structures, and in particular Pt and Pv, provide a minor contribution to the thalamo-hippocampal connection (Fig. 4). Re fibers innervate selectively the field CA1 and the subiculum (Herkenham, 1978;

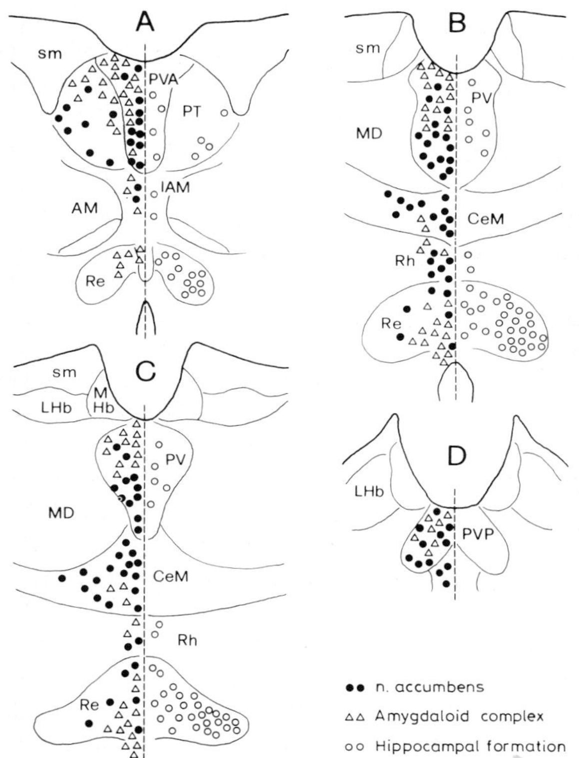

Fig. 4. Schematic representation of rostrocaudal (A-D) levels of the thalamic midline of the rat summarizing the distribution of neurons labeled retrogradely after multiple tracer injections in the amygdala, hippocampus and nucleus accumbens, Note in the paraventricular nucleus the dorsal prevalence of the neurons projecting to the amygdala and the ventral prevalence of those projecting to the nucleus accumbens; note in the nucleus reuniens the medial prevalence of the cells projecting to the amygdala and the lateral prevalence of those projecting to the hippocampal formation. (Reproduced with permission from Su and Bentivoglio, 1990).

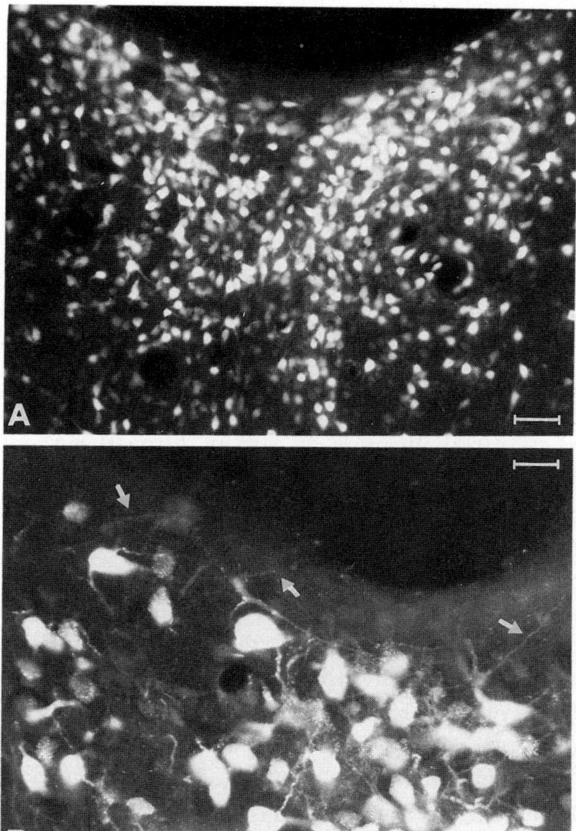

Fig. 5. Microphotographs of neurons retrogradely labeled in the paraventricular nucleus after fluorescent tracer injections in the amygdala of the rat; Fluoro-gold was injected on the right side and Fast Blue on the left side. (A) Note the dense labeling of cells in the most dorsal portion of the paraventricular nucleus, close to the border with the ventricle; scale bar: 50 μm. (B) Note that the dendrites of labeled cells (arrows) extend towards the ependymal lining; scale bar: 20 μm.

Wouterlood et al., 1990) where they form asymmetric synapses with small caliber dendrites or with dendritic spines (Wouterlood et al., 1990).

The strict relationship of the thalamic midline with rhinencephalic cortices is also supported by reports on the thalamo-entorhinal connection: dense projections of Re to the entorhinal cortex, and minor inputs from Rh, Pv and Pt as well as CeM, have been described in the rat (Segal, 1977; Beckstead, 1978; Herkenham, 1978, 1986), cat (Room and Groenewegen, 1986; Yanagihara et al., 1987) and monkey (Insausti et al., 1987). Re axons reach both superficial and deep layers of the entorhinal cortex and terminate in the parahippocampal region in layer I of the pre- and parasubiculum (Herkenham, 1978, 1986; Wouterlood et al., 1990). The pre- and parasubiculum are also innervated by the thalamic anterior nuclei, which do not seem to project upon the entorhinal cortex in rat and monkey (see Witter et al., 1989, for review). The perirhinal cortex receives thalamic input from the midline (where it originates, once again, predominantly from Re), as well as from posterior thalamic structures (Deacon et al., 1983; Witter et al., 1989). Altogether these data emphasize that the midline not only represents the main source of thalamic innervation of hippocampus and entorhinal cortex, but is also the only thalamic domain connected to wide portions of limbic cortices, and the Re nucleus stands out as the main thalamic source of this innervation. In the subdivision of the rat thalamic nuclei based on the laminar target of their cortical projections, Herkenham (1986) included Re in the "paralaminar" system, defined by a dense projection to layer I, on the basis of the Re connections with superficial layers of large portions of the limbic cortex.

The Re cells of origin of hippocampal projections are predominantly represented by neurons with radiating dendritic processes (Baisden and Hoover, 1979). This finding is in agreement with the Scheibels' (1967) observation, based on Golgi impregnation, that thalamic midline cells are mainly represented by radiating multipolar neurons which display, (especially in Re and Pv) an "open" dendritic field extending towards the neighbouring structures, in contrast with the apparent "closure" of the dendritic processes of adjacent thalamic structures, characterized by confluence of neuronal arborizations within the nuclear domain.

Midline connections with the cingulate cortex

Although no detailed investigations have been devoted to the relationships of the thalamic midline with the medial hemispheric wall, retrograde studies have consistently mentioned that the cingulate cortex receives afferents from the midline nuclei (rat: Finch et al., 1984. Thompson and Robertson, 1987; cat: Niimi et al. 1978; Robertson and Kaitz, 1981; Musil and Olson, 1988a; monkey: Jürgens, 1983; Vogt et al., 1979, 1987). Vogt et al. (1979) emphasized the differential distribution of afferent fibers to anterior and posterior cingulate cortex in the monkey. According to this study, the input from the midline (deriving mainly from Pv and Re) and the intralaminar nuclei represents a distinctive feature of the anterior cingulate cortex, possibly involved in pain-related transmission, whereas the posterior cingulate cortex is recipient of afferents from the thalamic anterior and laterodorsal nuclei. Musil and Olson (1988a) noted a dorsoventral gradient in the thalamic and cortical innervation of the anterior cingulate cortex in the cat: thalamic projections from the ventral anterior and rostral intralaminar nuclei, as well as cortical input from areas 4 and 6, were densest at dorsal levels, whereas thalamic midline afferents (from Pt, Pv and Re) and cortical input from prefrontal fields appeared strongest at ventral levels of the anterior cingulate cortex.

Midline relationships with the neocortex

The organization of the thalamocortical projections has been thoroughly re-examined with axonal tract tracing, but the relationship of the thalamic midline with the neocortex has been hitherto neglected. The information available up to now, and probably still incomplete, points to the prefrontal cortex as the main target of midline-neocortical projections: retrograde tracing studies in the cat (Niimi et al., 1981; Martinez Moreno et al., 1987; Musil and Olson, 1988b) and in the monkey (Preuss and Goldman-Rakic, 1987) have consistently mentioned afferents to the prefrontal cortex from cells scattered through the thalamic midline. In the cat these neurons are located mainly in Pv and Pt (Martinez-Moreno et al., 1987), with a preferential distribution upon the ventromedial part of the prefrontal cortex (Musil and Olsen, 1988b). In the rat Pt efferents have been traced anterogradely to the ventral surface of the frontal pole (Krettek and Price, 1977a), and Pv and Pt cells projecting to the ventromedial prefrontal cortex have been identified with retrograde tracers (Groenewegen, 1988). In the longitudinal bands of thalamo-frontal neurons, described in the monkey by Kievit and Kuypers (1977) on the basis of HRP retrograde transport, the most medial band, including the midline, was found to be related to the orbital cortex. Preliminary data based on anterograde and retrograde tracing (Friedman et al. 1987, 1989) suggest that in the monkey midline cells project upon layer I of a wide cortical territory.

Thalamic midline and extrapyramidal system

Intralaminar and midline nuclei represent the main source of thalamostriatal fibers, although neurons located in other thalamic structures also contribute to this connection (see Alheid et al., 1990 for review). Studies in rodents and cat reported that the thalamic innervation of the nucleus accumbens and ventral portion of the caudoputamen derives mainly from midline structures and from the medial portion of the posterior intralaminar complex (Groenewegen et al. 1980; Newman and Winans, 1980; Beckstead, 1984; Kelley and Stinus, 1984; Jayaraman, 1985; Phillipson and Griffiths, 1985; Berendse et al., 1988; Berendse and Groenewegen, 1990). These neurons are concentrated in the ventral part of Pv and in CeM, whereas Pt, Rh and Re provide only a minor contribution to this connection (Su and Bentivoglio, 1990; Fig. 4). Therefore, midline cell groups provide the thalamic access to the striatal sector heavily innervated by amygdaloid and hippocampal fibers (De Olmos and Ingram, 1972; Kelley and Domesick, 1982; Kelley et al., 1982; Groenewegen et al., 1987). Enhancement of the activity of Pv neurons by electrical stimulation or excitotoxin treatment was found to increase the utilisation of dopamine in the nucleus accumbens (Jones et al., 1989).

Different sets of thalamic afferents display a differential distribution in the complex compartmental organization of the striatum. In the cat midline terminals are distributed within the striosomes (the AChE-poor zones), whereas the intralaminar efferents terminate preferentially in the matrix which displays high AChE positivity (Ragsdale and Graybiel, 1988). In the rat, Pv efferents to the ventral striatum project selectively to the patch compartment and CeM to the matrix, as defined by enkephalin immunohistochemistry (Berendse et al., 1988).

The corticostriatal relationships and the return loops to the cortex through pallidothalamic and thalamocortical routes are organized in parallel systems subserving different functional roles (Alexander et al., 1986; Alheid et al., 1990). Through their output to the nucleus accumbens the midline nuclei have access to a circuit which is conveyed to the ventral pallidum and through ventral pallidal efferents to MD (Haber et al., 1985, 1990; Russchen et al., 1987; see also Heimer et al.'s contribution to this volume), whereas the output of the other thalamostriatal afferents is conveyed to the ventral thalamus.

The fine structure of the ventricular region of the thalamic midline

An unusual feature of the neurons retrogradely labeled from the amygdala in Pv is the presence of labeled dendrites extending towards the ependymal

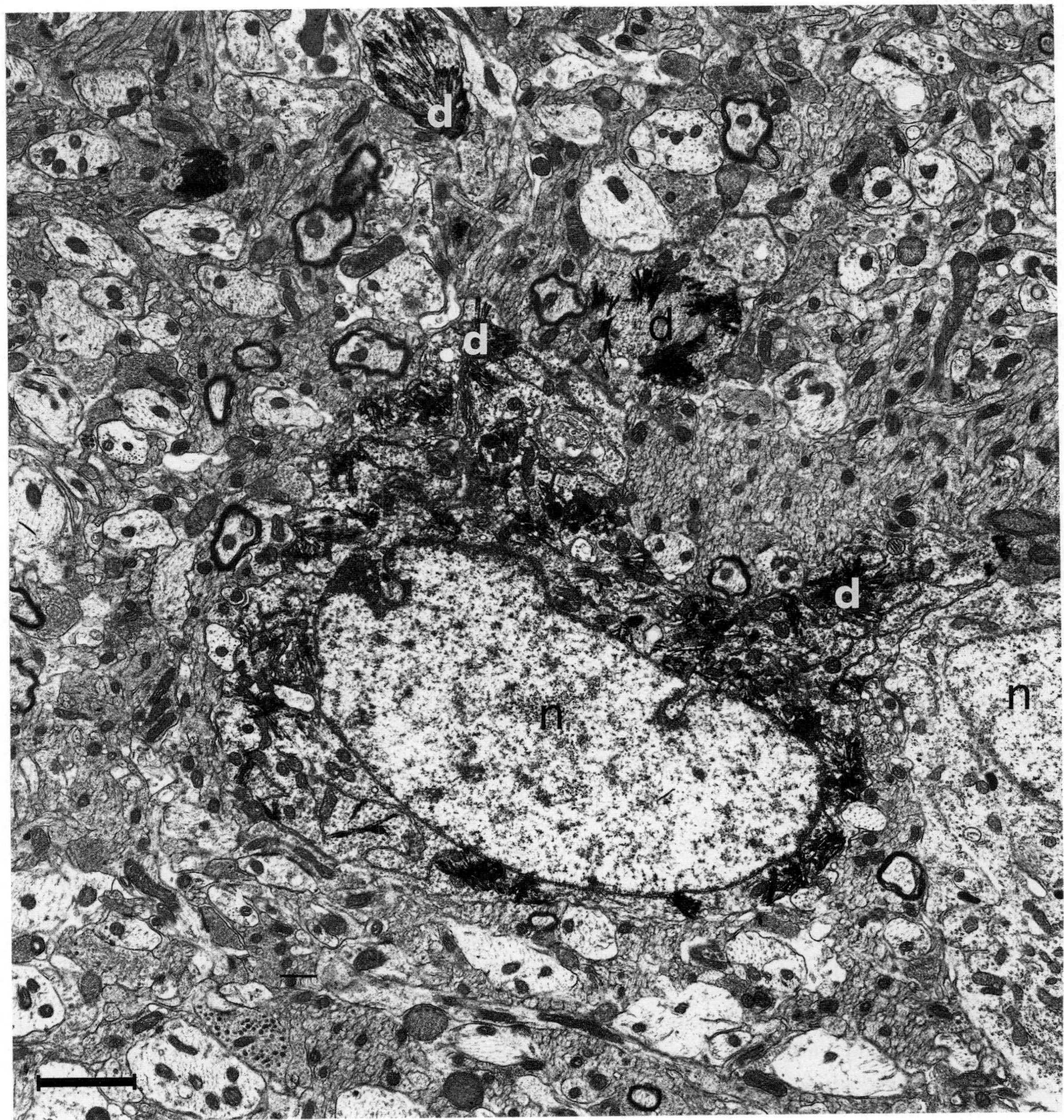

Fig. 6. Electron micrograph of a zone of neuropil in the thalamic paraventricular nucleus illustrating the retrograde neuronal labeling following injection of horseradish peroxidase into the ipsilateral amygdala in the rat. The labeled neuron (n, center) contains numerous clusters of crystalline tetramethylbenzidine reaction product, which can also be traced into the dendrites (d) and easily distinguished from unlabeled neurons (n, right). Scale bar: 2 μm.

surface (Fig. 5) in a pattern suggestive of a spatial relation to the overlying cerebrospinal fluid (Su and Bentivoglio, 1990), based on suggestive analogies of hypothalamic neurosecretory activity at the surface of the third ventricle. We have examined this region in some detail by electron

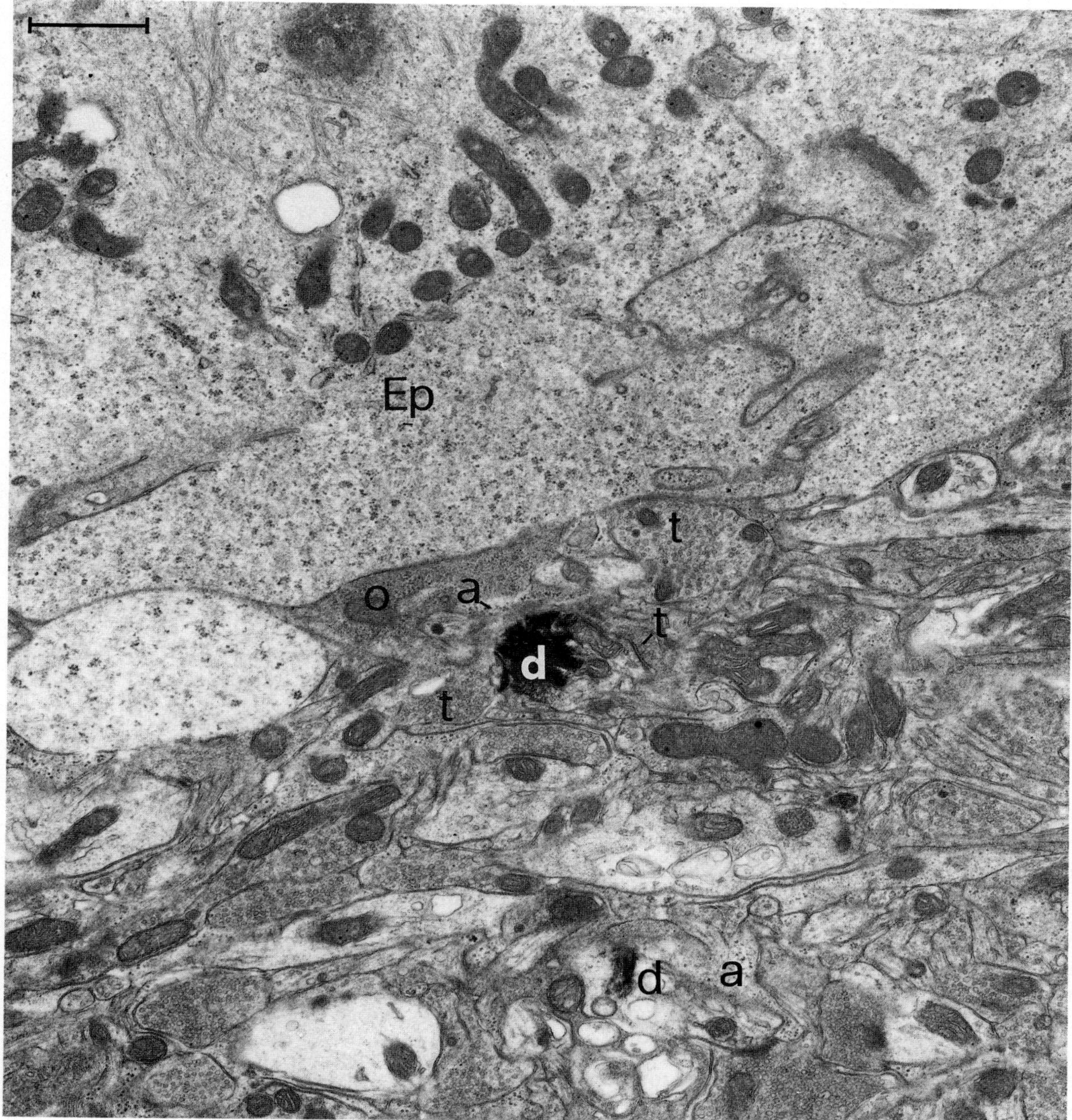

Fig. 7. A serially traced "terminal" dendrite of a neuron of the thalamic paraventricular nucleus of the rat, labeled by horseradish peroxidase injection in the amygdala. The labeled dendrite (d) is separated from the ependyma (Ep) by glycogen containing astrocyte (a) and oligodendrocyte (o) processes as well as axon terminals (t). Scale bar: 1 μm.

microscopy following retrograde labeling of Pv neurons (Fig. 6) after HRP injections in the amygdaloid complex (Balercia et al., 1990), and have successfully serially traced terminal dendrites to the base of the ependymal layer. Labeled dendrites are usually separated from ependymal cells by astrocyte processes containing glycogen microfilaments or thin, sinuous astrocyte leaflets (Fig. 7), which sometimes form membranous whorls. The labeled dendrites do not penetrate to the ependymal surface, although they may contact the basal portion of ependymal cells (Fig. 8). These studies also revealed cytological patterns of the ependymal and subependymal layers distinct from those of other specialized regions lining the third ventricle. Such cytological patterns include basal ependymal zones of intense vesicular activity. Putative neurosecretory and direct neuronal contact with the third ventricle seen in the hypothalamus, implicated in neuroendocrine interaction with the cerebrospinal fluid, were not observed in this highly specialized ependymal region of the thalamus.

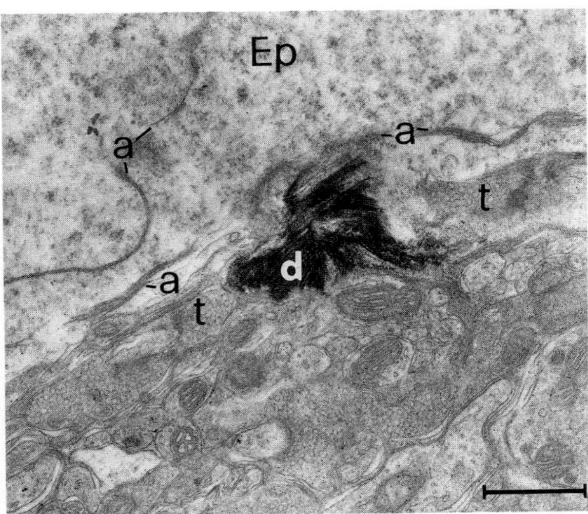

Fig. 8. A "terminal" dendrite of a projection neuron of the thalamic paraventricular nucleus of the rat, labeled after horseradish peroxidase injection in the amygdala. The dendrite (d) reaches the basal portion of an ependymocite (Ep) and is flanked by axonal terminals (t) and sinuous leaflets of astrocyte (a) processes. Scale bar: 0.5 μm.

Neurochemical features

Chemically-defined systems of innervation

Monoaminergic fibers

The afferents to the thalamus which derive from monoaminergic cell groups display regional zones of preferential innervation within the midline. Studies based on histofluorescence (Lindvall et al., 1974) and dopamine-beta-hydroxylase immunohistochemistry (Swanson and Hartman, 1975) have consistently shown that the midline, and in particular Pv, displays the densest adrenergic innervation in the thalamus, whereas the intralaminar and principal relay nuclei are lightly innervated. These afferents derive mostly from the noradrenergic cells of the locus coeruleus (Jones and Yang, 1985), as well as from noradrenergic neurons in the parabrachial nuclei (see earlier p. 58).

A dense plexus of dopamine-immunoreactive fibers has been observed in Pv, sparing the adjacent medial part of MD (Groenewegen 1988). This innervation may derive from the diencephalic dopamine-containing cell groups.

Serotonergic fibers, as shown by immunohistochemistry, are also concentrated within the midline (Steinbusch, 1981; Cropper et al., 1984) and derive from the dorsal and median raphe nuclei (Azmitia and Segal, 1978; Vertes and Martin, 1988). The serotonergic innervation spares Pt, is very dense in Pv, and serotonergic fibers are also distributed to Re and Rh.

Histamine-immunoreactive fibers, arising presumably from hypothalamic cell groups, are also densely distributed within the midline, where they predominate in Pv and Pt in the guinea pig thalamus (Airaksinen and Panula, 1988).

Cholinergic innervation

Both the midline and intralaminar nuclei display a high positivity to acetylcholinesterase (AChE) histochemistry (Jones, 1985). However, at variance with the intralaminar nuclei, which are characterized by intense AChE staining and strong choline-acetyl-transferase (CAT) immunoreactivity, the intense AChE staining of the thalamic midline corresponds to a low density of CAT-positive fibers, which are sparse in Pt and Re and even rarer in Pv (Levey et al., 1987; Houser et al., 1988). The significance of the discrepancy in the midline between high AChE and light cholinergic innervation is still unclear; the AChE-positivity could derive from AChE-containing cell groups of the brain stem, such as the locus coeruleus.

Peptidergic innervation

Immunohistochemical studies have shown that the midline region is heavily innervated by peptidergic fiber systems. Many of them are also distributed to the intralaminar nuclei but are either absent or rare in the rest of the thalamus, such that for most peptides the midline displays the densest thalamic innervation with regional zones of density. Cholecystokinin (CCK) is highly concentrated in Pv in the monkey (Molinari et al., 1987), more dispersed in the intralaminar nuclei and very moderate in other adjacent nuclear structures, such as the ventroposterior complex. In the rat the CCK innervation predominates in Pv and CeM (Hunt et al., 1987). Neuropeptide Y (NPY)- immunoreactive fibers are concentrated in Pv (monkey: Molinari et al., 1987; rat: De Quidt and Emson, 1986). Somatostatin-positive innervation, which also predominates in the midline (rat: Johansson et al., 1984), terminates densely in its ventral portion, mainly in Re and Rh, in the monkey (Molinari et al., 1987). Substance P (SP) immunoreactivity of bundles and puncta is denser in the thalamus than that of other peptides (rat: Cuello and Kanazawa 1978: Ljungdahl et al., 1978; Battaglia et al., 1988) and is heavily distributed within the midline which appears in the monkey as "an almost continuous sheet" of SP-positive fibers (Fig. 9; Molinari et al., 1987). Tachikinin-immunoreactive axons and terminals have also been detected in various regions of the human thalamus, especially in the midline and anterior intralaminar nuclei; the tachikinin innervation appears very dense in Pv (Hirai and Jones, 1989).

CCK-, NPY, somatostatin-, or SP-containing cell bodies were not detected in the monkey dorsal thalamus, indicating that these fiber systems derive from extrinsic sources; NPY, somatostatin and SP innervation is likely to ascend primarily to Pv from the hypothalamus, as part of the periventricular system arising from hypothalamic cell groups; however, most of these peptidergic fibers were seen to ascend to the thalamus from the lateral midbrain tegmentum (Molinari et al., 1987).

Neurotensin-positive innervation was also observed in the midline in the monkey (Makino et al., 1987), and appeared concentrated in the rat in Pv, sparing almost completely Pt (Jennes et al., 1982). Neurotensin-containing cell bodies have also been detected in midline structures (see further).

The midline thalamus is a preferential site of innervation of opioid peptides (beta-endorphin, enkephalin and dynorphin-containing fibers) in subprimates and primates, including humans (see Herkenham et al., 1988, for review, and Hirai and Jones, 1989). In subprimates and monkey, opiate receptors (of the Mu and K types) are also concentrated in thalamic midline regions, with regional predominance (in the rat, for example, the density of opiate receptors is higher in the dorsal part of Pv, throughout its extent, than in its ventral part). Although both opiate peptides and opiate receptors are very dense in the midline thalamus, their relative amounts, discrete patterns of distribution and phylogenetic variations, display a considerable disparity (see Herkenham et al., 1988 for review).

Neurochemical features of midline cell bodies

Neurotransmitters and neuromodulators

Very little is known about the molecules which characterize the neurotransmission or neuroregulation of thalamic midline cells. As indicated previously, most of the rich midline peptidergic innervation is extrinsic. Neurotensin-immunoreactive cells were observed in the dorsal portion of the midline (rat: Jennes et al., 1982; monkey: Makino et al., 1987) but the target of their efferents still needs to be identified. The amino acids glutamate and/or aspartate have been indicated as putative excitatory neurotransmitters of midline neurons projecting to the ventral striatum in the rat (Christie et al., 1987; Fuller et al., 1987; Robinson and Beart, 1988). The histochemical staining of cholinesterase (ChE) displays a very high positivity in Re in the rat, and its occurrence was verified in Re neurons projecting to the subiculum and retrosplenial cortex (Robertson and Gorenstein, 1987, indicating that ChE may play a role in these pathways.

Calbindin

The report that the calcium binding proteins calbindin D28k (Cb) and parvalbumin are highly expressed in the thalamus (Jones and Hendry, 1989; Celio, 1990) has raised considerable interest about their possible function in thalamic neurons, but the role fulfilled by these ''calcium buffering'' proteins is still unknown (see also Jones' chapter in this volume). In the rat, parvalbumin is expressed

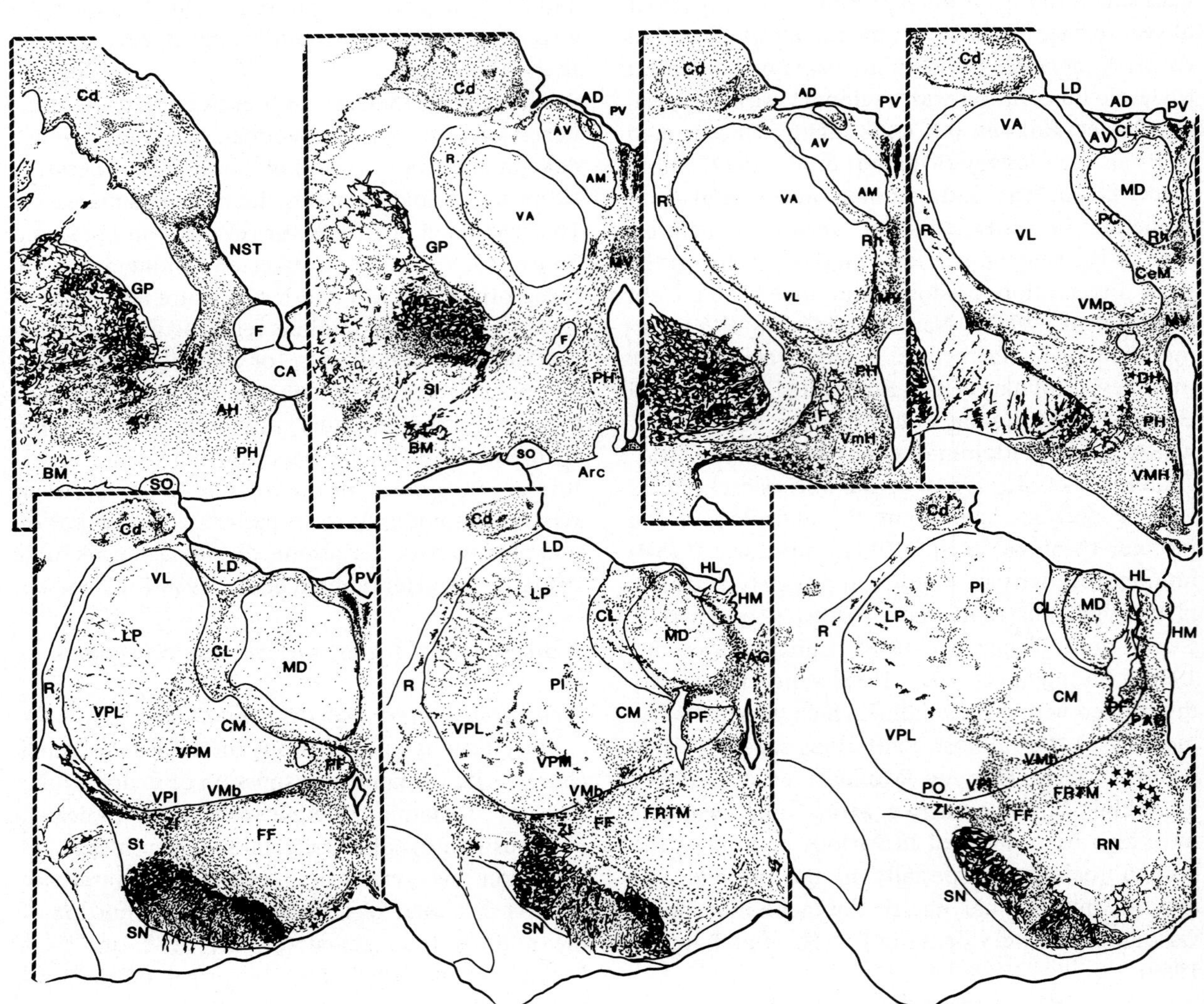

Fig. 9. Coronal sections in rostrocaudal order, showing the distribution of Substance P-immunoreactive fibers in the thalamus of a cynomolgous monkey. Note the dense staining of the midline. (Reproduced with permission from Molinari et al., 1987).

by cells of the reticular nucleus, whereas the dorsal thalamus is virtually devoid of positive cell bodies and, in particular, no parvalbumin-positive neurons are evident in the midline. On the other hand, the protein Cb has a striking distribution in the rat thalamus, where it appears concentrated in the midline, anterior intralaminar, and ventromedial nuclei (Fig. 10). The involvement of Cb-positive cells in the midline projections was investigated in the rat by means of immunocytochemistry combined with retrograde tracing (Bentivoglio and Schiff, 1989; Bentivoglio et al., 1989). The vast majority of midline-hippocampal neurons was found to express Cb, whereas the proportion of Cb-immunoreactive cells was much lower in the midline-amygdaloid cell population. This finding indicates that the information conveyed from the midline to different limbic targets not only takes origin from separate cell populations but is also characterized by a different neurochemical expression.

Selective distribution in the midline of the regulatory subunit of the cyclic AMP-dependent protein kinase (RII)

The second messenger RII, which is one of the two main cAMP-receptor proteins, may represent a multifunctional mediator of the intracellular action of cAMP (De Camilli et al., 1986, 1988). The distribution of RII-immunoreactivity in the nervous system is inhomogeneous (De Camilli et al., 1986). In the thalamus RII-positivity displays a strikingly selective distribution restricted to the midline, and appears concentrated in the neuropil of Pv and of the most medial portions of Rh and

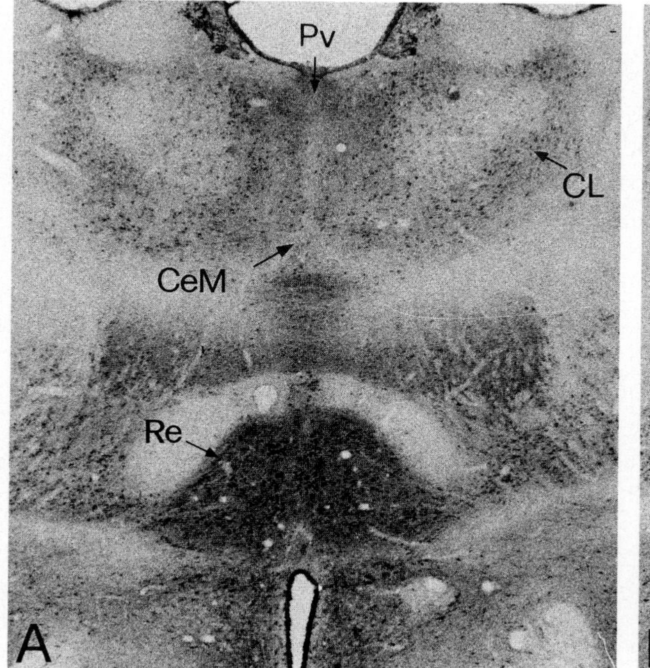

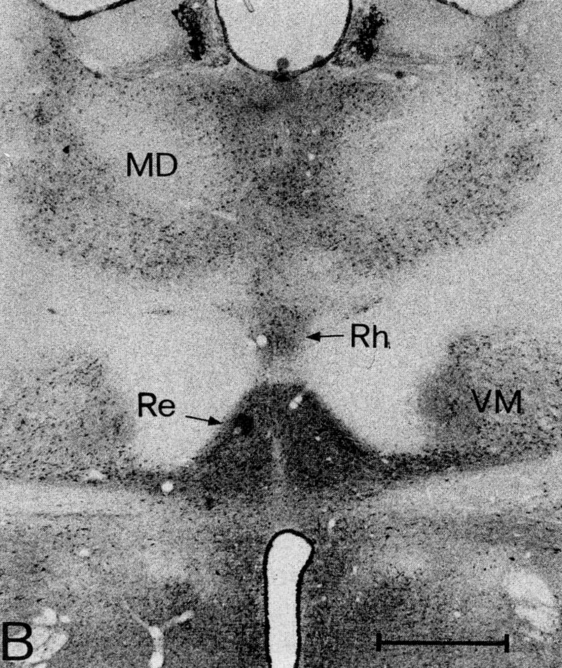

Fig. 10. Microphotographs of two coronal sections through the medial portion of the thalamus of the rat, showing calbindin – immunoreactive cell bodies. Note that in the thalamus positive cells are concentrated in midline, anterior intralaminar, and ventromedial nuclei. Positive cells are also evident in the medial habenula. Scale bar: 500 μm.

Re (Bentivoglio et al., 1988a). The RII-immunoreactive zone was compared to the midline sources of efferents to the amygdala and hippocampal formation by means of combined immunohistochemistry and retrograde tracing (Bentivoglio et al., 1988a). This study revealed that the Pv and Re territories projecting to the amygdala correspond selectively to the RII-immunoreactive zone, whereas RII-positivity is largely segregated from the midline areas projecting to the hippocampus. This finding supports the view that the thalamic midline is a collection of cell groups with distinct features. The possible role played by RII in the neuroregulation of thalamic midline cells still awaits clarification. However, it may be of interest to mention that this protein has been implicated in the molecular mechanisms of regulation of long-term memory (Schwarz and Greenberg, 1987).

Concluding remarks

The midline mosaic of thalamic cell groups

Retrograde and anterograde axonal transport of a variety of robust marker compounds has substantially enhanced available information on the projections to and from each thalamic nucleus, previously inferred from degeneration methods that were especially difficult to apply to the thalamic midline. Detecting a transported marker is usually less ambiguous than identifying distinct degeneration but both methods require critical scrutiny when small structures are analyzed with large lesions and large injection sites, even when the literature provides accordance among different workers. The accuracy of thalamic projections becomes clear when the topographical details of spatial relations can be determined; a feature that has been less successfully applied to the midline than to other thalamic nuclei. It is even sometimes implied that a zone to zone geometry is lacking by describing midline projections in global terms like "striatal" or "limbic" without resorting to spatial or architectural subdivision. Unifying features might be found in the distribution of specific neuronal proteins or neuropeptides, or perhaps the sites of gene expression for these substances can constitute the "key" for an organizing principle in the thalamic midline. Without knowing how to "weight" various criteria we must cautiously avoid haphazard mixing or arbitrary hierarchical ranking of each approach. Perhaps the lesson to be derived from anatomical studies is that a serious analysis of the connections of these thalamic nuclei has revealed a level of diversity and complexity that conflicts with the historical misuse of these data to subsume vastly different nuclear entities under the singular, misleading designation of "midline nuclei".

The data reviewed in this chapter point to two main considerations. Firstly, the midline is a collection of cell groups inserted in different circuits. The small size of midline structures and the difficulty in tracing precise spatial boundaries of the different cell populations renders difficult the task of recognizing their individuality. In some cases connectivity may provide a key of interpretation. For example, the injection of a retrogradely transported marker clearly distinguishes the potent amygdaloid projection of the cells of the dorsal paraventricular region, and the robust projection to the nucleus accumbens of the neurons grouped in the ventral paraventricular region, from the feebly visible paratenial projection to either the amygdala or the accumbens. On the other hand, the concentration of neurons projecting to the hippocampal formation in the nucleus reuniens distinguishes this ventral component from all the other midline cell groups as well as from adjacent thalamic structures. Even within the reuniens, the intranuclear mosaic of the medial cell populations projecting to the amygdala or the nucleus accumbens, inserted among lateral and dorsal neurons projecting to the hippocampus, emphasizes that a cellular, instead of nuclear, level of analysis is essential in the study of the thalamic midline. Many other features, such as the regional and even intranuclear differences in the chemically-signatured systems of innervation point to the midline as a highly ordered collection of neural territories.

Parallel output channels efferent from the thalamic midline

The multiareal distribution of ''nonspecific'' afferents to layer I described by Lorente de Nó (1938), the wide distribution of the ''recruiting'' response detected in electrophysiological studies, and the absence of retrograde degeneration after massive cortical ablations (see Introduction), all contributed to the hypothesis that a widely divergent collateralization could underlie the influence of the ''nonspecific'' thalamus on its multiple cortical and subcortical targets. However, the re-examination of intralaminar efferents (e.g. Bentivoglio et al., 1981; Macchi et al., 1984) provided evidence that different cortical areas, as well as cortical versus subcortical targets, are mainly innervated by separate intralaminar cell groups. A low degree of multiareal divergent collateralization was detected also in other systems of wide cortical innervation (e.g. deriving from the basal forebrain: Price and Stern, 1983; Walker et al., 1985). On the other hand, efferents of ''specific'' principal thalamic nuclei, such as sensory relays with two cortical representations (e.g. in the cat the projections of the ventrobasal complex to SI and SII, and of the dorsal lateral geniculate nucleus to striate and extrastriate fields) may be represented in part by bifurcating axons (Spreafico et al., 1981; Bullier et al., 1984). Altogether, these data strongly indicate that long distance axonal collateralization does not represent a distinguishing structural feature of ''nonspecific'' circuits, which appear, instead, organized in parallel output channels originating from separate cell collections. Thalamic midline efferents seem also to fit this orderly organization. Midline projections to the amygdaloid complex, hippocampal formation and nucleus accumbens display a very low degree of axonal collateralization in the rat (Su and Bentivoglio, 1990). Whether the same midline cells bifurcate upon the hippocampus and the entorhinal or perirhinal cortices still has to be verified. Nevertheless, there is now evidence that midline outputs to cortical and subcortical targets are also ''specifically'' organized in parallel output channels which derive from diverse cell groups in close proximity to one another.

Midline versus intralaminar cell circuits: structural differences and functional implications

As mentioned previously, midline and intralaminar cells are often grouped in a single ''midline and intralaminar'' entity, which is a misleading way to evade insight in these complex structures. Certainly, midline and intralaminar cell groups share important distinguishing features: both cell groups give origin to multiple sets of efferents towards cortical and subcortical targets; they both represent the main source of thalamo-subcortical projections; intralaminar and midline axons do not terminate in the cortex upon layer IV (see Herkenham, 1986, and Royce et al., 1989) at variance with most of the other thalamocortical axons. Intralaminar and midline efferents converge upon some cortical fields, such as the anterior portion of the medial wall of the hemisphere, as emphasized originally by Nauta and Whitlock (1954) and more recently by Vogt et al. (1987). Nevertheless, anatomical and functional scrutiny indicates that midline and intralaminar cell groups are involved in different kinds of information processing. The overall pattern of cortical areal distribution of midline and intralaminar efferents displays a striking diversity. Anterior intralaminar cells project heavily upon the neocortex, including primary motor and primary sensory fields which do not seem to be recipient of midline efferents. Conversely, midline cell groups display a strong preferential relationship with phylogenetically older cortical regions. The tight connections of anterior and posterior intralaminar structures with caudate and putamen, and the heavy connections of the midline with the nucleus accumbens indicate that these cell populations are inserted in distinct striatal efferent channels. The differential density of innervation from the reticular brain stem core and thalamic reticular nucleus indicates a different ''weight'' of these systems in the regulation of the activity of intralaminar and midline regions. The heavy input from cerebellum and spinal cord to the intralaminar thalamus, and the robust input from the hypothalamus and ''visceral'' brain stem cell groups to the thalamic midline provide other examples of a striking diversity in their afferent information. Quantitative and regional differences are evident in the peptidergic, monoaminergic and cholinergic innervation of intralaminar and midline regions. In the rat, calbindin-containing cell bodies are selectively concentrated in both the midline and anterior intralaminar structures, but this pattern displays great phylogenetic variations (Jones and Hendry, 1989). A considerable portion of the midline, but not of the intralaminar thalamus, is exposed to a contact with the ependymal lining, and could be influenced by molecules circulating in the cerebrospinal fluid. The list of differences in the intralaminar and midline organization could be much longer.

From the functional point of view, the inclusion of the midline in the ''nonspecific'' thalamus considered as one functional entity, has refocused attention on the midline as a site of subcortico-cortical activation. The intralaminar nuclei were considered to be the rostral pole of the reticular activating system since they could initiate widespread desynchronization of cortical activity (Moruzzi and Magoun, 1949). However, no detailed studies have been devoted to verify the participation of the midline in this function. The innervation of layer I of a wide cortical region indicates that midline efferents could be involved in general still unknown mechanisms of regulation of the cortical activity played by the most superficial layers. On the other hand, several features of organization suggest that midline cell groups could be involved also in other more defined functions, whose identification deserves greater effort and attention. Some midline cell groups could be involved in the relay of information from ''visceral'' periphery to the forebrain. Recent data in the rabbit (Buchanan et al., 1989) suggest that the midline nuclei could play a role in cardiovascular responses elicited during learning tasks and could therefore be involved in the regulation of sympathetically mediated autonomic adjustments.

Altogether, the efferent circuitry provides evidence that intralaminar and midline cells perform a different computation on cortical and subcortical processing: the midline thalamus may act as an interface between rhinencephalic structures, association cortices and the portion of the basal ganglia heavily innervated by hippocampus and amygdala, whereas the intralaminar cells could subserve different mechanisms of tonic activation of neocortical activity, as well as more specific roles of sensorimotor integration through connections with the neocortex and the neostriatum.

Midline cell groups as candidate in memory formation

Pathological damage along the walls of the third ventricle has been recognized for over a century from Wernicke's (1881) findings of a constellation of behavioral changes, including an amnesic component which later was recognized as essentially similar to Korsakoff's psychosis and currently known as the Wernicke-Korsakoff syndrome. Whether damage to the mammillary bodies and/or the medial region of the thalamus can be correlated specifically with retrograde amnesia remains a debatable subject due to insufficient congruent anatomical and behavioral information (see Victor et al., 1971; Squire, 1987, and Markowitsch, 1988 for review). Impairment of visual recognition memory has been observed in monkey after lesions which involved extensively the thalamic midline, but not after splitting of the massa intermedia (Aggleton and Mishkin, 1983a,b). However, these lesions extended also into the adjacent medial portions of MD and the anterior nuclei, and do not provide, therefore, a conclusive experimental evidence of the midline involvement in memory formation. Nevertheless, there is sufficient clinicopathological evidence to sustain the hypothesis that gliosis in the thalamic region underlying the third ventricle may account for a memory loss independent of mammillary nuclear pathology, and the combination of these lesions correlates with increased severity of memory defect (see Mair et al., 1979, for review). The two cases of Korsakoff's disease affected by a severe memory impairment in the absence of other cognitive defects described by Mair et al (1979) displayed a marked gliosis and shrinkage of the mammillary bodies, and in the thalamus the damage was limited to a thin band of gliosis in the midline nuclei. The same pathological picture was described more recently by Mayes et al. (1988) in two other cases of Korsakoff's syndrome.

The amygdala, hippocampus, entorhinal and perirhinal cortices have been found to play a role in the storage of experience in monkeys (Mishkin, 1978, 1982; Murray and Mishkin, 1986; Murray et al., 1989; Zola-Morgan et al., 1989) and they all receive a heavy input from thalamic midline cell populations. Hippocampus and amygdala are involved in different aspects of object recognition memory (Murray and Mishkin 1984, 1986; see also Murray, this volume). As previously emphasized, midline efferents to the hippocampus and amygdala originate from separate neuronal groups. Therefore, the cell mosaic of the thalamic midline could be involved in functionally distinct though interrelated systems, subserving differential roles in an integrated memory neural network. In the circuits involved in the retention of experience, the cortical encoding of sensory information is ''funneled'' through corticocortical circuits in the temporal cortex, and transferred from there to the hippocampus and amygdala (Mishkin, 1982). The anatomical substrate provided by the thalamus in memory formation has been related up to now mainly to the dense amygdalothalamic and hippocampothalamic innervation, returning to the neocortex through relays in MD and the anterior nuclei (see Amaral, 1987 for review). The midline nuclei, which are not main targets of amygdaloid and hippocampal fibers, but represent the main source of the thalamic return loop to hippocampus and amygdala, provide a major route for the transfer process from the thalamus to the limbic system, whose function merits further investigation.

Acknowledgements

This work was supported by the Italian Ministry of Public Education and NIH awards NS-5685 and TW 1530.

Abbreviations

AD	anterodorsal nucleus
AH	anterior hypothalamus
AM, Am	anteromedial nucleus
Arc	arcuate nucleus
AV, Av	anteroventral nucleus
BM	basal nucleus of Meynert
CA	anterior commissure
Cd	caudate nucleus
Cdc	central densocellular nucleus
CeM	central medial nucleus
CL, Cl	central lateral nucleus
Clc	central latocellular nucleus
CM	centre median nucleus
Cs	central superior nucleus
Csl	central superior lateral nucleus
D	nucleus Darkschewitsch
DH	dorsal hypothalamus
dm	dorsomedial hypothalamic nucleus
F, Fx	fornix
FF	fields of Forel
FRTM	mesencephalic reticular formation
GP	globus pallidus
Gm	medial geniculate nucleus
H	Forel's field H
Hb	habenular complex
HL, LHb	lateral habenular nucleus
HM,MHb	medial habenular nucleus
IAM	interanteromedial nucleus
ITP	inferior thalamic peduncle

LA	lateral hypothalamic area
LD, Ld	laterodorsal nucleus
LP, Lp	lateroposterior nucleus
mc	magnocellular medial geniculate nucleus
MD	mediodorsal nucleus
MV	medioventral nucleus
NST	nucleus of stria terminalis
PA, PV	paraventricular nucleus
PAG	periaqueductal gray
PC, pcn	paracentral nucleus
PH	posterior hypothalamus
Pl	lateral pulvinar nucleus
PO	posterior thalamic nucleus
pPd	peripeduncular nucleus
PF, Pf	parafascicular nucleus
Pt, pt	paratenial nucleus
PVA	anterior paraventricular nucleus
PVP	posterior paraventricular nucleus
Pulo	pulvinar nucleus, oral division
R	reticular thalamic nucleus
Re	nucleus reuniens
Rh	rhomboid nucleus
RN, NR	red nucleus
Rv	nucleus reuniens, ventral part
sm	stria medullaris
SN	substantia nigra
SO	supraoptic hypothalamic nucleus
spf	subparafascicular nucleus
St	subthalamic nucleus
TMT	mammillothalamic tract
VA	ventral anterior nucleus
Vim	nucleus ventralis intermedius
VL	ventrolateral nucleus
VM	ventromedial nucleus
vm, VHM	ventromedial hypothalamic nucleus
VMb	basal ventromedial nucleus
VMp	principal ventromedial nucleus
VP	ventroposterior nucleus
VPI	ventral posteroinferior nucleus
VPL	ventral posterolateral nucleus
Vplc	ventral posterolateral nucleus, caudal division
Vplo	ventral posterolateral nucleus, oral division
VPM, Vpm	ventral posteromedial nucleus
ZI	zona incerta

References

Aggleton, J.P. and Mishkin, M. (1983a) Visual recognition impairment following medial thalamic lesions in monkeys. *Neuropsychologia,* 21: 189 – 197.

Aggleton, J.P. and Mishkin, M. (1983b) Memory impairments following restricted medial thalamic lesions in monkey. *Exp. Brain Res.,* 52: 199 – 209.

Aggleton, J.P. and Mishkin, M. (1984) Projections of the amygdala to the thalamus in the cynomolgous monkey. *J. Comp. Neurol.,* 222: 56 – 68.

Aggleton, J.P., Burton, M.J. and Passingham, R.E. (1980) Cortical and subcortical afferents to the amygdala of the rhesus monkey *(Macaca mulatta). Brain Res.,* 190: 347 – 368.

Airaksinen, M.S. and Panula, P. (1988) The histaminergic system in the guinea pig central nervous system: An immunocytochemical mapping study using an antiserum against histamine. *J. Comp. Neurol.,* 273: 163 – 186.

Ajmone Marsan, C. (1965) The thalamus. Data on its functional anatomy and on some aspects of thalamocortical integration. *Arch. Ital. Biol.,* 103: 847 – 882.

Alexander, G.E., DeLong, M.R. and Strick, P.L. (1986) Parallel organization of functionally segregated circuits linking basal ganglia and cortex. *Ann. Rev. Neurosci.,* 9: 357 – 381.

Alheid, G.F., Heimer, L. and Switzer, R.C. III (1990) The basal ganglia. In G. Paxinos (Ed.), *Human Nervous System,* Academic Press, New York, pp. 483 – 583.

Altman, J. and Bayer, S.A. (1988) Development of the rat thalamus: II. Time and site of origin and settling pattern of neurons derived from the anterior lobule of the thalamic neuroepithelium. *J. Comp. Neurol.,* 275: 378 – 405.

Amaral, D.G. (1987) Memory: anatomical organization of candidate brain regions. In *Handbook of Physiology – The Nervous System, Vol. 5.* American Physiological Society, Bethesda, MD, pp. 211 – 294.

Amaral, D.G. and Cowan, W.M. (1980) Subcortical afferents to the hippocampal formation in the monkey. *J. Comp. Neurol.,* 189: 573 – 591.

Apkarian, A.V. and Hodge, C.J. (1989) Primate spinothalamic pathways: III. Thalamic terminations of the dorsolateral and ventral spinothalamic pathways. *J. Comp. Neurol.,* 288: 493 – 511.

Azmitia, E.C. and Segal, M. (1978) An autoradiographic analysis of the differential ascending projections of the dorsal and median raphe nuclei in the rat. *J. Comp. Neurol.,* 179: 641 – 667.

Baisden, R.H. and Hoover, D.B. (1979) Cells of origin of the hippocampal afferent projection from the nucleus reuniens thalami. A combined Golgi-HRP study in the rat. *Cell Tiss.*

Res. 203: 387 – 392.

Baisden, R.H., Hoover, D.B. and Cowie, R.J. (1979) Retrograde demonstration of hippocampal afferents from the interpeduncular and reuniens nuclei. *Neurosci. Lett.* 13: 105 – 109.

Balercia, G., Bentivoglio, M. and Kruger, L. (1990) The ependymal region of the thalamus. An electron microscopic study of the glial architecture and underlying labeled neurons of the rat paraventricular nucleus. *Europ. J. Neurosci.*, Supp. 3: 41.

Battaglia, G., Spreafico, R. and Rustioni, A. (1988) Substance P-immunoreactive fibers in the thalamus from ascending somatosensory pathways. In M. Bentivoglio and R. Spreafico (Eds.), *Cellular Thalamic Mechanisms,* Elsevier, Amsterdam, pp. 365 – 374.

Beckstead, R.M. (1978) Afferent connections to the entorhinal area in the rat as demonstrated by retrograde cell-labeling with horseradish peroxidase. *Brain Res.*, 152: 249 – 264.

Beckstead, R.M. (1984) The thalamostriatal projection in the cat. *J. Comp. Neurol.*, 223: 313 – 346.

Bentivoglio, M. and Schiff, D. (1989) Calbindin-immunoreactive neurons give origin to thalamolimbic pathways. *Europ. J. Neurosci.*, Suppl. 2: 270.

Bentivoglio, M., Cenci, M.A. and Su, H.-S. (1988a) The thalamic midline structures projecting to the amygdala display high immunoreactivity for the cAMP-receptor protein RII in the rat. *Soc. Neurosci. Abstr.* 14: 80.

Bentivoglio, M., Macchi, G. and Albanese, A. (1981) The cortical projections of the thalamic intralaminar nuclei, as studied in cat and rat with the multiple fluorescent retrograde tracing technique. *Neurosci. Lett.* 26: 5 – 10.

Bentivoglio, M., Minciacchi, D., Molinari, M., Granato, A., Spreafico, R. and Macchi, G. (1988b) The intrinsic and extrinsic organization of the thalamic intralaminar nuclei. In M. Bentivoglio and R. Spreafico (Eds.) *Cellular Thalamic Mechanisms,* Elsevier, Amsterdam, pp. 221 – 237.

Bentivoglio, M., Schiff, D. and Su, H.S. (1989) Differential expression of calbindin immunoreactivity in the thalamolimbic and thalamostriatal cell populations. *Soc. Neurosci. Abstr.* 15: 231.

Berendse, H.W., Voorn, P., te Kortschot, A. and Groenewegen, H.J. (1988) Nuclear origin of thalamic afferents of the ventral striatum determines their relation to patch/matrix configurations in enkephalin-immunoreactivity in the rat. *J. Chem. Neuroanat.*, 1: 3 – 10.

Berendse, H.W. and Groenewegen, H.J. (1990) Organization of the thalamostriatal projections in the rat, with special emphasis on the ventral striatum. *J. Comp. Neurol.*, 299: 187 – 228.

Buchanan, S.L., Thompson, R.H. and Powell, D.A. (1989) Midline thalamic lesions enhance conditioned bradycardia and the cardiac orienting reflex in rabbits. *Psychobiology,* 17: 300 – 306.

Bullier, J., Kennedy, H. and Salinger, W. (1984) Bifurcation of subcortical afferents to visual areas 17, 18, and 19 in the cat cortex. *J. Comp. Neurol.*, 228: 309 – 328.

Burton, H. and Craig, A.D. (1983) Spinothalamic projections in cat, raccoon and monkey: A study based on anterograde transport of horseradish peroxidase. In G. Macchi, A, Rustioni and R. Spreafico (Eds.) *Somatosensory Integration in the Thalamus,* Elsevier, Amsterdam, pp. 17 – 41.

Celio, M. (1990) Calbindin D28k and parvalbumin in the rat brain. *Neuroscience,* 35: 375 – 475.

Christie, M.J., Summers, R.J., Stephenson, J.A., Cook, C.J. and Beart, P.M. (1987) Excitatory amino acid projections to the nucleus accumbens septi in the rat: A retrograde transport study utilizing D-[^{3}H]aspartate and [^{3}H]GABA. *Neuroscience,* 22: 425 – 439.

Cornwall, J. and Philipson, O.T. (1988a) Afferent projections to the dorsal thalamus of the rat as shown by retrograde lectin transport. I. The mediodorsal nucleus. *Neuroscience,* 24: 1035 – 1049.

Cornwall, J. and Phillipson, O.T. (1988b) Afferent projections to the dorsal thalamus of the rat as shown by retrograde lectin transport. II. The midline nuclei. *Brain Res. Bull.*, 21: 147 – 161.

Cornwall, J., Cooper, J.D. and Phillipson, O.T. (1990) Projections to the rostral reticular thalamic nucleus in the rat. *Exp. Brain Res.*, 80: 157 – 171.

Cropper, E.C., Eisenman, J.S. and Azmitia, E.C. (1984) An immunocytochemical study of the serotonergic innervation of the thalamus of the rat. *J. Comp. Neurol.*, 224: 38 – 50.

Cuello, A.C. and Kanazawa, I. (1978) The distribution of substance P immunoreactive fibers in the rat central nervous system. *J. Comp. Neurol.*, 178: 129 – 150.

Deacon, T.W., Eichenbaum, H., Rosenberg, P. and Eckmann, K.W. (1983) Afferent connections of the perirhinal cortex in the rat. *J. Comp. Neurol.*, 220: 168 – 190.

De Camilli, P., Moretti, M., Denis Donini, S., Walter, U. and Lohmann, S.M. (1986) Heterogeneous distribution of the cAMP receptor protein RII in the nervous system: evidence for its intracellular accumulation in microtubules, microtubule-organizing centers, and in the area of the Golgi complex. *J. Cell Biol.*, 103: 189 – 203.

De Camilli, P., Solimena, M., Moretti, M. and Navone, F. (1988) Sites of action of second messengers in the neuronal cytomatrix. In *Intrinsic Determinants of Neuronal Form and Function,* Alan Liss, New York, pp. 487 – 520.

Dempsey, E.W. and Morison, R.S. (1942) The production of rhythmically recurrent cortical potentials after localized thalamic stimulation. *Am. J. Physiol.*, 135: 293 – 300.

De Olmos, J.S. and Ingram, W.R. (1972) The projection field of the stria terminalis in the rat brain. An experimental study. *J. Comp. Neurol.*, 146: 303 – 334.

De Quidt, M.A. and Emson, P.C. (1986) Distribution of neuropeptide Y-like immunoreactivity in the rat central nervous system. II. Immunohistochemical analysis. *Neuroscience,* 18: 545 – 618.

Eberhart, J.A., Morrell, J.I., Krieger, M.S. and Pfaff, D.W. (1985) An autoradiographic study of projections ascending from the midbrain central gray, and from the region lateral to it. *J. Comp. Neurol.,* 241: 285 – 310.

Edwards, S.B. and De Olmos, J.S. (1976) Autoradiographic studies of the projections of the midbrain reticular formation: Ascending projections of the nucleus cuneiformis. *J. Comp. Neurol.,* 165: 417 – 432.

Finch, D.M., Derian, E.L. and Babb, T.L. (1984) Afferent fibers to rat cingulate cortex. *Exp. Neurol.,* 83: 468 – 485.

Friedman, D.P., Bachevalier, J., Ungerleider, L.G. and Mishkin, M. (1987) Widespread thalamic projections to layer I of primate cortex. *Soc. Neurosci. Abstr.,* 13: 251.

Friedman, D.P., Li, L. and Ungerleider, L.G. (1989) Origins of thalamic projections to layer I of the cerebral cortex of the monkey. *Soc. Neurosci. Abstr.,* 15: 311.

Fuller, T.A., Russchen, F.T. and Price, J.L. (1987) Sources of presumptive glutamergic/aspartergic afferents to the rat ventral striatopallidal region. *J. Comp. Neurol.,* 259: 317 – 338.

Groenewegen, H.J. (1988) Organization of the afferent connections of the mediodorsal thalamic nucleus in the rat, related to the mediodorsal-prefrontal topography. *Neuroscience,* 24: 379 – 431.

Groenewegen, H.J., Vermeulen-Van der Zee, E., te Kortschot, A. and Witter, M.P. (1987) Organization of the projections from the subiculum to the ventral striatum in the rat. A study using anterograde transport of *Phaseolus vulgaris* leucoagglutinin. *Neuroscience,* 23: 103 – 120.

Groenewegen, H.J., Becker, N.E.H.M. and Lohman, A.H.M. (1980) Subcortical afferents of the nucleus accumbens septi in the cat, studied with retrograde axonal transport of horseradish peroxidase and bisbenzimid. *Neuroscience,* 5: 1903 – 1916.

Haber, S.N., Groenewegen, H.J., Grove, E.A. and Nauta, W.J.H. (1985) Efferent connections of the ventral pallidum: Evidence of a dual striato pallidofugal pathway. *J. Comp. Neurol.,* 235: 322 – 335.

Haber, S.N., Lynd, E., Klein, C. and Groenewegen, H.J. (1990) Topographic organization of the ventral striatal efferent projections in the rhesus monkey: an anterograde tracing study. *J. Comp. Neurol.,* 293: 282 – 298.

Hallänger, A.E. and Wainer, B.H. (1988) Ascending projections from the pedunculopontine tegmental nucleus and the adjacent mesopontine tegmentum in the rat. *J. Comp. Neurol.,* 274: 483 – 515.

Harris, R.M. (1987) Axon collaterals in the thalamic reticular nucleus from thalamocortical neurons of the rat ventrobasal thalamus. *J. Comp. Neurol.,* 258: 397 – 406.

Herkenham, M. (1978) The connections of the nucleus reuniens thalami: Evidence for a direct thalamo-hippocampal pathway in the rat. *J. Comp. Neurol.,* 177: 589 – 610.

Herkenham, M. (1986) New perspectives on the organization and evolution of nonspecific thalamocortical projections. In E.G. Jones and A. Peters (Eds.) *Cerebral Cortex, Vol. 5,* Plenum Press, New York, pp. 403 – 445.

Herkenham, M., McLean, S., Moon, S.L. and Pert, C.B. (1988) Autoradiography of receptor distributions suggests an endocrine function for neurotransmitters: Evidence from comparative anatomy of the opiate system. In M. Bentivoglio and R. Spreafico (Eds.) *Cellular Thalamic Mechanisms,* Elsevier, Amsterdam, pp. 417 – 432.

Hirai, T. and Jones, E.G. (1989) Distribution of tachykinin- and enkephalin-immunoreactive fibers in the human thalamus. *Brain Res. Reviews,* 14: 35 – 52.

Houser, C.R., Phelps, P.E. and Vaughn, J.E. (1988) Cholinergic innervation of the rat thalamus as demonstrated by the immunocytochemical localization of choline acetyltransferase. In M. Bentivoglio and R. Spreafico (Eds.) *Cellular Thalamic Mechanisms,* Elsevier, Amsterdam, pp. 387 – 398.

Hunt, C.A., Seroogy, K.B., Gall, C.M. and Jones, E.G. (1987) Cholecystokinin innervation of rat thalamus, including fibers to ventroposterolateral nucleus from dorsal column nuclei. *Brain Res.,* 426: 257 – 269.

Insausti, R. Amaral, D.G. and Cowan, W.M. (1987) The entorhinal cortex of the monkey: III. Subcortical afferents. *J. Comp. Neurol.,* 264: 396 – 408.

Jasper, H.H. (1949) Diffuse projection system: The integrative action of the thalamic reticular system. *Electroencephalogr. Clin. Neurophysiol.,* 1: 405 – 420.

Jennes, L., Stumpf, W.E. and Kalivas, P.W. (1982) Neurotensin: topographical distribution in rat brain by immunohistochemistry. *J. Comp. Neurol.,* 210: 211 – 224.

Jayaraman, A. (1985) Organization of thalamic projections in the nucleus accumbens and the caudate nucleus in cats and its relation with hippocampal and other subcortical afferent. *J. Comp. Neurol.,* 231: 396 – 420.

Johansson, O., Hökfelt, T. and Elde, R.P. (1984) Immunohistochemical distribution of somatostatin-like immunoreactivity in the central nervous system of the adult rat. *Neuroscience,* 13: 265 – 339.

Jones, E.G. (1985) *The Thalamus.* Plenum Press, New York.

Jones, E.G. and Hendry, S.H.C. (1989) Differential calcium binding protein immunoreactivity distinguishes classes of relay neurons in monkey thalamic nuclei. *Europ. J. Neurosci.,* 1: 222 – 246.

Jones, E.G. and Leavitt, R.Y. (1974) Retrograde axonal transport and the demonstration of non-specific projections to the cerebral cortex and striatum from thalamic intralaminar nuclei in the rat, cat and monkey. *J. Comp. Neurol.,* 154: 349 – 378.

Jones, B.E. and Yang, T.-Z. (1985) The efferent projections from the reticular formation and the locus coeruleus studied by anterograde and retrograde axonal transport in the rat. *J. Comp. Neurol.,* 242: 56 – 92.

Jones, M.W., Kilpatrick, I.C. and Phillipson, O.T. (1989) Regulation of dopamine function in the nucleus accumbens of the rat by the thalamic paraventricular nucleus and adjacent midline nuclei. *Exp. Brain Res.,* 76: 572 – 580.

Jürgens, U. (1983) Afferent fibers to the cingular vocalization region in the squirrel monkey. *Exp. Neurol.,* 80: 395 – 409.

Kelley, A.E. and Domesick, V.B. (1982) The distribution of the projection from the hippocampal formation to the nucleus accumbens in the rat: an anterograde and retrograde retrograde horseradish peroxidase study. *Neuroscience,* 7: 2321 – 2335.

Kelley, A.E. and Stinus, L. (1984) The distribution of the projection from the parataenial nucleus of the thalamus to the nucleus accumbens in the rat: An autoradiographic study. *Exp. Brain Res.,* 54: 499 – 512.

Kelley, A.E., Domesick, V.B. and Nauta, W.J.H. (1982) The amygdalostriatal projection in the rat: An anatomical study by anterograde and retrograde tracing methods. *Neuroscience,* 7: 615 – 630.

Kievit, J. and H.G.J.M. Kuypers (1977) Organization of the thalamocortical connexions to the frontal lobe in the rhesus monkey. *Exp. Brain Res.,* 29: 299 – 322.

Krettek, J.E. and Price, J.L. (1977a) The cortical projections of the mediodorsal nucleus and adjacent thalamic nuclei in the rat. *J. Comp. Neurol.,* 171: 157 – 192.

Krettek, J.E. and Price, J.L. (1977b) Projections from the amygdaloid complex to the cerebral cortex and thalamus in the rat and cat. *J. Comp. Neurol.,* 172: 687 – 722.

Kruger, L. (1959) The thalamus of the dolphin *(Tursiops truncatus)* and comparison with other mammals. *J. Comp. Neurol.,* 111: 133 – 194.

Kruger, L. and Mantyh, P.W. (1989) Gustatory and related chemosensory systems. In A. Björklund, T. Hökfelt and L.W. Swanson (Eds.) *Handbook of Chemical Neuroanatomy, Vol. 7, Part II,* Elsevier, Amsterdam, pp. 321 – 409.

Levey, A.I., Hallänger, A.E. and Wainer, B.H. (1987) Choline acetyltransferase immunoreactivity in the rat thalamus. *J. Comp. Neurol.* 257: 317 – 332.

Lindvall, A., Björklund, A., Nobin, A. and Stenevi, U. (1974) The adrenergic innervation of the rat thalamus as revealed by the glyoxylic acid fluorescence method. *J. Comp. Neurol.,* 154: 317 – 348.

Ljungdahl, A., Hökfelt, T. and Nilsson, G. (1978) Distribution of substance P-like immunoreactivity in the central nervous system of the rat. I. Cell bodies and nerve terminals. *Neuroscience,* 3: 861 – 943.

Lorente de Nó, R. (1938) Cerebral cortex: architecture, intracortical connections, motor projections. In J. Fulton (Ed.), *Physiology of the Nervous System,* Oxford University Press, London, pp. 291 – 340.

Macchi, G. and Bentivoglio, M. (1986) The thalamic intralaminar nuclei and the cerebral cortex. In A. Peters and E.G. Jones (Eds.) *Cerebral Cortex, Vol. 5,* Plenum Press, New York, pp. 355 – 401.

Macchi, G., Bentivoglio, M., Molinari, M. and Minciacchi, D. (1984) The thalamo-caudate versus thalamo-cortical projections as studied in the cat with fluorescent retrograde double labeling. *Exp. Brain Res.,* 54: 225 – 239.

Mair, W.G.P., Warrington, E.K. and Weiskrantz, L. (1979) Memory disorder in Korsakoff's psychosis. Neuropathological and neuropsychological investigation of two cases. *Brain,* 102: 749 – 783.

Makino, S., Okamura, H., Morimoto, N., Abe, J., Yanaihara, N. and Ibata, Y. (1987) Distribution of neurotensin-like immunoreactivity in the diencephalon of the Japanese monkey *(Macaca fuscata). J. Comp. Neurol.,* 260: 552 – 563.

Mantyh, P.W. (1983) The termination of the spinothalamic tract in the cat. *Neurosci. Lett.,* 38: 119 – 124.

Markowitsch, H.J. (1988) Diencephalic amnesia: A reorientation toward tracts? *Brain Res. Reviews,* 13: 351 – 370.

Martinez-Moreno, E., Llámas, A., Avendaño, C., Renes, E. and Reinoso-Suárez, F. (1987) General plan of the thalamic projections to the prefrontal cortex in the cat. *Brain Res.,* 407: 17 – 26.

Mayes, A.R., Meudell, P.R., Mann, D. and Pickering, A. (1988) Location of lesions in Korsakoff's syndrome: neuropsychological and neuropathological data on two patients. *Cortex,* 24: 367 – 388.

Mehler, W.R. (1980) Subcortical afferent connections of the amygdala in the monkey. *J. Comp. Neurol.,* 190: 733 – 762.

Meibach, R.C. and Siegel, A. (1977a) Efferent connections of the septal area in the rat: An analysis utilizing retrograde and anterograde transport methods. *Brain Res.,* 119: 1 – 20.

Meibach, R.C. and Siegel, A. (1977b) Thalamic projections of the hippocampal formation: Evidence for an alternate pathway involving the internal capsule. *Brain Res.,* 134: 1 – 12.

Minciacchi, D. and Granato, A. (1988) Developmental remodeling of thalamic projections to the frontal cortex in rats. In M. Bentivoglio and R. Spreafico (Eds.), *Cellular Thalamic Mechanisms,* Elsevier, Amsterdam, pp. 501 – 516.

Minciacchi, D. and Granato, A. (1989) Development of the thalamocortical system: Transient-crossed projections to the frontal cortex in neonatal rats. *J. Comp. Neurol.,* 281: 1 – 12.

Mishkin, M. (1978) Memory in monkeys severely impaired by combined but not separate removal of amygdala and hippocampus. *Nature,* 273: 297 – 298.

Mishkin, M. (1982) A memory system in the monkey. *Philos. Trans. R. Soc. Lond. B Biol. Sci.,* 298: 85 – 95.

Molinari, M., Hendry, S.H.C. and Jones, E.G. (1987) Distribution of certain neuropeptides in the primate thalamus. *Brain Res.,* 426: 270 – 289.

Morison, R.S. and Dempsey, E.W. (1942) A study of thalamocortical relations. *Am. J. Physiol.,* 135: 281 – 292.

Moruzzi, G. and Magoun, H.W. (1949) Brain stem reticular formation and activation of the EEG. *Electroencephalogr. Clin. Neurophysiol.* 1: 455 – 473.

Murray, E.A. and Mishkin, M. (1984) Severe tactual as well as memory deficits following combined removal of the amygdala and hippocampus in monkeys. *J. Neurosci.*, 4: 2565 – 2580.

Murray, E.A. and Mishkin, M. (1986) Visual recognition in monkeys following rhinal cortical ablations combined with either amygdalectomy or hippocampectomy. *J. Neurosci.*, 6: 1991 – 2003.

Murray, E.A., Bachevalier, J. and Mishkin, M. (1989) Effects of rhinal cortical lesions on visual recognition memory in rhesus monkeys. *Soc. Neurosci. Abstr.*, 15: 342.

Musil, S.Y. and Olson, C.R. (1988a) Organization of cortical and subcortical projections to anterior cingulate cortex in the cat. *J. Comp. Neurol.*, 272: 203 – 218.

Musil, S.Y. and Olson, C.R. (1988b) Organization of cortical and subcortical projections to medial prefrontal cortex in the cat. *J. Comp. Neurol.*, 272: 219 – 241.

Nauta, W.J.H. and Whitlock, D.G. (1954) An anatomical analysis of the non-specific thalamic projection system. In J.F. Delafresnaye (Ed.) *Brain Mechanisms and Consciousness*, Blackwell, Oxford, pp. 81 – 104.

Newman, R. and Winans, S.S. (1980) An experimental study of the ventral striatum of the golden hamster. I. Neuronal connections of the nucleus accumbens. *J. Comp. Neurol.*, 191: 167 – 192.

Niimi, K., Matsuoka, H., Aisaka, T. and Okada, Y. (1981) Thalamic afferents to the prefrontal cortex in the cat traced with horseradish peroxidase. *J. Hirnforsch.*, 22: 221 – 242.

Niimi, K., Niimi, M. and Okada, Y. (1978) Thalamic afferents to the limbic cortex in the cat studied with the method of retrograde axonal transport of horseradish peroxidase. *Brain Res.*, 145: 225 – 238.

Nissl, F. (1913) Die Grosshirnanteile des Kaninchens. *Arch. Psychiatr. Nervenkr.*, 52: 867 – 953.

Ottersen, O.P. and Ben-Ari, Y. (1979) Afferent connections to the amygdaloid complex of the rat and cat. I. Projections from the thalamus. *J. Comp. Neurol.*, 187: 401 – 424.

Peacock, J.H. and Combs, C.M. (1965a) Retrograde cell degeneration in diencephalic and other structures after hemidecortication of rhesus monkeys. *Exp. Neurol.*, 11: 367 – 399.

Peacock, J.H. and Combs, C.M. (1965b) Retrograde cell degeneration in adult cat after hemidecortication. *J. Comp. Neurol.*, 125: 329 – 336.

Phillipson, O.T. and Griffiths, A.C. (1985) The topographic order of inputs to nucleus accumbens in the rat. *Neuroscience*, 16: 275 – 296.

Porrino, L.J., Crane, A.M. and Goldman-Rakic, P.S. (1981) Direct and indirect pathways from the amygdala to the frontal lobe in rhesus monkeys. *J. Comp. Neurol.*, 198: 121 – 136.

Powell, T.P.S. and Cowan, W.M. (1956) A study on the thalamostriate relations in the monkey. *Brain*, 79: 364 – 390.

Preuss, T.M. and Goldman-Rakic, P.S. (1987) Crossed cortico thalamic and thalamo cortical connections of macaque prefrontal cortex. *J. Comp. Neurol.*, 257: 269 – 281.

Price, J.L. and Stern, R. (1983) Individual cells in the nucleus basalis-diagonal band complex have restricted axonal projections to the cerebral cortex in the rat. *Brain Res.*, 269: 352 – 356.

Ragsdale, C.W. Jr. and Graybiel, A.M. (1988) Multiple patterns of thalamostriatal innervation in the cat. in M. Bentivoglio and R. Spreafico (Eds.) *Cellular Thalamic Mechanisms*, Elsevier, Amsterdam, pp. 261 – 267.

Ricardo, J.A. and Koh, E.T. (1978) Anatomical evidence of direct projections from the nucleus of the solitary tract to the hypothalamus, amygdala, and other forebrain structures in the rat. *Brain Res.*, 153: 1 – 26.

Riley, J.N. and Moore, R.Y. (1981) Diencephalic and brainstem afferents to the hippocampal formation of the rat. *Brain Res. Bull.*, 6: 437 – 444.

Robertson, R.T. and Kaitz, S.S. (1981) Thalamic connections with limbic cortex. I. Thalamocortical projections, *J. Comp. Neurol.*, 195: 501 – 525.

Robertson, R.T. and Feiner, A.R. (1982) Diencephalic projections from the pontine reticular formation: Autoradiographic studies in the cat. *Brain Res.* 239: 3 – 16.

Robertson, R.T. and Gorenstein, C. (1987) "Non-specific" cholinesterase-containing neurons of the dorsal thalamus project to medial limbic cortex. *Brain Res.*, 404: 282 – 292.

Robinson, T.G. and Beart, P.M. (1988) Excitant amino acid projections from rat amygdala and thalamus to nucleus accumbens, *Brain Res. Bull.*, 20: 467 – 471.

Room, P. and Groenewegen, H.J. (1986) Connections of the parahippocampal cortex in the cat. II. Subcortical afferents. *J. Comp. Neurol.*, 251: 451 – 473.

Rose, J.E. (1942) The ontogenetic development of the rabbit's diencephalon. *J. Comp. Neurol.* 77: 61 – 129.

Rose, J.E. and Woolsey, C.N. (1943) A study of thalamocortical relations in the rabbit. *Bull. Johns Hopkins Hosp.*, 73: 65 – 128.

Rose, J.E. and Woolsey, C.N. (1949) Organization of the mammalian thalamus and its relationships to the cerebral cortex. *Electroencephalogr. Clin. Neurophysiol.*, 1: 391 – 403.

Royce, G.J., Bromley, S., Gracco, C. and Beckstead, R.M. (1989) Thalamocortical connections of the rostral intralaminar nuclei: An autoradiographic analysis in the cat. *J. Comp. Neurol.*, 288: 555 – 582.

Russchen, F.T. (1982) Amygdalopetal projections in the cat. II. Subcortical afferent connections. A study with retrograde tracing techniques. *J. Comp. Neurol.*, 207: 157 – 176.

Russchen, F.T., Amaral, D.G. and Price, J.L. (1987) The afferent input to the magnocellular division of the mediodorsal thalamic nucleus in the monkey, *Macaca fascicularis*. *J. Comp. Neurol.*, 256: 175 – 210.

Saper, C.B., Swanson, L.W. and Cowan, W.M. (1979) An autoradiographic study of the efferent connections of the lateral hypothalamic area in the rat. *J. Comp. Neurol.*, 183:

669 – 707.

Saper, C.B. and Loewy, A.D. (1980) Efferent connections of the parabrachial nucleus in the rat. *Brain Res.,* 197: 291 – 317.

Scheibel, M.E. and Scheibel, A.B. (1967) Structural organization of nonspecific thalamic nuclei and their projection toward cortex. *Brain Res.,* 1: 43 – 62.

Schwartz, J.H. and Greenberg, S.M. (1987) Molecular mechanisms for memory: second-messenger induced modifications of protein kinases in nerve cells. *Ann. Rev. Neurosci.,* 10: 459 – 476.

Segal, M. (1977) Afferents to the entorhinal cortex of the rat studied by the method of retrograde transport of horseradish peroxidase. *Exp. Neurol.,* 57: 750 – 765.

Sesack, S.R., Deutch, A.Y., Roth, R.H. and Bunney, B.S. (1989) Topographical organization of the efferent projections of the medial prefrontal cortex in the rat: An anterograde tract-tracing study with *Phaseolus vulgaris* leucoagglutinin. *J. Comp. Neurol.,* 290: 213 – 242.

Spreafico, R., Hayes, N.L. and Rustioni, A. (1981) Thalamic projection on the primary and secondary somatosensory cortices in cat: Single and double retrograde tracer studies. *J. Comp. Neurol.,* 203: 67 – 90.

Spreafico, R., Battaglia, G., De Curtis, M. and De Biasi, S. (1987) Morphological and functional aspects of nucleus reticularis thalami (RTN) of the rat. In J.-M. Besson, G. Guilbaud and M. Peschanski (Eds.), *Thalamus and Pain,* Elsevier, Amsterdam, pp. 111 – 126.

Squire, L.R. (1987) *Memory and Brain.* Oxford University Press, Oxford and New York.

Steinbusch, H.W.M. (1981) Distribution of serotonin-immunoreactivity in the central nervous system of the rat. Cell bodies and terminals. *Neuroscience,* 6: 557 – 618.

Steriade, M. and Deschênes, M. (1984) The thalamus as a neuronal oscillator. *Brain Res. Reviews,* 8: 1 – 63.

Steriade, M., Parent, A. and Hada, J. (1984) Thalamic projections of nucleus reticularis thalami of cat: A study using retrograde transport of horseradish peroxidase and fluorescent tracers. *J. Comp. Neurol.,* 229: 531 – 547.

Su, H.-S. and Bentivoglio, M. (1990) Thalamic midline cell populations projecting to the nucleus accumbens, amygdala and hippocampus in the rat. *J. Comp. Neurol.,* 297: 582 – 593.

Swanson, L.W. (1976) An autoradiographic study of the efferent connections of the preoptic region in the rat. *J. Comp. Neurol.,* 167: 227 – 256.

Swanson, L.W. and Cowan, W.M. (1979) The connections of the septal region in the rat. *J. Comp. Neurol.,* 167: 227 – 256.

Swanson, L.W. and Hartman, B.K. (1975) The central adrenergic system. An immunofluorescence study of the location of cell bodies and their efferent connections in the rat utilizing dopamine-β-hydroxylase as a marker. *J. Comp. Neurol.,* 163: 467 – 506.

Takada, M., Fishell, G., Li, Z.K., van der Kooy, D. and Hattori, T. (1987) The development of laterality in the forebrain projections of midline thalamic cell groups in the rat. *Dev. Brain Res.* 35: 275 – 282.

Thompson, S.M. and Robertson, R.T. (1987) Organization of the subcortical pathways for sensory projections to the limbic cortex. I. Subcortical projections to the medial limbic cortex in the rat. *J. Comp. Neurol.,* 265: 175 – 188.

Veening, J.G. (1978) Subcortical afferents of the amygdaloid complex in the rat: An HRP study. *Neurosci. Lett.,* 8: 197 – 202.

Velayos, J.L. and Reinoso-Suárez, F. (1985) Prosencephalic afferents to the mediodorsal thalamic nucleus. *J. Comp. Neurol.,* 206: 17 – 27.

Velayos, J.L., Jimeñez-Castellanos, J. Jr. and Reinoso-Suárez, F. (1989) Topographical organization of the projections from the reticular thalamic nucleus to the intralaminar and medial thalamic nuclei in the cat. *J. Comp. Neurol.,* 279: 457 – 469.

Vertes, R.P. and Martin, G.F. (1988) Autoradiographic analysis of ascending projections from the pontine and mesencephalic reticular formation and the median raphe nucleus in the rat. *J. Comp. Neurol.,* 275: 511 – 541.

Victor, M.R., Adams, R.D. and Collins, G.H. (1971) *The Wernicke-Korsakoff Syndrome.* Davis, Philadelphia, PA.

Vogt, B.A., Rosene, D.L. and Pandya, D.N. (1979) Thalamic and cortical afferents differentiate anterior from posterior cingulate cortex in the monkey. *Science,* 204: 205 – 207.

Vogt, B.A., Pandya, D.N., and Rosene, D.L. (1987) Cingulate cortex of the rhesus monkey: I. Cytoarchitecture and thalamic afferents. *J. Comp. Neurol.,* 262: 256 – 270.

Walker, A.E. (1938) *The Primate Thalamus.* University of Chicago Press, Chicago.

Walker, L.C., Kitt, C.A., DeLong, M.R. and Price, D.L. (1985) Noncollateral projections of basal forebrain neurons to frontal and parietal neocortex in primates. *Brain Res. Bull.,* 15: 307 – 314.

Wernicke, C. (1881) *Lehrbuch der Gehirnkrankheiten, Vol. II.* Theodore Fischer, Berlin.

Witter, M.P. and Groenewegen, H.J. (1986) Connections of the parahippocampal cortex in the cat. III. Cortical and thalamic efferents. *J. Comp. Neurol.,* 252: 1 – 31.

Witter, M.P., Groenewegen, H.J., Lopes da Silva, F.H. and Lohman, A.H.M. (1989) Functional organization of the extrinsic and intrinsic circuitry of the parahippocampal region. *Progr. Neurobiol.,* 33: 161 – 253.

Wouterlood, F.G., Saldana, E. and Witter, M.P. (1990) Projection from the nucleus reuniens thalami to the hippocampal region. A light and electron microscopic tracing study in the rat with the anterograde tracer *Phaseolus vulgaris-*leucoagglutinin. *J. Comp. Neurol.,* 296: 179 – 203.

Wyss, J.M., Swanson, L.W. and Cowan, W.M. (1979) A study of subcortical afferents to the hippocampal formation in the rat. *Neuroscience,* 4: 463 – 476.

Yanagihara, M., Niimi, K., and Ono, K. (1987) Thalamic projections to the hippocampal and entorhinal area in the cat. *J. Comp. Neurol.,* 266: 122 – 141.

Zola-Morgan, S., Squire, L.R., Amaral, D.G. and Suzuki, W.A. (1989) Lesions of perirhinal and parahippocampal cortex that spare the amygdala and hippocampal formation produce severe memory impairment. *J. Neurosci.,* 9: 4355 – 4370.

G. Holstege (Ed.)
Progress in Brain Research, Vol. 87

CHAPTER 5

The substantia nigra and its relations with the striatum in the monkey

Laura Feigenbaum Langer, Juan Jiménez-Castellanos and Ann M. Graybiel

Department of Brain and Cognitive Sciences, Massachusetts Institute of Technology, Cambridge, MA 02139, U.S.A.

Introduction

The relationship between the dopamine-containing neurons of the midbrain and the neurons of the striatum has been a matter of intense interest ever since the pathogenesis of Parkinson's disease was linked to the degeneration of dopamine-containing neurons in the nigral complex (Hassler, 1938; Greenfield and Bonsaquet, 1953; Ehringer and Hornykiewicz, 1960; Eadie, 1963; Barbeau, 1986; Jellinger, 1986; Gibb et al., 1990). It is now known that different sets of dopamine-containing neurons are affected in different clinical disorders (Uhl et al., 1985; Barbeau, 1986; Jellinger, 1986; Hirsch et al., 1988a; Waters et al., 1988). For example, in idiopathic Parkinson's disease and in certain other parkinsonian syndromes, including parkinsonism induced by metabolites of 1-methyl-4-phenyl-1,2,3,6-tetrahydropyridine (MPTP), the nigrostriatal pathway is much more severely affected than the mesolimbic pathway (Burns et al., 1983; Uhl et al., 1985; Deutch et al., 1986; Jellinger, 1986; German et al., 1988; Hirsch et al., 1988a). There are also other neurons damaged in these parkinsonian disorders, including neurons in the locus coeruleus and pedunculopontine region (Forno and Alvord, 1974; Barbeau, 1986; Hirsch et al., 1987; Zweig et al., 1987; Agid et al., 1990). However, the most consistent and severe damage in Parkinson's disease and MPTP-induced parkinsonism is in the nigral complex itself. Examining the functional relationship between the dopamine-containing midbrain neurons and the striatum could thus be crucial in understanding how the input-output processing of the striatum ultimately affects the control of voluntary motor behavior.

The cytoarchitectonic subdivisions of the nigral complex

From a strictly cytoarchitectonic point of view, the substantia nigra of the monkey can be divided into the classic pars compacta and pars reticulata on the basis of the different cell densities in these subdivisions, and into two other subdivisions: the dorsolateral pars lateralis and a fourth much more recently designated cell group, the "pars mixta" of François et al. (François et al., 1984); see Fig. 1. The pars mixta includes the dorsal part of the pars compacta of most earlier accounts (Crosby and Woodburne, 1943; Snider and Lee, 1961; Davis and Huffman, 1968; Kusama and Mabuchi, 1970; Schwyn and Fox, 1974; Szabo, 1980; Poirier et al., 1983) together with neurons of the adjoining tegmentum. The pars mixta probably in part corresponds to the pars gamma of the human substantia nigra as defined by Olszewski and Baxter, and it may even include part of their pars beta (Olszewski and Baxter, 1954).

The dopamine-containing A8, A9 and A10 cell groups first identified by Dahlström and Fuxe (Dahlström and Fuxe, 1964) in the rat overlap

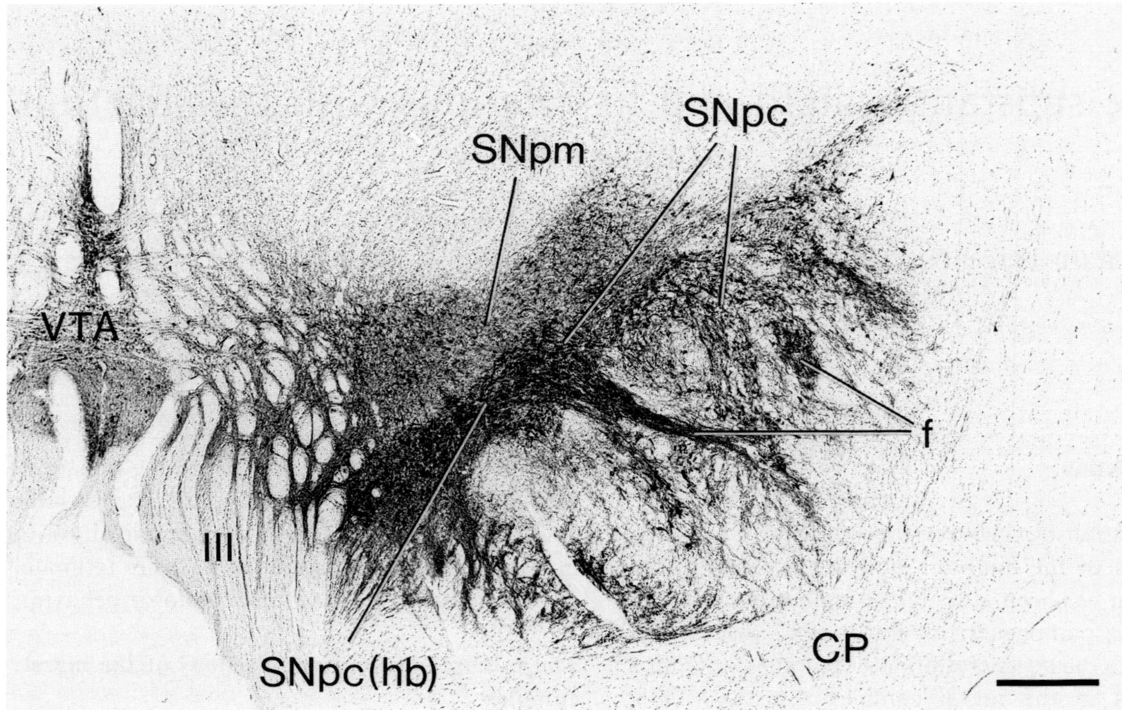

Fig. 1. Transverse section through nigral complex of a squirrel monkey, stained for tyrosine hydroxylase-like immunohistochemistry. The dopamine-containing cell groups shown are the median and paramedian ventral tegmental area of Tsai (VTA); the substantia nigra pars compacta (SNpc) with its main horizontal band SNpc (hb) and ventrally-extending fingers (examples marked by f); and the "pars mixta" of the substantia nigra (SNpm). Cell group A8 mainly lies caudal to the levels shown here. CP-cerebral peduncle; III-oculomotor nerve. Modified from Jimenéz-Castellanos and Graybiel, 1989a. Scale bar = 0.5 mm.

partly with these cytoarchitectonic subdivisions of the ventral midbrain. Cell group A9 largely corresponds to the substantia nigra pars compacta, but also includes the dopamine-containing neurons of the pars lateralis. Cell group A10 includes the median and paramedian cell groups of the ventral tegmental area of Tsai. The dopamine-containing neurons in the tegmentum that lie dorsal and caudal to the substantia nigra pars compacta form the less well known cell group A8. The rostral part of cell group A8 is found at the level of the red nucleus dorsal to the lateral part of the substantia nigra, in the ventrolateral reticular formation. In the primate, cell group A8 fuses with and partly overlaps with the "pars mixta" of François et al. (1984). Farther caudally, the neurons of cell group A8 form a smaller cluster medial to and within fibers of the medial lemniscus and in the ventral region of the lateral reticular formation (DiCarlo et al., 1973; Felton and Sladek, 1983). In their most caudal extent A8 neurons are scattered among the neurons of the pedunculopontine nucleus (Arsenault et al., 1988).

In some studies, alternative nomenclatures have been applied to these dopamine-containing cell groups in the non-human primate. For example, they have been referred to as the C8, C9, and C10 cell groups in the squirrel monkey (DiCarlo et al., 1973; Hubbard and DiCarlo, 1974) and as M8, M9, and M10 in the macacque monkey (Garver and Sladek, 1975). The original designations corresponding to Dahlström and Fuxe's A8, A9 and

A10 cell groups are retained here as this terminology directly links these dopamine-containing cell groups to the dopamine-containing cell groups of their original account. However, correspondences can only be approximated in comparing them in different species and in no species are these cell groups clearly delineated from each other.

Cytoarchitectonic subdivisions within the nigral pars compacta itself have also been identified. Fallon and co-workers (Fallon et al., 1978; Fallon and Moore, 1978; Fallon and Loughlin, 1987) described two distinct groups of neurons within the nigral pars compacta of the rat, and these are probably common to many mammalian species including primates. Fallon and colleagues found a dorsally situated subdivision in which neurons have horizontally oriented dendrites and a ventrally located tier of neurons that have vertically oriented dendrites, many extending into the pars reticulata (Fallon et al., 1978). A simple layered organization is not readily apparent in the nonhuman primate, but there is substantial evidence for the existence of segregated groups of neurons in the pars compacta including more dorsal and ventral parts (see below). It is not clear whether the horizontal tiers described by Fallon and coworkers are homologous to the pars alpha, beta and gamma cell layers described for the human substantia nigra (Olszewski and Baxter, 1954).

As a result of dual retrograde tracer studies of the nigrostriatal connection in the squirrel monkey combined with Nissl cytoarchitecture smaller subdivisions have also been identified in the monkeys's substantia nigra (Parent et al., 1983a,b; Jiménez-Castellanos and Graybiel, 1987a, Jiménez-Castellanos and Graybiel, 1989a). Injections of distinguishable retrograde tracers into the caudate nucleus and the putamen label conspicuous, nonoverlapping clusters of neurons within the substantia nigra pars compacta. Such clusters, about half of a millimeter wide, can be recognized in sections stained for Nissl substance. It would be of great interest to learn whether these correspond to any of the many cell groups of the pars compacta identified in the human substantia nigra (Hassler, 1938; Olszewski and Baxter, 1954; Braak and Braak, 1986).

Such heterogeneity in cellular composition suggests a degree of complexity in the substantia nigra far beyond its broad subdivision into the pars compacta and pars reticulata. This view is in good accord with evidence from studies of the afferent and efferent connections of the substantia nigra and the nigral distributions of the neurotransmitter-related compounds, all of which point to the nigral complex as a highly differentiated structure.

Histochemical heterogeneity of the substantia nigra

What is known of the neurochemical heterogeneity of the substantia nigra is largely based on evidence related to the neurotransmitters carried by afferents to the nigral complex. These afferent connections include fibers from the striatum and nucleus accumbens, the pallidum, the subthalamic nucleus, the amygdala, the lateral preoptico-hypothalamic region, the raphe nuclei, the pedunculopontine nucleus, and the cerebral cortex [see Mehler, 1981; Graybiel and Ragsdale, 1983; Parent, 1986]. With the striking exception of the large striatonigral projection to the pars reticulata, these inputs appear to be directed predominantly toward the pars compacta. The input to the substantia nigra from the cerebral cortex, most likely from the prefrontal cortex to the pars compacta (Künzle, 1978), is believed to be glutamatergic (Kornhuber et al., 1984). The candidate transmitter for the pallidonigral pathway to the pars compacta and pars reticulata is GABA (Hattori et al., 1973; Ribak et al., 1976; Brownstein et al., 1977; Ribak et al., 1980; Fisher, 1989). The neurochemical composition of the inputs from the subthalamic nucleus, amygdala and hypothalamic region have not yet been characterized. However, somatostatin-immunoreactive fibers have been observed within the nigral pars lateralis and may be derived from the subthalamic region (Chesselet and Graybiel, 1983a; Graybiel and Elde, 1983;

Chesselet, 1985) and glutamate has been identified in the subthalamic neurons (Smith and Parent, 1988; Albin et al., 1989). Connections from the raphe nuclei to the pars reticulata (Parent et al., 1981) and to the pars compacta (Bobillier et al., 1976; Azmitia and Segal, 1978) contain serotonin. The principal neurotransmitter in the projection to the substantia nigra from the pedunculopontine nucleus is believed to be acetylcholine (Graybiel, 1977; Moon-Edley and Graybiel, 1983; Scarnati et al., 1986; Beninato and Spencer, 1987a,b; Henderson and Greenfield, 1987; Gould et al., 1989; Martinez-Murillo et al., 1989).

The majority of the intrinsic neurons of the substantia nigra's pars compacta are distinguished by their content of dopamine (Andén et al., 1964; Dahlström and Fuxe, 1964), and subpopulations of these intrinsic neurons contain the calcium binding protein calbindin D-$_{28k}$ (Gerfen et al., 1985) as discussed below. It is also known that many dopamine-containing neurons of the substantia nigra pars compacta (Butcher and Marchand, 1978) and nigral interneurons (Henderson and Greenfield, 1987) contain acetylcholinesterase (AChE), and that this substance can be released with dopamine (Greenfield et al., 1980; Greenfield et al., 1981; Greenfield et al., 1989). Cholecystokinin has been shown to be colocalized in subpopulations of mesencephalic dopamine-containing neurons, but these apparently are almost exclusively in the ventral tegmental area (Hökfelt et al., 1980, 1984; Zaborszky et al., 1985; Palacios et al., 1989). Neurons of the nigral pars reticulata (excepting ventrally displaced dopamine-containing neurons) are GABAergic and some also appear to contain enkephalin (Emson et al., 1980; Oertel et al., 1982; Taquet et al., 1982; Gaspar et al., 1983; Nagai et al., 1983; Inagaki and Parent, 1984; Mugnaini and Oertel, 1985; Inagaki et al., 1986; Smith et al., 1987; Waters et al., 1988). The pars lateralis of the substantia nigra can be distinguished in the monkey by its relatively high content of cytochrome oxidase activity (Ma, 1989) and in other species, including human, by its content of somatostatin-immunoreactive fibers (Graybiel and Elde, 1983; Hirsch et al., 1988b); it contains a mixture of dopaminergic and non-dopaminergic neurons.

Of all known afferent connections to the substantia nigra, the most massive one, predominantly directed toward the pars reticulata, is from the striatum (Schwyn and Fox, 1974; Szabo, 1979). Striatonigral fibers have been shown to contain GABA, substance P and other tachykinins and dynorphin (Kim et al., 1971; Hattori et al., 1973; Brownstein et al., 1977; Gale et al., 1977; Hong et al., 1977; Kanazawa et al., 1977; Fonnum et al., 1978; Jessell et al., 1978; Nagy et al., 1978; Kanazawa et al., 1980; Walaas and Fonnum, 1980; Oertel et al., 1981; Chesselet and Graybiel, 1983b; Kanazawa et al., 1984; Palkovits et al., 1984; Zamir et al., 1984; Quirion et al., 1985; Haber and Watson, 1985; Arai and Emson, 1986; Chesselet et al., 1987). Enkephalin-immunoreactive fibers also pervade parts of the pars reticulata, and some are found in the pars compacta. The origin of extrinsic enkephalinergic fiber systems is uncertain (Haber and Elde, 1982; Chesselet and Graybiel, 1983a,b; Bouras et al., 1984; Inagaki and Parent, 1984, 1985).

Many of these neurotransmitter-related compounds have been shown to be organized in a nonhomogeneous manner within the substantia nigra (Inagaki and Parent, 1984, 1985; Jiménez-Castellanos and Graybiel, 1987a; Waters et al., 1988; Jiménez-Castellanos and Graybiel, 1989a). It is probable that these heterogeneous fiber patterns represent distinct anatomical subdivisions having different patterns of connectivity. Regional subdivisions within the substantia nigra have been demonstrated by autoradiographic binding for receptor-related ligands (Martres et al., 1985; Dubois et al., 1986; Pazos et al., 1987a,b; Beckstead et al., 1988; Besson et al., 1988; Graybiel et al., 1989). These undoubtedly are related also to differential distributions of afferent fibers and of intrinsic nigral neurons as indicated below for striatonigral and nigrostriatal projection neurons.

In 1972, two groups independently discovered

that the dopamine-containing innervation of the striatum first develops in distinct "islands" in the caudoputamen (Olson et al., 1972; Tennyson et al., 1972) and only later extends diffusely across the striatum as a whole. Acute depletion of dopamine in the mature rat's striatum by treatment with alpha-methylparatyrosine, an inhibitor of the catecholamine synthetic enzyme, tyrosine hydroxylase, results in a comparable islandic pattern (Olson et al., 1972; see also Fukui et al., 1986 and Ryan et al., 1988). This evidence was the first to suggest that the nigrostriatal tract might have different components (islandic and diffuse), that these might have different metabolic properties (dopamine turnover being slower in islandic fibers), and that these might even originate in different neurons of the nigral complex.

The suggestion that there are subdivisions in the nigrostriatal projection has been strongly supported by work in a number of species including, most recently, the primate. First, the regions of termination of dopaminergic fibers were shown (Graybiel, 1984) to correspond to striosomes, the histochemically distinct zones in the striatum first identified on the basis of their low AChE activity and later shown to be distinct from the surrounding extrastriosomal matrix on the basis of a large number of neurotransmitter-related distributions

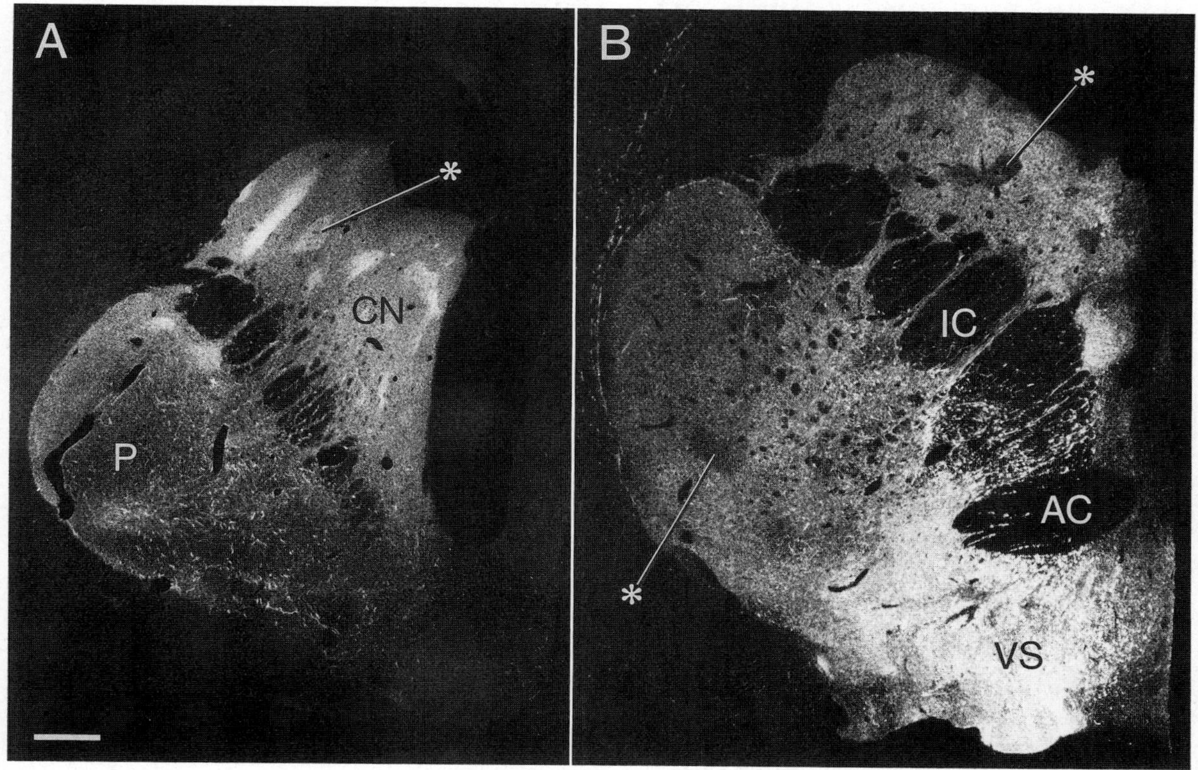

Fig. 2. Nigrostriatal innervation of striosomes and matrix in the squirrel monkey. A shows autoradiogram through the striatum in a case (SMRN8) in which the anterograde tracer ^{35}S-methionine was injected into the substantia nigra pars compacta so as to involve mainly the lateral part of the main horizontal band and especially the associated ventrally-extending fingers (see Fig. 1). There is predominant labeling of striosomes (example marked by asterisk) in the caudate nucleus and medial putamen with much weaker labeling of the matrix. B shows an autoradiogram through the striatum in another squirrel monkey (SMRN5) in which a deposit of ^{35}S-methionine involved cell group A8 and the pars mixta. There is predominant labeling of the extrastriosomal matrix so that striosomes in the field of terminal labeling (examples marked by asterisks) appear weakly labeled. CN-caudate nucleus; P-putamen; VS-ventral striatum; IC-Internal capsule; AC-anterior commissure. Scale bar = 1 mm.

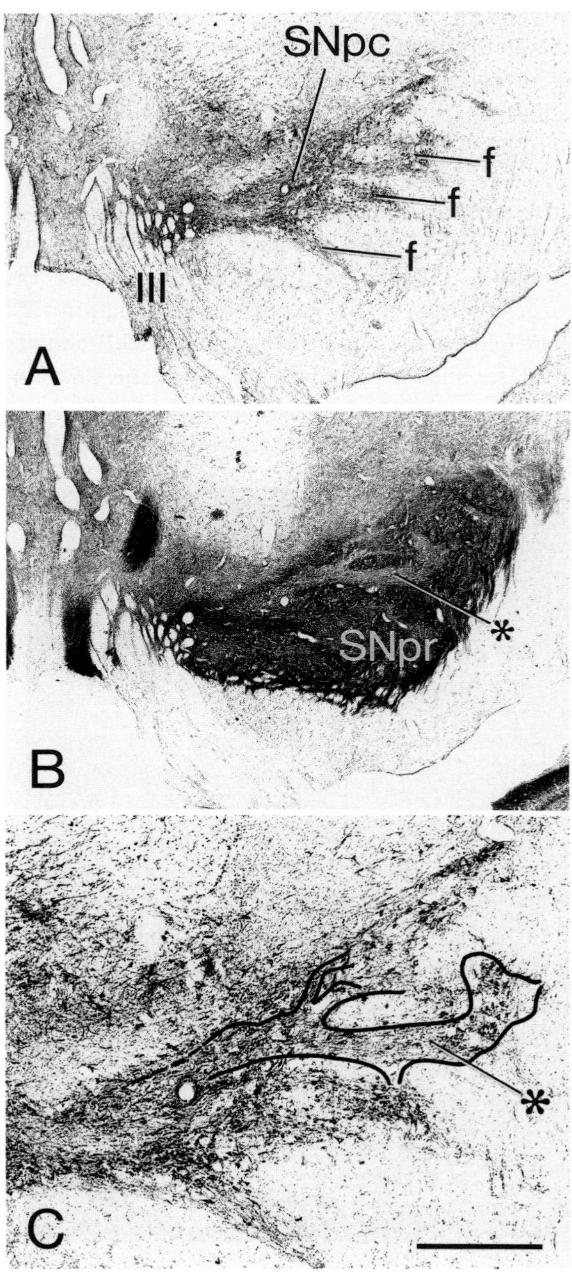

Fig. 3. A and B show adjacent transverse sections through the substantia nigra of the squirrel monkey stained by tyrosine hydroxylase (TH)-like immunoreactivity (A) and acetylcholinesterase (AChE) activity (B). In B, there is a prominent AChE-poor ventrally-extending zone marked by an asterisk that corresponds to some of the ventrally-extending clusters of TH-positive neurons and neuropil shown in A (see TH-positive fingers marked by f's) but not to all of them. C illustrates the extent of overlap at higher magnification (scale bar indicates 0.5 mm) with a photograph of the TH-stained cells onto which the borders of the AChE-poor finger (asterisk) have been drawn. III- oculomotor nerve; SNpc- substantia nigra, pars compacta; SNpr- substantia nigra, pars reticulata.

[see Graybiel and Ragsdale, 1978; Graybiel, 1986, 1989]. In a series of studies in the rat (Moon-Edley and Herkenham, 1983; Gerfen, 1985; Gerfen et al., 1987) and cat (Jiménez-Castellanos and Graybiel, 1985, 1987b) it was then demonstrated that the nigrostriatal projection (and more generally all of the mesostriatal projections from cell groups A8, A9 and A10 terminating in the caudoputamen) can be divided into components having preferred terminal sites in striosomes or in the matrix. Most recently, this plan of subdivision has been documented in the monkey (Feigenbaum and Graybiel, 1988; Langer and Graybiel, 1989); see Fig. 2. In each species studied, cell group A8 appears to project more strongly to the matrix than to striosomes. The weak projection from A10 to the caudoputamen also terminates mainly in the matrix. A specialized part of cell group A9 projects more to striosomes than to matrix. In the rat, the striosome-projecting part of the substantia nigra corresponds to ventral cells of the pars compacta (Gerfen et al., 1987). In the cat, the striosome-projecting zone corresponds to a hypercellular ventromedial part of the pars compacta, the densocellular zone (Jiménez-Castellanos and Graybiel, 1987b). In the squirrel monkey, available evidence suggests that there is also a specialized part of the substantia nigra that projects predominantly to striosomes (Feigenbaum and Graybiel, 1988; Langer and Graybiel, 1989).

The striosome-projecting zone of the substantia nigra is neurochemically specialized. In the rat this zone has been reported to contain neurons low in calbindin D_{28k}-like immunoreactivity (Gerfen et al., 1985). In the cat, the striosome-projecting densocellular zone is rich in sigma receptor binding sites (Graybiel et al., 1989) and has low AChE activity (Jiménez-Castellanos and Graybiel, 1987b).

The densocellular zone is also low in D1 binding sites and is abutted ventrally by a zone of high D1 binding (Besson et al., 1988). Heterogeneous patterns of D1 binding and sigma binding have also been shown in the monkey, as have heterogeneous binding characteristics of a number of receptor ligands and calbindin D_{28k} (Gerfen et al., 1985; Pazos et al., 1987a,b; Jiménez-Castellanos and Graybiel, 1987b; Beckstead et al., 1988; Besson et al., 1988; Graybiel et al., 1989). Whether these preferential distributions delimit the striosome- and matrix-projecting subdivisions of the primate substantia nigra, however, is not yet clear.

In the squirrel monkey, AChE staining, which in the cat reveals the densocellular zone as a zone of reduced staining, has a striking compartmental distribution in the primate substantia nigra (Fig. 3). In AChE-stained sections through the substantia nigra, dorsoventral zonations and mediolateral subdivisions of the pars compacta are readily demonstrable, and there is also a local compartmentalization in which regions of differentially low or high AChE staining are apparent. Particularly prominent are elongated finger-like zones of low AChE activity that extend ventrally from the main horizontal tier of the pars compacta. These AChE-poor fingers in most instances match similar TH-immunostained streamers seen in adjacent sections, but not all TH-positive neurons lie in the ventrally extending AChE-poor fingers (Fig. 3). There thus are marked differences in the AChE environment of different sets of TH-positive (dopaminergic) neurons of the substantia nigra pars compacta in this primate.

It is not clear whether such histochemical compartmentalization in the substantia nigra pars compacta relates to heterogeneous afferent connections of the substantia nigra or to local differences in the interneurons, projection neurons or glia of the nigral complex. However, the AChE seen in histochemical preparations apparently largely reflects membrane-associated ectoenzyme derived from release by cells or fibers, so that the histochemical compartmentalization may well reflect a functional compartmentalization. AChE-containing pathways from the striatum and pedunculopontine nucleus have been suggested (Olivier et al., 1970; Beninato and Spencer, 1987a,b; Henderson and Greenfield, 1987), yet kainic acid injections into the rat's substantia nigra produce a severe reduction of AChE staining, suggesting a relative poverty of this enzyme within nigral afferents (Nagy et al., 1978). Other experiments (Lehmann et al., 1979) indicate that after kainic acid lesions of the rat's striatum there is an insignificant reduction of nigral AChE activity. If the AChE activity in the substantia nigra is related to a pedunculopontine input to the substantia nigra pars compacta, it could reflect the presence of a direct cholinergic innervation of the substantia nigra thought, on the basis of experiments in the rat and cat, to originate in the pedunculopontine nucleus and also possibly the lateral dorsal tegmental nucleus (Beninato and Spencer, 1987a,b). Such a pathway could be important for cholinergic-dopaminergic interactions noted in the substantia nigra in pharmacological and physiological studies (Dray and Straughan, 1976; Lichtensteiger et al., 1976; Dray, 1979; Greenfield et al., 1981). Interestingly, in the cat, the striosome-projecting densocellular zone is a region of particularly reduced muscarinic ligand binding (Nastuk and Graybiel, 1990).

At least part of the AChE activity in the substantia nigra is cellular and two types of AChE-positive nigral neurons have been described (Henderson, 1981). The smaller of the two AChE-containing cell types probably respresents the interneuron described in Golgi studies (Juraska et al., 1977; François et al., 1979). Most, if not all, nigrostriatal dopamine-containing neurons are thought to contain AChE in the rat (Butcher and Marchand, 1978; Lehmann and Fibiger, 1978; Henderson, 1981) in accord with evidence for an AChE-containing pathway from the substantia nigra to the striatum (Shute and Lewis, 1963, 1967). Cholinesterase activity has also been observed in astrocytes in the cat's substantia nigra (Kreutzberg and Graybiel, unpublished observations).

Strict proof for coexistence of AChE and

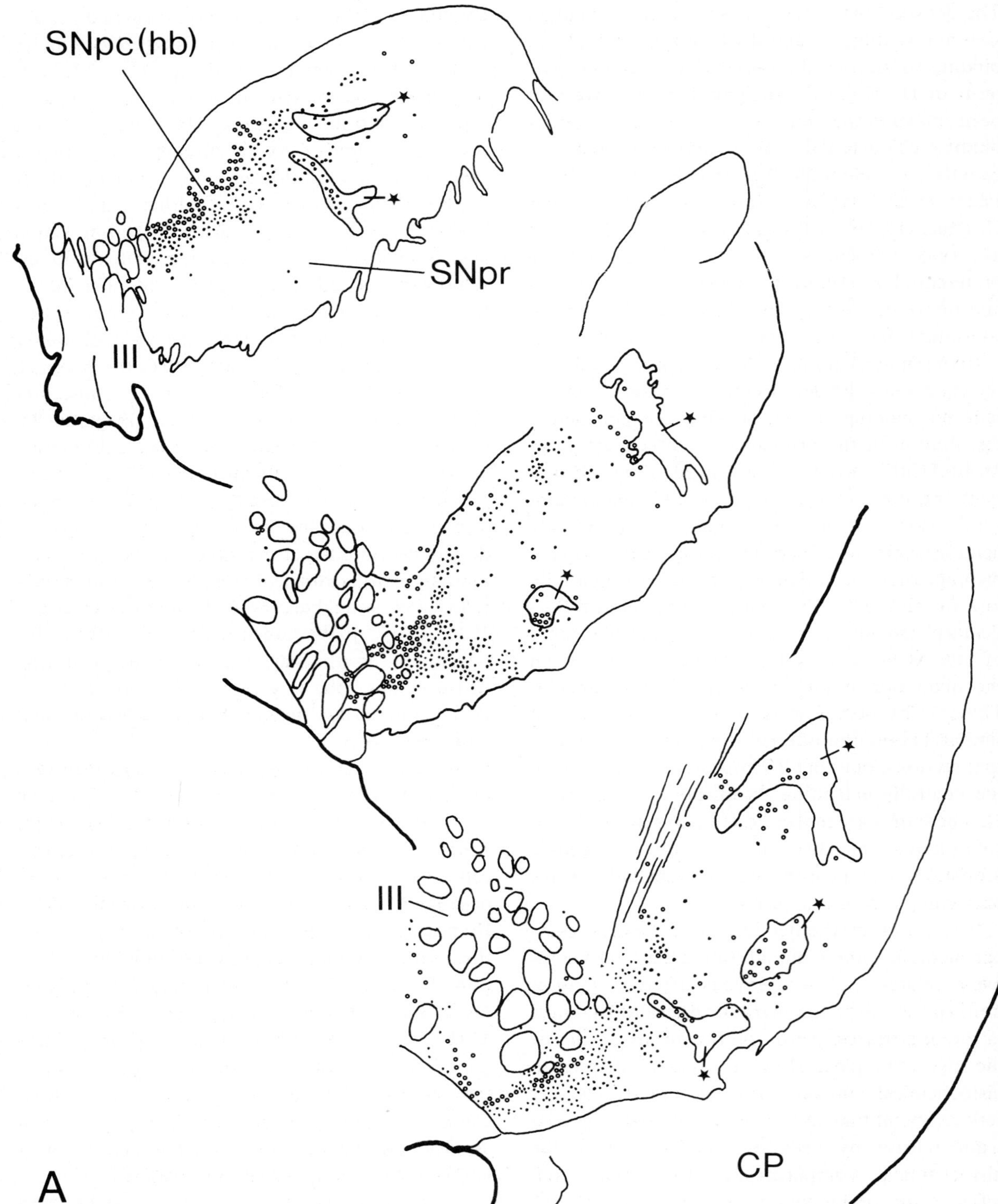
SNpc(hb)
SNpr
III
III
CP
A

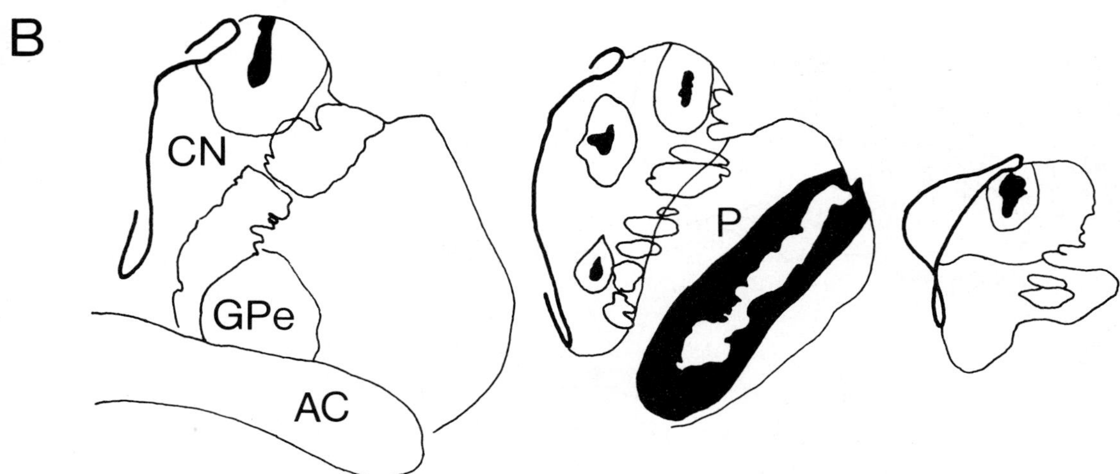

Fig. 4. A. Distribution of retrogradely labeled nigrostriatal neurons (large and small dots) plotted in relation to locations in AChE-poor zones (stars) of the substantia nigra of a squirrel monkey (SMHN-1). In the same hemisphere, several injections of horseradish peroxidase-wheatgerm agglutinin (HRP-WGA) were made in the caudate nucleus and a single large injection of fast blue was placed in the putamen as shown in B. Caudate nucleus-projecting neurons shown by large dots, putamen-projecting neurons by small dots. No double-labeled neurons were observed. The fast-blue labeled neurons were plotted directly from the AChE-stained section; HRP-WGA-stained neurons were plotted from the serially adjacent section. Note, in horizontal band of the substantia nigra's pars compacta SNpc (hb), that putamen-projecting neurons lie dorsal to caudate nucleus-projecting neurons. Most of the retrogradely labeled neurons situated in the AChE-poor ventrally extending fingers (stars) are putamen-projecting neurons; but these also occur outside the AChE-poor fingers. SNpc(hb)- horizontal band of substantia nigra pars compacta; SNpr-substantia nigra pars reticulata; CP-cerebral peduncle; III-oculomotor nerve; CN-caudate nucleus; P-putamen; GPe-globus pallidus, external segment; AC-anterior commissure.

dopamine in nigral neurons has not been obtained in the monkey by double staining. However, tracer injections placed either in the caudate nucleus or in the putamen elicit labeling in the substantia nigra that is organized according to borders visible with AChE histochemistry (Jiménez-Castellanos and Graybiel, 1989a). Retrogradely labeled nigrostriatal neurons are located in the AChE-poor fingers after some injections, but in other experiments the fingers are devoid of labeling (Figs. 4 and 5). These neuronal clusters may be related to the reported segregation of subpopulations of nigral neurons projecting either to the caudate nucleus or to the putamen in the squirrel monkey (Parent et al., 1983a; Parent et al., 1983b; Smith and Parent, 1986), but the correspondence does not appear to be complete, because both nigrocaudatal and nigroputamenal projection neurons can be found in the same AChE-poor finger (Jiménez-Castellanos and Graybiel, 1989a). At the level of the main horizontal band, clusters of putamen-projecting neurons tend to lie dorsal to caudate nucleus-projecting neurons (Fig. 4), but in some cases clusters of nigroputamenal projection neurons do seem to be related to AChE-poor zones (Fig. 5).

Given that AChE histochemistry can be used to demonstrate the striosome-projecting zone in the pars compacta of the cat's substantia nigra, an attractive possibility is that the compartmentalization seen in AChE-stained preparations in the monkey is related to the subdivision of the striatum into striosomes and extrastriosomal matrix. However, HRP-WGA injection sites presumably involving both the striosomal and matrix compartments can give rise to neuronal labeling almost confined to single AChE-poor ventrally extending fingers of the pars compacta (see

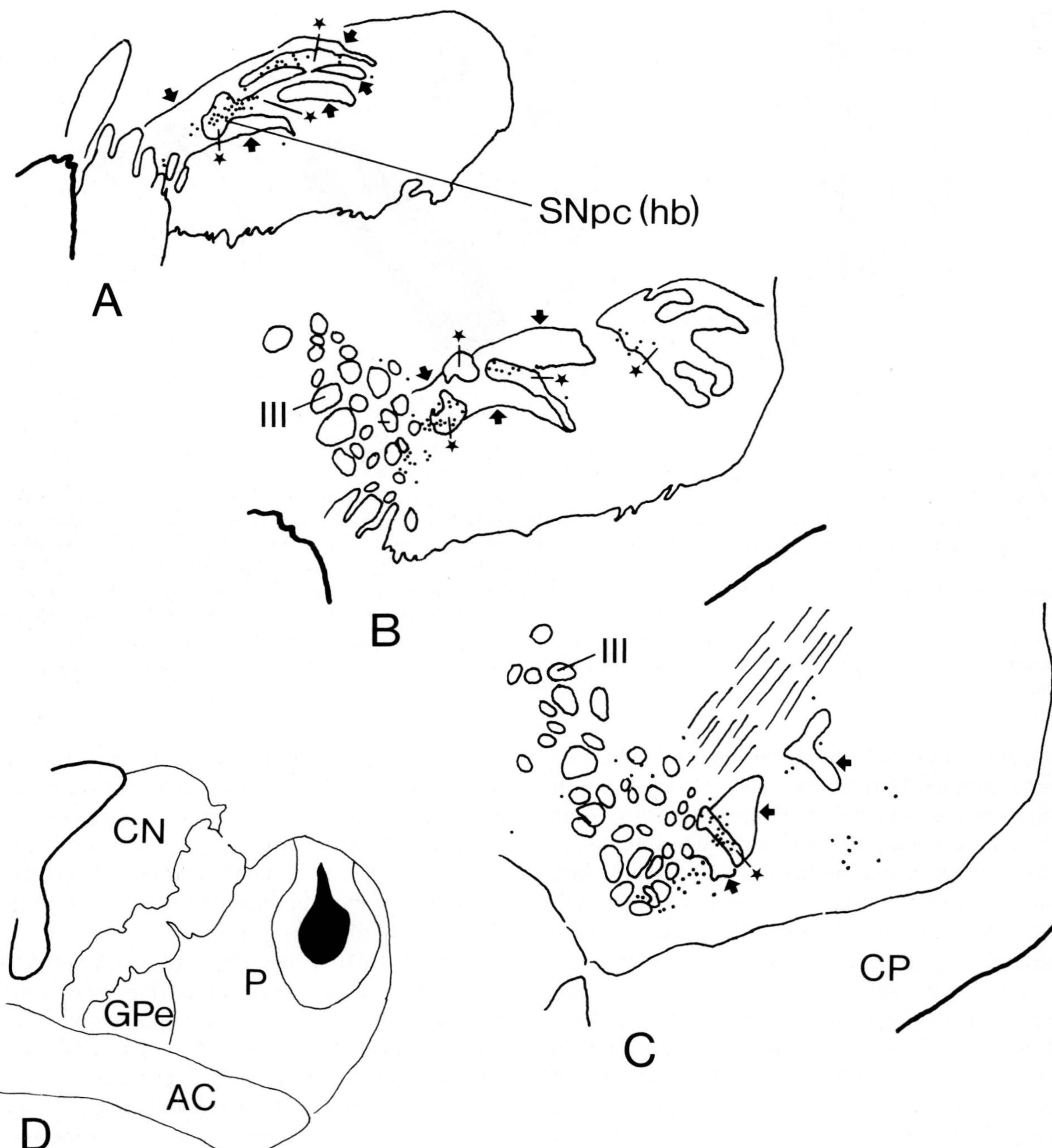

Fig. 5. A-C. Relation between AChE-poor zones of substantia nigra pars compacta (stars) and clusters of nigrostriatal neurons (dots) retrogradely labeled by an injection of horseradish peroxidase into the putamen (D). Arrows point to regions of high AChE activity. Note that most of the retrogradely labeled neurons lie in AChE-poor zones. SNpc(hb)- substantia nigra pars compacta; CP- cerebral peduncle; III-oculomotor nerve; CN-caudate nucleus; P- putamen; GPe-globus pallidus, external segment; AC-anterior commissure.

Jiménez-Castellanos and Graybiel, 1989a). Conversely, intranigral injections of anterograde tracer involving both ventrally-extending AChE-poor fingers and the zones around them can lead to predominant labeling of striosomes (Langer and Graybiel, 1989). Still untested is the possibility that the nigral compartments are related not to striosomes and matrix but to efferent-neuron compartments recently identified in the striatal matrix (Desban et al., 1989; Jiménez-Castellanos and Graybiel, 1989b; Giménez-Amaya and Graybiel, 1990). The retrogradely labeled nigrostriatal neurons lying outside the AChE-poor fingers could also correspond to a nondopaminergic population of nigrostriatal neurons (Ljungdahl et al., 1975; Guyenet and Aghajanian, 1978; Guyenet and Crane, 1981; Van der Kooy et al., 1981; Gerfen et al., 1987).

Functional and clinical considerations

The functional circuitry of the basal ganglia is organized as a system of discrete channels apparently differentiating among broad classes of afferent information both on a regional basis and on a local, compartmental basis. The evidence reviewed here suggests that there is a comparable complexity in the organization of the midbrain dopamine-containing cell groups. Different parts of the nigral complex in the primate brain project preferentially to the caudate nucleus and to the putamen. Different parts project preferentially to striosomes and matrix. In the squirrel monkey, a further histochemical compartmentalization in the substantia nigra has been discovered that may relate to yet other features of nigrostriatal terminal fields.

At the first level of nigrostriatal organization, the separation of caudate nucleus-projecting and putamen-projecting neurons in the substantia nigra is of special interest in relation to evidence that in Parkinson's disease, nigral neurons projecting to the putamen may be more vulnerable than neurons projecting to the caudate nucleus (Bernheimer et al., 1973; Kish et al., 1988). This fits with the classic notion that idiopathic Parkinson's disease is a "putamenal disease". Much evidence in the primate suggests that the putamen is more closely related to sensorimotor mechanisms and the caudate nucleus to associative types of behavior (Künzle, 1975; Goldman and Nauta, 1977; DeLong and Georgopoulos, 1981; Goldman-Rakic, 1984; Parent et al., 1984; Smith and Parent, 1986).

The behavioral significance of the striosome-matrix subdivisions and consequently of the nigrostriatal systems related to these two compartments is not known. Interestingly, however, this compartmentalization appears to relate to a global trend for sensory and motor and some association cortex to project mainly to the matrix compartment of the striatum and for some parts of prefrontal and insulotemporal cortex, as well as basolateral amygdala, to project to striosomes within at least part of the striatum (Ragsdale and Graybiel, 1981; Donoghue and Herkenham, 1986; Alexander et al., 1988; Ragsdale and Graybiel, 1988). This separation of information coming into the striatum suggests that striosomal ordering minimally segregates channels having more to do with the processing of primary sensorimotor information from some channels associated with functions at a cognitive level. Because the extrastriosomal matrix is also known to receive some limbic-associated inputs, for example from the cingulate gyrus and parts of the amygdala (Donoghue and Herkenham, 1986; Ragsdale and Graybiel, 1988) an absolute compartmental segregation of sensorimotor and limbic-associated functions is not likely (Graybiel, 1989). Moreover, in the rat, different layers of the same cortical region (limbic or not) can project, respectively, to striosomes and matrix (Gerfen, 1989). The distinction between striosomes and matrix is observed not only by corticostriatal inputs, but by every other class of afferent fiber known to project to the striatum. This arrangement suggests that dopamine-containing striatal afferents selectively innervating striosomes and matrix would be in a position to act at least partly independently as local tuning mechanisms for compartmentalized channels of information flow through the striatum.

The fact that different groups of neurons give rise to the mesostriatal projection to striosomes and to the matrix not only suggests that these projection systems may have different functional impacts on the control of behavior, but also raises the possibility that they may have different vulnerabilities in pathological conditions affecting dopaminergic neurons. If so, there might be new opportunities for therapies based on differential targeting of drugs to these subsystems or on reconstructing specific circuits by transplanting particular neuronal types to the damaged regions. For pharmacological studies of the basal ganglia, the differentiation between nigrostriatal inputs to striosomes and to matrix may have particular functional significance. Markers for many classes of dopaminergic and cholinergic function including receptor binding sites, uptake sites and enzymes have systematically different distributions in striosomes and matrix (Graybiel and Ragsdale, 1978; Nastuk and Graybiel, 1985; Joyce et al., 1986; Lowenstein et al., 1987; Ferrante and Kowall, 1987; Richfield et al., 1987; Beckstead et al., 1988; Besson et al., 1988; Nastuk and Graybiel, 1988; Graybiel and Moratalla, 1989; Hirsch et al., 1989; Marshall et al., 1989). Differences in dopamine release in and out of regions enriched in striosomal tissue also have been reported (Kemel et al., 1989).

These findings suggest that drugs affecting either dopamine or acetylcholine in the striatum could have different effects in striosomes and in the matrix. There are hints that these distinctions may also prove significant clinically (Graybiel et al., 1990a). MPTP-induced degeneration of fibers innervating the matrix has been reported in dogs acutely treated with MPTP (Wilson et al., 1987; Turner et al., 1988). Differential vulnerability of striosome-directed mesostriatal fibers has also been reported in the weaver mutant mouse in which there is a dramatic loss of the dopamine-containing innervation of the caudoputamen (Graybiel et al., 1988, 1990b). In idiopathic Parkinson's disease, damage to mesencephalic cell groups is non-uniform with, for example, the strongly matrix-projecting A8 cell group only about half as vulnerable as the substantia nigra pars compacta considered as a whole (Hirsch et al., 1988a). Both in Parkinson's disease and MPTP-induced parkinsonism in the monkey, ventrally situated neurons of the substantia nigra pars compacta have been reported more vulnerable than dorsal neurons (Hassler, 1938; Jellinger, 1986; Gibb et al., 1990; German et al., 1989).

Ultimately, the effects of these dopaminergic mesostriatal systems are transmitted to the projection neurons of the striatum. Both regional and local aspects of striatal organization also govern these output systems. Much, but not all, of the putamenofugal projection in the monkey is destined for the globus pallidus, whereas the caudate nucleus projects strongly (but not exclusively) to the substantia nigra (Parent et al., 1984; Giménez-Amaya and Graybiel, 1988, 1990; Graybiel, 1989). Striosome-matrix compartmentalization is reflected in the local targeting of the fibers from each of these striatal nuclei. Neurons of the matrix project strongly to the pallidum and substantia nigra pars reticulata, an outflow that is distinctly sensorimotor in character. The striosomes may project in small volume to the pallidum (Giménez-Amaya and Graybiel, 1990), but the main output of striosomes is to the substantia nigra. Within the substantia nigra, the target of this striosomal projection is either to the pars compacta itself [reported in the rat (Gerfen et al., 1987)] or to regions in or near the zone specifically projecting to striosomes [reported in the cat: Jiménez-Castellanos and Graybiel, 1987b]. This last finding suggests that striosomes might function in a reciprocal loop to control dopaminergic nigral neurons. Conceivably then, the release of dopamine within the substantia nigra and in the striatum may depend on the coordination of nigral and striatal subsystems reflecting the striosome and matrix subdivisions of the striatum.

Acknowledgements

The work reported here was supported by a Javits Neuroscience Investigator Award [NS25529-02], the Seaver Institute and a Whitaker Health Sciences Fund Fellowship. We are grateful to Ms. Diane Watson-Mitchell for her help with word processing, to Bruce Quinn for his comments on the manuscript and to Mr. Henry F. Hall, who is responsible for the photography.

References

Agid, Y., Graybiel, A.M., Ruberg, M., Hirsch, E., Blin, J., Dubois, B. and Javoy-Agid, F. (1990) The efficacy of levodopa treatment declines in the course of Parkinson's disease: do non-dopaminergic lesions play a role? In M.B. Streifler, A.D. Korczyn, E. Melmed and M.B.H. Youdin (Eds.). *Advances in Parkinson's Disease: Anatomy, Pathology and Therapy. Advances in Neurology,* Vol. 53. Raven Press, New York, pp. 83 – 100.

Albin, R.L., Aldridge, J.W., Young, A.B. and Gilman, S. (1989) Feline subthalamic nucleus neurons contain glutamate-like but not GABA-like or glycine-like immunoreactivity. *Brain Res.,* 491: 185 – 188.

Alexander, G.E., Koliatsos, V.E., Martin, L.J., Hedreen, J., Hamada, I., and DeLong, M.R. (1988) Organization of the primate basal ganglia motor circuit: 1. Motor cortex and supplementary motor area project to complementary regions within matrix compartment of putamen. *Soc. Neurosci. Abstr.,* 14: 287.

Andén, N.E., Carlsson, A., Dahlström, A., Fuxe, K., Hillarp, N.A., and Larsson, K. (1964) Demonstrating and mapping out nigro-neostriatal dopamine neurons. *Life Sci.,* 3: 523 – 530.

Arai, H. and Emson, P.C. (1986) Regional distribution of neuropeptide K and other tachykinins [neurokinin A, neurokinin B and substance P] in rat central nervous system. *Brain Res.,* 399: 240 – 249.

Arsenault, M.-Y., Parent, A., Seguela, P. and Descarries, L. (1988) Distribution and morphological characteristics of dopamine-immunoreactive neurons in the midbrain of the squirrel monkey *[Saimiri sciureus]. J. Comp. Neurol.,* 267: 489 – 506.

Azmitia, E.C. and Segal, M. (1978) An autoradiographic analysis of the differential ascending projections of the dorsal and median raphe nuclei in the rat. *J. Comp. Neurol.,* 179: 641 – 668.

Barbeau, A. (1986) Parkinson's Disease: Clinical features and etiopathology. In P.J. Vinken, G.W. Bruyn and H.L. Klawans (Eds.). *Handbook of Clinical Neurology,* Vol. 49. Elsevier Press, Amsterdam, pp. 87 – 152.

Beckstead, R.M., Wooten, G.F., Trugman, J.M. (1988) Distribution of D1 and D2 dopamine receptors in the basal ganglia of the cat determined by quantitative autoradiography. *J. Comp. Neurol.,* 268: 131 – 145.

Beninato, M. and Spencer, R.F. (1987) The cholinergic innervation of the rat substantia nigra: a light and electron microscopic immunohistochemical study. *Exp. Brain Res.,* 72: 178 – 184.

Beninato, M. and Spencer, R.F. (1987) A cholinergic projection to the rat substantia nigra from the pedunculopontine tegmental nucleus. *Brain Res.,* 412: 169 – 174.

Bernheimer, H., Birkmayer, W., Hornykiewicz, O., Jellinger, K., Seitelberger, F. (1973) Brain dopamine and the syndromes of Parkinson and Huntington. *J. Neurol. Sci.,* 20: 415 – 455.

Besson, M.J., Graybiel, A.M. and Nastuk, M.A. (1988) [3H]-SCH23390 binding to D1 dopamine receptors in the basal ganglia of the cat and primate: delineation of striosomal compartments and pallidal and nigral subdivisions. *Neuroscience,* 26: 101 – 119.

Bobillier, P., Sequin, S., Petitjean, F., Salvert, D., Touret, M., and Jouvet, M. (1976) The raphe nuclei of the cat brain stem: a topographical atlas of their efferent projections as revealed by autoradiography. *Brain Res.,* 113: 449 – 486.

Bouras, C., Taban, C.H., and Constantinidis, J. (1984) Mapping of enkephalin in human brain. An immunofluorescence study on brains from patients with senile and presenile dementia. *Neuroscience,* 12: 179 – 190.

Braak, H. and Braak, E. (1986) Nuclear configuration and neuronal types of the nucleus niger in the brain of the human adult. *Human Neurobiol.,* 5: 71 – 82.

Brownstein, M.J., Mroz, E.A., Tappaz, M.L. and Leeman, S.E. (1977) On the origin of substance P and glutamic acid decarboxylase (GAD) in the substantia nigra. *Brain Res.,* 135: 315 – 323.

Burns, R.S., Chiueh, C.C., Markey, S.P., Ebert, M.H., Jacobowitz, D.M. and Kopin, I.J. (1983) A primate model of parkinsonism: selective destruction of dopaminergic neurons in the pars compacta of the substantia nigra by N-methyl-4-phenyl-1,2,3,6-tetrahydropyridine. *Proc. Natl. Acad. Sci. U.S.A.,* 80: 4546 – 4550.

Butcher, L.L. and Marchand, R. (1978) Acetylcholinesterase is synthesized and transported by dopamine neurons in the pars compacta of the substantia nigra: functional significance and histochemical correlations on the same brain section. In L. Usdin (Ed.), *Catecholamines: basic and clinical frontiers,* Pergamon Press, Oxford, pp. 223 – 240.

Chesselet, M.-F. (1985) Somatostatinergic inputs to the region of the A8 cell group. *Soc. Neurosci. Abstr.,* 11: 208.

Chesselet, M.-F. and Graybiel, A.M. (1983) Subdivisions of the pallidum and the substantia nigra demonstrated by immunohistochemistry. *Soc. Neurosci. Abstr.,* 8: 9.

Chesselet, M.-F. and Graybiel, A.M. (1983) Met-enkephalin-like and dynorphin-like immunoreactivity of the basal ganglia of the cat. *Life Sci.,* 33: 37 – 40.

Chesselet, M.-F., Weiss, L., Wuenschell, C., Tobin, A.J. and Affolter, H.-U. (1987) Comparative distribution of mRNAs for glutamic acid decarboxylase, tyrosine hydroxylase and tachykinins in the basal ganglia: An in situ hybridization study in the rodent brain. *J. Comp. Neurol.,* 262: 125 – 140.

Crosby, E.C. and Woodburne, R.T. (1943) The nuclear pattern of the non-tectal portions of the midbrain and isthmus in primates. *J. Comp. Neurol.,* 78: 441 – 482.

Dahlström, A. and Fuxe, K. (1964) Evidence for the existence of monoamine-containing neurons in the central nervous system. I. Demonstration of monoamines in the cell bodies of brain stem neurons. *Acta Physiol. Scand.,* 62: 1 – 55.

Davis, R. and Huffman, R.D. (1968) *A Stereotaxic Atlas of the Brain of the Baboon [Papio].* Univ. Texas Press, Austin.

DeLong, M.R. and Georgopoulos, A.P. (1981) Motor functions of the basal ganglia. In *APS Handbook of Physiology. The Nervous System,* Vol. 2 Williams and Wilkins, Baltimore, pp. 1017 – 1061.

Desban, M., Gauchy, C., Kemel, M.L., Besson, M.J. and Glowinski, J. (1989) Three-dimensional organization of striosomal compartments and patchy distribution of striatonigral projections in the matrix of the cat caudate nucleus. *Neuroscience,* 29: 551 – 566.

Deutch, A.Y., Elsworth, J.D., Goldstein, M., Fuxe, K., Redmond, D.E., Jr., Sladek, J.R., Jr. and Roth, R.H. (1986) Preferential vulnerability of A8 dopamine neurons in the primate to the neurotoxin 1-methyl-4-phenyl-1,2,3,6-tetrahydropyridine. *Neurosci. Lett.,* 68: 51 – 56.

DiCarlo, V., Hubbard, J.E. and Pate, P. (1973) Fluoresence histochemistry of monoamine-containing cell bodies in the brain stem of the squirrel monkey *Saimiri sciureus. J. Comp. Neurol.,* 152: 347 – 372.

Donoghue, J.P. and Herkenham, M. (1986) Neostriatal projections from individual cortical fields conform to histochemically distinct striatal compartments in the rat. *Brain Res.,* 365: 397 – 403.

Dray, A. (1979) The striatum and the substantia nigra: a commentary on their relationships. *Neuroscience,* 4: 1407 – 1439.

Dray, A. and Straughan, D.W. (1976) Synaptic mechanisms in the substantia nigra. *J. Pharm. Pharmacol.,* 228: 400 – 405.

Dubois, A., Savasta, M., Curet, O. and Scatton, B. (1986) Autoradiographic distribution of the D1 agonist 3H-SKF38393 in the rat brain and spinal cord. Comparison with the distribution of D2 dopamine receptors. *Neuroscience,* 19: 125 – 137.

Eadie, M.J. (1963) Pathology of certain medullary nuclei in Parkinsonism. *Brain,* 86: 781 – 792.

Ehringer, H. and Hornykiewicz, O. (1960) Verteilung von Noradrenalin und Dopamine [3-hydroxytyramin] in Gehirn des Menschen und ihr Verhalten bei Erkrankugen des extrapyramidalen Systems. *Klin. Wschr.,* 38: 1236 – 1239.

Emson, P.C., Arregui, A., Clement-Jones, V., Sandberg, B.E. and Rossor, M. (1980) Regional distribution of met-enkephalin and substance P immunoreactivity in normal human brain and in Huntington's disease. *Brain Res.,* 199: 147 – 160.

Fallon, J.H. and Loughlin, S.E. (1987) Monoamine innervation of cerebral cortex and a theory of the role of monoamines in cerebral cortex and basal ganglia. In E.G. Jones and A. Peters (Eds.), *Cerebral Cortex,* Vol. 6. Plenum, New York, pp. 41 – 127.

Fallon, J.H. and Moore, R.Y. (1978) Catacholamine innervation of the basal forebrain. IV. Topography of the dopamine projection to the basal forebrain and neostriatum. *J. Comp. Neurol.,* 180: 545 – 580.

Fallon, J.H., Riley, J. and Moore, R.Y. (1978) Substantia nigra dopamine neurons: separate populations project to neostriatum and allocortex. *Neurosci. Lett.,* 7: 157 – 162.

Feigenbaum, L.A., and Graybiel, A.M. (1988) Heterogeneous striatal afferent connections from distinct regions of the dopamine-containing midbrain of the primate. *Soc. Neurosci. Abstr.,* 14: 156.

Felton, D.L. and Sladek, Jr. J.R. (1983) Monoamine distribution in primate brain. V. Monoaminergic nuclei: anatomy, pathways and local organization. *Brain Res. Bull.,* 10: 171 – 284.

Ferrante, R.J. and Kowall, N.W. (1987) Tyrosine hydroxylase-like immunoreactivity is distributed in the matrix compartment of normal and Huntington's disease striatum. *Brain Res.,* 416: 141 – 146.

Fisher, R.S. (1989) GABAergic pallidonigral and accessory striatonigral connections demonstrated in cats by double peroxidase labeling. *Synapse,* 4: 165 – 167.

Fonnum, F., Gottesfeld, Z., and Grofová, I. (1978) Distribution of glutamate decarboxylase, choline acetyltransferase and aromatic amino acid decarboxylase in the basal ganglia of normal and operated rats. Evidence for striatopallidal, striatoentopeduncular and striatonigral gabaergic fibers. *Brain Res.,* 143: 125 – 138.

Forno, L.S. and Alvord, E.C. (1974) Depigmentation in the nerve cells of the substantia nigra and locus coeruleus in Parkinsonism. *Adv. Neurol.,* 5: 195 – 202.

François, C., Percheron, G., Yelnik, J. and Heyner, S. (1979) Demonstration of the existence of small local circuit neurons in the Golgi-stained primate substantia nigra. *Brain Res.,* 172: 160 – 164.

François, C., Percheron, G. and Yelnik, J. (1984) Localization of nigrostriatal, nigrothalamic and nigrotectal neurons in ventricular coordinates in macaques. *Neuroscience,* 13: 61 – 76.

Fukui, K., Kariyama, H., Kashiba, A., Kato, N. and Kimura, H. (1986) Further confirmation of heterogeneity of the rat striatum: different mosaic patterns of dopamine fibers after administration of methamphetamine or reserpine. *Brain Res.,* 382: 81 – 86.

Gale, K., Hong, J.S. and Guidotti, A. (1977) Presence of

substance P and GABA in separate striatonigral neurons. *Brain Res.*, 136: 371 – 375.

Garver, D.L. and Sladek, J.R. Jr. (1975) Monoamine distribution in primate brain. I. Catecholamine-containing perikarya in the brain stem of Macaca speciosa. *J. Comp. Neurol.*, 159: 289 – 304.

Gaspar, P., Berger, B., Gay, M., Hammon, M., Cesselin, F., Vigny, A., Javoy-Agid, R. and Agid, Y. (1983) Tyrosine hydroxylase and methionine-enkephalin in the human mesencephalon. *J. Neurol. Sci.*, 58: 247 – 267.

Gerfen, C.R. (1985) The neostriatal mosaic. I. Compartmental organization of projections from the striatum to the substantia nigra in the rat. *J. Comp. Neurol.*, 236: 454 – 476.

Gerfen, C.R. (1989) The neostriatal mosaic: striatal patch-matrix organization is related to cortical lamination. *Science*, 246: 385 – 387.

Gerfen, C.R., Baimbridge, K.G. and Miller, J.J. (1985) The neostriatal mosaic: Compartmental distribution of calcium-binding protein and parvalbumin in the basal ganglia of the rat and monkey. *Proc. Natl. Acad. Sci. USA*, 82: 8780 – 8784.

Gerfen, C.R., Herkenham, M. and Thibault, J. (1987) The neostriatal mosaic. II. Patch- and matrix-directed mesostriatal dopaminergic and non-dopaminergic systems. *J. Neurosci.*, 7: 3915 – 3934.

German, D.C., Dubach, M., Askari, S., Speciale, S.G. and Bowden, D.M. (1988) 1-methyl-4-phenyl-1,2,3,6-tetrahydropyridine-induced parkinsonism syndrome in *Macaca fascicularis:* which midbrain dopaminergic neurons are lost? *Neuroscience*, 24: 161 – 174.

German, D.C., Manaye, K., Smith, W.K., Woodward, D.J. and Saper, C.B. (1989) Midbrain dopaminergic cell loss in Parkinson's disease: computer visualization. *Ann. Neurol.*, 26: 507 – 514.

Gibb, W.R.G., Fearnley, J.M. and Lees, A.J. (1990) The anatomy and pigmentation of the human substantia nigra in relation to selective neuronal vulnerability. In M.B. Streifler, A.D. Korczyn, E. Melmed and M.B.H. Youdin (Eds.).*Advances in Parkinson's Disease: Anatomy, Pathology and Therapy. Advances in Neurology*, Vol. 53. Raven Press, New York, pp. 31 – 34.

Giménez-Amaya, J.M. and Graybiel, A.M. (1988) Compartmental origins of the striatopallidal projection in the primate. *Soc. Neurosci. Abstr.*, 14: 156.

Giménez-Amaya, J.M. and Graybiel, A.M. (1990) Compartmental origins of the striatopallidal projection in the primate. *Neuroscience*, 34: 111 – 126.

Goldman, P.S. and Nauta, W.J.H. (1977) An intricately patterened prefronto-caudate projection in the rhesus monkey. *J. Comp. Neurol.*, 177: 369 – 386.

Goldman-Rakic, P.S. (1984) Modular organization of prefrontal cortex. *Trends Neurosci.*, 7: 419 – 424.

Gould, E., Woolf, N.J. and Butcher, L.L. (1989) Cholinergic projections to the substantia nigra from the pedunculopontine and lateral tegmental nuclei. *Neuroscience*, 28: 611 – 623.

Graybiel, A.M. (1977) Direct and indirect preoculomotor pathways of the brainstem: an autoradiographic study of the pontine reticular formation in the cat. *J. Comp. Neurol.*, 175: 37 – 78.

Graybiel, A.M. (1984) Correspondence between the dopamine islands and striosomes of the mammalian striatum. *Neuroscience*, 13: 1157 – 1187.

Graybiel, A.M. (1986) Neuropeptides in the basal ganglia. In J.B. Martin and J.D. Barchas (Eds.), *Neuropeptides in Neurologic and Psychiatric Disease*, Raven Press, New York, pp. 135 – 161.

Graybiel, A.M. (1989) Dopaminergic and cholinergic systems in the striatum. In A.R. Crossman and M.A. Sambrook (Eds.), *Neural mechanisms in disorders of movement*, Libbey, London, pp. 3 – 15.

Graybiel, A.M. and Elde, R.P. (1983) Somatostatin-like immunoreactivity characterizes neurons of the nucleus reticularis thalami in the cat and monkey. *J. Neurosci.*, 3: 1308 – 1321.

Graybiel, A.M. and Moratalla, R. (1989) Dopamine uptake sites in the striatum are distributed differentially in striosome and matrix compartments. *Proc. Natl. Acad. Sci., U.S.A.*, 86: 9020 – 9024.

Graybiel, A.M. and Ragsdale, C.W. (1978) Histochemically distinct compartments in the striatum of human, monkey and cat demonstrated by acetylcholinesterase staining. *Proc. Natl. Acad. Sci. USA*, 75: 5723 – 5726.

Graybiel, A.M. and Ragsdale, C.W. (1983) Biochemical anatomy of the striatum. In P.C. Emson (Ed.), *Chemical Neuroanatomy*, Raven Press, New York, pp. 427 – 504.

Graybiel, A.M., Ohta, K. and Roffler-Tarlov, S. (1988) Toward a genetic analysis of the striosomal system: patterns of nigrostriatal loss in mutant weaver mouse. *Soc. Neurosci. Abstr.*, 14: 1066.

Graybiel, A.M., Besson, M-J., and Weber, E. (1989) Neuroleptic-sensitive binding sites in the nigrostriatal system: Evidence for differential distribution of sigma sites in the substantia nigra, pars compacta of the cat. *J. Neurosci.*, 9: 326 – 338.

Graybiel, A.M., Hirsch, E.C. and Agid, Y.A. (1990) The nigrostriatal system in Parkinson's disease. In M.B. Streifler, A.D. Korczyn, E. Melmed and M.B.H. Youdin (Eds.). *Advances in Parkinson's Disease: Anatomy, Pathology and Therapy. Advances in Neurology*, Vol. 53. Raven Press, New York, pp. 17 – 24.

Graybiel, A.M., Ohta, K. and Roffler-Tarlov, S. (1990) Patterns of cell and fiber vulnerability in the mesostriatal system of mutant mouse weaver: I. Gradients and compartments. *J. Neurosci.*, 10: 720 – 733.

Greenfield, J.G. and Bonsaquet, F.D. (1953) The brainstem lesions in Parkinsonism. *J. Neurol. Neurosurg. Psychiatry*, 16: 213 – 226.

Greenfield, S., Cheramy, A., Leviel, V., and Glowinski, J. (1980) *In vivo* release of acetylcholinesterase in cat substantia nigra and caudate nucleus. *Nature,* 284: 355 – 357.

Greenfield, S.A., Stein, J.F., Hodgson, A.J., and Chubb, I.W. (1981) Depression of nigral pars compacta cell discharge by exogenous acetylcholinesterase. *Neuroscience,* 6: 2287-2295.

Greenfield, S.A., Nedergaard, S., Webb, C., and French, M. (1989) Pressure ejection of acetylcholinesterase within the guinea pig substantia nigra has non-classical actions on the pars compacta cells independent of selective receptor and ion channel blockade. *Neuroscience,* 29: 21 – 25.

Guyenet, P.G. and Aghajanian, G.K. (1978) Antidromic identification of dopaminergic and other output neurons of the rat substantia nigra. *Brain Res.,* 150: 69 – 84.

Guyenet, P.G. and Aghajanian, G.K. (1981) Non-dopaminergic nigrostriatal pathway. *Brain Res.,* 213: 291 – 305.

Haber, S. and Elde, R. (1982) The distribution of enkephalin immunoreactive fibers and terminals in the monkey central nervous system: An immunohistochemical study. *Neuroscience,* 7: 1049 – 1095.

Haber, S.N. and Watson, S.J. (1985) The comparative distribution of enkephalin, dynorphin and substance P in the human globus pallidus and basal forebrain. *Neuroscience,* 14: 1011 – 1024.

Hassler, R. (1938) Zur Pathologie der Paralysis Agitans und des post-encephalitischen Parkinsonismus. *J. Psychol. Neurol.,* 48: 387 – 476.

Hattori, T., McGeer, P.L., Fibiger, H.C., and McGeer, E.G. (1973) On the source of GABA containing terminals in the substantia nigra. Electron microscopic, autoradiographic and biochemical studies. *Brain Res.,* 54: 103 – 114.

Henderson, Z. (1981) Ultrastructure and acetylcholinesterase content of neurons forming connections between the striatum and substantia nigra of rat. *J. Comp. Neurol.,* 197: 185 – 196.

Henderson, Z. and Greenfield, S.A. (1987) Does the substantia nigra have a cholinergic innervation? *Neurosci. Lett.,* 73: 109 – 113.

Hirsch, E.C., Graybiel, A.M., Duyckaerts, C. and Javoy-Agid, F. (1987) Neuronal loss in the pedunculopontine tegmental nucleus in Parkinson's disease and in progressive supranuclear palsy. *Proc. Natl. Acad. Sci., U.S.A.,* 84: 5976 – 5980.

Hirsch, E., Graybiel, A.M. and Agid, Y.A. (1988) Melanized neurons are differentially susceptible to degeneration in Parkinson's disease. *Nature,* 334: 345 – 348.

Hirsch, E.C., Graybiel, A.M., Javoy-Agid, F., Cervera, P., Hauw, J.J., Duyckaerts, C., Agid, Y. (1988) Distribution of seven different neuropeptides in human substantia nigra of control and parkinsonian brains. *Ninth Intl. Symposium on Parkinson's Disease,* June.

Hirsch, E.C., Graybiel, A.M., Hersh, L.B., Duyckaerts, C. and Agid, Y. (1989) Striosomes and extrastriosomal matrix contain different amounts of immunoreactivecholine acetyltransferase in the human striatum. *Neurosci. Lett.,* 96: 145 – 150.

Hökfelt, T., Skirboll, L., Rehfeld, J.F., Goldstein, M., Markey, K. and Dann, O. (1980) A subpopulation of mesencephalic dopamine neurons projecting to limbic areas contains a cholecystokinin-like peptide: Evidence from immunohistochemistry combined with retrograde tracing. *Neuroscience,* 5: 2093 – 2124.

Hökfelt, T., Everitt, B.J., Theodorsson-Norheim, E., and Goldstein, M. (1984) Occurrence of neurotensin-like immunoreactivity in subpopulations of hypothalamic, mesencephalic and medullary catecholamine neurons. *J. Comp. Neurol.,* 222: 543 – 559.

Hong, J.S., Yang, H.-Y.T., Racagni, G., and Costa, E. (1977) Projections of substance P containing neurons from neostriatum to substantia nigra. *Brain Res.,* 122: 541 – 544.

Hubbard, J.E. and DiCarlo, V. (1974) Fluoresence histochemistry of monoamine-containing cell bodies in the brain stem of the squirrel monkey *Saimiri sciureus. J. Comp. Neurol.,* 153: 369 – 384.

Inagaki, S. and Parent, A. (1984) Distribution of substance P and enkephalin-like immunoreactivity in the substantia nigra of the rat, cat and monkey. *Brain Res. Bull.,* 13: 319 – 329.

Inagaki, S. and Parent, A. (1985) Distribution of enkephalin-immunoreactive neurons in the forebrain and upper brainstem of the squirrel monkey. *Brain Res.,* 359: 267 – 280.

Inagaki, S., Kubota, Y. and Kito, S. (1986) Ultrastructural localization of enkephalin immunoreactivity in the substantia nigra of the monkey. *Brain Res.,* 362: 171 – 174.

Jellinger, K. (1986) Pathology of parkinsonism. In S. Fahn (Ed.), *Recent Developments in Parkinson's Disease,* Raven Press, New York, pp. 33 – 66.

Jessell, T.M., Emson, P.C., Paxinos, G. and Cuello, A.C. (1978) Topographic projections of substance P and GABA pathways in the striato- and pallido-nigral system: A biochemical and immunohistochemical study. *Brain Res.,* 152: 487 – 498.

Jiménez-Castellanos, J. and Graybiel, A.M. (1985) The dopamine-containing innervation of striosomes: nigral subsystems and their striatal correspondents. *Soc. Neurosci. Abstr.,* 11: 1249.

Jiménez-Castellanos, J. and Graybiel, A.M. (1987) Subdivisions of the primate substantia nigra pars compacta detected by acetylcholinesterase activity. *Brain Res.,* 437: 349 – 354.

Jiménez-Castellanos, J. and Graybiel, A.M. (1987) Subdivisions of the dopamine-containing A8-A9-A10 complex identified by their differential mesostriatal innervation of striosomes and extrastriosomal matrix. *Neuroscience,* 23: 223 – 242.

Jiménez-Castellanos, J. and Graybiel, A.M. (1989) Evidence that histochemically distinct zones of the primate substantia nigra pars compacta are related to patterned distributions of nigrostriatal projection neurons and striatonigral fibers.

Expl. Brain Res., 74: 227 – 238.

Jiménez-Castellanos, J. and Graybiel, A.M. (1989) Compartmental origins of striatal efferent projections in the cat. *Neuroscience,* 32: 297 – 321.

Joyce, J.N., Sapp, D.W. and Marshall, J.F. (1986) Human striatal dopamine receptors are arranged in compartments. *Proc. Natl. Acad. Sci. USA,* 83: 8002 – 8006.

Juraska, J.M., Wilson, C.J. and Groves, P.M. (1977) The substantia nigra of the rat: A Golgi study. *J. Comp. Neurol.,* 172: 585 – 600.

Kanazawa, I., Emson, P.C., and Cuello, A.C. (1977) Evidence for the existence of substance P-containing fibers in the striatonigral and pallidonigral pathways in the rat brain. *Brain Res.,* 119: 447 – 453.

Kanazawa, I., Mogaki, S., Muramoto, O. and Kuzuhara, S. (1980) On the origin of substance P-containing fibers in the entopeduncular nucleus and substantia nigra in the rat. *Brain Res.,* 184: 481 – 485.

Kanazawa, I., Ogawa, T., Kimura, S., and Munekata, E. (1984) Regional distribution of substance P, neurokinin α and neurokinin β in rat central nervous system. *Neurosci. Res.,* 2: 111 – 120.

Kemel, M.L., Desban, M., Glowinski, J., and Gauchy, C. (1989) Distinct presynaptic control of dopamine release in striosomal and matrix areas of the cat caudate nucleus. *Proc. Natl. Acad. Sci., U.S.A.,* 86: 9006 – 9010.

Kim, J.S., Bak, I.J., Hassler, R. and Okada, Y. (1971) Role of gamma-aminobutyric acid (GABA) in the extrapyramidal motor system. 2. Some evidence for the existence of a type of GABA-rich strionigral neuron. *Exp. Brain Res.,* 14: 95 – 104.

Kish, S.J., Shannah, K., Hornykiewicz, O. (1988) Uneven patterns of dopamine loss in the striatum of patients with idiopathic Parkinson's disease. Pathophysiologic and clinical implications. *N. Engl. J. Med.,* 318: 876 – 880.

Kornhuber J., Kim, J.S., Kornhuber, M.E., and Kornhuber, H.H. (1984) The cortico-nigral projection: Reduced glutamate content in the substantia nigra following frontal cortex ablation in the rat. *Brain Res.,* 322: 124-126.

Künzle, H. (1975) Bilateral projections from precentral motor cortex to the putamen and other parts of the basal ganglia. *Brain Res.,* 88: 195 – 210.

Künzle, H. (1978) An autoradiographic analysis of the efferent connections from premotor and adjacent prefrontal regions [areas 6 and 9] in *Macaca fascicularis. Brain Behav. Evol.,* 15: 185 – 234.

Kusama, T. and Mabuchi, M. (1970) *Stereotaxic Atlas of the Brain of Macaca fuscata.* Univ. Tokyo Press, Tokyo.

Langer, L.F. and Graybiel, A.M. (1989) Distinct nigrostriatal projection systems innervate striosomes and matrix in the primate striatum. *Brain Res.,* 498: 344 – 350.

Lehmann, J. and Fibiger, H.C. (1978) Acetylcholinesterase in the substantia nigra and caudate-putamen of the rat: properties and localization in dopaminergic neurons. *J. Neurochem.,* 30: 615 – 624.

Lehmann, J., Fibiger, H.C. and Butcher, L.L. (1979) The localization of acetylcholinesterase in the corpus striatum and substantia nigra of the rat following kainic acid lesions of the corpus striatum: a biochemical and histochemical study. *Neuroscience,* 4: 217 – 225.

Lichtensteiger, W., Felix, D., Leinhart, R. and Hefti, F. (1976) A quantitative correlation between single unit activity and fluorescence intensity of dopamine neurons in zona compacta of substantia nigra as demonstrated under the influence of nicotine and physostigmine. *Brain Res.,* 117: 85 – 103.

Ljungdahl, Å., Hokfelt, T., Goldstein, M. and Park, D. (1975) Retrograde peroxidase tracing of neurons combined with transmitter histochemistry. *Brain Res.,* 84: 313 – 319.

Lowenstein, P.R., Slesinger, P.A., Singer, H.S., Walker, L.C., Casanova, M.F., Price, D.L. and Coyle, J.T. (1987) An autoradiographic study of the development of [^{3}H]hemicholinium-3 binding sites in human and baboon basal ganglia: a marker for the sodium-dependent high-affinity choline uptake system. *Devel. Brain Res.,* 34: 291 – 297.

Ma, T.P. (1989) Identification of the substantia nigra pars lateralis in the macaque using cytochrome oxidase and fiber stains. *Brain Res.,* 480: 305 – 311.

Marshall, J.F., Navarrete, R. and O'Dell, S.J. (1989) Striosomal and gradient pattern of dopamine high-affinity and monoamine synaptic vesicle sites in rabbit caudate. *Soc. Neurosci. Abstr.,* 15: 906.

Martinez-Murillo, R., Villalba, R., Montero-Cabellero, M.I. and Rodrigo, J. (1989) Cholinergic somata and terminals in the rat substantia nigra: an immunocytochemical study with optical and electron microscopic techniques. *J. Comp. Neurol.,* 281: 397 – 415.

Martres, M.P., Bouthenet, M.L., Sales, N., Sokoloff, P. and Schwartz, J.C. (1985) Widespread distribution of brain dopamine receptors evidenced with [^{125}I]iodosulpiride, a highly selective ligand. *Science,* 228: 752 – 754.

Mehler, W.R. (1981) The basal ganglia – circa 1982. A review and commentary. *Appl. Neurophysiol.,* 44: 261 – 290.

Moon-Edley, S. and Graybiel, A.M. (1983) The afferent and efferent connections of the feline nucleus tegmenti, pedunculopontinus, pars compacta. *J. Comp. Neurol.,* 217: 187 – 215.

Moon-Edley, S. and Herkenham, M. (1983) Heterogeneous dopaminergic projections to the neostriatum of the rat: nuclei of origin dictates relationship to opiate receptor patches. *Anat. Rec.,* 205: 120A.

Mugnaini, E. and Oertel, W.H. (1985) Atlas of the distribution of GABAergic neurons and terminals in the rat CNS as revealed by GAD immunohistochemistry. In A. Bjorklund and T. Hokfelt (Eds.), *Handbook of Chemical Neuroanatomy,* Vol. 4 Elsevier, Amsterdam, pp. 436 – 595.

Nagai, T., McGeer, P.L. and McGeer, E.G. (1983) Distribution of GABA-T-intensive neurons in the rat forebrain and midbrain. *J. Comp. Neurol.*, 218: 220 – 238.

Nagy, J.I., Carter, D.A., and Fibiger, H.C. (1978) Anterior striatal projections to the globus pallidus, entopeduncular nucleus and substantia nigra in the rat: the GABA connection. *Brain Res.*, 158: 15 – 29.

Nastuk, M.A., and Graybiel, A.M. (1985) Patterns of muscarinic cholinergic binding in the striatum and their relation to dopamine islands and striosomes. *J. Comp. Neurol.*, 237: 176 – 194.

Nastuk, M.A. and Graybiel, A.M. (1988) Autoradiographic localization and biochemical characteristics of M1 and M2 muscarinic binding sites in the striatum of the cat, monkey and human. *J. Neurosci.*, 8: 1052 – 1062.

Nastuk, M.A. and Graybiel, A.M. (1990) M1 and M2 muscarinic cholinergic binding sites in the cat's substantia nigra: development and status at maturity. *Dev. Brain Res.* (in press).

Oertel, W.H., Schmechel, D.E., Brownstein, M.J., Tappaz, M.L., Ransom, D.H. and Kopin, I.J. (1981) Decrease of glutamate decarboxylase (GAD)-immunoreactive nerve terminals in the substantia nigra after kainic acid lesion of the striatum. *J. Histochem. Cytochem.*, 29: 977 – 980.

Oertel, W.H., Tappaz, M.L., Berod, A. and Mugnaini, E. (1982) Two-color immunohistochemistry for dopamine and GABA neurons in rat substantia nigra and zona incerta. *Brain Res. Bull.*, 9: 463 – 474.

Olivier, A., Parent, A., Simard, H. and Poirier, L.J. (1970) Cholinesterasic striatopallidal and striatonigral efferents in the cat and monkey. *Brain Res.*, 18: 273 – 282.

Olson, L., Seiger, Å. and Fuxe, K. (1972) Heterogeneity of striatal and limbic innervation: highly fluorescent islands in developing and adult rats. *Brain Res.*, 44: 283 – 288.

Olszewski, J. and Baxter, D. (1954) *Cytoarchitecture of the Human Brain Stem.* Karger, Basel.

Palacios, J.M., Savasta, M. and Mengod, G. (1989) Does cholecystokinin colocalize with dopamine in human substantia nigra? *Brain Res.*, 488: 369 – 375.

Palkovits, M., Brownstein, M.J. and Zamir, N. (1984) On the origin of dynorphin and alpha-neo-endorphin in the substantia nigra. *Neuropeptides,* 4: 193 – 199.

Parent, A. (1986) Mammalian substantia nigra: a dual structure. In *Comparative Neurobiology of the Basal Ganglia* Wiley, New York, pp. 199 – 226.

Parent, A., Descarries, L. and Beaudet, A. (1981) Organization of ascending serotonin systems in the adult rat brain. An autoradiographic study after intraventricular administration of [^{3}H]-5-hydroxytryptamine. *Neuroscience,* 6: 115 – 138.

Parent, A., Mackey, A. and De Bellefeuille, L. (1983) The subcortical afferents to caudate nucleus and putamen in primate: a fluorescence retrograde double labeling study. *Neuroscience,* 10: 1137 – 1150.

Parent, A., Mackey, A., Smith, Y. and Boucher, R. (1983) The output organization of the substantia nigra in primate as revealed by a retrograde double labeling method. *Brain Res. Bull.*, 10: 529 – 537.

Parent, A., Bouchard, C. and Smith, Y. (1984) The striatopallidal and striatonigral projections: two distinct fiber systems in primate. *Brain Res.*, 303: 385 – 390.

Pazos, A., Probst, A. and Palacios, J.M. (1987) Serotonin receptors in the human brain- III. Autoradiographic mapping of serotonin-1 receptors. *Neuroscience,* 21: 97 – 122.

Pazos, A., Probst, A. and Palacios, J.M. (1987) Serotonin receptors in the human brain- IV. Autoradiographic mapping of serotonin-2 receptors. *Neuroscience,* 21: 123 – 139.

Poirier, L.J., Giguere, M. and Marchand, R. (1983) Comparative morphology of the substantia nigra and ventral tegmental area in monkey, cat and rat. *Brain Res. Bull.*, 11: 371 – 397.

Quirion, R., Gaudreau, P., Martel, J-C., St.-Pierre, S. and Zamir, N. (1985) Possible interactions between dynorphin and dopaminergic systems in rat basal ganglia and substantia nigra. *Brain Res.*, 331: 358 – 362.

Ragsdale, C.W. and Graybiel, A.M. (1981) The fronto-striatal projection in the cat and monkey and its relationship to inhomogeneities established by acetylcholinesterase histochemistry. *Brain Res.*, 208: 259 – 266.

Ragsdale, C.W. and Graybiel, A.M. (1988) Fibers from the basolateral nucleus of the amygdala selectively innervate striosomes in the caudate nucleus of the cat. *J. Comp. Neurol.*, 269: 506 – 522.

Ragsdale, C.W. and Graybiel, A.M. (1990) A simple ordering of neo-cortical areas established by the compartmental organization of their striatal projections. *Proc. Natl. Acad. Sci., U.S.A.*, 87: 6196 – 6199.

Ribak, C.E., Vaughn, J., Saito, K., Barber, R. and Roberts, E. (1976) Immunocytochemical localization of glutamate decarboxylase in rat substantia nigra. *Brain Res.*, 116: 287 – 298.

Ribak, C.E., Vaughn, J.E. and Roberts, E. (1980) GABAergic nerve terminals decrease in the substantia nigra following hemitransections of the striatonigral and pallidonigral pathways. *Brain Res.*, 192: 413 – 420.

Richfield, E.K., Young, A.B. and Penney, J.B. (1987) Comparative distribution of dopamine D1 and D2 receptors in the basal ganglia of turtles, pigeons, rats, cats and monkeys. *J. Comp. Neurol.*, 262: 446 – 463.

Ryan, L.J., Martone, M.E., Linder, J.C. and Groves, P.M. (1988) Continuous amphetamine administration induces tyrosine hydroxylase immunoreative patches in the adult rat striatum. *Brain Res. Bull.*, 21: 133 – 137.

Scarnati, E., Proia, A., Campana, E. and Pacitti, C. (1986) A microiontophoretic study on the nature of the putative synaptic neurotransmitter involved in the pedunculopontine-substantia nigra pars compacta excitatory pathway of the rat. *Exp. Brain Res.*, 62: 470 – 478.

Schwyn, R.C. and Fox, C.A. (1974) The primate substantia nigra: a Golgi and electron microscopic study. *J. Hirnforsch,* 15: 95 – 126.

Shute, C.C.D. and Lewis, P.R. (1963) Cholinesterase-containing systems of the brain of the rat. *Nature,* 199: 1160–1164.

Shute, C.C.D. and Lewis, P.R. (1967) The ascending cholinergic reticular system: neocortical, olfactory and subcortical projections. *Brain,* 90: 197–220.

Smith, Y. and Parent, A. (1986) Differential connections of caudate nucleus and putamen in the squirrel monkey *Saimiri sciureus. Neuroscience,* 18: 347–371.

Smith, Y. and Parent, A. (1988) Neurons of the subthalamic nucleus in primates display glutamate but not GABA immunoreactivity. *Brain Res.,* 453: 353–356.

Smith, Y., Parent, A., Seguela, P. and Descarries, L. (1987) Distribution of GABA-immunoreactive neurons in the basal ganglia of the squirrel monkey [*Saimiri sciureus*]. *J. Comp. Neurol.,* 259: 50–64.

Snider, R.S. and Lee, J.C. (1961) *A Stereotaxic Atlas of the Monkey Brain [Macaca mulatta].* Univ. Chicago Press, Chicago.

Szabo, J. (1979) Striatonigral and nigrostriatal connections. *Appl. Neurophysiol.,* 42: 9–12.

Szabo, J. (1980) Organization of the ascending striatal afferents in monkeys. *J. Comp. Neurol.,* 189: 307–321.

Taquet, H., Javot-Agid, F., Cesselin, F., Haman, M., Legrand, J.C. and Agid, Y. (1982) Microtopography of met-enkephalin, dopamine, and noradrenaline in the ventral mesencephalon of human control and parkinsonian brains. *Brain Res.,* 235: 303–314.

Tennyson, V.M., Barrett, R.E., Cohen, G., Cote, L., Heikkila, R. and Mytilineou, C. (1972) The developing neostriatum of the rabbit: correlation of fluoresence histochemistry, electron microscopy, endogeneous dopamine levels and [^{3}H]-dopamine uptake. *Brain Res.,* 46: 251–285.

Turner, B.H., Wilson, J.S., McKenzie, J.C. and Richtand, N. (1988) MPTP produces a pattern of nigrostriatal degeneration which coincides with the mosaic organization of the caudate nucleus. *Brain Res.,* 473: 60–64.

Uhl, G.R., Hedreen, J.C. and Price, D.L. (1985) Parkinson's disease: loss of neurons from the ventral tegmental area contralateral to therapeutic surgical lesions. *Neurology,* 35: 1215–1218.

Van der Kooy, D., Coscina, D.V. and Hattori, T (1981) Is there a non-dopaminergic nigrostriatal pathway? *Neuroscience,* 6: 345–357.

Walaas, I. and Fonnum, F. (1980) Biochemical evidence for gamma-aminobutyrate containing fibers from the nucleus accumbens to the substantia nigra and ventral tegmental area in the rat. *Neuroscience,* 5: 63–72.

Waters, C.M., Peck, R., Rossor, M., Reynolds, G.P. and Hunt. S.P. (1988) Immunocytochemical studies on the basal ganglia and substantia nigra in Parkinson's disease and Huntington's chorea. *Neuroscience,* 25: 419–438.

Wilson, J.S., Turner, B.H., Morrow, G.D. and Hartman, P.J. (1987) MPTP produces a mosaic-like pattern of degeneration in the caudate nucleus of dog. *Brain Res.,* 423: 329–332.

Zaborszky, L., Alheid, G.F., Beinfeld, M.C., Eiden, L.E., Heimer, L. and Palkovits, M. (1985) Cholecystokinin innervation of the ventral striatum: A morphological and radioimmunological study. *Neuroscience,* 14: 427–453.

Zamir, N., Palkovits, M., Weber, E., Mezey, E. and Brownstein, M.J. (1984) A dynorphinergic pathway of Leu-enkephalin production in rat substantia nigra. *Nature,* 307: 643–645.

Zweig, R.M., Whitehouse, P.J., Casanova, M.F., Walker, L.C., Jankel, W.R. and Price, D.L. (1987) Loss of pedunculopontine neurons in progressive supranuclear palsy. *Ann. Neurol.,* 22: 18–25.

G. Holstege (Ed.)
Progress in Brain Research, Vol. 87

CHAPTER 6

Role of the forebrain in oculomotor function

Okihide Hikosaka

National Institute for Physiological Sciences, Okazaki 444, Japan

Introduction

Eye movement is relatively simple yet requires many calculations. At every moment three pairs of extraocular muscles must cooperate; motor innervation to these muscles must be finely tuned. Furthermore, we must move right and left eyes in an almost identical manner. However, we probably do not need the forebrain to do such sophisticated jobs; the brainstem can take care of them. What does the forebrain do then? Its main job is probably "decision-making". But how is a decision made? This is what I have been trying to answer.

Cortical eye fields

Stimulation of the cerebral cortex of an alert animal produces a variety of movements depending on where the stimulation is applied. In a pioneering experiment in the 19th century using alert monkeys, Ferrier was able to demonstrate that skeletal movements were elicited from a restricted area around the central sulcus, which is now regarded as the sensory-motor cortex. This was the first step toward the understanding of the functional organization of the cerebral cortex. Eye movements, however, can be evoked from wider areas including the frontal, parietal and temporal cortices.

Since Ferrier's experiment, interest has been focussed on a smaller region in the frontal cortex, which is now widely known as the frontal eye field. This is the area from which eye movements are elicited with minimal thresholds. Robinson and Fuchs (1969) have shown that the evoked eye movements were the same as normal saccadic eye movements. The stimulus-evoked saccades are directed to the side contralateral to the stimulation. Their direction and amplitude are dependent on where in the frontal eye field the stimulus is applied, but are independent of how strong the stimulus is. This result suggests that there is a retinotopic map inside the frontal eye field. Neurons in the frontal eye field discharge before a saccade, but only before the saccade is similar to the movement evoked by stimulation applied to the point where the cell is recorded, as demonstrated first by Bruce et al. (1985).

Interestingly, the presaccadic discharge is also dependent on how the saccade is initiated. If the monkey works hard and makes a saccade to a visual target to obtain a reward, the frontal eye field cell will discharge before the saccade. If he makes the same saccade but without such urgent needs outside the tasks, the same cell shows no or little activity (Bruce and Goldberg, 1985). Such behavioral dependency of presaccadic neuronal activity is generally seen in the cerebral cortex and the basal ganglia, and points to a fundamental feature regarding the role of the forebrain in behavior: only purposive eye movements may involve the forebrain; less intentional or reflex-like movements may be completed within the brainstem containing the superior colliculus.

Recently, another saccade-related area was discovered by Schlag and Schlag-Rey (1987) in the mesial side of the frontal cortex. This region is called the supplementary eye field, since its location appears to be the rostral extension of the supplementary motor area. As in the frontal eye field, weak stimulation in this area evokes contralateral saccades. However, the amplitude and direction of the evoked saccades seem to be affected by the initial eye position.

It is not yet clear why there are two eye fields in the frontal cortex. There is some evidence, however, suggesting that neurons in the supplementary eye field tend to be more active before voluntary, non-visually guided saccades (Schlag and Schlag-Rey, 1987). The existence of two eye fields in the frontal cortex is reminiscent of the two premotor areas, arcuate and supplementary motor areas, which are both involved in the initiation of skeletal movements (Tanji and Kurata, 1985).

The cerebral cortex is not the only area in the forebrain that is related to eye movements. In the central thalamus and the basal ganglia neurons are found that change their spike activity before saccadic eye movements. We now know that these forebrain oculomotor areas are intimately interconnected.

A key structure in the oculomotor system is the superior colliculus, which is not a part of the forebrain but is located more downstream. It receives signals from the cerebral cortex and the basal ganglia, and sends its saccadic motor outputs to the brainstem saccade generators.

Superior colliculus

The superior colliculus is a phylogenetically old structure and is called the optic tectum in the lower vertebrates. It is thought to control the prey-catching behavior in which the animal orients its eye, head or body to its target (Ewert, 1980). Its superficial layer receives direct fiber connections from the retina in a retinotopic manner, while the intermediate and deep layers emit descending fibers to the lower brainstem (see Holstege, Chapter 14 this volume).

If an object appears in the visual field, a group of visual cells in the superficial layer respond to it. The animal will then move its eye, head, or body to the object. Such orienting movements are controlled by the descending projection; neurons in the intermediate layer, just beneath the previously active visual cells, emit a burst of spikes, and their signal is transmitted downstream to the brainstem reticular formation and is shaped up to be a pulse output to the extraocular muscles (Sparks, 1986).

The oculomotor function of the superior colliculus can fully be appreciated by the experiment in which a GABA agonist, muscimol, is injected into the superior colliculus of the monkey (Hikosaka and Wurtz, 1985a). Following this treatment, the monkey was unable to make a saccade.

The suggestion that the basal ganglia might be related to eye movements came from the discovery that the substantia nigra pars reticulata has fiber connection to the superior colliculus (Faull and Mehler, 1978; Jayaraman et al., 1977).

Substantia nigra pars reticulata

In order to investigate the mechanism in which the basal ganglia might participate in the initiation of saccadic eye movements, Robert Wurtz and I first trained the monkey to make saccadic eye movements and inserted a microelectrode into the substantia nigra. We found a number of neurons that changed their discharge rate before saccades (Hikosaka and Wurtz, 1983a-c). They were found exclusively in the pars reticulata which is non-dopaminergic, not in the pars compacta which is dopaminergic. A striking feature common to pars reticulata neurons is that they fire continually with very high frequency mostly between 50 and 100 spikes/sec. The presaccadic activity in those neurons was always a decrease in discharge rate; they may stop firing before a saccade.

Many of these presaccadic nigra neurons send their axons to the superior colliculus; they were found to be activated antidromically by local electrical stimulation of the superior colliculus (Hikosaka and Wurtz, 1983d). We then compared the activities of thus identified neuron pairs to see the relationship between the substantia nigra and the superior colliculus. Before a saccade, the substantia nigra neurons stopped discharging while the colliculus neurons showed a burst of spike activity. This result strongly suggested that the nigro-collicular connection is inhibitory. This was in line with other studies suggesting that the nigro-collicular connection is GABAergic (Di Chiara, 1979). Once the substantia nigra neurons stop discharging and the tonic inhibition is removed, the superior colliculus neurons get ready to be excited and therefore are likely to produce a saccade.

It was still uncertain, however, whether this nigro-collicular inhibition is necessary for normal eye movements. One way to answer this question is to remove the nigro-collicular connection and see what happens to eye movements. It turned out to be very difficult to make a selective lesion in the substantia nigra, however. We finally came to the idea of a functional and reversible blockade; the idea was to inject a GABA agonist into the substantia nigra to suppress the high frequency, tonic discharges of substantia nigra neurons thereby functionally disconnecting the nigro-collicular connection. The substantia nigra is ideally suited to this experiment since it contains abundant GABA receptors, probably more than any other brain structures (Fahn and Cote, 1968). Following this procedure, the monkey became unable to fixate his gaze on a spot of light on the screen and made saccades continually to the side contralateral to the injection (Hikosaka and Wurtz, 1985b). This experiment suggested that the substantia nigra exerts a tonic inhibition on the superior colliculus, and this is necessary to prevent unwanted saccades.

A functional scheme is drawn from this experiment (Fig. 1). When the monkey is not making an eye movement, substantia nigra neurons keep inhibiting superior colliculus neurons with their high background activity. In fact, the relationship is probably reversed: because of the tonic inhibition, the superior colliculus neurons are disenabled so that no saccade is elicited. Once the substantia nigra neurons stop discharging and the tonic inhibition is removed, the superior colliculus neurons get either excited or ready to be excited, therefore producing a saccade.

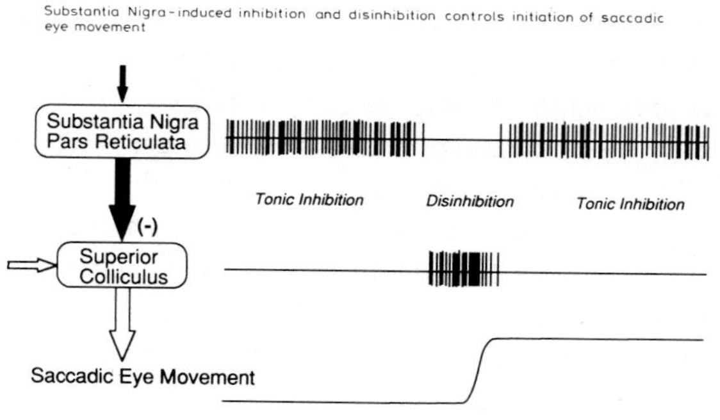

Fig. 1. The basal ganglia exert inhibitory control over the oculomotor portion of the superior colliculus.

The next question was obviously how the substantia nigra neurons stop discharging. The substantia nigra is one of the two major output stations in the basal ganglia, and is known to receive fiber connections from other parts of the basal ganglia (DeLong and Georgopoulos, 1981). The caudate nucleus is one of these areas.

Caudate nucleus

Unlike the substantia nigra the caudate nucleus is an extremely quiet area. Among such quiet neurons, we found saccade-related cells in a relatively restricted area (Hikosaka et al., 1989a-c). Fig. 2 shows frontal sections of the caudate nucleus from rostral (a) to caudal (f). Circles indicate neurons that were somehow related to the saccade tasks; dots are neurons unrelated to the tasks. The task-related cells were clustered in the central part of the caudate and the clustered region was elongated rostro-caudally. Although classified as saccade-related, their activity was generally dependent on how and in what situation the saccade was initiated.

Movements can occur in different situations. An eye movement may be guided by visual information, as in the saccade task (Wurtz and Goldberg, 1972). If the monkey presses the lever on the chair, a small spot of light comes on at the center of the screen. After a random period of time the spot becomes slightly dim and the monkey has to release his hand as soon as possible to get rewarded. This forces the monkey to fixate on the spot of light all the time. If the light spot steps from the center to another location, the monkey naturally moves his line of sight by making a saccade. This is the saccade guided by visual information.

However, we do not behave just by reacting changes in our environment, but may anticipate

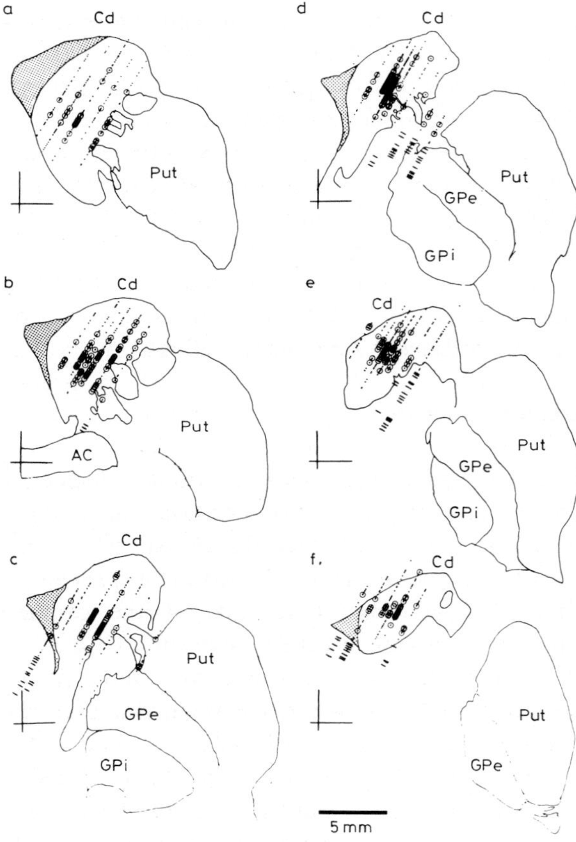

Fig. 2. Locations of saccade-related neurons (circles) and other recorded neurons (dots) in the monkey caudate nucleus. They are plotted on representative histological sections from rostral (*a*) to caudal (*f*). Bars: neurons with high-frequency discharges. Cd, caudate nucleus; Put, putamen; GPe, globus pallidus, external segment; GPi: globus pallidus, internal segment; AC, anterior commissure. (From Hikosaka et al., 1989a).

the change in environment on the basis of experience or memory and initiate a movement before something actually happens. Delayed saccade task was devised to realize such memory-guided, anticipatory behavior as an eye movement task (Hikosaka and Wurtz, 1983a). In contrast to the saccade task the peripheral target spot comes on after a time gap following the central fixation spot. The position of the target is indicated at each trial while the monkey is fixating. Therefore, the monkey remembers the position and makes a saccade before the target actually appears. This is a saccade guided be the memory of visual target location and at the same time anticipating the upcoming target. We did not force the monkey to make such anticipatory movements; it is a natural behavior. Interestingly, a large portion of saccade-related cells in the caudate nucleus or the substantia nigra are selectively related to this type of saccade.

Fig. 3 shows one of the typical caudate nucleus neurons related to saccades. In the delayed saccade task (left), the neuron started discharging near the end of the fixation period, and the discharge peaked with a saccade to the remembered position of the target. However, the neuron showed no discharge when saccades were made to the same target which was now actually present (right). The difference was rather surprising since the saccades in these two situations were nearly identical.

The similarity in saccade-related activity between the substantia nigra and the caudate nucleus suggested that the saccade-related signals are transmitted from the caudate to the substantia nigra. In order to examine this possibility we again performed stimulation experiments (Hikosaka and Sakamoto, in preparation). We inserted two microelectrodes into the caudate and the substantia nigra through guide tubes. While recording spike activity of a single substantia nigra neuron, we moved the caudate electrode up and down and passed a pulse of currents to see if the nigral cell activity changed.

The effect of stimulation was clear and in most cases inhibitory if the stimulating electrode was

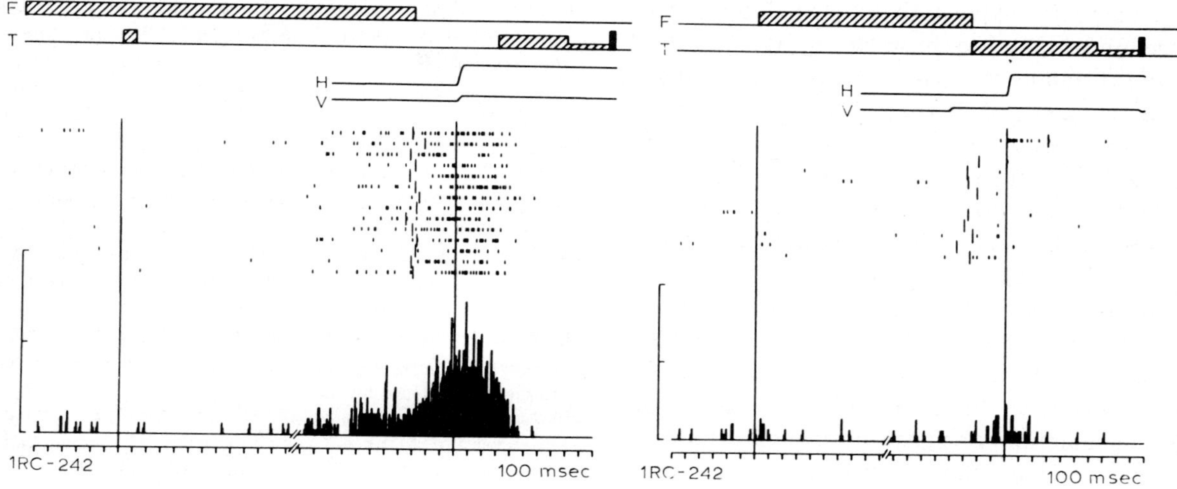

Fig. 3. A caudate nucleus neuron specifically related to memory-guided saccade. (Right) neuron showed no activity if saccades were made from the fixation (F) to a visual target (T) (saccade task). (Left) same neuron showed vigorous activity starting before saccade to the remembered position of the same visual target (delayed saccade task); its position was indicated by a cue stimulus (first hatched area on scheme line T) while the monkey was fixating. Cell activity is shown as a raster display, each dot indicating a single action potential and each line indicating a single trial of task. Averaged activities are shown below as spike time histograms. Vertical bar on each raster line indicates offset of fixation point. H and V, examples of horizontal and vertical eye positions. (Modified from Hikosaka et al., 1989a).

within the saccade-related area in the caudate nucleus. Single pulse stimulation of 100 μA produced a clear suppression of spike discharges in substantia nigra neurons. The nigra neurons decreased spike activity before purposive saccades, while caudate neurons recorded close to the stimulating electrode fired before similar saccades. This experiment supports the hypothesis that the saccade-related decrease in nigra cell activity is caused by a phasic inhibition originating from the caudate nucleus.

Inhibition and disinhibition in basal ganglia control saccades

The caudate nucleus and the substantia nigra are both included in the basal ganglia. They constitute two serial inhibitions: caudate-nigral and nigro-collicular. The nigro-collicular inhibition is tonically active whereas the caudate-nigral inhibition becomes active only phasically. The tonic component acts to suppress the output. The stronger the tonic component, the more effective is the suppression. The second, phasic component opens the inhibitory gate, producing an output. Interestingly, the effectiveness of the phasic component depends on the strength of the tonic component: the stronger the tonic inhibition, the more effective and more clear-cut becomes the output which is released from the tonic inhibition. In short, *disinhibition* is the way in which the basal ganglia act on the superior colliculus.

Interaction of cortical and basal ganglia inputs in the superior colliculus

The superior colliculus is the site where many different types of information converge. Reflex-inducing inputs from the retina, information related to spatial attention from the parietal cortex and visually guided motor signals from the frontal eye fields. These inputs, as a whole, may facilitate the production of saccadic eye movements. What is special about the basal ganglia then? The basal ganglia input is unique in that it is inhibitory while all the other inputs are considered to be excitatory. Excitatory inputs are basically additive. If there are various kinds of signals going on in the brain, the superior colliculus may become in the state of overflow and consequently the animal would be forced to move eyes and other body parts incessantly. This was actually shown in our experiments in which the GABAergic nigro-collicular transmission was blocked (Hikosaka and Wurtz, 1985a,b). By contrast, inhibitory input is essentially interactive. It acts to suppress other excitatory inputs. Therefore, the basal ganglia may control or modulate other motor signals by changing the level of the tonic inhibition. Furthermore, the basal ganglia could play an important role in the initiation of movements by removing the inhibition.

Another important aspect is that the basal ganglia are relatively dominated by memory-dependent information, as shown for the caudate nucleus saccadic discharge, whereas the cerebral cortex is dominated by sensory information. A saccadic eye movement is most likely to occur if it is anticipated and at the same time a trigger signal is given; this is presumably because the anticipation activates the basal ganglia pathway leading to disinhibition and the trigger signal activates the direct cortical pathways leading to excitation. By contrast, a saccade may not occur even in the presence of a trigger signal if the movement is not anticipated or prepared; this is because the basal ganglia-induced inhibition remains high.

References

Bruce, C.J. and Goldberg, M.E. (1985) Primate frontal eye fields, I. Single neurons discharging before saccades. *J. Neurophysiol.,* 53: 603 – 635.

Bruce, C.J., Goldberg, M.E., Bushnell, M.C. and Stanton, G.B. (1985) Primate frontal eye fields. II. Physiological and anatomical correlates of electrically evoked eye movements. *J. Neurophysiol.,* 54: 714 – 732.

DeLong, M.R. and Georgopoulos, A.P. (1981) Motor functions of the basal ganglia. In: Handbook of Physiology, The Nervous System, edited by V.B. Brooks. Bethesda, MD: Am. Physiol. Soc., sect. 1, part 2, vol. II, chapt. 21, pp. 1017 – 1061.

Di Chiara, G., Porceddu, M.L., Morelli, M.L., Mulas, M.L. and Gessa, G.L. (1979) Evidence for a GABAergic projection from the substantia nigra to the ventromedial thalamus and to the superior colliculus of the rat. *Brain Res.,* 176: 273 – 284.

Ewert, J-P. (1980) Neuroethology. Springer. Berlin.

Fahn, S. and Cote, L. (1968) Regional distribution of g-aminobutyric acid (GABA) in brain of the rhesus monkey. *J. Neurochem.,* 15: 209 – 213.

Faull, R.L.M. and Mehler, W.R. (1978) The cells of origin of nigrotectal, nigrothalamic and nigrostriatal projections in the rat. *Neuroscience,* 3: 989 – 1002.

Hikosaka, O., Sakamoto, M. and Usui, S. (1989a) Functional properties of monkey caudate neurons. I. Activities related to saccadic eye movements. *J. Neurophysiol.,* 61: 780 – 798.

Hikosaka, O., Sakamoto, M. and Usui, S. (1989b) Functional Properties of Monkey Caudate Neurons. II. Visual and Auditory Responses. *J. Neurophysiol.,* 61: 799 – 813.

Hikosaka, O., Sakamoto, M. and Usui, S. (1989c) Functional Properties of Monkey Caudate Neurons. III. Activities Related to Expectation of Target and Reward. *J. Neurophysiol.,* 61: 814 – 832.

Hikosaka, O. and Wurtz, R.H. (1983a) Visual and oculomotor functions of monkey substantia nigra pars reticulata. I. Relation of visual and auditory responses to saccades. J. *Neurophysiol., 49:* 1230-1253.

Hikosaka, O. and Wurtz, R.H. (1983b) Visual and oculomotor functions of monkey substantia nigra pars reticulata. II. Visual responses related to fixation of gaze. *J. Neurophysiol.,* 49: 1254 – 1267.

Hikosaka, O. and Wurtz, R.H. (1983c) Visual and oculomotor functions of monkey substantia nigra pars reticulata. III. Memory-contingent visual and saccade responses. *J. Neurophysiol.,* 49: 1268 – 1284.

Hikosaka, O. and Wurtz, R.H. (1983d) Visual and oculomotor functions of monkey substantia nigra pars reticulata. IV. Relation of substantia nigra to superior colliculus. *J. Neurophysiol.,* 49: 1285 – 1301.

Hikosaka, O. and Wurtz, R.H. (1985a) Modification of saccadic eye movements by GABA-related substances. I. Effect of muscimol and bicuculline in the monkey superior colliculus. *J. Neurophysiol.,* 53: 266 – 291.

Hikosaka, O. and Wurtz, R.H. (1985b) Modification of saccadic eye movements by GABA-related substances. II. Effects of muscimol in the monkey substantia nigra pars reticulata. *J. Neurophysiol.,* 53: 292 – 308.

Holstege, G. (1991) Descending motor pathways and the spinal motor system. Limbic and non-limbic components. In: G. Holstege (Ed.), *Role of the forebrain in sensation and behavior, Progress in Brain Research Vol. 87,* Elsevier, Amsterdam, pp. 000 – 000.

Jayaraman, A., Batton, R.R. and Carpenter, M.B. (1977) Nigrotectal projections in the monkey: and autoradiographic study. *Brain Res.,* 135: 147 – 152.

Robinson, D.A. and Fuchs, A.F. (1969) Eye movements evoked by stimulation of frontal eye fields. *J. Neurophysiol.*, 32: 637 – 648.

Schlag, J. and Schlag-Rey, M. (1987) Evidence for a supplementary eye field. *J. Neurophysiol.*, 57: 179 – 200.

Sparks, D.L. (1986) Translation of sensory signals into commands for control of saccadic eye movements: role of primate superior colliculus. *Physiol. Rev.*, 66: 118 – 171.

Tanji, J. and Kurata, K. (1985) Contrasting neuronal activity in supplementary and precentral motor cortex of monkeys. I. Responses to instructions determining motor responses to forthcoming signals of different modalities. *J. Neurophysiol.*, 53: 129 – 141.

Wurtz, R.H. and Goldberg, M.E. (1972) Activity of superior colliculus in behaving monkey: III. Cells discharging before eye movements. *J. Neurophysiol.*, 35: 575 – 586.

G. Holstege (Ed.)
Progress in Brain Research, Vol. 87

CHAPTER 7

"Perestroika" in the basal forebrain: Opening the border between neurology and psychiatry

Lennart Heimer, Jose de Olmos[1], George F. Alheid, and László Záborszky

University of Virginia, Charlottesville, VA 22908, U.S.A. and [1]Instituto de Investigacion Medica, Cordoba, Argentina

Introduction

"Schizophrenia is arguably the worst disease affecting mankind, even AIDS not excepted" (editorial in *Nature,* Vol. 336, November 10, 1988, p. 95). This quote from a prestigious science magazine reflects a growing desire to understand the cause of insanity and to come to grips with the social ramifications of mental illness. The timing seems well chosen as we are approaching one of the most commemorative bicentennials in the annals of Psychiatry. In 1792 the French psysician, Phillippe Pinel, literally unlocked the chains and shackles of the mentally deranged and let them out of their dungeons. Thus started the slow process in which the bestial treatment of individuals with serious mental disorder gradually became more humane. But the cause of schizophrenia is still shrouded in mystery and serious mental illness still carries a significant stigma. On the other hand, there have been impressive advances in the neurosciences in recent years, in basic subjects of anatomy, physiology, pharmacology, and molecular biology, and in imaging techniques for the study of the human brain in vivo, and an increasing number of research programs are now being pursued with great expectations of one day finding a cure for schizophrenia and other crippling brain disorders. But the task is enormous, and only a concerted collaborative research effort into the pathophysiological mechanisms of neuropsychiatric disorders is likely to lead to the design of rational and efficient therapies. The purpose of this communication is to focus the attention on recent advances in our understanding of basal forebrain organization. Such knowledge forms the necessary conceptual framework for physiologic, behavioral and clinical studies of forebrain functions relevant to neuropsychiatric disorders.

The report of cortical cholinergic deficits in Alzheimer patients (Davis and Maloney, 1976), coupled with neuroanatomical studies indicating that a large part of the cholinergic innervation of the cortex is derived from neurons in basal forebrain (Divac, 1975; Kievit and Kuypers, 1975; Mesulam and Van Hoesen, 1978; Mesulam et al., 1983; Saper 1984), as well as the observation that this disease is often accompanied by degenerative changes in the basal nucleus of Meynert (Whitehouse et al., 1981), focused attention on the basal forebrain and provided a new incentive for its scientific exploration. From an historical perspective, these clinical-anatomical correlations appear to confirm what some clinicians, neuroanatomists, and pathologists had long emphasized; i.e., that the basal nucleus of Meynert is especially vulnerable in the aging process (e.g., Brockhaus, 1942; Hassler, 1938; Kodama, 1929; Macchi, 1951). More recent studies provide ample support for this proposition (e.g., Arendt et al., 1983; 1986; Candy et al., 1983; Etienne et al., 1986; Jellinger, 1985; McGeer et al., 1984; Nakano and

Hirano, 1983; Perry et al., 1983; Riederer and Jellinger, 1983; Rossor et al., 1982; Tagliavini et al., 1984; Tagliavini and Pilleri 1983; Wilcock et al., 1983).

The basal nucleus of Meynert is located in a region of the mediobasal forebrain that is most often termed the "substantia innominata"* and the nucleus itself is occasionally called the "nucleus of the substantia innominata", or simply substantia innominata (Foix and Nicolesco, 1925; Friedemann, 1911; Vogt and Vogt, 1952; see also Brockhaus, 1942). This, however, is unsuitable for two reasons. On the one hand, the basal nucleus is only one of the neuronal cell groups in this territory, and on the other hand, neurons with all the characteristics of cells in the basal nucleus of Meynert are located, singularly or in groups, in many forebrain regions outside the general region referred to as the substantia innominata.

The morphology of the basal forebrain has been notoriously difficult to analyze, and students of basal forebrain organization and function have been frequently confronted by poorly defined anatomical systems and controversial boundaries. True to its "name", this is nowhere more evident than in the general region termed the substantia innominata. Nonetheless, as a result of intense efforts by neuroscientists using modern tracer techniques and histochemical methods in every conceivable combination, the more prominent functional-anatomical systems of the mediobasal forebrain, including the basal nucleus of Meynert, have come into sharper focus.

Based on our own investigations spanning the past two decades, and the data provided by many others in this "golden age" of neuroanatomy, it is clear that major portions of this enigmatic region belong to nearby and better defined anatomical systems. It is for this reason that attempts to define precise anatomical boundaries of the substantia innominata are often frustrating or misleading. Indeed, it seems that the time has come to abandon the term in favor of more appropriate designations for those parts that can be clearly identified. These include ventral aspects of the basal ganglia; i.e., the ventral striatopallidal system (Alheid and Heimer, 1988; Heimer et al., 1985;), and the medial extension of the centromedial amygdaloid area into and including the bed nucleus of the stria terminalis; i.e., the extended amygdala (Alheid and Heimer, 1988; de Olmos et al., 1985) As indicated above, a third important component of this region is the basal nucleus of Meynert (Kölliker, 1896; Meynert, 1872), a collection of generally large and mostly cholinergic neurons with prominent projections to the cerebral cortex (Divac, 1975; Jones et al., 1976; Kievit and Kuypers, 1975; Mesulam et al., 1983; Mesulam and Van Hoesen, 1978), but also with axons innervating amygdala and thalamus (Butcher and Woolf, 1986; Carlsen et al., 1985; Hallanger et al., 1987; Levey et al., 1987; Parent et al., 1988; Price et al., 1988; Steriade et al., 1987; Woolf et al., 1984). The basal nucleus of Meynert is part of a more widespread complex of aggregated and nonaggregated corticopetal cells which are found within or adjacent to many anatomical structures in the basal forebrain, including the septal-diagonal band complex, the ventral striatopallidal system, and extended amygdala. The ventral striatopallidal system, the extended amygdala, and the basal nucleus of Meynert are interwoven in a complex topography that we will first depict in a series of drawings as a prelude to a more detailed discussion of their morphological features, interrelations with other brain structures, and clinically relevant considerations.

Pictorial survey of the human basal forebrain in frontal sections

Although the schematic diagrams in Figs. 1 and 12 – 15 of the basal forebrain refer primarily to the

* Although this region is sometimes called the substantia innominata of Reichert (1859-1861), it is more appropriate to credit Reil (1809), who referred to the area as "die ungenannte Mark-Substanz." (See also Alheid and Heimer, 1988, page 4).

human brain, the concept of the ventral striatopallidal system (red-pink colors) and the extended amygdala (yellow-green colors) are derived from a variety of normal-anatomical and experimental studies primarily in the rat and primate brain. These studies have been reviewed in detail in several recent papers and book chapters (e.g., Alheid and Heimer, 1988; Alheid et al., 1990; de Olmos, 1990; de Olmos et al., 1985). The location of the mostly large cortico-, thalamo-, and amygdalopetal neurons generally identified with the basal nucleus of Meynert is indicated by solid black triangles. One black triangle indicates the presence of many cholinergic cells and the topographic distribution of these cells is based on recent Nissl and histochemical studies of the human brain (Hedreen et al., 1984; Mesulam and Geula 1988; Mufson et al., 1989; Saper, 1990; Saper and Chelimsky, 1984; Ulfig, 1989). It should be noted that although the majority of the large corticopetal neurons in the basal forebrain areas referred to in this article are cholinergic, a significant number of generally smaller non-cholinergic corticopetal cells are known to exist in this region (see below); these are depicted in Fig. 13 but not in schematic drawings in Fig. 1. Another set of cholinergic neurons, which are located throughout the striatum, has been indicated by white triangles. Although they are also large, they are interneurons and generally considered to constitute a distinct cell population from the other large cholinergic basal forebrain neurons represented by solid black triangles. However, the extent to which the two sets of cholinergic neurons differ is not quite clear. Discussions of the neuropathology of Alzheimer's disease have focused primarily on the cholinergic basal forebrain neurons, and only recently has there been some indication that also the striatal cholinergic interneurons may be compromised in Alzheimer's disease (Oyanagi et al., 1987).

Rostral section through the caudal part of the nucleus accumbens (Fig. 1A; see also Figs. 4A – D). A prominent landmark at this level is the lateral extension of the anterior commissure (ac) which has been cut parallel to its laterally coursing axons (compare Fig. 4B). The caudate nucleus (C) and the putamen (P) are continuous with each other through striatal cell-bridges across the anterior limb of the internal capsule (ic). Together with the globus pallidus (GP), these two parts of the striatum, the caudate and putamen, constitute the dorsal parts of the basal ganglia above the temporal limb of the anterior commissure. However, the basal ganglia extend ventrally below the anterior commissure and into a region which has sometimes been referred to as the subcommissural substantia innominata (Miodonski, 1967). That the putamen extends to the ventral surface of the human brain can be clearly seen in AChE-stained sections (Figure 4D) or for that matter in any histochemical procedure that preferentially stains striatal areas. This ventral extension of the putamen is continuous medially with the caudomedial part of the accumbens, forming what is often referred to as fundus striati in the human brain (Fig. 4A). The medial part of the ventral striatum at this level, represented by the caudomedial accumbens, seems to differ from the rest of the ventral striatum in the sense that it has neurochemical features and connections that are reminiscent not only of striatum (red color), but also of the bed nucleus of the stria terminalis (BST) and the remainder of the extended amygdala, as indicated by yellow-green color (Alheid and Heimer, 1988; Candy et al., 1985). Although the ventral striatum is primarily populated by lightly stained, rounded neurons of medium size, it is nevertheless quite heterogenous (see below). Globus pallidus also extends well below the anterior commissure and since it forms a ventral complement to ventral striatum it has been referred to as "ventral pallidum" or VP (Heimer and Wilson, 1975). In the extreme medial part of the sections in Fig. 1A, we have depicted the large hyperchromic cells which constitute the nucleus of the diagonal band (Hedreen et al., 1984; see also Fig. 4B). This nucleus, which can be followed in progressively more rostral sections, where it is continuous with the medial septum (Fig. 4A), is generally recogniz-

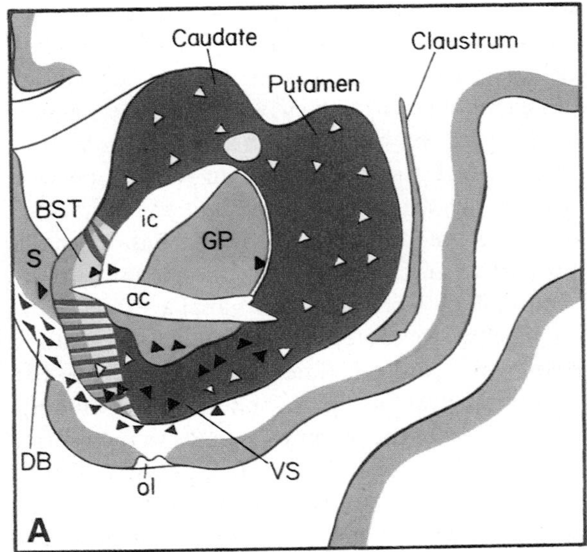
Caudate
Putamen
Claustrum
BST
ic
GP
S
ac
DB
ol
VS
A

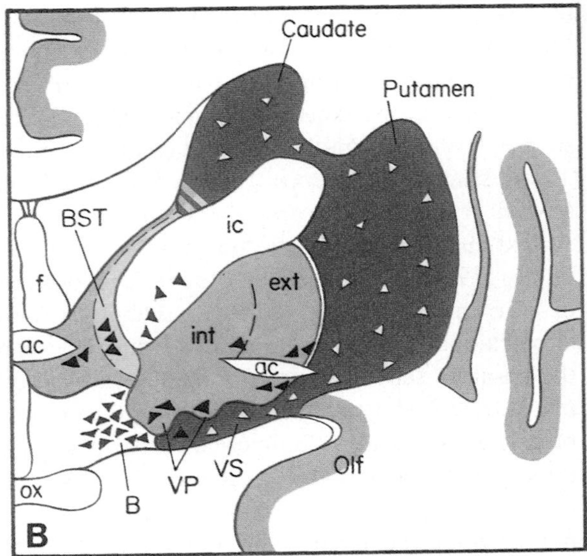
Caudate
Putamen
BST
ic
f
ext
ac
int
ac
ox
B
VP
VS
Olf
B

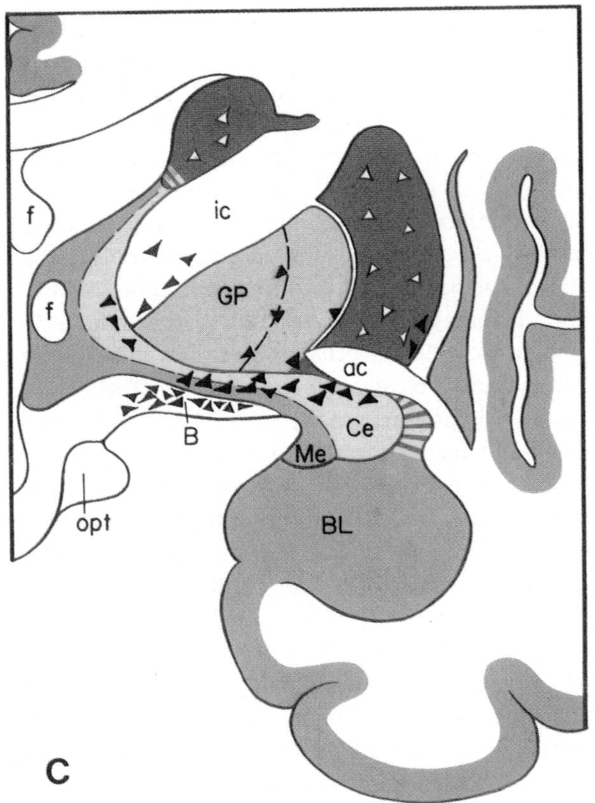
f
ic
f
GP
ac
B
Ce
Me
opt
BL
C

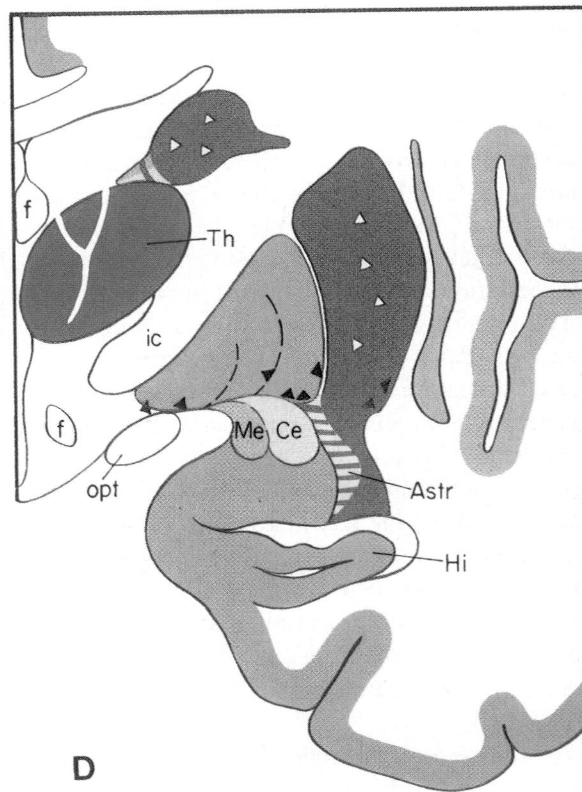
f
Th
ic
f
Me
Ce
opt
Astr
Hi
D

ed as the nucleus of the vertical limb of the diagonal band, whose cholinergic cell population has been referred to as "Ch2" by Mesulam et al., (1983). Although the nucleus of the diagonal band is the most prominent component of the magnocellular corticopetal system at this level there are scattered groups of large hyperchromic neurons (solid black triangles) found in other parts of the basal forebrain, including the external capsule, ventral and dorsal pallidum and the bed nucleus of stria terminalis, and many of these are undoubtedly cholinergic (e.g., Mesulam and Geula, 1988; Perry et al., 1984; Saper, 1990).

Section through the optic chiasm and maximal extent of ventral pallidum (Fig. 1B). In this slightly more caudal section, the anterior commissure crosses the midline, and the temporal limb of the anterior commissure is positioned further laterally. Globus pallidus (GP), which at this level consists of two segments, is significantly larger in size and occupies a large area above the temporal limb of the anterior commissure. However, it is apparent both from Nissl-stained preparations and from sections stained with a variety of pallidal markers, that the pallidal complex occupies a considerable area also beneath the temporal limb of the anterior commissure (Fig. 5). Striatal tissue, in continuity with putamen, still extends far ventrally toward the surface where it occupies part of the anterior perforated space. Although the accumbens has disappeared at this level, the bed nucleus of stria terminalis (BST), which is one of the main components of the "extended amygdala" has reached a considerable size (See also Fig. 8A). The diagonal band nucleus with numerous large cholinergic cells has gradually moved to a more lateral position, and it is more often labeled as the basal nucleus of Meynert at this level, where its main part is still confined just medial to the ventral striatopallidal complex. The part labeled "B" (basal nucleus) in Fig. 1B corresponds to the anteromedial part of Ch4 in the nomenclature introduced by Mesulam et al., (1983). As indicated in the drawing, however, a significant number of cholinergic neurons are scattered in other forebrain areas including ventral striatum and ventral pallidum, dorsal pallidum (mainly in the medullary laminae), bed nucleus of stria terminalis and the internal capsule (Mesulam and Geula, 1988; Perry et al., 1984; Saper and Chelimsky, 1984). Bed nucleus of stria terminalis (yellow-green) can be easily identified at this level where it envelopes the mid-portion of the anterior commissure in a characteristic fashion.

Section through the amygdaloid body and the extended amygdala (Fig. 1C). Whereas at this slightly more caudal level, the topography of the dorsal basal ganglia and the internal capsule is very similar to the situation in Fig. 1B, dramatic changes occur ventrally. The ventral striatopallidal system has disappeared and been replaced in large part by the extended amygdala (yellow-green color), which represents an impressive forebrain structure. This drawing constitutes a highly simplified sketch of this complicated and highly differentiated structure (de Olmos, 1990). As indicated by the diagram, the "extended amygdala" refers to an extension of the central and medial amygdaloid nuclei, rather than of the amygdaloid body as a whole. The larger part of the amygdaloid body, the basolateral complex, which has many

Fig. 1. Schematic drawings showing the human basal forebrain in a series of frontal sections starting rostrally at the level of the septum-accumbens (A) and ending at the caudal aspect of the amygdaloid body (D). Striatum (caudate nucleus, putamen and ventral striatum) is indicated with red color, globus pallidus and ventral pallidum with pink color, and the extended amygdala with yellow (extension of the central amygdaloid nucleus) and green (extension of the medial amygdaloid nucleus) colors. ac = anterior commissure; Astr = amygdalostriatal transition area; B = basal nucleus of Meynert; BST = bed nucleus of stria terminalis; Ce = central amygdaloid nucleus; DB = diagonal band; f = fornix; GP = globus pallidus; Hi = hippocampus; ic = internal capsule; Me = medial amygdaloid nucleus; opt = optic tract; ox = optic chiasm; VP = ventral pallidum; VS = ventral striatum. © Dr. L. Heimer.

similarities with the overlying cerebral cortex, is not included in the concept of the extended amygdala. The drawing encapsulates features of the extended amygdala occurring at several rostrocaudal levels. The area bridged by cell-columns between the centromedial amygdala (Ce-Me) and bed nucleus of stria terminalis (BST) has been referred to as the "sublenticular substantia innominata" by Miodonski (1967). An area lateral to the central amygdaloid nucleus is indicated by yellow-red stripes. This poorly studied territory which, like the medial (shell) region of the accumbens, is most closely related to the striatum, nonetheless may represent a transition zone between striatum and extended amygdala, and as indicated in the various levels of Fig. 1, similar transition zones may also occur adjacent to the bed nucleus of the stria terminalis and alongside the entire course of the stria terminalis. The cluster of large hyperchromatic cells which represent the basal nucleus of Meynert is more compact and shows its greatest mediolateral extent at this level.

Section through the caudal parts of basal ganglia and amygdaloid body (Fig. 1D). Compared to the slightly more rostral level in Fig. 1C, this level is notable for several reasons. Of the extended amygdala, only the central and medial amygdaloid nuclei remain; both the bed nucleus of the stria terminalis, which has been replaced by the thalamus, and the sublenticular part of the extended amygdala have disappeared. The area of the basolateral amygdaloid complex has likewise been reduced in size and the very rostral tip of the hippocampus is now visible. The globus pallidus still appears voluminous, and the accessory medullary lamina appears to almost divide the internal pallidal segment into two parts. In addition, at this level and caudally, as the cerebral peduncle becomes adjacent to the optic tract, numerous neurons may be found scattered within the fibers of the human cerebral peduncle (Alheid et al., 1990). This does not appear to be the case for other primate brains (macaque, squirrel monkey, marmoset) that we have examined, but is reminiscent of the entopeduncular nucleus of most other mammals. Some of these cells are in the midst of a substance P-rich neuropil, and probably represent ectopic cells of the internal pallidal segment. Other cells within the myelin-rich areas adjacent to the pallidum may not receive any substance P terminals (Alheid et al., 1990), and therefore might represent an additional specialization within the pallidal complex. A discussion follows of three major functional-anatomical systems interdigitating in the mediobasal forebrain.

Three major functional-anatomical systems interdigitate in the mediobasal forebrain

The ventral striatopallidal system

The terms ventral striatum and ventral pallidum were introduced mare than 10 years ago in the rat brain to emphasize the fact that the main parts of the basal ganglia; i.e., the caudate-putamen (striatum) and the globus pallidus extend ventrally to the surface of the brain in the region of the olfactory tubercle (Heimer and Wilson, 1975). Indeed, the olfactory tubercle itself has unmistakable striatal and pallidal characteristics, although it is often identified as part of the olfactory cortex (e.g., Ramon y Cajal, 1955; Danner and Pfister, 1981; Luskin and Price, 1983; Meyer et al., 1989; Price and Slotnick, 1983; Stephan, 1975). This, however, is not surprising. It receives direct olfactory bulb input and it has traditionally been described, at least in macrosmatic mammals, as a

Fig. 2. Nissl and acetylcholinesterase stained frontal sections through the rat brain demonstrating ,,striatal cell bridges'' (curved arrows) between the main dorsal part of the striatal complex and the superficial dense cell layer of the olfactory tubercle. Note also the sharp border (straight arrows) between the olfactory tubercle and the laterally situated olfactory or piriform cortex. White triangles delineate the border between the shell and the core regions of the nucleus accumbens in A. ac = anterior commissure; Acb = nucleus accumbens; lo = lateral olfactory tract.

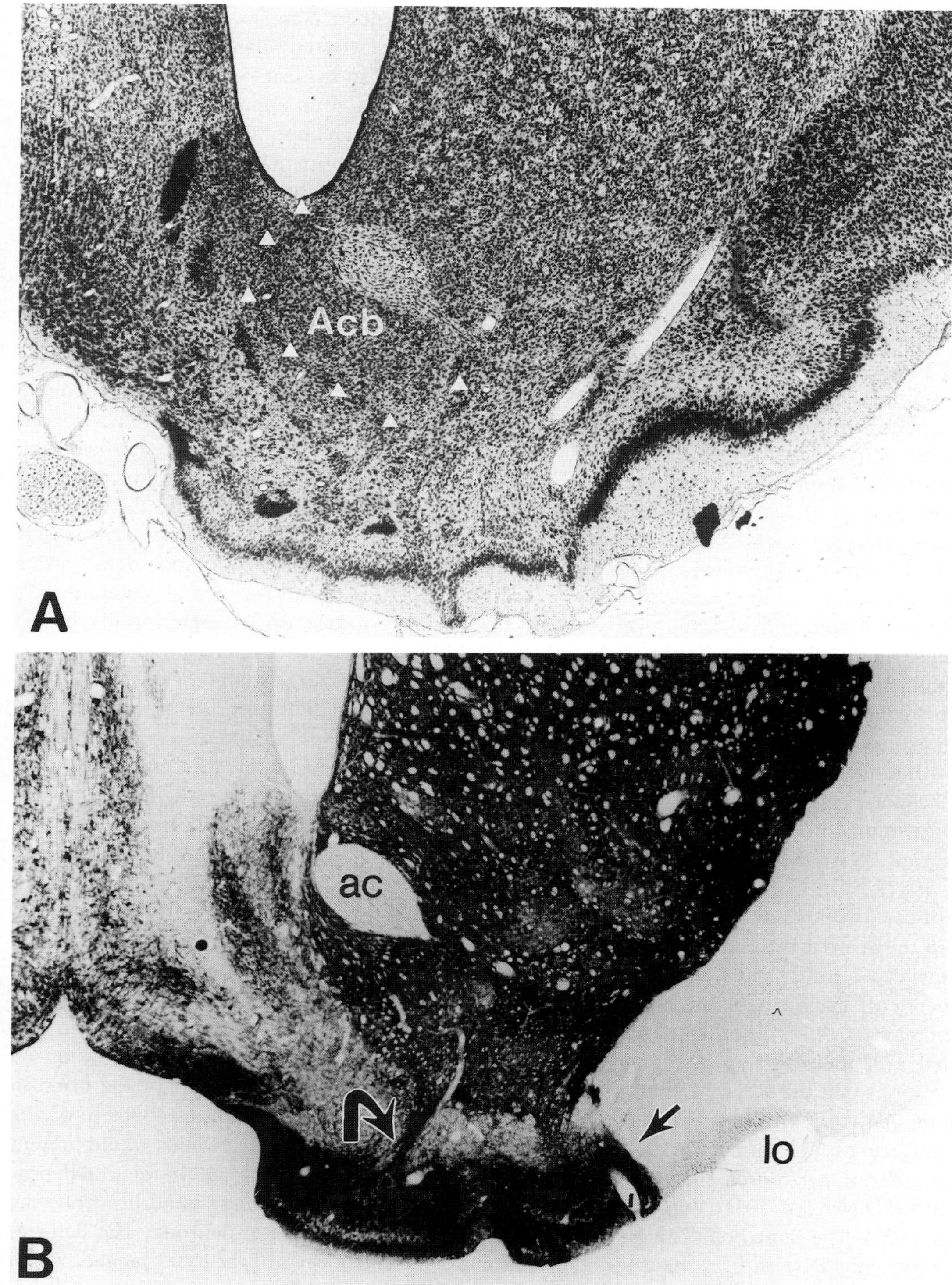
Acb
A
ac
lo
B

laminated structure with three layers, although, as Ramon y Cajal (1955) observes: ". . . the second zone containing pyramids which are more irregular than in any other cortical region." Furthermore, Blackstad (1967), points out that even if the olfactory tubercle of macrosmatic mammals is reminiscent of a cortical structure, it does not conform in any significant degree to a pattern of radial and tangential organization characteristic of a "cortical" structure. A detailed study of regular Nissl or acetylcholinesterase sections (Fig. 2), furthermore, indicates a direct continuity in the form of "striatal cell bridges" (curved arrows in Fig. 2) between the main dorsal part of the striatal complex (caudate-putamen) and the superficial dense cell layer of the olfactory tubercle. In addition, there is little doubt about the sharp boundary (straight arrow in Fig. 2) between the olfactory tubercle and the olfactory cortex. With the advantages offered by modern anatomical tracing and histochemical methods it is clear that the olfactory tubercle has more in common with the overlying striatal complex than with the neighboring olfactory cortex, and it can be best understood as a ventral extension of the striatal complex, or, indeed, as a ventral extension of the basal ganglia including both striatal and pallidal components (Fig. 3; see also Alheid and Heimer, 1988; Heimer et al., 1987; Millhouse and Heimer, 1984; Switzer et al., 1982; Young et al., 1984; Zahm et al., 1987; Zahm and Heimer, 1987).

A paucity of cortical characteristics is even more pronounced in the primate or human anterior perforated space which is sometimes equated with the olfactory tubercle of macrosmatic mammals (see, however, Heimer et al., 1977). For instance, it can be appreciated even in regular cell and myelin-stained preparations that the accumbens or fundus striati and putamen (Fig. 4A, 4B, and 4C) reach the ventral surface of the human brain in the region of the anterior perforated space (see also Beccari, 1910, 1911; Macchi, 1951; Von Economo and Koskinas, 1925). The same point can be made even more convincingly by the aid of a striatal marker; e.g., acetylcholinesterase (Fig. 4D). The fact that the pallidal complex accompanies the ventral parts of the striatum towards the surface of the primate brain can be seen in regular Nissl stain, if the section is cut at an appropriate angle (see Fig. 7 in Alheid and Heimer, 1988) and it can be appreciated even more clearly in histochemical preparations stained for pallidal markers such as glutamic acid decarboxylase, substance-P, enkephalin, or epidermal growth factor (Alheid et al., 1990; Alheid and Heimer, 1988; Beach and McGeer, 1984; DiFiglia et al., 1982; 1984; Fallon et al., 1984; Haber and Elde, 1981; Haber and Nauta, 1983; Haber and Watson, 1985; Mai et al., 1986) or, as illustrated in the sections from a human brain in Fig. 5, by a stain for endogenous iron (Alheid et al., 1989b; 1990; Alheid and Heimer, 1988; Dwork et al., 1988; Francois et al., 1981; Hill and Switzer, 1984; Spatz, 1922; Switzer et al., 1982), all of which stain particularly densely in pallidal areas. Such preparations demonstrate finger-like extensions of the ventral pallidum (VP) close to the surface of the anterior perforated space (Fig. 6), where they interdigitate with ventral striatal tissue (see also Sakamoto et al., 1988). This pronounced interdigitation of ventral striatal and ventral pallidal tissue components seems to be a prominent feature in many mammals, including the rat (Fig. 3) and the human (Fig. 5). Since iron can be detected with magnetic resonance imaging (MRI), it is also possible to visualize some of these pallidal features in vivo (e.g., Fig. 28 in Alheid et al., 1990).

The interdigitation between ventral pallidal components and magnocellular corticopetal cells, which constitutes another important feature in the ventral part of the basal forebrain is demonstrated in Fig. 7 (see also Fig. 1B). While reviewing the complicated anatomy of this part of the brain in Nissl preparations, it is useful to conceive of the additional level of complexity which would present itself in preparations showing the neuronal processes including the long dendrites of the magnocellular corticopetal neurons. The delineation of the ventral parts of the basal ganglia, which was originally aided by a combination of classic

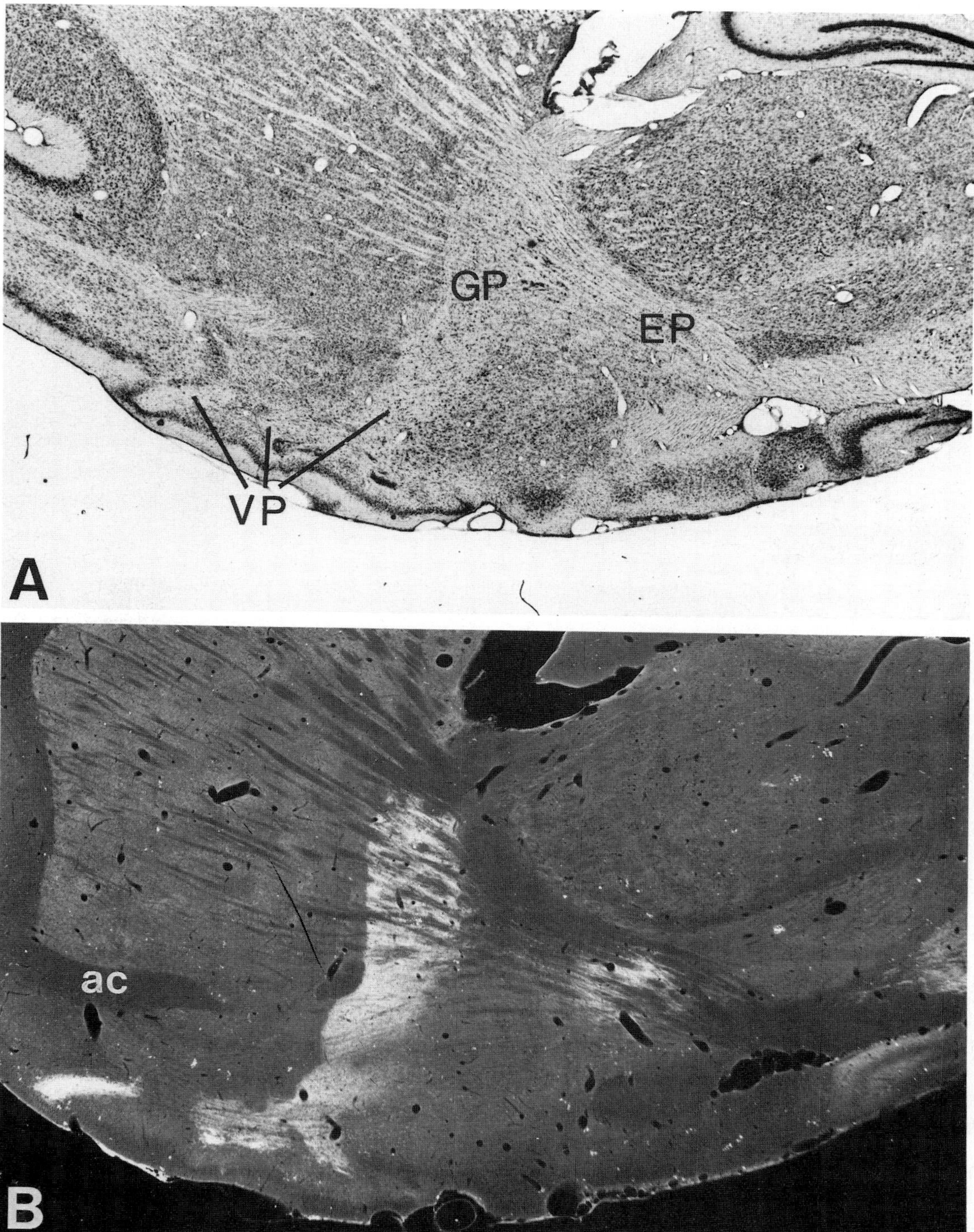

Fig. 3. Adjacent sagittal sections from the rat brain stained with the Nissl method (A) and with an immunostain for epidermal growth factor (B). Although the main parts of the pallidal complex can be appreciated in the Nissl stained section, its borders and especially its ventral extensions in the deep part of the olfactory tubercle can be more easily seen with a pallidal marker, e.g., epidermal growth factor. Note the immunostaining of the entopeduncular nucleus (EP) corresponding to the internal pallidal segment in primates. ac = anterior commissure; GP = globus pallidus; VP = ventral pallidum.

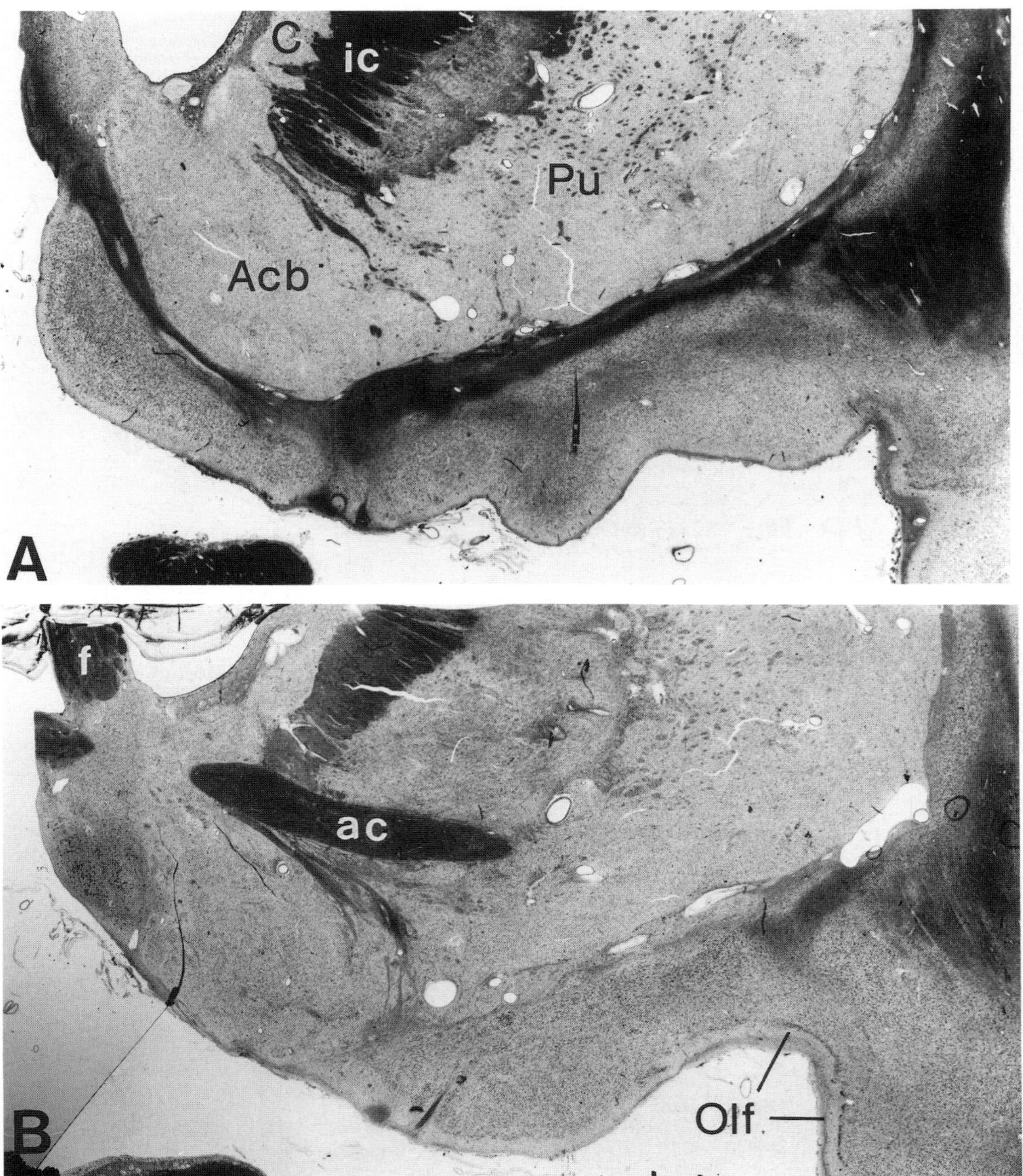

Fig. 4. Frontal sections through the rostral part of the human basal forebrain stained with the Klüver-Barrera method for cells and myelinated fibers (A-C) and with a histochemical stain for acetylcholinesterase (D). The figure in A demonstrates how the caudate nucleus (C) and the putamen (Pu) is in direct continuity with each other underneath the rostral part of the internal capsule (ic) in a region called accumbens (Acb) or fundus striati, which is part of ventral striatum. Note how ventral striatum reaches the ventral surface of the brain in B and C. This fact can be appreciated even more clearly in the acetylcholinesterase-stained section in D, which

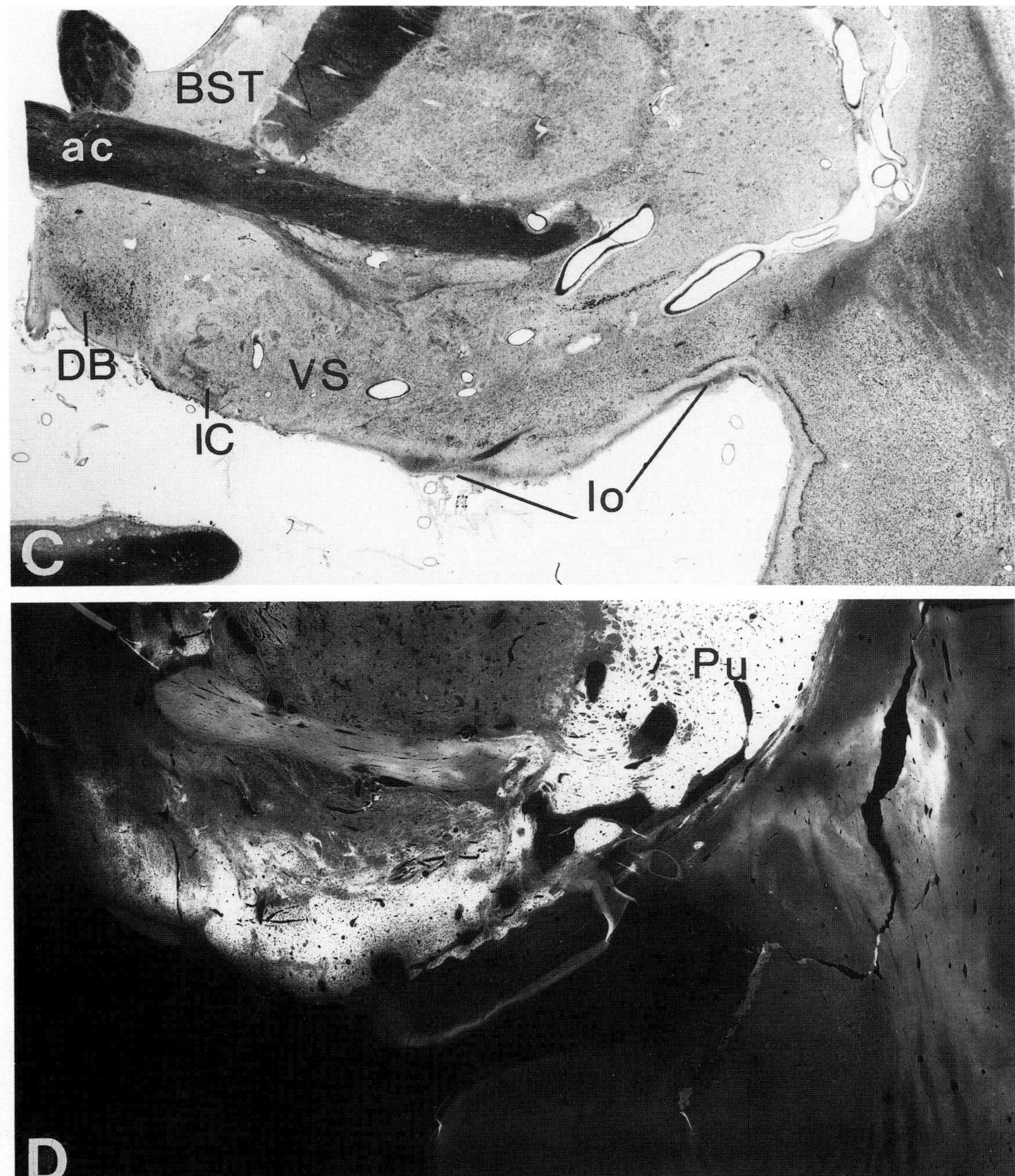

demonstrates the ventral extension of the putamen (Pu) towards the ventral surface just medial to the frontal olfactory area. Figs. A and C from Alheid et al., 1990 with permission of Academic Press; Fig. D was kindly provided by Dr. Robert Brashear. ac = anterior commissure; DB = nucleus of the diagonal band of Broca; f = fornix; IC = island of Calleja; lo = lateral olfactory tract; Olf = olfactory cortex; VS = ventral striatum.

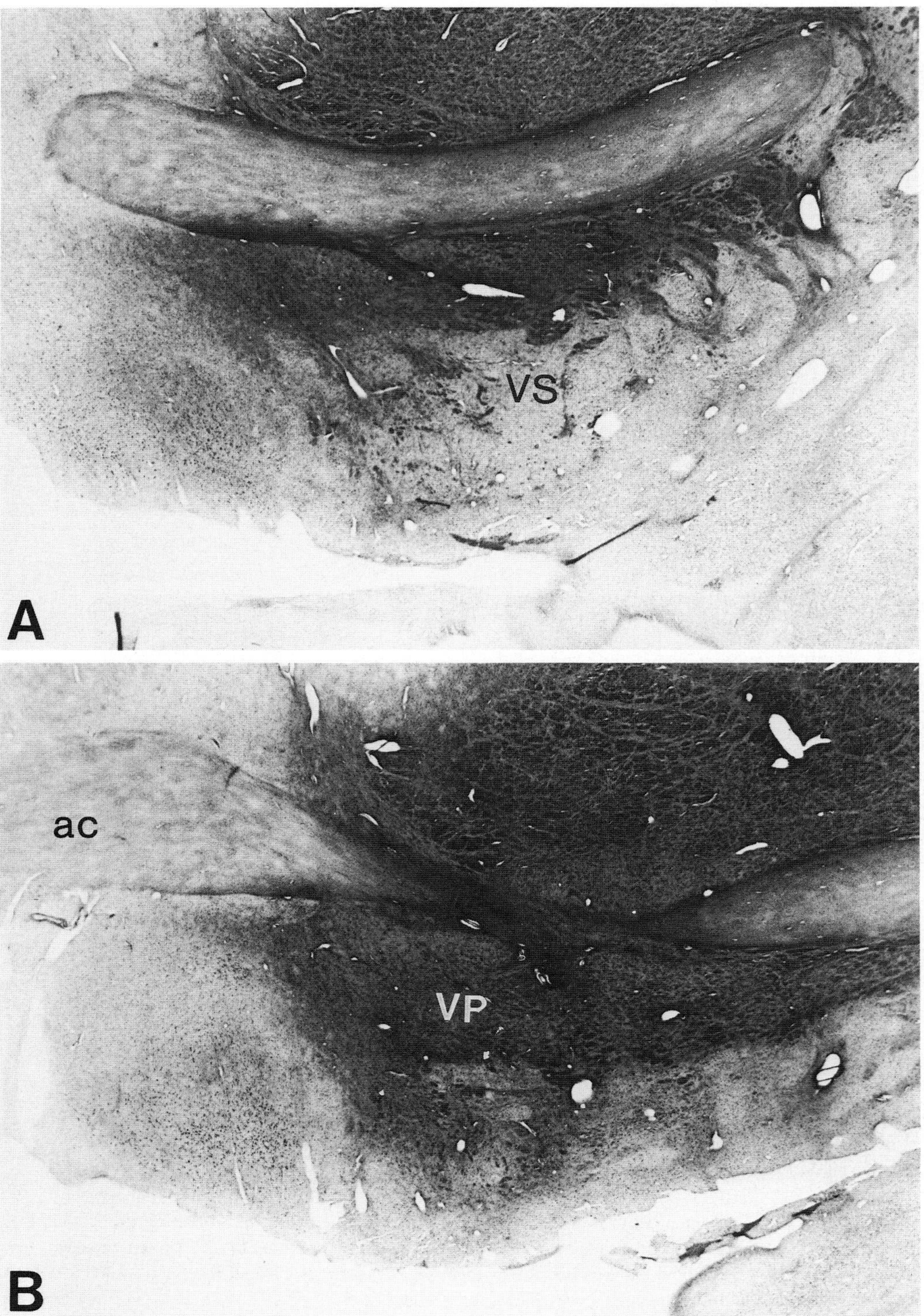

Fig. 5. A and B demonstrate the extent of the ventral pallidum (VP) underneath the anterior commissure (ac) in two nearby frontal sections of the human brain stained for iron. Note the interdigitation of ventral pallidal and ventral striatal tissue components. Fig.

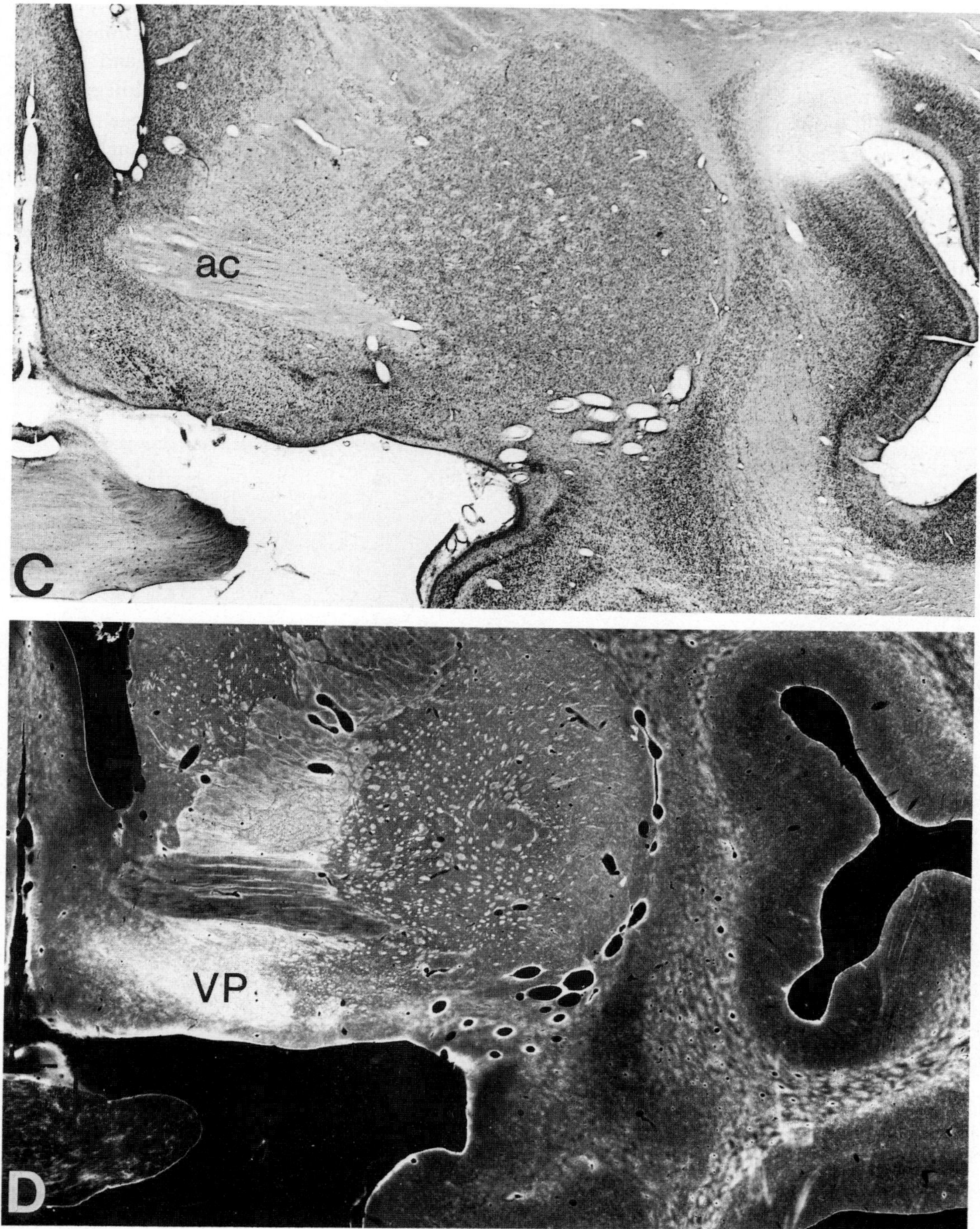

B is from Alheid et al., 1990 with permision from Academic Press. The extent of the ventral pallidum in cynomolgus (macaca fascicularis) monkey is demonstrated in photographs C (from a Nissl stained section) and D (from an iron-stained section).

Nissl preparations and hodological studies in experimental animals, has now proceeded by the aid of a variety of morphological and histochemical techniques both in non-primates and primates, including the human brain (Alheid and Heimer, 1988; Alheid et al., 1990; Fallon, 1987; Groenewegen, 1988; Haber and Nauta, 1983; Haber et al., 1985; Heimer, 1978; Heimer et al., 1985; Newman and Winans, 1980a,b).

The notion of the ventral striatopallidal system drew attention to some important anatomical relations, which have led to a fundamental reevaluation of forebrain organization. Well-known forebrain regions including not only the accumbens and the olfactory tubercle, but also significant portions of the substantia innominata, which have unmistakable striatal and pallidal characteristics, can be considered as integral parts of the basal ganglia. The telencephalic input to these ventral parts of the basal ganglia comes primarily from frontal and temporal association cortex, periallo- and allocortical areas; e.g., entorhinal cortex, hippocampus and olfactory cortex, as well as from the cortical-like basolateral amygdala (Beckstead, 1979; Groenewegen et al., 1982; 1987; Kelley and Domesick, 1982; Krayniak et al., 1981; Newman and Winans, 1980a,b; Ragsdale and Graybiel, 1988; Russchen and Price,

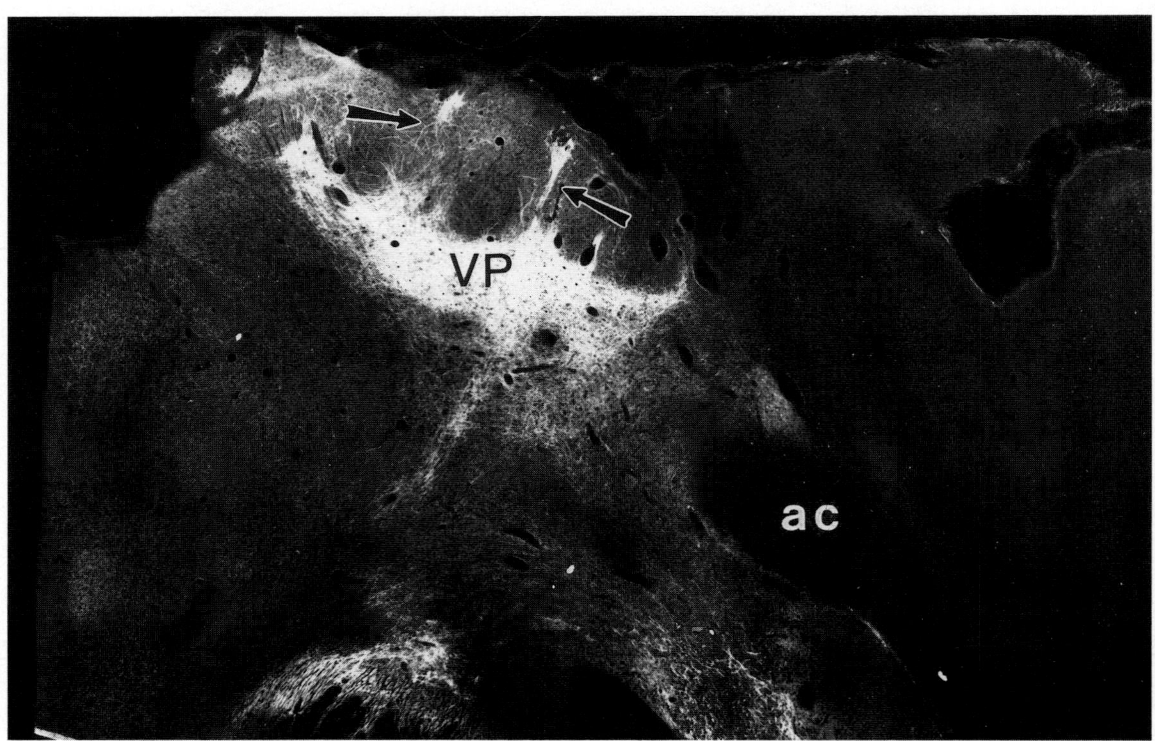

Fig. 6. Substance P-stained horizontal section through the olfactory tubercle close to the ventral surface of a marmoset monkey demonstrates substance P-positive finger-like extensions (arrows) of ventral pallidum (VP) interdigitating with ventral striatal tissue compartments in the tubercle. ac = anterior commissure.

Fig. 7. Adjacent horizontal sections through the ventral extension of the ventral pallidum in the marmoset stained with the Nissl method. Note the interdigitation of ventral pallidal (VP) elements with the large, hyperchrome cells belonging to the magnocellular corticopetal cell system (arrows). ac = anterior commissure; ot = optic tract.

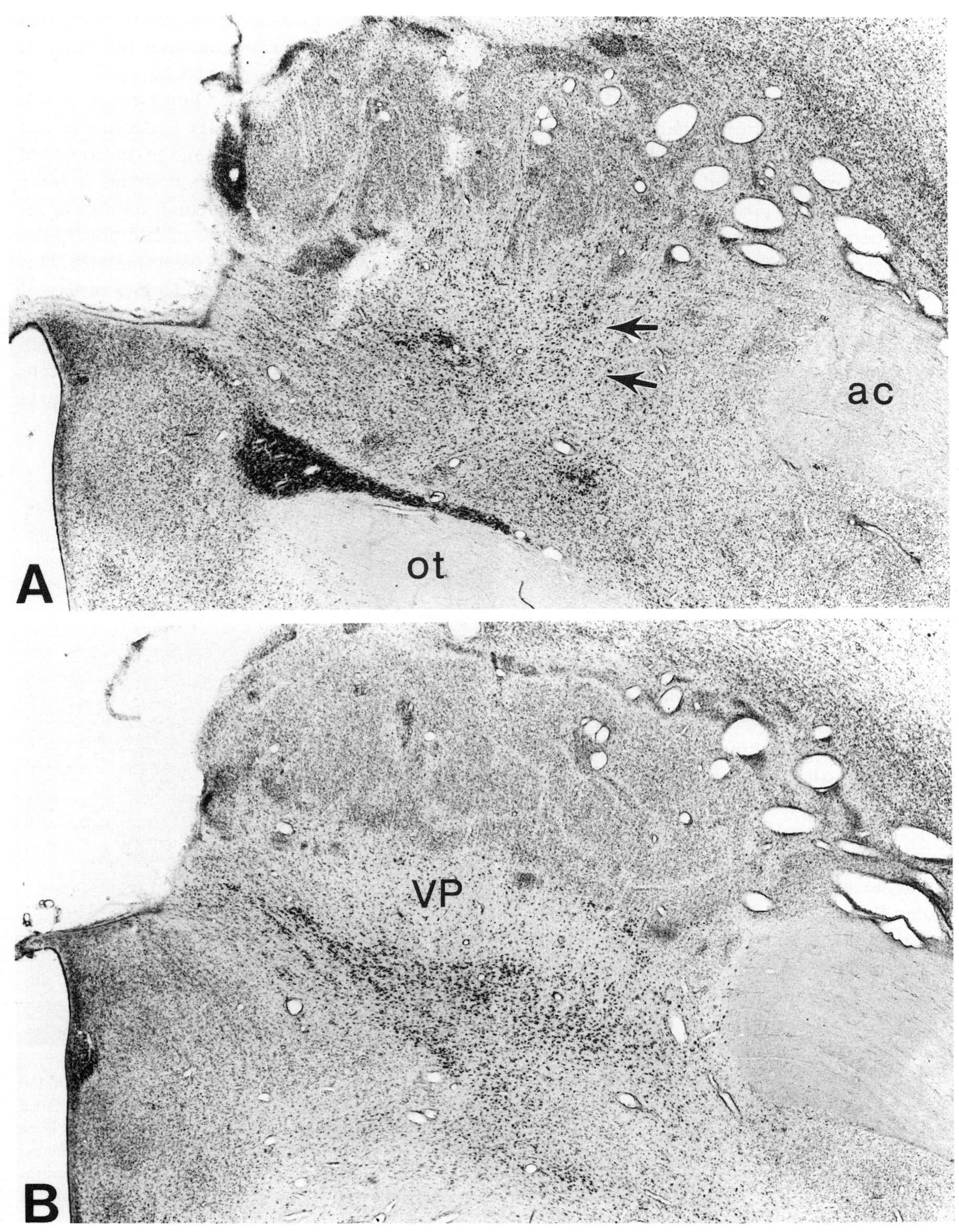
ac
ot
A
VP
B

1984; Russchen et al., 1985a,b; Zaborszky et al., 1985). These structures are usually considered components of the elusive "limbic system" and as such, they were often characterized by their relations to the hypothalamus rather than to the basal ganglia, which is most often considered a key structure in the "extrapyramidal" motor system.

A lingering problem is posed by the nucleus accumbens and perhaps by the medial portion of the olfactory tubercle. We have suggested that the medial part of the accumbens, or the entire extent of the shell area of the accumbens (Zaborszky et al., 1985), although certainly striatal in character, may also contain elements of the extended amygdala (Alheid and Heimer, 1988; Alheid et al., 1990; de Olmos et al., 1985; Heimer et al., 1985). For example, in most histochemical stains, the rostral border of the bed nucleus of the stria terminalis merges in a graded fashion with the caudomedial nucleus accumbens. Moreover, the medial part of the accumbens sends projections, not only to typical basal ganglia structures, but also to the entire extent of the lateral preoptic-hypothalamic continuum, and part of the shell region even sends some fibers to the medial sectors of the hypothalamus (Groenewegen and Russchen, 1984; Heimer et al., 1990; Nauta et al., 1978). Such connections are typical features of the extended amygdala, rather than any other part of the striatopallidal system.

The extended amygdala

In his classic study of the forebrain, Johnston (1923) noted that the nucleus accumbens, the bed nucleus of the stria terminalis, and the central and medial amygdaloid nuclei appear to constitute an anatomical entity. Jonhston argued that these structures evolved from gray matter enveloping the longitudinal association bundle between forebrain and temporal areas of embryos and lower vertebrates. In his view, pockets of gray matter accompanying the stria terminalis in mammals, represent remnants of this continuous column of neurons. Although Johnston's idea found favor for a time, it eventually fell from current awareness until a few anatomists incorporated this view in their discussions of the basal forebrain or amygdala. The idea was revived especially by de Olmos (1969; 1972; 1990; de Olmos et al., 1985), who argued that the continuity between the bed nucleus of the stria terminalis and the centromedial amygdala (Fig. 8) also includes columns of gray matter located in the sublenticular substantia innominata (Fig. 1C, 9, and 10), in addition to the scattered cells alongside the stria terminalis. This proposition is reinforced by data from a variety of laboratories that have noted the morphological, hodological, or histochemical similarities between the bed nucleus of the stria terminalis and the central and medial nuclei of the amygdala (Holstege et

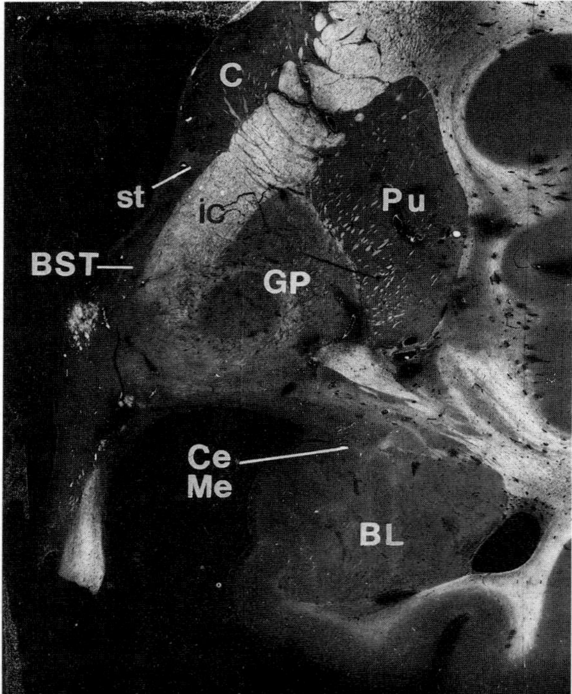

Fig. 8. Direct print of myelin-stained frontal section of the human brain cut at an angle to show the bed nucleus of the stria terminalis (BST) and the amygdaloid body in one plane. Note the dorsal extension of the BST alongside the stria terminalis. BL = basolateral amygdala; C = caudate nucleus; Ce = central amygdaloid nucleus; GP = globus pallidus; Me = medial amygdaloid nucleus; Pu = putamen; st = stria terminalis.

al., 1985; McDonald, 1983; Price et al., 1987; Woodhams et al., 1983), as well as the continuity of these structures across the sublenticular territory intervening between them (see also Alheid

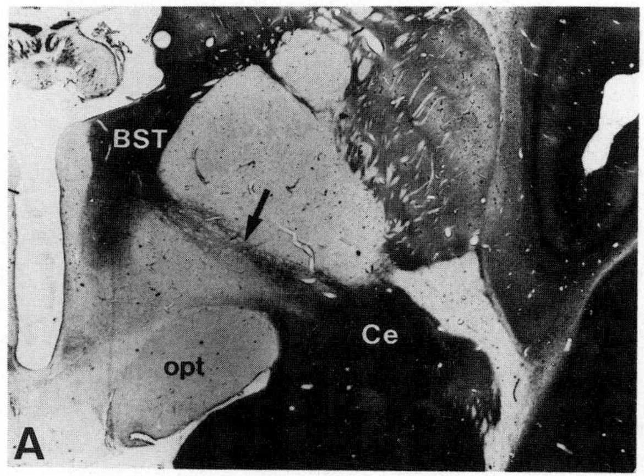

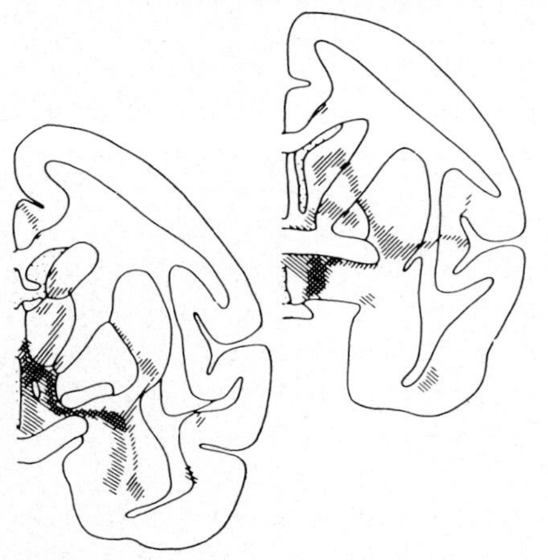

Fig. 9. (A) The extended amygdala demonstrated in a coronal section through the basal ganglia of the marmoset stained with a modified Timm's method for zinc (Danscher, 1982). Note the continuity (arrow) between the bed nucleus of the stria terminalis (BST) and the centromedial amygdala (Ce) (from Alheid et al., 1990; with permission from Academic Press). (B) Picture showing subcortical vocalization areas in the squirrel monkey (from Müller-Preuss and Jürgens, 1976; with permission). The area of heavy cross-hatching which corresponds to the region of the extended amygdala, represents an area of convergence for several pathways originating in vocalization areas of the anterior limbic cortex (Jürgens and Ploog, 1970). Electrical stimulation of the heavily cross-hatched areas yields species-specific vocalization.

and Heimer, 1988; Alheid et al., 1990; Gray, 1988; Grove, 1988a,b; Michel et al., 1988; Moga et al., 1989; Schwaber et al., 1982).

The continuum formed by the centromedial amygdala, sublenticular substantia innominata and bed nucleus of stria terminalis has recently been termed the "extended amygdala" (Alheid and Heimer, 1988). This formidable forebrain structure can be easily appreciated in appropriate sections (Fig. 9; see also Fig. 12 in Alheid and Heimer, 1988 and Fig. 6 in Amaral et al., 1989; see also Bennett-Clarke and Joseph, 1986; Mufson et al., 1988). At both ends of the extended amygdala, i.e., in the bed nucleus of stria terminalis and in the amygdaloid body respectively (Fig. 8; see also Figs. 1C, 12, 13, 14, and 15), are expanded collections of cells compared with the attenuated interconnecting collumns. As indicated earlier, the caudomedial part of the accumbens, which is undoubtedly part of the striatal complex, also has many features typical of the extended amygdala. In fact, in the rat, the shell area of the accumbens (Zaborszky et al., 1985) and even the medial part of the ventral pallidum can be seen to be directly continuous with the rest of the extended amygdala in sections stained with immunohistochemical techniques for a variety of peptides, including cholecystokinin (Zaborszky et al., 1985), neurotensin (Emson et al., 1985; Zahm, 1989), angiotensin II (Alheid and Heimer, 1988; Lind et al., 1985), vasoactive intestinal peptide (Abrams et al., 1985), and proopiomelanocortin (POMC) (Khachaturian et al., 1985). This situation is demonstrated in Fig. 10, using angiotensin II as a marker for the extended amygdala. The shell of the accumbens, likewise, is characterized not only by projection to the ventral pallidum, but to hypothalamus and associative connections to other parts of the extended amygdala (Alheid et al., 1989a; Groenewegen and Russchen, 1984; Heimer et al., 1990; Mogenson et al., 1983). Therefore, the territory of the extended amygdala seems to include as its most rostromedial component, elements of the shell area of the accumbens. To what extent the ventral striatal and extended amygdaloid components interact in the

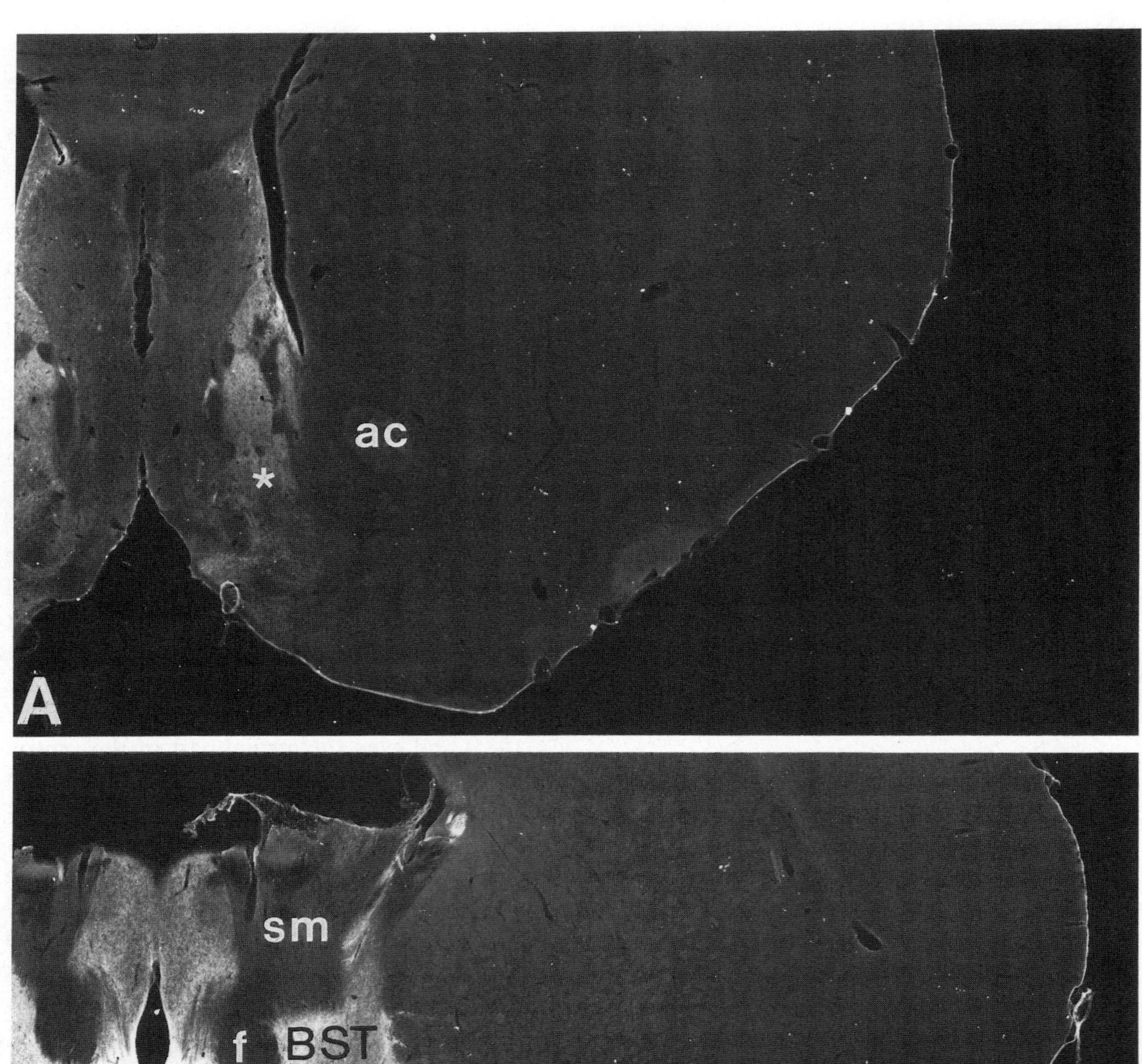
ac
*
A
sm
f
BST
B

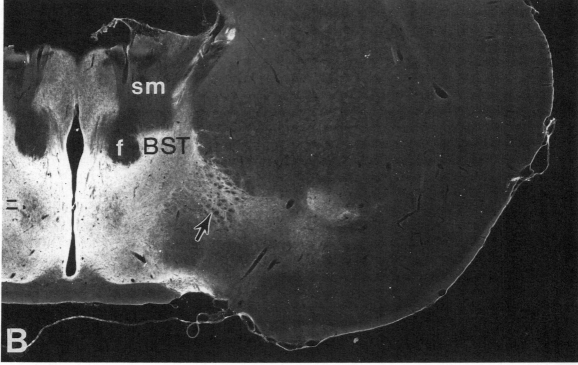

shell of the accumbens is not known.

It should be noted that the term extended amygdala is only applied to cell groups related to the central and medial amygdaloid nuclei. While this may apply to elements of the basomedial amygdala (de Olmos et al., 1985), it does not include the large basolateral complex (Fig. 1C) which is characterized by very different anatomical attributes, when compared with the centromedial amygdala and the rest of the extended amygdala. The large basolateral amygdaloid complex is, in many ways, reminiscent of a cortical structure and its cortical features have often been emphasized (Carlsen and Heimer, 1988; Crosby and Humphrey, 1941; de Olmos et al., 1985; Hall 1972a,b; Lauer, 1945; McDonald, 1984; Millhouse and de Olmos, 1983). Except for its lack of any obvious lamination, its cortical nature is suggested by histochemistry, connections, and cell morphology. The basolateral amygdala is reciprocally connected with a variety of cortical areas (e.g., de Olmos, 1990; Price et al., 1987), including motor or premotor cortex (Avendano et al., 1983; Sripanidkulchai et al., 1984), and it receives direct cholinergic and non-cholinergic input from the magnocellular basal forebrain system (Carlsen et al., 1985; Nagai et al., 1982; Woolf and Butcher, 1982). The basolateral amygdaloid complex is also connected to the thalamus, projecting to the mediodorsal nucleus while receiving afferents from the midline and intralaminar nuclei (Aggleton and Mishkin, 1984; Otterson and Ben Ari, 1979; Price et al., 1987; Russchen et al., 1987), and like the rest of the cerebral cortex, it projects directly to the striatum (e.g., Kelley et al., 1982; Russchen and Price, 1984; Russchen et al., 1985b). It is also closely related to the extended amygdala in the sense that it projects massively into this structure (de Olmos, 1972; 1990; Kelley et al., 1982; Krettek and Price, 1978; Ragsdale and Graybiel, 1988; Russchen and Price, 1984; Russchen et al., 1985a).

Compared to the basolateral amygdaloid complex, the central and medial amygdaloid nuclei have very different anatomical affiliations and neurochemical characteristics, and these have been reviewed in detail in several recent chapters (e.g., de Olmos et al., 1985; de Olmos, 1990; Price et al., 1987). Along with the histochemical similarities, the parallels in the connections between corresponding portions of the bed nucleus of the stria terminalis and the centromedial amygdala, as well as with cells in the interconnecting sublenticular areas, have provided the impetus for the notion of an extended amygdala.

In the following account, several of the more striking features that support the proposition of an amygdala-related forebrain continuum are briefly surveyed. In 1977, Novotny described a specific sublenticular pathway between the amygdaloid body and the bed nucleus of stria terminalis in the primate. The first indication of a significant sublenticular neuronal continuum between the amygdaloid body and the bed nucleus of the stria terminalis was provided in normal rats by the Cupric-silver method (de Olmos, 1969; 1972) which revealed a substantial bridge of granular argyrophilic neuropil and neurons between the central amygdaloid nucleus and the lateral bed nucleus of stria terminalis. More recent reports of normal-anatomical and experimental material, primarily in the rat, but also in the primate, substantiate this original notion of a sublenticular neuronal continuum between the amygdaloid body and the bed nucleus of stria terminalis, and support an expansion of the concept to include the medial amygdala, medial bed nucleus of the stria terminalis, and interconnecting cell groups (Alheid and Heimer, 1988; Alheid et al., 1989b; Amaral et

Fig. 10. Immunostained frontal sections through the rat brain showing the distribution of angiotensin II in the medial shell of the accumbens (asterisk) and medial olfactory tubercle (A), and in a more caudal section (B) in hypothalamus and the bed nucleus of the stria terminalis (BST) and its extension into the sublenticular part of the extended amygdala (arrow). ac = anterior commissure; f = fornix; sm = stria medullaris.

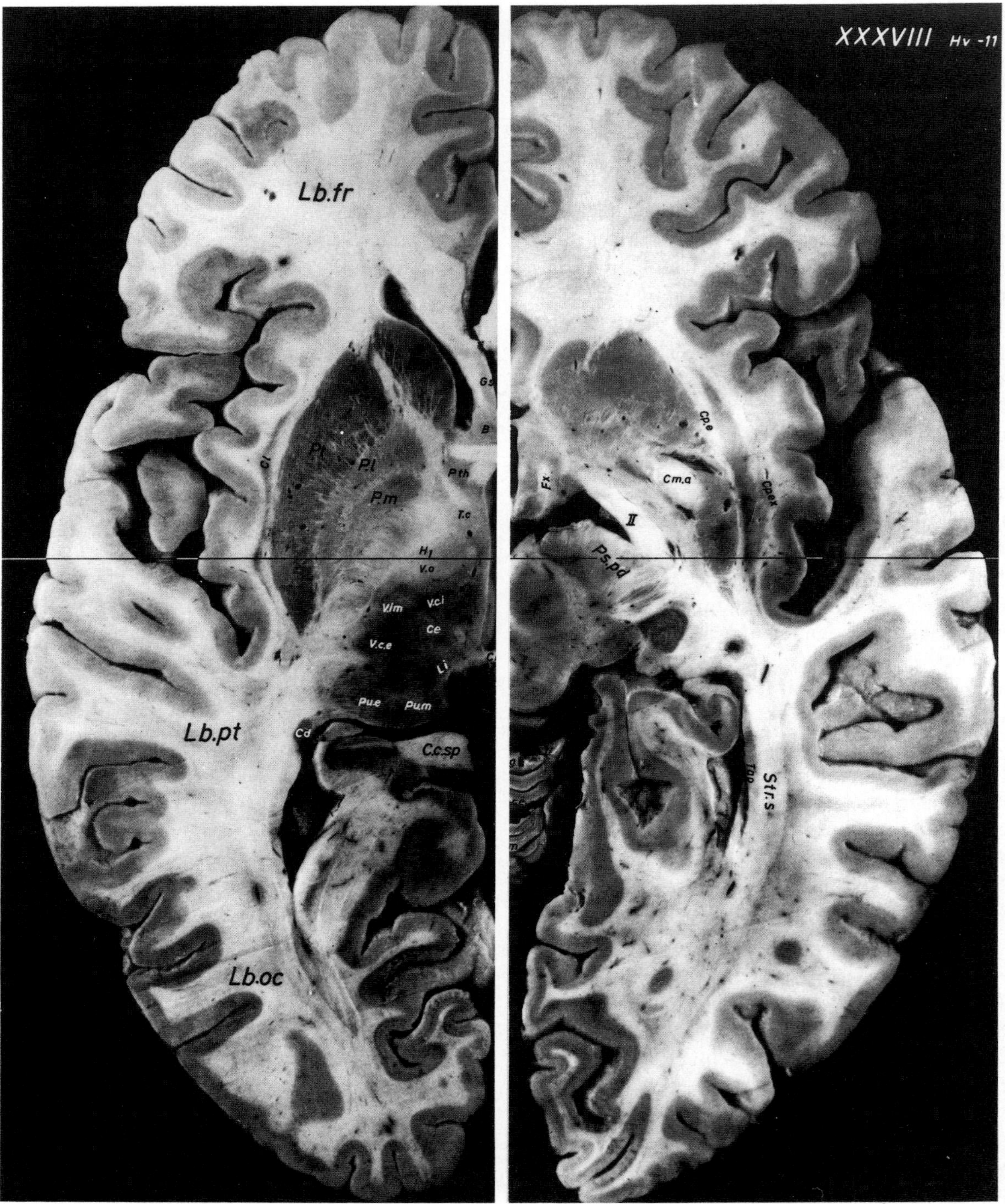

Fig. 11. Horizontal sections through the human brain. The hemisection to the left, which demonstrates the different parts of the dorsal striatopallidal system, represents a more dorsal level than the section to the right, which cuts through the ventral parts of the striatopallidal system and part of the extended amygdala. These two photographs have served as models for the drawings in Figs. 12A and 12B in which the abbreviations reflect a modern nomenclature (from Schaltenbrand and Bailey, 1959 with permission from Georg Thieme Verlag, Stuttgart).

al., 1989; de Olmos et al., 1985; Grove, 1988a,b; Lind et al., 1985; Michel et al., 1988; Moga et al., 1989; Mufson et al., 1988; Price et al., 1987; Schwaber et al., 1982; Zaborszky et al., 1985).

The term "extended amygdala" (Alheid and Heimer, 1988) is suggested to encompass this entire macrostructure, since one might expect that the role of this forebrain continuum should resemble the physiology of the rather more well-studied central and medial amygdaloid nuclei. It should be emphasized, however, that the extended amygdala is formed by two major subdivisions (Fig. 1C and 12B). One consists of the central amygdaloid nucleus, cell columns in the dorsal or anterodorsal sublenticular substantia innominata, and the lateral bed nucleus of stria terminalis (yellow color). The other division consists of the medial amygdaloid nucleus, cell columns in the ventral or posteroventral sublenticular substantia innominata, and the medial bed nucleus of the stria terminalis (green color).

One of the more striking anatomical features that distinguishes these two territories from one another is their connections with the hypothalamus, brainstem and spinal cord; brainstem and more caudal connections are by and large most characteristic of the central extended amygdaloid group. Both territories have close relations to lateral and medial hypothalamus, although the central amygdaloid group is characterized by especially extensive connections with the lateral hypothalamus, while the medial amygdaloid group seems to be more particularly interconnected with several of the nuclear groups in the medial sector of the hypothalamus. On the same basis, several additional nuclei within the amygdala might be loosely grouped with either of the major subdivisions of the "extended amygdala." For example, the intercalated cell islands of the amygdala (Fig, 12C) are found scattered throughout the centromedial amygdala, but also in association with the stria terminalis, the bed nucleus of the stria terminalis, and the posterolateral portions of the anterior commissure. These cell islands appear to have several projections in common with the central amygdaloid group, and we have included them with the central amygdaloid group (de Olmos et al., 1985; de Olmos, 1990). On much the same grounds, the amydalo-striatal transition area (Figs. 1C, 1D, 12A, and 13A) may be associated with the central amygdaloid portions of the extended amygdala, rather than with the medial amygdaloid group. Since this zone does appear to have as much in common with the striatum as it does with the amygdala, we have generally suggested this "mixed nature" by the mixed-color coding in our diagrams.

In a similar vein, the ventral cortical nucleus in primates (e.g., de Olmos, 1990; i.e., the posterolateral cortical nucleus of the rodent according to de Olmos et al., 1985, or portions of the periamygdaloid cortex according to Price et al., 1987), as well as the basomedial nucleus (i.e., basal accessory nucleus of Price et al., 1987), and the amygdalo-hippocampal transition area, appear to be more closely associated with the medial hypothalamus and by analogy, with the medial amygdaloid group of the extended amygdala (Fig. 12D). However, one should keep in mind that the basomedial amygdala has as many similarities with the adjacent basolateral amygdala as it does with the medial amygdaloid portion of the extended amygdala, so that in the case of this nucleus, and perhaps also for the primate ventral cortical nucleus and amygdalohippocampal transition area, the borders of the medial portions of the extended amygdala cannot be precisely drawn.

In primates, the sublenticular portions of the extended amygdala can best be followed in continuity between the centromedial amygdala and the bed nucleus of stria terminalis in coronal sections (Fig. 9). The picture in the human of the extended amygdala is sometimes interrupted, in part, by myelinated fiber bundles. Many of the cells in the sublenticular extended amygdala of the human are medium-sized and elongated, with the larger diameter uniformly diagonally-directed along the orientation of the interconnecting fiber bundles. This feature is usually enough to distinguish the extended amygdaloid cell columns from cells in the

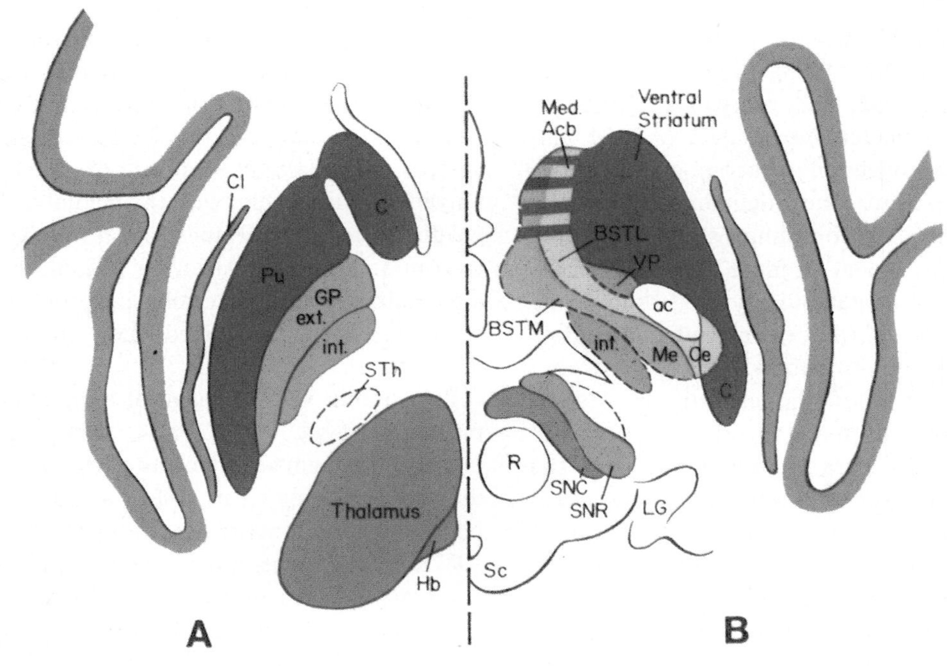

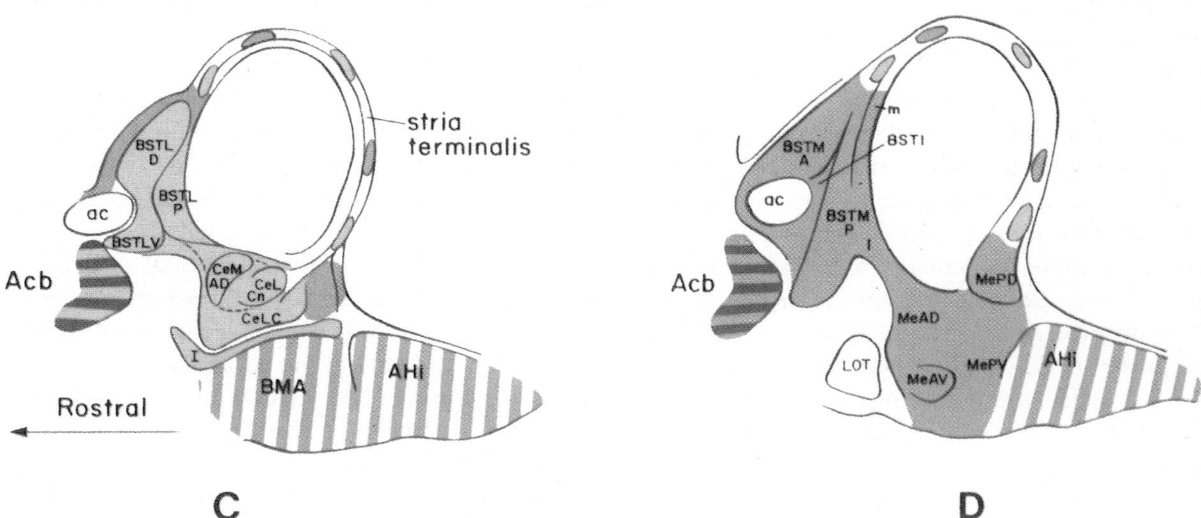

Fig. 12. The drawings in A and B represent a close rendition of the topographical anatomy shown in the two horizontal sections in Fig. 11, although with some artistic liberty especially in regard to the delineation of the extended amygdala and the ventral striatopallidal complex in the more ventrally located section to the right. C and D represent drawings of the two main components of the rat extended amygdala in the sagittal plane with special emphasis on the various subdivisions within the two main extended amygdaloid components. With stria terminalis making a dorsally convex detour above the internal capsule, the extension of the

ventral striatopallidal system, or from the polymorphic hyperchromic cells of the magnocellular corticopetal cell system, which interdigitates to a significant degree with the extended amygdala (Fig. 1C).

The extended amygdala has many features that distinguishes it from surrounding neuronal systems, including a high degree of internal associative connections as well as widespread connections with a large number of structures in various parts of the brain and brainstem, including, presumably, the spinal cord (see below). However, there are also a number of distinctive characteristics for each of the major subdivisions of the extended amygdala. As already indicated, the more dorsally located extension of the central amygdaloid nucleus, for instance, is characterized by argyrophilic neuropil (de Olmos, 1969) and by immunoreactivity for a large number of neuropeptides, most of which are also found in the adjacent basal ganglia. One possible exception to this is angiotensin II immunoreactivity, which is rather dense in both divisions of the extended amygdala, but almost non-existent within the basal ganglia. This immunoreactivity does not, however, have a distinctive border with adjacent territories of the diencephalon (Fig. 10). In contrast, zinc containing terminals are found in the striatum and are especially dense in both divisions of the extended amygdala, but for the most part, are very scarce in adjacent portions of the diencephalon (Fig. 9A).

The basal nucleus of Meynert and the magnocellular corticopetal forebrain complex

Morphological studies over the past 20 years have revealed that the cerebral cortex, amygdaloid body, and thalamus receive projections from a widely dispersed, more or less continuous collection of aggregated and non-aggregated cells which occupy extensive territories in the basal forebrain, but in particular the medial septum, diagonal band of Broca (vertical and horizontal limbs), sublenticular substantia innominata (much of which constitutes the extended amygdala), and peripallidal regions (Amaral and Kurtz, 1985; Butcher and Woolf, 1986; Carlsen et al., 1985; Mesulam et al., 1983; Paxinos and Butcher, 1985; Rye et al., 1984; Schwaber et al., 1987; Sofroniew et al., 1985; Woolf et al., 1984). Although close to 90% of the neurons projecting to the neocortex in rat and monkeys are cholinergic (Everitt et al., 1988; Mesulam et al., 1983; Saper and Chelimsky, 1984), many of the neurons projecting to allocortical areas including the hippocampus, olfactory cortex, olfactory bulb, and the amygdala are non-cholinergic using either GABA, and possibly a number of peptides as transmitters (Caffé et al., 1989; Fisher et al., 1988; Melander et al., 1985; Ulfig et al., 1990; Vincent et al., 1985; Walker et al., 1989; Zaborszky et al., 1986). This system of cholinergic and non-cholinergic corticopetal neurons, which are intermingled to varying degree, has been referred to as the "magnocellular corticopetal cell complex" or "magnocellular basal forebrain system" (e.g., Alheid and Heimer, 1988; Divac, 1975; Hedreen et al., 1984; Saper, 1987; Walker et al., 1989).

The magnocellular basal forebrain system is a prominent feature in all mammals, although there are some inter-specific differences in regard to the

central and medial amygdaloid groups do in fact appear as a ring formation around the internal capsule. ac = anterior commissure; Acb = accumbens; AHI = amygdalo-hippocampal transition area; BMA = basomedial amygdaloid nucleus, anterior part; BSTI = bed nucleus of the stria terminalis, intermediate division; BSTLD, BSTLP, BSTLV = bed nucleus of the stria terminalis, lateral division, dorsal, posterior, ventral parts; BSTMA, BSTMPI, BSTMPm = bed nucleus of the stria terminalis, medial division, anterior, posterolateral, posteromedial parts; C = caudate nucleus; Ce = central amygdaloid nucleus; CeLC, CelCn = central amygdaloid nucleus, lateral division, capsular, central parts; CeMAD = central amygdaloid nucleus, medial division, anterodorsal part; GPext = globus pallidus, external segment; Hb = habenula; int = globus pallidus, internal segment; LG = lateral geniculate nucleus; LOT = nucleus of the lateral olfactory tract; MeAD, MeAV, MePD, MePV = medial amygdaloid nucleus, anterodorsal, anteroventral, posterodorsal, posteroventral parts; Pu = putamen; R = red nucleus; Sc = superior colliculus; SNC = substantia nigra, pars compacta; SNR = substantia nigra, pars reticulata; STh = subthalamic nucleus; VP = ventral pallidum.

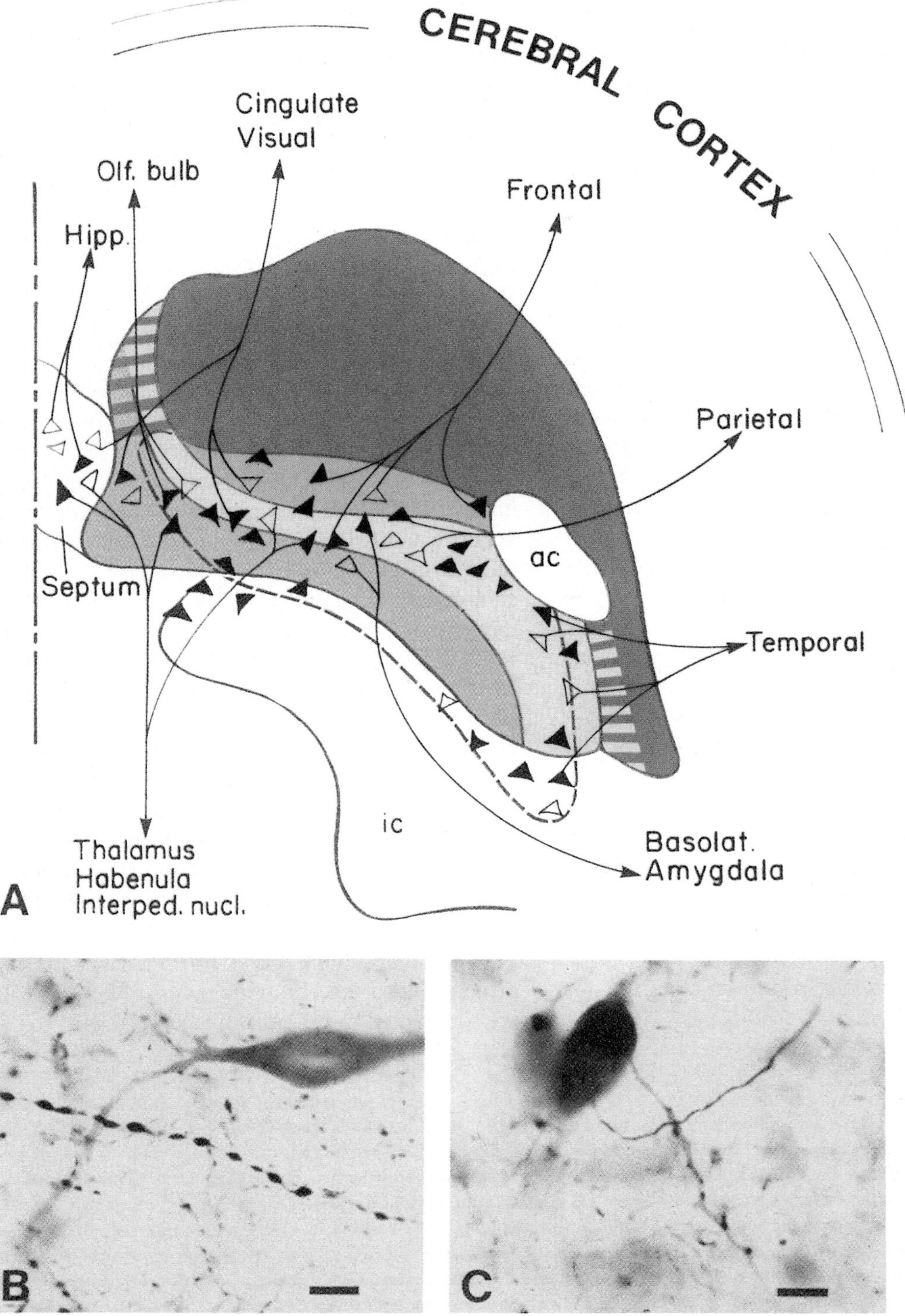
CEREBRAL CORTEX
Cingulate
Visual
Olf. bulb
Frontal
Hipp.
Parietal
ac
Septum
Temporal
ic
Thalamus
Habenula
Interped. nucl.
Basolat.
Amygdala
A
B
C

extent to which individual cells aggregate into more or less confined nuclear groups. This tendency towards cellular aggregation is most pronounced in the primate, where one of the major components with prominent projections to neocortex and amygdala is identified as the basal nucleus of Meynert (Kölliker, 1896; Meynert, 1872). Even so, the cells projecting to the neocortex occupy an extensive territory and the boundaries for this dispersed group of cells are so diffuse as to defy the very term "nucleus". Rather, the basal nucleus of Meynert directly continues rostromedially with the nucleus of the diagonal band and its cells invade extensively and to varying degrees, other basal forebrain structures including the basal ganglia and the extended amygdala as indicated in the drawings (Figs. 1 and 13A).

The intermingling of large cholinergic neurons with the pallidal complex is most obvious at the base of the primate brain (Fig. 7) in an area which has only recently been shown to contain ventral extensions of the pallidal complex referred to as ventral pallidum (Alheid and Heimer, 1988; Alheid et al., 1990; Haber, 1987). This situation is schematically depicted in Fig. 1B, where ventral pallidal "fingers" can be seen to interdigitate with ventral striatal tissue. Just dorsally, the magnocellular cells are primarily located in the medullary laminae of the globus pallidus, and interestingly, not seldom within the interal capsule (Fig. 1B). Caudal to the ventral pallidum, in the region of the sublenticular substantia innominata (Fig. 1C), the magnocellular complex is rather more segregated from the pallidum, except for the peripallidal cells located in the medullary laminae and internal capsule. On the other hand, a significant part of the magnocellular complex at this level interdigitates with elements of the extended amygdala. In the primate, the extent of this widely dispersed complex of a more or less well-defined cell group can be best illustrated in horizontal sections (Fig. 13A; see also Figs. 95 – 97 in Johnston, 1923; Fig. 4 in Jones et al., 1976; and Figs. 19, 32 in Alheid et al., 1990).

As indicated earlier, the different subpopulations of the cholinergic system have been designated as "Ch1-4" by Mesulam and his colleagues in primates (Mesulam et al., 1983), and the basal nucleus of Meynert corresponds to cell group Ch4 in Mesulam's nomenclature.*

Experimental neuroanatomical methods in monkeys have shown that different cortical areas receive their major cholinergic input from individual sectors of the nucleus basalis complex (Fig. 13A), and indirect evidence has suggested the existence of a topographic arrangement also in the human brain from postmortem examination of brains of Alzheimer's Disease patients (Mesulam and Geula, 1988). Individual cholinergic corticopetal axons have a rather restricted zone of termination (Eckenstein et al., 1988), concordant with a general absence of divergent collaterals to remote cortical or subcortical areas (Koliatsos et

* It seems to be a general consensus that the Ch-nomenclature applies best to primates. It does not seem to be useful in rodents (e.g., Carlsen et al., 1985) where it may even be misleading (Butcher and Semba, 1989).

Fig. 13. (A) Schematic drawing of a horizontal section (see Fig. 12B) to show the topographic distribution of the magnocellular cortico-, amygdalo-, and thalamopetal system containing both cholinergic (solid black triangles) and noncholinergic (open triangles) neurons. In this figure, extra effort was made to depict the overall outline of the extended amygdala and globus pallidus (dotted lines) as they actually might appear in a horizontal section of the human brain. The close correspondence of the magnocellular complex with the ventral parts of the pallidal complex and the body of the extended amygdala should be appreciated. B and C photomicrographs of double-immunostained sections from rat brain to show the relationship between cholinergic neurons (brown; stained with an antibody against choline acetyltransferase) and noradrenergic/adrenergic axons (black-purple; stained with an antibody against dopamine-β-hydroxylase; DAB DAB-nickel technique). The neuron in (B), located in the bed nucleus of the stria terminalis, is surrounded by different types of monoaminergic fibers showing a large number of varicosities, presumable representing endstructures. The neuron in (C) is located in the sublenticular part of the extended amygdala. Note the numerous catecholaminergic varicosities alongside the dendrite, reminiscent of a climbing fiber. © Dr. L. Heimer.

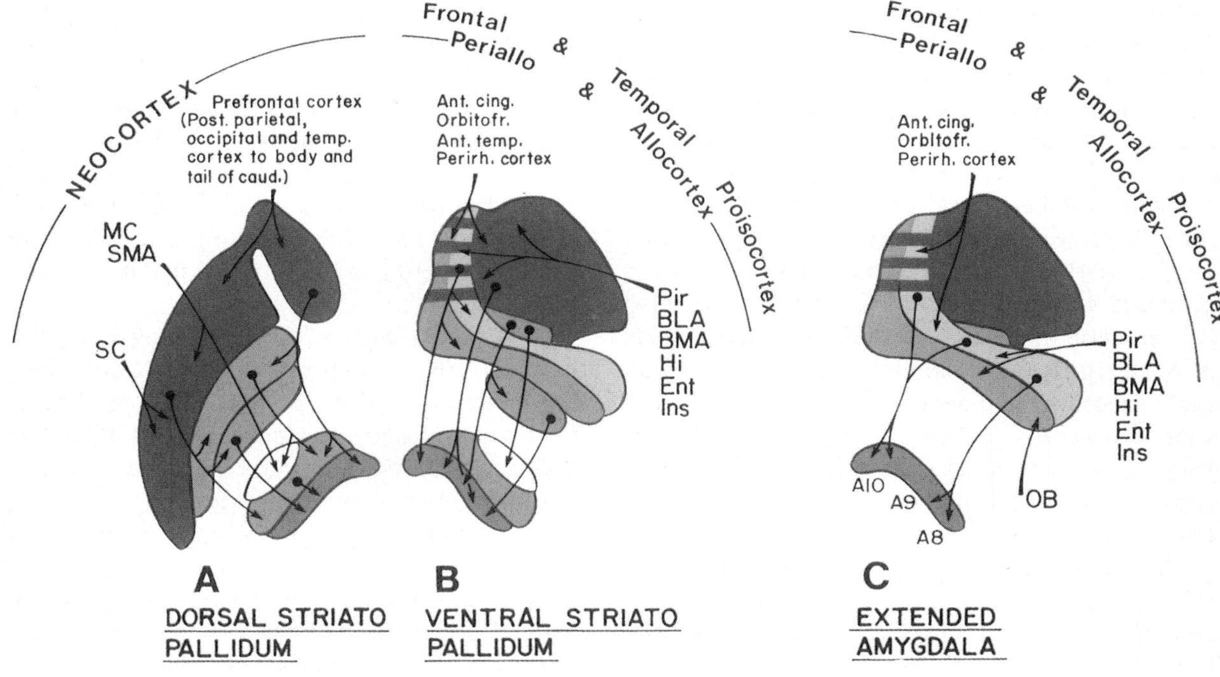
NEOCORTEX
Prefrontal cortex
(Post. parietal, occipital and temp. cortex to body and tail of caud.)
MC
SMA
SC
Frontal
Periallo
&
Temporal
&
Allocortex
Proisocortex
Ant. cing.
Orbitofr.
Ant. temp.
Perirh. cortex
Pir
BLA
BMA
Hi
Ent
Ins
Ant. cing.
Orbitofr.
Perirh. cortex
A10
A9
A8
OB
A
DORSAL STRIATO PALLIDUM
B
VENTRAL STRIATO PALLIDUM
C
EXTENDED AMYGDALA

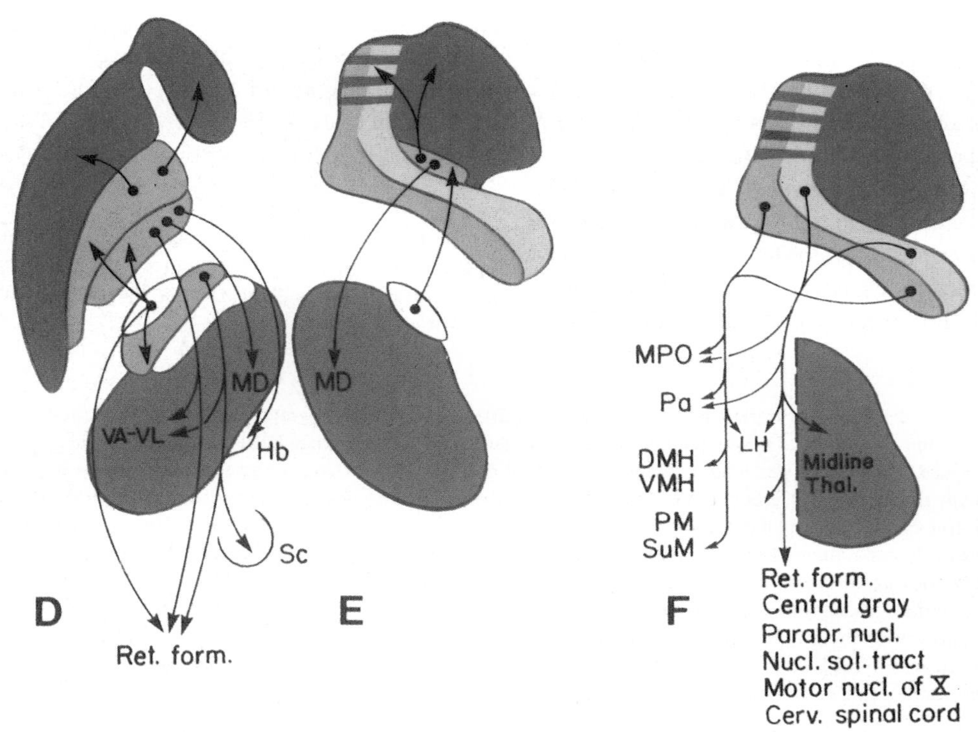
MD
VA-VL
Hb
Sc
Ret. form.
D
MD
E
MPO
Pa
DMH
VMH
PM
SuM
LH
Midline Thal.
F
Ret. form.
Central gray
Parabr. nucl.
Nucl. sol. tract
Motor nucl. of X
Cerv. spinal cord

al., 1988; Price and Stern, 1983; Walker et al., 1985). Subpopulations of cholinergic neurons, therefore, may be able to selectively influence restricted cortical areas. This is consistent with postmortem studies, which have shown that the disease process in Alzheimer's disease often differentially affects individual sectors of Ch4, correlating with the pathological changes in the cortex (Arendt et al., 1985). In contrast to this relative specificity in the efferent projections of the cholinergic system, is the apparent diffuse array of afferents to regions containing cholinergic projection neurons (see below).

Highlights of the neuronal circuitry in basal forebrain

Documenting the systematic organization of basal forebrain connections presents a significant challenge. While the afferents and efferents of the dorsal parts of the striatum are rather well understood (e.g., Alexander et al., 1986; Alheid et al., 1990; Carpenter, 1986; 1981; Gerfen, 1988; Graybiel and Ragsdale, 1979; 1983; Heimer et al., 1985; Kitai, 1981; Mehler, 1982; Mehler and Nauta, 1974; Nauta and Domesick, 1984; Nauta and Mehler, 1966), the connections of the ventral parts of the basal forebrain appear as a tangled web, particularly as a result of the interwoven aspect of the ventral striatopallidal system and the extended amygdala with the cells belonging to the corticopetal complex of neurons. In particular, the close contiguity of the magnocellular corticopetal complex and the central amygdaloid subdivision of the extended amygdala mitigates against the identification of specific afferents to the corticopetal cells, except when they occur in isolated clusters, such as in the diagonal band nuclei or in the compact part of the basal nucleus of Meynert in primates. Even in these latter instances it is likely that the afferent systems are underestimated since the extensive dendritic arborizations of these large hyperchromic cells may extend their receptive zone well beyond the obvious accumulation of cell bodies.

Since we have in several recent papers considered the connections of the ventral forebrain in detail (Alheid and Heimer, 1988; Alheid et al., 1989b, 1990; de Olmos 1990; de Olmos et al., 1985; Heimer et al., 1985; Zaborszky 1989), we will only discuss here the comparison between the afferents and efferents of the different systems in basal forebrain in order to aid in the discrimination between them and to facilitate our subsequent discussion of clinical-anatomical correlations. A visual summary is provided in the schematic Figs. 13 – 15 of basal forebrain connections.

Descending corticofugal pathways

While practically the entire cortical mantle participates in the formation of a cortico-striato-pallidal complex (Figs. 14A and 14B) only a subset of these cortical areas provide innervation to the extended amygdala (Fig. 14C), and directly or indirectly, to the magnocellular corticopetal complex of the basal forebrain.

The striatopallidal system. In general, for dorsal striatum, neocortical (isocortical) afferents predominate with somatomotor areas of cortex

Fig. 14. Upper row: schematic drawings of the cortical input to the main dorsal parts of the basal ganglia (A), the ventral striatopallidal system (B), and the extended amygdala (C), and their descending projections to the subthalamic nucleus and substantia nigra. Lower row: descending projections from dorsal (D) and ventral (E) parts of the basal ganglia and from the extended amygdala (F). BLA = basolateral amygdala; BMA = basomedial amygdala; DMH = dorsomedial hypothalamic nucleus; Ent = entorhinal area; Hb = habenula; Hi = hippocampus; Ins = insula; LH = lateral hypothalamus; MC = motor cortex; MD = mediodorsal thalamic nucleus; MPO = medial preoptic area; Pa = paraventricular nucleus; Pir = piriform cortex; PM = premamillary region; OB = olfactory bulb; Sc = superior colliculus; SC = somatosensory cortex; SMA = supplementary motor area; SuM = supramamillary region; VA-VL = ventral anterior and ventral lareral thalamic complex; VMH = ventromedial hypothalamic nucleus. © Dr. L. Heimer.

particularly projecting to the putamen, while sensory and association areas including prefrontal cortex, send their afferents to the caudate nucleus (see reviews by Alexander et al., 1986; Alheid et al., 1990; Goldman-Rakic and Selemon, 1986). An exceptional input vis- à- vis the generally neocortical aspect of dorsal striatum, is represented by the afferents from the basolateral amygdaloid complex (Kelley et al., 1982; Ragsdale and Graybiel, 1988; Russchen et al., 1985b) which, however, project more heavily to the ventral striatum. Nonetheless, the basolateral amygdala together with the neocortical areas in the temporal lobe and the anterior cingulate cortex are territories that appear to innervate both dorsal and ventral striatum (Van Hoesen et al., 1976; 1981). Olfactory afferents, either directly from the olfactory bulb or indirectly from olfactory (piriform) cortex, as well as afferents from hippocampus, entorhinal area, anterior cingulate, and insular cortices also contribute to the innervation of the ventral striatum (see review by Alheid et al., 1990).

The subthalamic nucleus which appears to reciprocate connections with both the dorsal and ventral pallidum is remarkable in that it receives direct afferents from motor-premotor cortex (Hartmann-Von Monakow et al., 1978; Kitai and Deniau, 1981; Künzle, 1976; 1978; Künzle and Akert, 1977; Petras, 1969; Rinvik et al., 1979; Romansky et al., 1979). The dopaminergic cells in the substantia nigra-ventral tegmental area, likewise receive direct cortical input from prefrontal and premotor cortices (e.g., Beckstead, 1979; Bunney and Aghajanian, 1976; Gerfen et al., 1982; Künzle, 1978; Phillipson, 1979; Room et al., 1985; Sakai, 1988; Wyss and Sripanidkulchai, 1984; and reviews by Alheid et al., 1990; Fallon and Loughlin, 1987).

The extended amygdala. Cortical afferents to the extended amygdala to a degree mirror those of the ventral striatum, and include axons originating in the olfactory bulb, olfactory cortex, hippocampus, entorhinal cortex, perirhinal cortex, insula, orbitofrontal cortex and the anterior cingulate cortex, as well as afferents from the basolateral amygdaloid complex (Fig. 14C; for reviews see de Olmos, 1990; de Olmos et al., 1985; Price et al., 1987). For the extended amygdala, afferents from the olfactory bulb in the primate only reach the medial amygdaloid subdivision (Price, 1990; Turner et al., 1978), whereas cortical afferents from frontal cortex and from perirhinal cortex terminate preferentially in the central amygdaloid subdivision of the extended amygdala (Van Hoesen, 1981).

The magnocellular forebrain complex. Cortical afferents to the magnocellular forebrain complex are, as we have suggested above, difficult to resolve. Moreover, few of the reported experiments to date are of sufficient resolution to discriminate between afferents to corticopetal cells themselves, or to any possible associated interneuronal system, or to adjacent portions of the extended amygdala. Because of the proximity of these structures, direct synaptic contacts need to be verified by electron microscopy combined with immunohistochemical and/or tracing techniques (e.g., Lemann and Saper, 1985; Zaborszky et al., 1984). In general, the same areas that innervate the extended amygdala are identified as candidate afferents to the magnocellular complex. While this does not provide much leverage in discriminating whether exactly the same cortical areas project to both neuronal substrates, it is notable that many of the neocortical areas that receive innervation from the magnocellular neurons of basal forebrain do not seem to directly reciprocate these inputs (Mesulam and Mufson, 1984). For example, primary sensory and motor cortex, as well as parietal association areas do not project to the vicinity of the magnocellular complex.

An exception to the general problem of the afferents to the magnocellular complex are the corticopetal cells in the medial septum/diagonal band complex, which are, for the most part, clear of the nearby striatopallidal and extended amygdaloid territories. The cells in the septum-diagonal band complex receive reciprocating projections from the hippocampus, although the bulk of the hippocampal feedback appears to occur via a relay in the lateral septum, and it appears likely that no direct afferents from hippocampus synapse on cholinergic neurons (Leranth and Frotscher, 1989). Other cortical afferents potentially targeting the diagonal band complex come from orbitofrontal cortex, anterior cingulate areas, retrosplenial cortex, insular, piriform, and entorhinal cortex (for review see Zaborszky, 1989).

Descending projections from the basal forebrain systems

The striatopallidal system. Within the striatopallidal system, striatal areas are the main recipient of cortical input, and the striatal output is directed toward the external pallidal segment, the internal pallidal segment, including pars reticulata of the substantia nigra, as well at to the dopaminergic cells in the pars compacta of substantia nigra (Fig. 14A). Each one of these projections come mainly from separate striatal cell populations (Beckstead and Cruz, 1986; Féger and Crossman, 1984; Parent et al., 1984; Smith and Parent, 1986). The external pallidum receives striatal input from a more or less distinct population of neurons that use GABA and met-enkephalin as cotransmitters, and which may in some instances also contain neurotensin (e.g. Aronin et al., 1984; Haber and Elde, 1981; Sugimoto and Mizuno, 1987; Zahm et al., 1985) while another population of striatal neurons which use at least substance P and GABA as cotransmitters (Penny et al., 1986), send projections to the internal pallidal segment and to the closely related pars reticulata. The distribution of efferents from the striatum is such that the main source of efferents to the primate dorsal pallidum appears to be from the putamen while the caudate projects more massively to the substantia nigra pars reticulata (Féger and Crossman, 1984; Parent et al., 1984; Smith and Parent, 1986).

The ventral striatum presents a rather more complicated problem insofar as the components of the ventral pallidum corresponding to the external and internal segment of dorsal pallidum seem to occur in a mixed fashion with both substance P and met-enkephalin immunoreactivities (coexisting with GABAergic markers) appearing rather dense in the subcommissural pallidal zone (Alheid and Heimer, 1988; Alheid et al., 1990; Haber and Nauta, 1983; Haber and Watson, 1985; Heimer et al., 1985; Mai et al., 1986; Mai and Cuello, 1990). This overlap, however, is not complete since substance P appears to be more dense ventrally and medially, while met-enkephalin immunoreactivity appears more dense dorsolaterally (see discussion in Alheid and Heimer 1988; Alheid et al., 1990; see also Sakamoto et al., 1988). The nucleus accumbens is the main source of afferents to the immediately subcommissural portion of the ventral pallidum, (Heimer and Wilson, 1975; Mogenson et al., 1983; Swanson and Cowan, 1975) while the olfactory tubercle projects directly to the pallidal fingers that help to from the deep polymorph layers of the olfactory tubercle, but also, at least in the rat, to a deeper lateral portion of the immediate subcommisural ventral pallidum (Heimer et al., 1987). Interestingly, in the primate the nucleus accumbens projects also to the medial tip of the internal pallidal segment, (Alheid et al., 1989a; 1990; Hedreen and DeLong, 1986, cited in Alexander et al., 1986; Lynd et al., 1988) so that the accumbens appears to be well integrated in the better known pallidofugal systems represented by the output of the internal pallidal segment. It does appear likely that separate populations of cells in the accumbens and olfactory tubercle give rise to the enkephalinergic or substance P projections to ventral pallidal areas.

One additional complication in ventral striatum is the existence of a small projection to the area of the midline thalamus involving the paraventricular nucleus of the thalamus and perhaps the most medial portions of the mediodorsal thalamic nucleus (Alheid et al., 1989a; Groenewegen, 1988). Striatothalamic projections are not generally recognized, but projections to the paraventricular nucleus have been reported for the rat globus pallidus (see below).

The external pallidal segment plays a rather

complicated role in the organization of basal ganglia output, for aside from the direct projections of this nucleus to the internal pallidal segment-substantia nigra pars reticulata and subthalamic nucleus, connections have been observed between the external segment and the thalamus (Groenewegen, 1988; Hattori and Sugimoto, 1983; Young et al., 1984). At least in the rat, several of the projection systems from the external pallidal segment have been shown to be collateralized in the sense that individual neurons may project to the internal pallidal segment and in addition send a recurrent branch to striatum (Kitai and Kita, 1984), whereas other neurons project to both substantia nigra and striatum (Staines and Fibiger, 1984). Still other neurons apparently have branching axons with terminations both in thalamus and striatum (Takada et al., 1986). In the ventral pallidum similar projections have been observed; neurons projecting to mediodorsal thalamus are more numerous than their counterpart in the dorsal pallidum (Hreib et al., 1988; Mogenson et al., 1987; Price and Slotnick, 1983; Young et al., 1984) and we have in the past likened the output from these cells to the pallidothalamic projection from the internal pallidal segment and pars reticulata substantia nigra. However, the fact that accumbens efferents reach both ventral pallidum and the internal pallidal segment, suggests that the pallidal efferents to mediodorsal thalamus from both dorsal and ventral pallidum might represent an additional circuit in striatopallidal processing. Ventral pallidum also appears to send a significant projection to the nucleus accumbens (Beckstead, 1983; Haber et al., 1985) which originates in noncholinergic cells, and appears quite massive when retrogradely labeled and compared with the dorsal pallidostriatal pathway (Alheid, unpublished observations), so that the likelihood is high that ventral pallidothalamic and pallidostriatal projections originate from single neurons with bifurcating axons.

Projections from the internal pallidal segment, from pars reticulata substantia nigra, and perhaps equivalent neurons in the ventral pallidum appear to represent the major exit pathway from the basal ganglia (Figs. 14D and 14E). These include a variety of targets, including the ventral anterior ventrolateral thalamus, the lateral habenula, the mesencephalic dopamine cell complex, the superior colliculus, and the brainstem reticular formation. Efferents to the thalamus including the internal and ventral pallidal projections to the mediodorsal thalamus appear to quickly reenter the basal ganglia via a transthalamic, transcortical route that by and large should carry the information back to the original parallel corridors within the striatum and pallidum (e.g. see Alexander et al., 1986). Similarly, pallidal efferents directed at dopaminergic targets also appear to result in reentry to basal ganglia via direct projections back to striatum, but perhaps also through dopaminergic synapses in cortex. Efferents to the lateral habenula are of unknown significance but appear to be subsequently referred to brainstem areas such as the raphe nuclei which in turn project to the basal ganglia but also to widespread areas of the telencephalon. Following the pioneering study of the projection of the lentiform nucleus by Nauta and Mehler (1966), basal ganglia projections to the brainstem reticular formation have now been well established (see discussion in Alheid et al., 1990). Axons reaching the superior colliculus and reticular formation appear to target motor zones, with the former involved in the oculomotor control system while at least some of the latter efferents seem to be related to locomotion (Garcia-Rill et al., 1981; Garcia-Rill et al., 1983a,b).

The extended amygdala. We cannot, at the present time, present a coherent picture of synaptic links internal to the extended amygdala that are in any way comparable to the fine detail available for the striatopallidal system. Nonetheless, distinctive subterritories exist within each of the two subdivisions of the extended amygdala (e.g., Figs. 12C and 12D) and it will be a challenge for future research to define the fine grain of synaptic processing intrinsic to these structures. The central amygdaloid portion of the extended amygdala is in many respects superficially similar to a simplified version of the striatopallidal system (Alheid and Heimer, 1988; Alheid et al., 1989b; 1990; Fallon and Loughlin, 1987) with medium-sized densely spiny cells in the lateral portions of the central nucleus and in the lateral portions of the bed nucleus of the stria terminalis resembling those in the mass of the striatum. Aspiny fusiform cells in the medial part of the central amygdaloid nucleus, in the interconnecting sublenticular parts of the extended amygdala, and in the ventral and posterior portions of the lateral bed nucleus of the stria terminalis, superficially resemble pallidal cells. Both spiny and aspiny cell types, however, give rise to descending projections to the brainstem (Fig. 14F; Moga and Gray, 1985a,b). These important pathways reach the ventral tegmental area, pars compacta substantia nigra, and peripeduncular nucleus but also the midbrain reticular formation, the central gray, parabrachial nucleus, nucleus of the solitary tract, dorsal motor nucleus of the vagus, nucleus ambiguous, trigeminal nucleus, probably the locus coeruleus, as well as other brainstem catecholamine cells and the cervical spinal cord (Danielson et al., 1989; de Olmos et al., 1985; Gray and Magnuson, 1987; Grove, 1988b; Holstege et al., 1985; Hopkins, 1975; Hopkins and Holstege, 1978; Mizuno et al., 1985; Moga and Gray, 1985a,b; Moga et al., 1989; Price and Amaral, 1981; Price et al., 1987; Sandrew et al., 1986; Schwaber et al., 1982; Veening et al., 1984).

Distinctive from the striatopallidal system, the extended amygdala demonstrates a striking amount of internal collaterals. That is, long axons interconnect the rostral and caudal parts of the extended amygdala. In general, the topography of the two main subdivisions of the extended amygdala are maintained in this system of collaterals insofar as internal projections from the central amygdaloid nucleus or from the lateral bed nucleus of the stria terminalis seem to stay within the central amygdaloid division, and internal projections from the medial amygdaloid nucleus and medial bed nucleus of the stria terminalis are more directed within the medial amygdaloid division (see reviews by de Olmos et al., 1985; Grove, 1988b; Price et al., 1987). A larger contingent of projections, however, are directed from the medial amygdaloid subdivision to the central amygdaloid zones, and in fact, most other amygdaloid nuclei provide afferents to the central subdivision of the extended amygdala. In this respect the latter represents an important nexus for amygdaloid information directed caudal to the hypothalamus and as an indirect influence on the ascending efferents of the central subdivision directed toward the magnocellular corticopetal cells in basal forebrain (see below). The extensive system of collaterals within the extended amygdala appears to represent a functionally important distinction between this structure and the striatum which seems to be rather tightly organized in parallel channels (see above, and reviews in Alexander et al., 1986; Alheid et al., 1990; Percheron et al., 1984).

At the level of the hypothalamus, the central amygdaloid portion of the extended amygdala gives rise to a dense field of terminals in the lateral hypothalamus, but also appears to innervate the medial preoptic-anterior hypothalamic area, the paraventricular nucleus, dorsal hypothalamus and dorsomedial nuclei and the premammillary and supramammillary regions as well as the tuberomammillary nuclei (Gray et al., 1989; Grove, 1988b; Krettek and Price, 1978; Price and Amaral, 1981; see also de Olmos, 1990; de Olmos et al., 1985; Price et al., 1987). The medial subdivision of the extended amygdala targets particularly the medial territories of the hypothalamus including the medial preoptic area, the anterior hypothalamic area, the ventromedial and dorsomedial hypothalamic nuclei, and areas in and around the paraventricular hypothalamic nucleus and the premammillary nuclei (de Olmos et al., 1985; Gray et al., 1989; Grove, 1988b; Kevetter and Winans, 1981a,b; Krettek and Price, 1978; Price et al., 1987). The medial subdivision of the extended amygdala also sends a moderate number of axons to the brainstem, reaching the ventral tegmentum, and the area in and just adjacent to the central gray (de Olmos et al., 1985; see also de

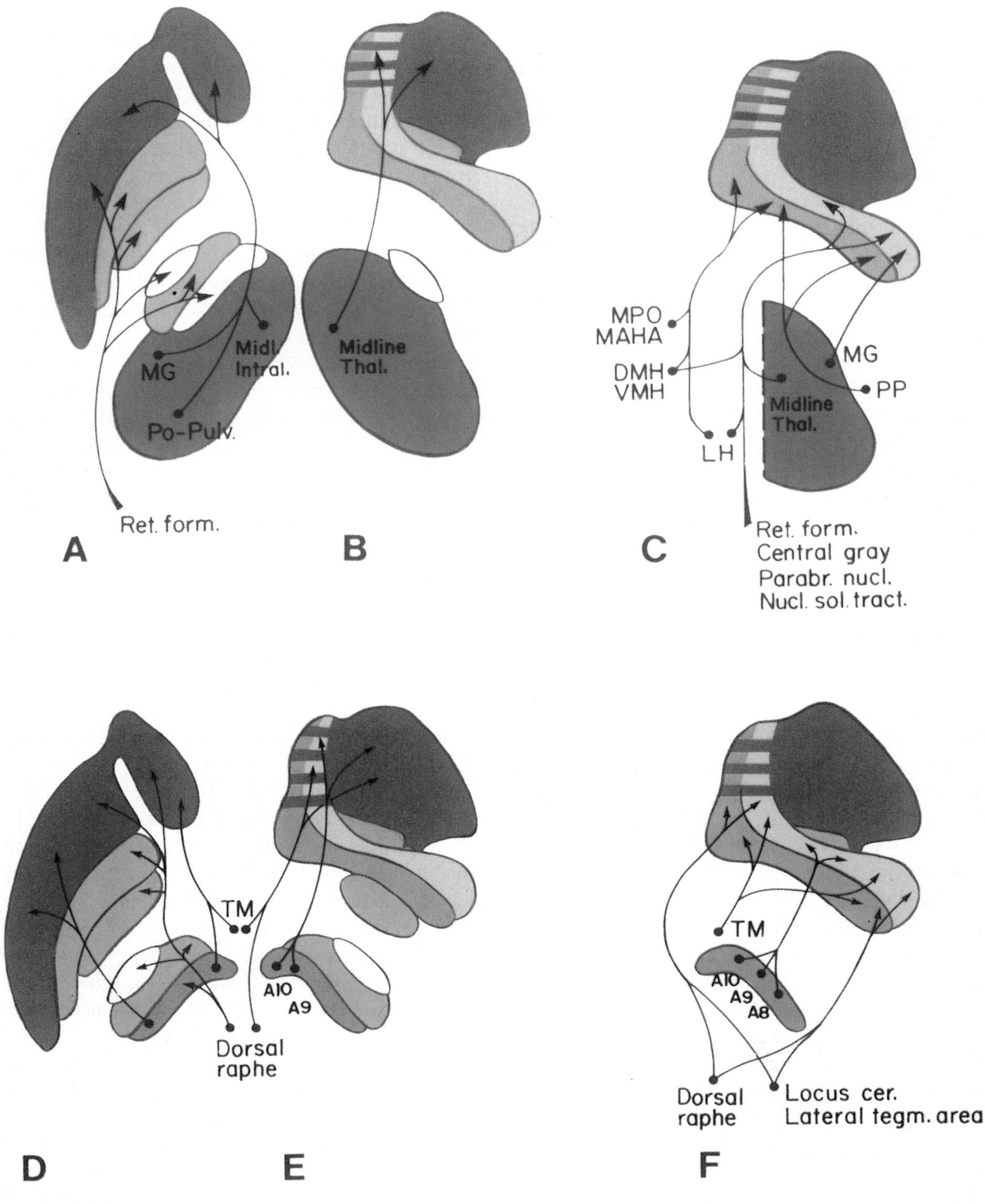

Fig. 15. Upper row: thalamic and brainstem projections to the dorsal (A) and ventral (B) parts of the basal ganglia, and to the extended amygdala (C). Lower row: ascending monoaminergic and histaminergic pathways to the dorsal (D) and ventral (E) parts of the

Olmos, 1990).

Thalamic targets of the extended amygdala are found in the midline nuclei, i.e. nucleus reuniens, the rhomboid nucleus (or central nuclear complex), and medial pulvinar, but in contrast to other amygdaloid areas, apparently no axons reach the mediodorsal thalamus from either the central or medial amygdaloid nuclei, although terminals do reach mediodorsal thalamus from the basomedial nucleus and from the amygdalohippocampal area, two zones that are rather more closely related to the medial subdivision of the extended amygdala (see Price et al., 1987 for review).

The magnocellular forebrain complex. The magnocellular complex of the basal forebrain does not appear to give rise to widespread descending projections but among these are projections to the thalamus, epithalamus and interpeduncular nucleus. Projections to thalamus from the magnocellular complex have attracted recent attention and include projections to the mediodorsal thalamus and reticular nucleus of the thalamus (Asanuma, 1989; Hallanger et al., 1987; Parent et al., 1988) with the main projection directed at the reticular nucleus of the thalamus. Both cholinergic and non-cholinergic cells have been identified as participating in the innervation of this structure so that it is not clear at the present time whether all of these cells should be assigned to the magnocellular complex, or whether parallel circuits could be derived from the other major structures in basal forebrain. Such efferents do not seem to be characteristic of the extended amygdala. However, some of the cells projecting to the reticular nucleus of the thalamus do seem to be confined to pallidal areas. Significantly, at least in the rat, some cholinergic and non-cholinergic neurons apparently send collaterals to both the reticular thalamic nucleus and to the cortex (Jourdain et al., 1989).

Ascending pathways from the brainstem

The striatopallidal system. Ascending projections to the striatopallidal system come from the brainstem and thalamus (Fig. 15). Virtually every subdivision of the striatopallidal system receives some serotonergic input from the serotonin containing cells of the midbrain, principally from the dorsal raphe. In contrast to this widespread input from the raphe, no afferents from the noradrenergic cells in the brainstem have been identified (for review see Alheid et al., 1990).

Another source of afferents, at least to the dorsal striatopallidal system, is from the midbrain reticular formation in or around the pedunculopontine tegmental nucleus (e.g., Jackson and Crossman, 1983; Lee et al., 1988). However, some controversy exists as to the exact source of these afferents. In recent times many investigators have come to exclusively associate the pars compacta of the pedunculopontine tegmental nucleus with the large cholinergic neurons that help to form this nucleus, and it has been tacitly assumed that many of the afferents to the striatopallidal system originate in these cells. In contrast, several reports (Lee et al., 1988; Rye et al., 1987) have offered evidence that it is non-cholinergic cells in an area medial, rostral, and ventral to the cholinergic neurons that are reciprocally connected with the striatopallidal system, and have termed this territory, the midbrain extrapyramidal area. Despite the evidence generally favoring this view, it does appear that cholinergic afferents terminate in pars compacta substantia nigra, and may reach pars reticulata as well (Gould et al., 1989).

The extended amygdala. A rich variety of afferents reach the extended amygdala from the brainstem (Fig. 15C). In addition to axons from the raphe nuclei (dorsal but also median and

basal ganglia and to the extended amygdala (F). DMH = dorsomedial hypothalamic nucleus; LH = lateral hypothalamus; MAHA = medial anterior hypothalamic area; MG = medial geniculate nucleus; MPO = medial preoptic area; PP = peripeduncular nucleus; TM = tuberomamillary area; VMH = ventromedial hypothalamic nucleus. © Dr. L. Heimer.

caudal linear nuclei), noradrenergic cells in the locus coeruleus, and noradrenergic and adrenergic neurons in the lateral tegmentum, all provide axons terminating in both subdivisions of extended amygdala (Fallon, 1981). Well documented pathways also exist from the nucleus of the solitary tract, the parabrachial nuclei, and from the central gray. The nucleus of the solitary tract and peribrachial nuclei seem to have particularly close reciprocal relations with the central amygdaloid division of the extended amygdala (see Grove, 1988a; Holstege et al., 1985; Moga et al., 1989; Schwaber et al., 1982; and reviews in de Olmos, 1990; de Olmos et al., 1985; Price et al., 1987; Russchen, 1986).

The magnocellular forebrain complex. As we have discussed above, the close proximity of the extended amygdala to the magnocellular complex complicates attempts to identify particular afferents to the cholinergic and non-cholinergic cells that project to cortex. Nonetheless, dopamine-β-hydroxylase terminals have been suggested or identified on cholinergic cells in basal forebrain at the light and ultrastructural level (Jones and Cuello, 1989; Zaborszky et al., 1990), while serotonergic terminals on cholinergic cells seem likely from light microscopic experiments (Jones and Cuello, 1989; Zaborszky et al., 1990). A variety of afferents from the brainstem reach the diagonal band complex where terminations on corticopetal cells are less ambivalent (Semba et al., 1988). However, many of these have not been confirmed ultrastructurally to preclude the possibility that synapses might be confined to neurons with descending projections. Brainstem structures afferent to the diagonal band include the parabrachial nuclei, laterodorsal tegmental nucleus, locus coeruleus, ventrolateral medulla and the raphe nuclei (for review see Zaborszky, 1989).

Dopaminergic afferents to basal forebrain. Dopamine terminals are found in both the striatum and the extended amygdala with the major part of the afferents to dorsal striatum originating in the A9 cell groups of the pars compacta substantia nigra, while the ventral tegmental area (A10) provides the major input to the ventral striatum (Figs. 15D, 15E, and 15F). Afferents from the retrorubral area (A8) and ventral tegmental area provide the major input to the extended amygdala and this includes afferents from dopamine cells in the so-called "dorsal tier" of substantia nigra pars compacta (for reviews see Alheid et al., 1990; Fallon and Loughlin, 1987). Some medial to lateral topography is seen in the dopamine afferents to forebrain, with striatal dopamine afferents spread out over extended rostral-caudal terminal fields (e.g., Beckstead et al., 1979). This is in some respects complementary to the extended rostral-caudal terminations seen in the cortico-striatal projection (e.g., Selemon and Goldman-Rakic, 1985). Using double immunohistochemical techniques, both at light and EM levels, we found (Zaborszky et al., 1990) that tyrosine hydroxylase (TH)-containing axons establish synapses with cholinergic neurons in the basal forebrain. Since TH is the first enzyme in the catecholamine biosynthetic pathway, the TH immunoreactivity observed in these terminals could represent dopamine, noradrenaline or adrenaline. However, differences in both the forebrain distribution of TH versus dopamine-beta-hydroxylase (the enzyme containing noradrenergic or adrenergic terminals) axon terminals, and different morphological features of DBH-positive versus TH-positive axon types, suggest that at least TH contacts on cholinergic cells in the ventromedial globus pallidus and internal capsule represent dopaminergic terminals. According to retrograde tracing experiments these putative dopaminergic afferents may originate in the substantia nigra (Martinez-Murillo et al., 1988).

Hypothalamic afferents

The striatopallidal system. Hypothalamic connections, in general, are not characteristic of the striatopallidal system, however, some recent evidence suggests that a slight peptidergic projection (α-MSH) may reach the dorsal and ventral striatum from a large complex of cells in the perifornical-lateral hypothalamic-zona incerta area (Khachaturian et al., 1985, 1986; Köhler and Swanson, 1984; Köhler et al., 1984; Umegaki et al., 1983), and that afferents from neurons in the tuberomammillary area (histamine, GABA, substance P, met-enkephalin, galanin, met-enk-Arg^6-Phe^7 heptapeptide) might also contribute axons to the dorsal and ventral striatum (Inagaki et al., 1988; Köhler et al., 1985; Steinbusch et al., 1986; Watanabe et al., 1984).

The extended amygdala. Hypothalamic afferents are characteristic of the extended amygdala (Fig. 15C) and serve as an additional distinction from adjacent striatopallidal areas. Both the medial and lateral hypothalamus give rise to amygdalopetal fibers. Thus, the central subdivision mainly receives afferents from the lateral-preoptic-anterior hypothalamic continuum, from dorsal hypothalamus and from the ventromedial hypothalamic nucleus. These areas also contribute axons to the medial subdivision of the extended amygdala, while additional sources of afferents to the medial subdivision include the medial preoptic area, anterior hypothalamus, paraventricular nucleus, and premammillary nuclei (for reviews see de Olmos, 1990; de Olmos et al., 1985; Grove, 1988a, and Price et al., 1987).

The magnocellular forebrain complex. Hypothalamofugal axons course in and around the corticopetal cells so that a large number of potential afferents exist. In light microscopic experiments with phaseolus vulgaris leucoagglutinin, terminal varicositites abutting cholinergic cells and dendrites have been identified from the lateral hypothalamus and from a variety of medial hypothalamic nuclei, and these have been confirmed ultrastructurally as synaptic contacts (Zaborszky and Cullinan, 1989). The hypothalamic projection to the cholinergic neurons appear from light microscopic analysis to follow a medial-to-lateral topography; i.e., medial hypothalamic neurons project to the medial septum diagonal band complex, while progressively more lateral areas of the hypothalamus project to more lateral and caudal cholinergic neurons within the sublenticular areas.

Thalamic afferents

The striatopallidal system. Thalamic afferents to the striatum have generally been ascribed to the intralaminar nuclei (Figs. 15A and 15B) which project more or less topographically to the striatum. It has been argued (Beckstead, 1984) that, at least in the cat, this is a dual topography with projections from rostral intralaminar nuclei (central lateral, paracentral, central medial and rhomboid nuclei, including the paraventricular nuclei) covering the entire striatal mass including ventral striatum, and a duplicate projection from the caudal intralaminar nuclei (centromedio-parafascicular nucleus and subparafascicluaris). A number of other posterior thalamic nuclei have been identified as afferent to the striatum, suggesting that the striatum receives an almost complete set of sensory afferents either directly (see below) or via the thalamic relay, and that these target similar areas of the striatum as those which receive the most direct transcortical sensory input. Visual (lateral posterior-pulvinar), auditory (medial geniculate), and somatosensory (medial posterior and suprageniculate nuclei) information reach the striatum from thalamus, while as we have seen olfactory information enters the ventral striatum directly from olfactory bulb, or indirectly from olfactory (piriform) cortex. In the cat, Yasui et al. (1987) have argued that afferents also reach the striatum from the caudal trigeminal nucleus. Other thalamic areas projecting to the striatum include the ventral anterior-ventral lateral complex, and the paratenial nucleus. This latter nucleus in the rat appears to particularly target the medial ventral part of the ventral striatum (medial accumbens and medial olfactory tubercle, Carlsen and Heimer, 1986).

The extended amygdala. A variety of afferents

reach the extended amygdala from the thalamus (Fig. 15C; e.g., Aggleton, et al., 1980; Mehler, 1980; Otterson and Ben Ari, 1979; and reviews in de Olmos, 1990; de Olmos et al., 1985; Price et al., 1987; Russchen, 1986). The midline nuclei; i.e., the paraventricular nucleus, the paratenial nucleus, nucleus reuniens, and the rhomboid nucleus provide afferents especially to the central division of the extended amygdala, but also to some extent to the medial amygdaloid division. The paraventricular, paratenial, and rhomboid nuclei apparently project to the medial nucleus accumbens and olfactory tubercle as well (Beckstead, 1984). Caudally, the subparafascicular nucleus also sends projections to the medial and central subdivisions of extended amygdala and to the tubercle, while the ventral part of the parafascicular nucleus sends projections to the nucleus accumbens as well as to the central division of the extended amygdala. Caudolaterally, the medial division of the medial geniculate and the peripeduncular nucleus also send projections into the extended amygdala with the central amygdaloid nucleus and amygdalostriatal transition area receiving the main terminations of the geniculate, and the peripeduncular nucleus terminations more densely distributed within the medial subdivision (Jones et al., 1976).

The magnocellular forebrain complex. Only a limited number of thalamic nuclei appear to be potential afferents to the magnocellular complex. These include the midline and intralaminar nuclei, and possibly the mediodorsal thalamus both of which appear to innervate the diagonal band and sublenticular areas (Fuller et al., 1986; Irle and Markowitsch, 1986; Russchen et al., 1985a). A particularly dense termination around the hyperchromic cells of the magnocellular complex is provided by the peripeduncular nucleus (Jones et al., 1976).

Ascending projections from the basal forebrain systems

The striatopallidal sytem. Most ascending afferents of the striatopallidal system represent intrinsic connections between the various subdivisions that comprise this major forebrain structure. A particular exception is perhaps the mesencephalic dopamine complex which in addition to dense projections to the striatum, also sends afferents to broad territories of the cortex, amygdala and basal forebrain. It is somewhat problematic, however, determining to what degree the particular dopaminergic cells that receive descending projections of the striatopallidal system also project to extrastriatal structures. It has been suggested that the dopaminergic complex might be conceived of as a dual structure with ventral pars compacta neurons receiving striatal inputs as well as pallidal inputs from internal pallidal areas (including pars reticulata) and projecting back to striatum, while the "dorsal" layer of cells extending from the ventral tegmental area across the pars compacta and into the retrorubral area receives input from areas extrinsic to the striatum, including, but not limited to the extended amygdala, and projects back to the territory of the extended amygdala, diagonal band and cortex, as well as to the striatum itself (Fallon and Loughlin, 1987; Fallon and Moore, 1978; Feigenbaum-Langer and Graybiel, 1989; Gerfen et al., 1987).

In non-primates ascending projections to the cortex have also been reported from the external pallidal segment and from the striatum itself, however, these do not appear to be a feature of the primate brain (for review, see Alheid et al., 1990). The only cortically projecting cells observed in primate pallidal areas appear to be hyperchromic cells of the magnocellular complex that are mainly found compressed within the confines of the medullary laminae, or embedded within the internal capsule (e.g., Mesulam et al., 1983).

The extended amygdala. As we have discussed earlier, many of the subcortical projections of the extended amygdala to telencephalic areas might be considered as intrinsic axons within the rostral-caudal extent of this macrostructure. However, additional efferents to subcortical areas are observed and include projections to the remaining nuclei of the amygdala. The extended amygdala projects to varying degrees from the medial or central subdivision, to the cortical amygdaloid nuclei including also the amygdalo-piriform transition area. In the rat, a substantial projection from both divisions of the extended amygdala apparently reaches the anterior amygdaloid area, and a similar projection seems likely in the primate. The anterior amygdala from one point of view could be considered as ancillary to the magnocellular complex since it is adjacent with this structure laterally, and has dense projections to olfactory cortex (Saper, 1984). Similarly, the extended amygdala apparently sends afferents to the magnocellular forebrain complex, with the greater contribution arriving from the central division (Kelley et al., 1982; Krettek and Price, 1978; Price and Amaral, 1981; Russchen et al., 1985a; see also summary by Zaborszky, 1989). These efferents are mainly targeted to magnocellular neurons in the sublenticular areas adjacent to the extended amygdala including the horizontal limb of the diagonal band, but not to the cells in the medial septum-vertical limb of the diagonal band. However, the medial subdivision of extended amygdala also sends axons to the septum, including the medial septum-vertical limb of the diagonal band (see discussion by de Olmos et al., 1985).

Cortical projections from the extended amygdala are sparse; these include projections to the hippocampus, entorhinal cortex, temporal cortex, and insula, and originate mainly in the medial subdivision of extended amygdala. From one point of view the non-cholinergic corticopetal cells within the sublenticular areas (including anterior amygdala) tend to project to those cortical areas that are afferent to the extended amygdala, so that they might be considered as the substrate for the reciprocal symmetry from the extended amygdala (de Olmos et al., 1985) analogous to that which characterizes so many brain systems. On the other hand, the extended amygdala also appears to reach cholinergic cells in these forebrain areas, which project to a broader field of cortical targets, and whether these might be considered in the same category remains an interesting possibility (e.g., see Alheid and Heimer, 1988; Alheid et al., 1990). In any case, hippocampopetal cells within the medial septum-diagonal band may have a similar relation with the lateral septum (Alheid and Heimer, 1988; Alheid et al., 1989; 1990; Leranth and Froscher, 1989).

The magnocellular forebrain complex. The magnocellular complex in addition to its widespread cortical projections also innervates other portions of the forebrain. In particular, afferents reach the quasi-cortical basolateral complex in the amygdala which appears to receive some of the densest terminations of the cholinergic neurons, but which also receives non-cholinergic inputs from adjacent forebrain cells (Carlsen et al., 1985). Other less dense projections reach the olfactory group of nuclei in the amygdala, as well as in varying degrees to the central and medial subdivisions of the extended amygdala.

The corticopetal projections of the magnocellular complex are intriguing in that outside of the thalamus, few of the broadly projecting corticopetal areas of the brain can be said to have such a specific topography (Fig. 13A). In general, there is a rostral-caudal and medio-lateral topography, of course, the most anterior portions of this complex, if one includes the medial septal-diagonal band nuclei, projects to the hippocampus and entorhinal cortex. The areas immediately adjacent and caudal project to prefrontal areas of cortex, while more caudal and lateral parts of the complex project to parietal and temporal cortex and to the amygdala (see Mesulam et al., 1983). The projections to primary visual cortex are an exception in that cells targeting this area are found rostrally in the diagonal band and in the rostral most portions of the sublenticular areas (Woolf et al., 1984).

The search continues for the anatomical locus of neuropsychiatric disorders

Alzheimer's disease, Parkinson's disease, Huntington's chorea, mood disorders and schizophrenia constitute a major share of all chronically disabling brain disorders. Each one of these disease categories has distinctive features, but they are also characterized by a certain communality in regard to symptomatology. Although the overlap in symptoms is more or less pronounced from patient to patient, a review of the clinical literature reveals that all of these disorders are characterized by cognitive impairments, abnormal movements, psychoses, and depression. A striking example of apparent convergence in symptomatology is provided by the Parkinson patient with cognitive impairments and dementia (Growdon and Corkin, 1986; Korczyn et al., 1986) associated with cholinergic deficit reminiscent of an Alzheimer dementia (Boller et al., 1980; Gaspar and Gray, 1984; Hornykiewicz and Kish, 1984; Horvath et al., 1989; Nakano and Hirano, 1984; Perry et al., 1983; Ruberg et al., 1982; Yoshimura, 1988). Another comparison is the Alzheimer patient with Parkinsonian symptoms including myoclonus rigidity, bradykinesia, and gait abnormalities (Fisher et al., 1985; Leverenz and Sumi, 1984; Mayeux and Stern, 1985; Mölsa et al., 1984; Pearce, 1974). In fact, the suggestion has been made that these two disorders, Parkinson's and Alzheimer's disease, may form two extremes on a spectrum (Appel, 1981; Korczyn et al., 1986; Rossor, 1981) where a significant number of patients appear somewhere on a continuum between the two prototypical pictures of Alzheimer's disease and Parkinsonism. Many other examples of such converging features can be mentioned; e.g., the Huntington patient with symptoms reminiscent of manic-depressive disorders or schizophrenia (McHugh and Folstein, 1975), and the Parkinson patient with depressive symptoms (Fibiger, 1984; Mayeux et al., 1984; Robins, 1976; Warburton, 1967). The occurrence of motor disturbances in schizophrenic patients is a well-known phenomenon (e.g., Grebb and Cancro, 1989; Marsden et al., 1975), as are neurologic abnormalities in general in this large group of patients (e.g., Stevens, 1989). Although tardive dyskinesia, attributed to antipsychotic treatment, is one of the most notorious motor disturbances in schizophrenics, similar dyskinesias along with a variety of other motor abnormalities, were described already by Kraepelin (1919) as an integral part of the schizophrenic symptom complex well before the advent of antidopaminergic neuroleptics (see also Crow et al., 1984; Trimble, 1981). The distinction, finally, between Alzheimer's disease, mood disorders, and schizophrenia is also blurred in many instances with potential overlap in a number of symptoms including those related to affect and motivation, as well as in the general area of distorted perceptions and thought processes (e.g., Grebb and Cancro, 1989; Horvath et al., 1989).

Even this short survey of the clinical literature leaves the distinct impression that these disorders affect, in many cases at least, some strategically located anatomical systems, which can explain the multifarious and often strikingly converging symptomatology. The three partly interdigitating systems that have been discussed in some detail on the previous pages; i.e., the ventral striatopallidal system, the extended amygdala, and the corticopetal magnocellular forebrain system are obvious candidates, and an examination of the neuropathologic literature does support this proposition. More specifically, pathologic changes in the basal forebrain, often defined in a more restricted fashion as the basal nucleus of Meynert or substantia innominata, is a prominent feature in Alzheimer's disease (Arendt et al., 1983; Davis and Maloney, 1976; Etienne et al., 1986; Jacobs and Butcher, 1986; Mann et al., 1984; Price et al., 1987; Whitehouse et al., 1981), Parkinson's disease (Arendt et al., 1983; Candy et al., 1983; Chui et al., 1986; Hassler, 1938; Lewy, 1912; 1913; Nakano and Hirano, 1983; 1984; Tagliavini et al., 1984; Ulfig, 1989; Von Buttlar-Brentano, 1952; Whitehouse et al., 1983), Korsakoff's psychosis (Arendt et al., 1983; Butters, 1985; Crosson, 1986), and schizophrenic disorders (Averback, 1981; Bogerts et al., 1985; Nieto and Escobar, 1972; Stevens, 1982; Von Buttlar-Brentano, 1952). Although the changes are often dramatic, they are also characterized by great variability and there is still some controversy in regard to the specific pathology encountered. This is especially the case in regard to schizophrenia, where the variability in regard to the location of the brain lesion is especially great (Berman and Weinberger, 1989; Stevens, 1982) and where reports of degenerative changes in, for instance, the basal nucleus of Meynert have been severely criticized (see discussion in Jellinger, 1985).

Admittedly, the pathology in these various disorders is by no means limited to the ventromedial parts of the basal forebrain. Parkinson's disease and Huntington's chorea, for instance, are typical basal ganglia disorders with primary involvement of the mesotelencephalic dopamine system in Parkinson's disease (Crossman, 1987; Hornykiewicz, 1977; Javoy-Agid et al., 1981) and an equally pronounced degeneration and progressive neuronal loss in striatum in Huntington's chorea (Bruyn, 1968; Martin, 1984; see also Clark et al., 1983). As indicated previously, the basal ganglia extend to the ventral surface of the human brain and the mesencephalic dopamine system, which is primarily involved in Parkinson's disease, projects prominently, not only to the dorsal striatum but also to the ventral striatum and extended amygdala (Fig. 15D, 15E, and 15F), and presumably also to the magnocellular corticopetal forebrain neurons (e.g., Jones and Cuello, 1989; Semba et al., 1988; Zaborszky et al., 1990; see also Figs. 13B and 13C). Therefore, no great leap in imagination is required to understand how degeneration of the ascending mesencephalic dopamine system, especially if it includes the fibers from medial substantia nigra and ventral tegmental area (Javoy-Agid and Agid, 1980; Rinne et al., 1989), can play havoc with all three of these basal forebrain systems.

The neuropathology of Alzheimer's disease and schizophrenia is noteworthy for the heterogeneity of anatomical sites affected (e.g., Berman and Weinberger, 1989; Stevens, 1982; 1983; Van Hoesen and Damasio, 1987). However, considerable attention has focused on medial temporal lobe structures; i.e., the hippocampus formation, including the entorhinal area, and the amygdaloid body. The behavioral significance of these temporal lobe structures is well documented in the clinical literature. For instance, temporal lobe lesions or tumors have a tendency to produce psychotic symptoms (e.g., Davison and Bagley, 1969; Emsley and Paster, 1985; Malamud, 1967; see also Lishman, 1987), and from several studies of epileptic patients (e.g., Flor-Henry, 1969; Hill, 1962; Perez et al., 1985; Slater and Bear, 1963; Stevens, 1986; Trimble and Bolwig, 1986) the conclusion seems inescapable that there is a relationship between schizophrenic symtoms and temporal lobe pathology (Stevens, 1989). During the last few decades a number of studies using histologic techniques and imaging methods have confirmed the importance of these structures both in Alzheimer's disease (e.g., Herzog and Kemper, 1980; Hopper and Vogel, 1976; Hyman et al., 1989; Mann et al., 1988; Van Hoesen and Damasio, 1987) and in schizophrenia (e.g., Bogerts et al., 1985; Brown et al., 1986; Falkai and Bogerts, 1986; Hopper and Vogel, 1976; Jakob and Beckman, 1986; Kovelman and Scheibel, 1984).

As for the functional role of the two major temporal lobe structures; i.e., the hippocampus and the amygdala, it is generally appreciated that the hippocampus formation is crucially involved in memory functions (Damasio, 1984; Scoville and Milner, 1957; Zola-Morgan et al., 1986), whereas the amygdaloid body is well known for its many functions related to emotionally colored experiences or events. It serves in a sense as a "sensory-emotional" interface (Le Doux, 1986; 1987) as it seems to be decisively involved in evaluating the significance of external events or in evaluating sensory stimuli in terms of their emotional and motivational significance (Gloor, 1978; Gloor et al., 1982).

The hippocampus and amygdaloid body, although markedly different in structural organization, have one strikingly important feature in common; i.e., they both receive highly processed sensory information through a series of transcortical pathways (see for example the reviews by Price et al., 1987; Turner, 1981; Van Hoesen, 1981; 1985). This information, no doubt, is instrumental for the functional integrity of these structures in the interrelated fields of memory, learning, and sensory-affective associations (Aggleton and Mishkin, 1986; Mishkin, 1978; Mishkin et al., 1984; Squire, 1987). As if to underscore the close association between the hippocampus formation and the amygdaloid body, a number of reciprocal connections have recently been discovered between the two structures in several animals, including the monkey (Amaral, 1986; Aggleton, 1986; see also discussions by Price et al., 1987; Van Hoesen, 1981). Importantly, and as shown in Figs. 14B and 14C, the subcortical projections of both the hippocampus formation and the basolateral amygdaloid body, and for that matter most of the anterior temporal cortex, involve significantly the ventral striatopallidal system and the extended amygdala. Therefore, it is reasonable to suggest that pathologic changes in the medial temporal lobe structures, which seem to be significantly involved in at least some patients with Alzheimer's disease and schizophrenia, can disturb the physiology or change the anatomical circuits in the ventral striatopallidal system, extended amygdala, and the magnocellular corticopetal forebrain system with subsequent disruption of a number of areas ranging from motor functions, basic drives like eating, drinking, and sexual behavior, to personality changes involving stress, mood, and higher cognitive functions (e.g., Alheid et al., 1977; Gallagher, 1990; Gray, 1988; Kapp et al., 1984; Kelley et al., 1977; Le Doux, 1987; Mogenson et al., 1980; Price et al., 1987; Richardson et al., 1988; Rolls et al., 1979).

Although the ventromedial temporal lobe may be especially vulnerable to a variety of both perinatal and postnatal traumatic events (e.g., de Lisi et al., 1988; McNeil, 1988; the special vulnerability of the hippocampus to anoxic-ischemic insults is infamous), other telencephalic regions, notably the prefrontal-orbitofrontal cortex, has also figured prominently in discussions of the pathogenesis of schizophrenia (e.g., Andreasen et al., 1986; Benes et al., 1986; Ingvar and Franzen, 1974; Müller, 1985; Weinberger, 1986). As if to underscore the importance of the ventral striatopallidal system and the extended amygdala in the generation of schizophrenic symptoms, one is reminded of the fact that the prefrontal-orbitofrontal cortex represents, besides the temporal lobe, the major area of origin for telencephalic projections to these basal forebrain systems. Weinberger (1986; Weinberger and Berman, 1988) has suggested that prefrontal hypometabolism in schizophrenia may, at least in part, be a secondary result of medial temporal lobe pathology. The fact that the medial temporal lobe structures, including the entorhinal area, have widespread and significant relations with other cortical areas, not least prefrontal areas (Barbas and de Olmos, 1990; Price et al., 1987; Rosene and Van Hoesen, 1977; Swanson and Köhler, 1986; Swanson et al., 1987) becomes important in this context. Finally, it is interesting to contemplate the fact that subfrontal cortical areas and the anterior temporal lobe are remarkably vulnerable in closed head injuries (Courville, 1937), and psychiatric sequelae following head trauma may include changes in behavior, affect, and emotion not seldom resembling schizophrenia and affective psychoses (e.g., Lishman, 1987; Nasrallah et al., 1981).

The "plasticity" hypothesis of mental illness

In 1979, Gerald Schneider speculated that plastic changes in the catecholamine pathways to the basal forebrain following a lesion in the hippocampus formation or amygdala might be the cause of schizophrenia (Schneider, 1979), and this idea has recently been revived by Stevens (1990). The basal forebrain structures and neuronal assemblies discussed in this paper would be likely targets for anatomical, physiological or biochemical changes that may result from primary lesions in the temporal lobe. Such secondary changes are often referred to with the broad term "neuronal plasticity''. The ''plasticity'' hypothesis of schizophrenia (e.g., Haracz, 1985; Van Praag, 1981), or of any other multisystem disorder for that matter, is especially attractive to anatomically oriented scientists, since it can be tested in a number of ways by the aid of modern anatomical and immunohistochemical methods. Of course, the changes can be of a functional nature and amenable to physiologic and biochemical techniques rather than to classic neuroanatomical methodologies. Nonetheless, the anatomical details related to the ventral striatopallidal system and extended amygdala become relevant in this context, because these systems represent two of the major subcortical targets for direct projections from the temporal lobe structures; i.e., the hippocampus formation and the amygdaloid body that have figured so prominently in discussions of the pathogenesis of schizophrenia and Alzheimer's disease. For proponents of the dopamine theory of schizophrenia (Carlsson, 1988; Carlsson and Lindquist, 1963; Randrup and Munkvad, 1974; Van Rossen, 1986), special note should be taken from the fact that the dopaminergic pathway from the ventral tegmental area, which is believed to play a pivotal role in schizophrenia, projects not only to the ventral striatum including the accumbens but also to the extended amygdala, as well as to the hippocampus formation and the entorhinal area, although it seems that separate groups of dopamine cells project to each terminal field (Fallon and Moore, 1978; Swanson, 1982). Nonetheless, a primary lesion in the hippocampus formation or amygdaloid body may well result in transneuronal effects which in turn might change the release of dopamine and other transmitters in the ventral striatum and extended amygdala. For instance, it is well documented that the peptide content in striatal neurons is subject to trans-synaptic regulation of dopamine containing afferent systems (Bean et al., 1989; Eggerman and Zahm, 1988; Zahm, 1990; Zahm and Johnson, 1989). In fact the potential for secondary changes are innumerable, but an understanding of the basal forebrain anatomical circuits and their transmitter content provides some guidelines of what to look for, and where to look for plasticity changes following localized lesions in various parts of the amygdala or the hippocampus formation.

The pathophysiologic mechanisms resulting in schizophrenia may vary between different groups of diseased individuals, but the fact that traumatic or degenerative lesions in medial temporal lobe structures have a tendency to produce schizophrenia-like symptoms is important, because it suggests a model for schizophrenia which is likely to throw light on this dreaded disease, regardless of etiology. Indeed, the details of neuronal connections are crucially important in a number of current notions regarding degenerative brain disorders (Appel, 1981; Ferreyra-Moyano and Barragan, 1989; Mann et al., 1988; Pearson et al., 1985; Saper et al., 1987). As a further elaboration of the classic notion that viruses or toxins can spread through peripheral nerves to the central nervous system through axoplasmic transport, these authors have suggested that the anatomical pattern of degeneration in disorders like Parkinson's disease and Alzheimer's disease, known as ''system degenerations'', may be predetermined by the anatomical connections, in the sense that the spread of the disease occurs through axonal and transneuronal transport of a toxic substance, or by the failure or absence of a normally transported trophic factor.

The opening of the border between neurology and psychiatry

The conclusion seems inescapable; the disorders discussed in this commentary are characterized in large part by the same symptoms, and the sites of pathology, or at least the functional-anatomical systems affected by the pathological process, are in large part the same. Furthermore, and regardless of pathogenesis, these disorders seem to pay little attention to the functional-anatomical schemes (e.g., extrapyramidal and limbic systems) that have been devised to facilitate functional and clinical considerations. As alluded to previously, this point is repeatedly being emphasized by many of the most debilitating brain disorders like Alzheimer's and Parkinson's disease, Huntington's chorea, and the schizophrenic disorders, all of which have clinical features that tend to smudge the boundaries between neurology and psychiatry. Neurologic abnormalities, for instance, are found in about half the patients with schizophrenic disorders (Grebb and Cancro, 1989), but they are often subtle (Cadet et al., 1986), and Grebb and Cancro have suggested that a psychiatrist "should be capable of performing an even more refined neurological examination than a neurologist usually performs." Likewise, the neurologists caring for patients with typical basal ganglia symptoms e.g., parkinsonism, should, it seems, be as alert to mental symptoms as the psychiatrist-in-charge, because the overt motor symptoms may well overshadow more discrete cognitive and emotional symptoms. The unfortunate dichotomy between neurology and psychiatry, that has characterized much of this century has admittedly been counter-productive for many patients with brain disease (Geschwind, 1975). However, with the increasingly rapid developments in various fields of neuroscience, and as reflected in modern textbooks (e.g., Comprehensive Textbook of Psychiatry, edited by Kaplan and Sadock, Williams Wilkins, 1989; Diseases of the Nervous System, edited by Asbury, McKhann and McDonald, W.B. Saunders Company, 1986; Neurology and Psychiatry: A Meeting of Minds, edited by Müller, Karger, 1990), the "no man's land" between neurology and psychiatry (Geschwind, 1975) is gradually disappearing. Maybe the opening of the borders between neurology and psychiatry will eventually lead to a close alliance between the two disciplines? This would make sense from a functional-anatomical point of view. Instead of debating the boundaries of the limbic system, neuroanatomists are increasingly directing their attention to the unique characteristics of individual neuronal circuits or systems that often cross the changing boundaries of the "limbic system" (e.g., Poletti, 1986). To identify anatomical units and neuronal assemblies with similar afferent and efferent connections and a certain uniformity in their intrinsic organization has become a desirable pursuit, and the anatomical viewpoint presented in this article is part of such an effort.

In their stimulating article entitled "Schizophrenia and the Limbic System", Torrey and Peterson (1974) refer to a book on schizophrenia that was pubished in 1957 in which an author notes that ". . . it is difficult to envisage how an alteration of as unspecific a region as this (the substantia innominata) could have the systemic effects presumably required to induce schizophrenic behaviors." With the advantages offered by modern neuroanatomical techniques, the substantia innominata is no longer the "terra incognita" of the telencephalon. The anatomy of the basal forebrain is unfolding under the persistent expeditions of anatomical exploration. The boundaries and the topography of the separate territories that comprise this fundamentally important part of the brain have been identified. Hopefully, this new anatomy will serve as a framework for a more detailed analysis of basal forebrain anatomical systems and neuron circuits, thereby facilitating physiological studies and clinical-anatomical correlations in part of the brain that is implicated in such a wide variety of neurologic and psychiatric disorders.

Although much exploration is still needed, the new anatomy of the basal forebrain has emphasized some fundamental organizational principles which are of immediate clinical relevance.

First, the basal ganglia (i.e., striatal and pallidal components), best known for their motor functions, reach the ventral surface of the human brain in the region of the anterior perforated space. These ventral parts of the basal ganglia; i.e., the ventral striatopallidal system, receives its cortical input from allo- and periallocortical formations, the basolateral amygdaloid body, and some prefrontal-temporal neocortical areas. Whatever motor functions are related to the ventral striatopallidal system, they are likely to be elaborate behaviors that reflect the complex association areas that are afferent to this part of the striatopallidal system. However, regardless of the type of functions the ventral striatopallidal system normally subserves, a disruption of the functional integrity of this part of the basal ganglia is likely to have repercussions in the form of inappropriate or abnormal movements.

Second, a significant part of the ventral striatal territories in the region of the medial accumbens interdigitates with another major forebrain structure, the "extended amygdala." The notion of the extended amygdala which incorporates the bed nucleus of the stria terminalis and the centromedial amygdala with several little known parts of the sublenticular forebrain areas, is based on a certain uniformity in the internal organization of these structures, and by striking parallels in their afferent and efferent connections. Unlike the basal ganglia, the extended amygdala is characterized by a high degree of internal associative connections, but much like the ventral striatopallidal system, it receives cortical input from hippocampus and basolateral amygdala and from other higher order multimodal association areas in prefrontal and anterior temporal lobe. Widespread, but highly organized projections to a number of neuroendocrine, autonomic, and somatomotor centers in hypothalamus, brainstem and even the spinal cord, is a hallmark of this system, and one might expect a constellation of motor and affective symptoms, endocrine and autonomic abnormalities whenever the functions of the extended amygdala are significantly compromised. In particular, the close relation that the extended amygdala has with the monoaminergic systems and the endocrine centers in the hypothalamus should be of special interest in mood disorders.

Third, the cholinergic and noncholinergic neurons of the magnocellular cortico-, amygdalo-, and thalamopetal basal forebrain systems interdigitate significantly with the basal ganglia, and especially with the extended amygdala. Through its intimate relations with the widespread cortical projections of the magnocellular forebrain complex, the extended amygdala may well serve as an important anatomical substrate for the well-known influence of motivational and emotional states on cognition.

Concluding remarks

For the sake of brevity, this description of the anatomy of the basal forebrain has touched only peripherally on closely related areas of septal and hypothalamic neuronal systems (e.g., Swanson, 1987; Swanson et al., 1987; Swanson, Chapter 9, this volume) or the many aspects of diffuse ascending brainstem projections (e.g., Saper, 1987). Nevertheless, considering the strategic position of the three basal forebrain systems discussed at length is this review, and the intimate relation that they have with each other and with other parts of the neuraxis, it is not difficult to envision how disruption of the functional integrity of any one of these systems can easily present itself with a multitude of symptoms that show little regard for traditional boundaries of neurologic and psychiatric disciplines.

Acknowledgements

Supported by USPHS Grants 17743 (LH), 23945 (LZ), and by Consejo Nacional de Investigaciones Cientificas y Tecnicas of Argentina (J. de O.). The authors wish to thank Mr. Lee Snavely and Ms. Linda S. Vega for skillfull assistance, and Drs, Jack Grebb and Gary Van Hoesen for reading the manuscript and making valuable suggestions.

References

Abrams G.M., Nilaver G. and Zimmerman E.A. (1985) VIP-containing neurons. In: A. Bjorklund and T. Hkfelt (Eds.), *Handbook of Chemical Neuroanatomy, Vol. 4, Part 1*. Elsevier Science Publishers, Amsterdam, pp. 335 – 354.

Aggleton J.P. (1986) Description of the amygdalo-hippocampal interconnections in the macaque monkey. *Exp. Brain Res.*, 64: 515 – 526.

Aggleton J.P., Burton M.J. and Passingham R.E. (1980) Cortical and subcortical afferents to the amygdala of the rhesus monkey (*Macaca mulatta*). *Brain Res.*, 190: 347 – 368.

Aggleton J.P. and Mishkin M. (1984) Projections of the

amygdala to the thalamus in the cynomolgus monkey. *J. Comp. Neurol.*, 222: 56 – 68.

Aggleton J.P. and Mishkin M. (1986) The amygdala; sensory gateway to the emotions. In: R. Plutchick and H. Kellerman (Eds.). *Biological foundations of emotion.* Academic Press, New York, pp. 281 – 299.

Alexander G.E., DeLong M.R. and Strick P.L. (1986) Parallel organization of functionally segregated circuits linking basal ganglia and cortex. *Ann. Rev. Neurosci.*, 9: 357 – 381.

Alheid G., Heimer L. and Switzer R.C. (1990) The basal ganglia. In: G. Paxinos (Ed.), The human nervous system. Academic Press, San Diego, pp. 483 – 582.

Alheid G.F., Haselton C.L. and Heimer L. (1989a) Accumbens projections to dorsal and ventral pallidum and to the extended amygdala in the monkey using PHA-L. *Soc. Neurosci. Abstr.*, 15: 904.

Alheid G.F. and Heimer, L. (1988) New perspectives in basal forebrain organization of special relevance for neuropsychiatric disorders; the striatopallidal, amygdaloid, and corticopetal components of substantia innominata. *Neuroscience,* 27: 1 – 39.

Alheid G.F. McDermott L., Kelly J., Halaris A. and Grossman S.P. (1977) Deficits in food and water intake after knife cuts that deplete striatal DA or hypothalamic NE in rats. *Pharmac. Biochem. Behav.*, 6: 273 – 287.

Alheid G.F., Van Hoesen G. and Heimer L. (1989b) Functional neuroanatomy. In: H.I. Kaplan and J. Sadock: (Eds.), *Comprehensive Textbook of Psychiatry, V.* Williams & Wilkins, Baltimore; pp. 26 – 45.

Amaral D.G. (1986) Amygdalohippocampal and amygdalocortical projections in the primate brain. In: R. Schwarcz and Y. Ben-Ari (Eds.), *Excitatory Amino Acids and Epilepsy.* Plenum Press, New York, pp. 3 – 18.

Amaral D.G., Avendano C. and Benoit R. (1989) Distribution of somatostatin-like immunoreactivity in the monkey amygdala. *J. Comp. Neurol.*, 284: 294 – 313.

Amaral D.G. and Kurtz J. (1985) An analysis of the origins of the cholinergic and non-cholinergic septal projections to the hippocampal formation in the rat. *J. Comp. Neurol.*, 240: 37 – 59.

Andreasen N., Nasrallah H.A., Dunn V., Olson S.C., Grove W.M., Ehrhardt J.C., Coffman J.A. and Crossett J.H.W. (1986) Structural abnormalities in the frontal system in schizophrenia. *Arch. Gen. Psychiatry,* 43: 136 – 144.

Appel S.H. (1981) A unifying hypothesis for the cause of amyotrophic lateral sclerosis, Parkinsonism, and Alzheimer disease. *Ann. Neurol.*, 10: 499 – 505.

Arendt T., Bigl V., Arendt A. and Tennstedt A. (1983) Loss of neurons in the nucleus basalis of Meynert in Alzheimer's disease, paralysis agitans and Korsakoff's disease. *Acta Neuropathol.*, 61: 101 – 108.

Arendt T., Bigl V., Tennstedt A. and Arendt A. (1985) Neuronal loss in different parts of the nucleus basalis is related to neuritic plaque formation in cortical target areas in Alzheimer's disease. *Neuroscience,* 14: 1 – 14.

Arendt T., Zvegintseva H.G. and Leontovich T.A. (1986) Dendritic changes in the basal nucleus of Meynert and in the diagonal band nucleus in Alzheimer's disease; a quantitative Golgi investigation. *Neuroscience,* 19: 1265 – 1278.

Aronin N., Di Figlia M., Graveland G.A., Schwartz W.F. and Wu J.Y. (1984) Localization of immunoreactive enkephalins in GABA synthesizing neurons of the rat neostriatum. *Brain Res.*, 300: 276 – 380.

Asanuma C. (1989) Axonal arborizations of a magnocellular basal nucleus input and their relation to the neurons in the thalamic reticular nucleus of rats. *Proc. Natl. Acad. Sci. USA,* 86: 4746 – 4750.

Avendano C., Price J.L. and Amaral D.G. (1983) Evidence for an amygdaloid projection to pre-motor cortex but not to motor cortex in the monkey. *Brain Res.*, 264: 111 – 117.

Averback, P. (1981) Lesions of the nucleus ansae peduncularis in neuropsychiatric disease. *Arch. Neurol.*, 38: 230 – 235.

Barbas H. and de Olmos J. (1990) Projections from the amygdala to basoventral and mediodorsal prefrontal regions in the rhesus monkey. *J. Comp. Neurol.*, 300: 549 – 571.

Beach T.G., McGeer E.G. (1984) The distribution of substance P in the primate basal ganglia; an immunohistochemical study of baboon and human brain. *Neuroscience,* 13: 29 – 52.

Bean, A.J., During, M.J., Deutch, A.Y. and Roth, R.H. (1989) Effects of dopamine depletion on striatal neurotensin: biochemical and immunohistochemical studies. *J. Neurosci.*, 9: 4430 – 4438.

Beccari N. (1910) Il lobo parolfattoro neí mammiferi. *Arch Ital. Anat. Embryol.*, 9, 173 – 220.

Beccari, M. (1911) La sostanza perforata anteriore e i suoi rapporti col rinencefalo nel cervello dell'uomo. *Arch. Ital. Anat. Embryol.*, 10: 261 – 328.

Beckstead, R.M. (1979) An autoradiographic examination of corticocortical and subcortical projections of the mediodorsal-projection (prefrontal) cortex in the rat. *J. Comp. Neurol.*, 184: 43 – 62.

Beckstead R.M. (1983) A pallidostriatal projection in the cat and monkey. *Brain Res. Bull.*, 11: 629 – 632.

Beckstead R.M. (1984) The thalamostriatal projection in the cat. *J. Comp. Neurol.*, 223: 313 – 346.

Beckstead R.M. and Cruz C.J. (1986) Striatal axons to the globus pallidus, entopeduncular nucleus and substantia nigra come mainly from separate populations in cat. *Neuroscience,* 19: 147 – 158.

Beckstead R.M., Domesick V.B. and Nauta W.J.H. (1979) Efferent connections of the substantia nigra and ventral tegmental area in the rat. *Brain Res.*, 175: 191 – 217.

Benes F.M., Davidson J. and Bird E.D. (1986) Quantitative cytoarchitectural studies of the cerebral cortex of schizophrenics. *Arch. Gen. Psychiatry,* 43: 31 – 35.

Bennett-Clarke C.A. and Joseph S.A. (1986) Immunocytochemical localization of somatostatin in human brain. *Peptides,* 7: 877 – 884.

Berman K.F. and Weinberger D.R. (1989) Schizophrenia: Brain structure and function. In: H.I. Kaplan and J. Sadock (Eds.), *Comprehensive Textbook of Psychiatry, V.* Williams & Wilkins, Balimore, pp. 705 – 717.

Blackstad T. (1967) Cortical gray matter- A correlation of light and electron microscopic data. In: H. Hyden (Ed.), *The neuron.* Elsevier, Amsterdam, pp. 49 – 118.

Bogerts B., Meertz E. and Schnfeldt-Bausch R. (1985) Basal ganglia and limbic system pathology in schizophrenia; a morphometric study of brain volume and shrinkage. *Arch. Gen. Psychiatry,* 42: 784 – 791.

Boller F., Mizutani R. and Roessman U. (1980) Parkinson's disease, dementia and Alzheimer's disease; clinicopathological correlations. *Ann. Neurol.,* 7: 329 – 355.

Brockhaus, H. (1942) Vergleichend-anatomische Untersuchungen über den Basalkernkomplex. *J. Psychol. Neurol.,* 51: 57 – 95.

Brown R., Colter N. Corsellis J.A.N., Crow T.J., Frith C.D., Jagoe R., Johnstone E.C. and Marsh L. (1986) Postmortem evidence of structural brain changes in schizophrenia; differences in brain weight, temporal horn area, and parahippocampal gyrus compared with affective disorder. *Arch. Gen. Psychiatry,* 43: 36 – 42.

Bruyn G.W. (1968) Huntington's chorea: Historical, clinical and laboratory synopsis. In: P.J. Vinken and G.W. Bruyn (Eds.), *Handbook of Clinical Neurology, vol 6,* Elsevier, Amsterdam, pp. 298 – 378.

Bunney B.S. and Aghajanian G.K. (1976) The precise localization of nigral afferents in the rat as determined by retrograde tracing technique. *Brain Res.,* 117: 423 – 435.

Butcher L.L. and Semba K. (1989) Reassessing the cholinergic basal forebrain: Nomenclature, schemata, and concepts. *Trends Neurosci.,* 12: 483 – 485.

Butcher L.L. and Woolf N.J. (1986) Central cholinergic systems; synopsis of anatomy and overview of physiology and pathology. In: A.B. Scheibel and A.F. Wechsler (Eds.), *The Biological Substrates of Alzheimer's Disease.* New York: New York, pp. 73 – 86.

Butters N. (1985) Alcoholic Korsakoff's syndrome; some unresolved issues concerning etiology, neuropathology, and cognitive deficits. *J. Clin. Exper. Neuropsych.,* 7: 181 – 210.

Cadet J.L., Rickler K.C. and Weinberger D.R. (1986) The neurological examination in schizophrenia (Ch1). In: H.A. Nasrallah and D.R. Weinberger (Eds.), *Handbook of Schizophrenia (Vol 1): The Neurology of Schizophrenia.* New York: Elsevier Science Publishers, New York, pp. 1 – 47.

Caffé A.R., Van Ryen P.C. Van der Woude T.P. and Van Leeuwen F.W. (1989) Vasopressin and oxytocin systems in the brain and upper spinal cord of macaca fascicularis. *J. Comp. Neurol.,* 287: 302 – 325.

Candy J.M., Perry R.H., Perry E.K., Irving D., Blessed G., Fairbairn A.F. and Tomlinson B.E. (1983) Pathological changes in the nucleus of Meynert in Alzheimer's and Parkinson's disease. *J. Neurolog. Sci.,* 54: 277 – 289.

Candy J.M., Perry R.H., Thompson J.E., Johnson M. and Oakley A.E. (1985) Neuropeptide localisation in the substantia innominata and adjacent regions of the human brain. *J. Anat.,* 140: 309 – 327.

Carlsen J. and Heimer L. (1986) The projection from the parataenial thalamic nucleus, as demonstrated by the Phaseolus vulgaris-leucoagglutinin (PHA-L) method, identifies a subterritorial organization of the ventral striatum. *Brain Res.,* 374: 375 – 379.

Carlsen J., Heimer L. (1988) The basolateral amygdaloid complex as a cortical-like structure. *Brain Res.,* 441: 377 – 380.

Carlsen J., Zaborszky L. and Heimer, L. (1985) Cholinergic projections from the basal forebrain to the basolateral amygdaloid complex: A combined retrograde fluorescent and immunohistochemical study. *J. Comp. Neurol.,* 234: 155 – 167.

Carlsson A. (1988) The current status of the dopamine hypothesis of schizophrenia. *Neuropsychopharm.,* 1: 179 – 186.

Carlsson A., Lindquist M. (1963) Effect of chlorpromazine or haloperidol on formation of 3-methoxytyramine and normetanephrine in mouse brain. *Acta. Pharmacol.,* 20: 140 – 144.

Carpenter M.G. (1981) Anatomy of the corpus striatum and brainstem integrating systems. In: V. Brooks (Ed.), *Handbook of Physiology; The Nervous System, Motor Control (Vol. II).* Bethesda, MD: Amer. Physiol. Soc., pp. 947 – 955.

Carpenter M.B. (1986) Anatomy of the basal ganglia. In: P.J. Vinken, G.W. Bruyn, and H.L. Klawans (Eds.), *Extrapyramidal Disorders: Handbook of Clinical Neurology, Vol. 49* (Rev Series 5). Elsevier Science Publishers, Amsterdam; pp. 1 – 18.

Chui H.C., Mortimer J.A., Slager U., Zarow C., Bondareff W. and Webster D.D. (1986) Pathologic correlates of dementia in Parkinson's disease. *Arch. Neurol.,* 43: 991 – 995.

Clark A.W., Parhad I.M., Folstein S.E., Whitehouse P.J., Hedreen J.C., Price D.L. and Chase G.A. (1983) The nucleus basalis in Huntington's disease. *Neurobiology,* 33: 1262 – 1266.

Courville C.B. (1937) Pathology of the Central Nervous System, Part 4. Pacific, Mountainview, California.

Crosby E.C. and Humphrey T. (1941) Studies of the vertebrate telencephalon. II. The nuclear pattern of the anterior olfactory nucleus, tuberculum olfactorium and the amygdaloid complex in adult man. *J. Comp. Neurol.,* 121 – 213.

Crossman A.R. (1987) Parkinsonism degeneration of dopamine cells in pars compacta and ventral tegmental area. *Neuroscience,* 21: 1 – 40.

Crosson B. (1986) On localization versus systemic effects in alcoholic Korsakoff's syndrome; a comment on Butters (1985). *J. Clin. Exp. Neuropsychol.,* 8(6) Dec: 744 – 748.

Crow T.J., Bloom S.R., Cross A.J., Ferrier I.N., Johnstone

E.C., Owen F., Owens D.G.C. and Roberts G.W. (1984) Abnormal involuntary movements in schizophrenia; neurochemical correlates and relation to the disease process. In: E. Usdin, A. Carlsson, A. Dahlstrom, and J. Engel (Eds.), *Catecholamines. Part C: Neuropharmacology and Central Nervous System: Therapeutic Aspects.* Liss, New York; pp. 61 – 67.

Damasio A.R. (1984) The anatomic basis of memory disorders. *Seminars in Neurology, Vol. 4,* pp. 223 – 224.

Danielson E.H., Magnuson D.J. and Gray T.S. (1989) The central amygdaloid nucleus innervation of the dorsal vagal complex in rat; a *phaseolus vulgaris* leucoagglutinin lectin anterograde tracing study. *Brain Res. Bull.,* 22: 705 – 715.

Danner H. and Pfister C. (1981) Untersuchungen zur Zytoarchitectonik des Tuberculum Olfactorium der Ratte. *J. Hirnforsch.* 22: 685 – 696.

Danscher G. (1982) Exogenous selenium in the brain; a histochemical tecnique for light and electron microscopical localization of catalytic selenium bonds. *J. Histochem.,* 76: 281 – 293.

Davis P. and Maloney A.J. (1976) Selective loss of cholinergic neurons in Alzheimer's disease. *Lancet, II:* 1403.

Davison K. and Bagley C.R. (1969) Schizophrenia-like psychoses associated with organic disorders of central nervous system; a review of the literature. Br. J. Psychiat. (Special Publication No. 4). In: E. Herrington (Ed.), *British Journal of Psychiatry,* Headley Bros. Ltd, Ashford, U.K. 113 – 184.

de Lisi L.E., Dauphinais I.D., Gershon E.S. (1988) Perinatal complications and reduced size of brain limbic structures in familial schizophrenia. *Schizophrenia Bull.,* 14: 185 – 191.

de Olmos J.S. (1969) Distribution of the granular argyrophilic neurons in normal cat and monkey brains. *82nd Ann. Ses. AAA. Anat. Rec.,* 163: 177 – 78.

de Olmos J.S. (1972) The amygdaloid projection field in the rat as studied with the cupric-silver method. In: B.E. Elefteriou (Ed.), The Neurobiology of the Amygdala. Plenum Press, New York; pp. 145 – 204.

de Olmos J.S., Alheid G.F. and Beltramino C.A. (1985) Amygdala. In G. Paxinos (Ed.), *The Rat Nervous System.* Academic Press, Sydney; pp. 223 – 334.

de Olmos, J. (1990) The amygdaloid body. In G. Paxinos (Ed): *The Human Nervous System.* Academic Press, San Diego, pp. 583 – 710.

DiFiglia M., Aronin M. and Martin J.B. (1982) Light and electron microscopic localization of immunoreactive leu-enkephalin in the monkey basal ganglia. *J. Neurosci.,* 2: 303 – 320.

DiFiglia M., Graveland G.A., Schwartz W.F. and Wu J.Y. (1984) Localization of immunoreactive enkephalins in GABA synthesizing neurons of the rat neostriatum. *Brain Res.,* 300: 276 – 380.

Divac I. (1975) Magnocellular nuclei of the basal forebrain project to neocortex, brainstem and olfactory bulb; review of some functional correlates. *Brain Res.,* 93: 385 – 398.

Dwork A.J., Schon E.A. and Herbert J. (1988) Nonidentical distribution of transferrin and ferric iron in human brain. *Neuroscience,* 27: 333 – 345.

Eckenstein F.P., Baughman R.W. and Quinn J. (1988) An anatomical study of cholinergic innervation in rat cerebral cortex. *Neuroscience,* 25: 457 – 474.

Emson P.C., Goedert M. and Mantyh P.W. (1985) Neurotensin-containing neurons. In: A. Björklund, T. Hökfelt (Eds.), *Handbook of chemical neuroanatomy, Vol. 4, part 1.* Elsevier Science Publishers, Amsterdam, pp. 355 – 405.

Emsley R.A. and Paster L. (1985) Lipoid proteinosis presenting with neuropsychiatic manifestations. *J. Neurol.,* 48: 1290 – 1292.

Eggerman, K. W. and Zahm, D.S. (1988). Numbers of neurotensin-immuno-reactive neurons in the rat ventral striatum selectively increased following acute haloperidol administration. Neuropeptides 11: 125 – 132.

Etienne P., Robitaille Y., Wood P., Gauthier S., Nair N.P.V. and Quirion R. (1986) Nucleus basalis neuronal loss, neuritic plagues and choline acetyltransferase activity in advanced Alzheimer's disease. *Neuroscience,* 19: 1279 – 1291.

Everitt B.J., Sirkiä T.E., Roberts A.C., Jones G.H. and Robbins T.W. (1988) Distribution and some projections of cholinergic neurons in the brain of the common marmoset, *Callithrix jacchus. J. Comp. Neurol.,* 271: 533 – 558.

Falkai P. and Bogerts B. (1986) Cell loss in the hippocampus of schizophrenics. *Eur. Arch. Psychiat. Neurol. Sci.,* 236: 154 – 161.

Fallon J.H. (1981) Histochemical characterization of dopaminergic, noradrenergic and serotonergic projections to the amygdala. In: Y. Ben-Ari (Ed.), *The Amygdaloid Complex.* Elsevier Biomedical, Press, Amsterdam, pp. 175 – 184.

Fallon J.H. (1987) Growth factors in the basal ganglia. In: M.B. Carpenter and A. Jayaraman (Eds.), *Advances in Behavioral Biology, Vol. 32, The Basal Ganglia II.* Plenum Press, New York, pp. 247 – 281.

Fallon J.H. and Loughlin S.E. (1987) Monoamine innervation of cerebral cortex and a theory of the role of monoamines in cerebral cortex and basal ganglia. In: E.G. Jones and A. Peters (Eds.), *Cerebral Cortex (Vol. 6).* Plenum, New York, pp. 41 – 127.

Fallon J.H. and Moore R.Y. (1978) Catecholamine innervation of the basal forebrain. IV. Topography of the dopamine projection to the basal forebrain and neostriatum. *J. Comp. Neurol.,* 180: 545 – 580.

Fallon J.H. Seroogy K.B., Loughlin S.E., Morrison R.S., Bradshaw R.A., Knauer D.J. and Cunningham D.D. (1984) Epidermal growth factor immunoreactive material in the central nervous system: Location and development. *Science,* 224: 1107 – 1109.

Féger J. and Crossman A.R. (1984) Identification of different subpopulations of neostriatal neurones projecting to globus pallidus or substantia nigra in the monkey; a retrograde fluorescence double-labelling study. *Neurosci. Lett.,* 49:

7 – 12.

Feigenbaum-Langer L. and Graybiel A.M. (1989) Distinct nigrostriatal projection systems innervate striosomes and matrix in the primate striatum. *Brain Res.,* 498: 344 – 350.

Ferreyra-Moyano, H. and Barragan, E. (1989) The olfactory system and Alzheimer disease. *Int. J. Neurosci. 49:* 157 – 197.

Fibiger H.C. (1984) The neurobiological substrates of depression in Parkinson's disease; a hypothesis. *J. Can. Sci. Neurol.* 11: 105 – 107.

Fisher R.S. Buchwald N.A., Hull C.D. and Levine M.S. (1988) GABAergic basal forebrain neurons project to the neocortex: The localization of glutamic acid decarboxylase and choline acetyltransferase in feline corticopetal neurons. *J. Comp. Neurol.,* 272: 489 – 502.

Fisher A., Hanin I, and Lachman, C. (1985) *Alzheimer's and Parkinson's Diseases: Advances in Behavioral Biology (Vol. 29).* Plenum Press, New York.

Flor-Henry P. (1969) Psychosis and temporal lobe epilepsy. *Epilepsia,* 10: 363 – 395.

Foix C. and Nicolesco J. (1925) Anatomie cerebrale; les noyaux gris centraux et la region mesencephalo-sous-optique; suivi d'un appendice sur l'anatomie pathologique de la maladie de parkinson. Masson, Paris, p. 581.

Francois C., Nguyen-Legros J. and Percheron G. (1981) Topographical and cytological localization of iron in rat and monkey brains. *Brain Res.,* 215: 317 – 322.

Friedemann M. (1911) Die Cytoarchitektonik des Zwischenhirns der Cercopitheken mit besonderer Berücksichtigung des thalamic opticus. *J. Psychol. Neurol. (Leipzig),* 18: 309 – 378.

Fuller T.A., Carnes K.M. and Price J.L. (1986) Afferents to the horizontal diagonal band of rat. *Soc. Neurosci. Abstr.,* 12: 315.

Gallagher M. (1990) The amygdala central nucleus and appetitive pavlovian conditioning; lesions impair one class of conditioned behavior. *J. Neurosci.,* 10: 1906 – 1911.

Garcia-Rill E., Skinner R.D. and Gilmore S.A. (1981) Pallidal projections at the mesencephalic locomotor region (MLR) in the cat. *Am. J. Anat.,* 161: 311 – 321.

Garcia-Rill E., Skinner R.D., Gilmore S.A. and Owings R. (1983a) Connections of the mesencephalic locomotor region (MLR). II. Afferents and efferents. *Brain Res. Bull.,* 10: 63 – 71.

Garcia-Rill E., Skinner R.D., Jackson M.B. and Smith M.M. (1983b) Connections of the mesencephalic locomotor region (MLR) I. Substantia nigra afferents. *Brain Res. Bull.,* 10: 57 – 62.

Gaspar P. and Gray, F. (1984) Dementia in idiopathic Parkinson's disease. *Acta. Neuropathol. (Berlin),* 64: 43 – 52.

Gerfen C.R. (1988) Synaptic organization of the striatum. *J. Electron. Microsc. Tech.,* 10: 265 – 281.

Gerfen C.R., Herkenham M. and Thibault J. (1987) The neostriatal mosaic. II. Compartmental organization of mesostriatal dopaminergic and non-dopaminergic systems. *J. Neurosci.,* 7: 3915 – 3934.

Gerfen C.R., Staines W.A., Arbuthnott G.W. and Fibiger H.D. (1982) Crossed connections of the substantia nigra in the rat. *J. Comp. Neurol.,* 207: 283 – 303.

Geschwind N. (1975) The borderland of neurology and psychiatry; some common misconceptions. In: D.F. Benson and D. Blumer (Eds.), *Psychiatric Aspects of Neurologic Disease.* Grune and Stratton, New York, pp. 1 – 9.

Gloor M.D. (1978) Inputs and outputs of the amygdala; what the amygdala is trying to tell the rest of the brain. In: K.E. Livingston and O. Hornykiewicz (Eds.), Limbic Mechanisms; The Continuing Evolution of the Limbic System Concept. Plenum Press, New York, pp. 189 – 209

Gloor P., Olivier A., Quesney L.F., Andermann F. and Horowitz S. (1982) The role of the limbic system in experiential phenomena of temporal lobe epilepsy. *Ann. Neurol.,* 12: 129 – 144.

Goldman-Rakic P.S. and Selemon L.D. (1986) Topography of corticostriatal projections in nonhuman primates and implications for functional parcellation of the neostriatum. In: E.G. Jones and A. Peters (Eds.), *Cerebral Cortex Vol. 5.* Pleunum Press, New York pp. 447 – 466.

Gould E., Woolf N.J., Butcher L.L. (1989) Cholinergic projections to the substantia nigra from the pedunculopontine and laterodorsal tegmental nuclei. *Neuroscience,* 28: 611 – 623.

Gray T.S. (1987) The organization and possible function of amygdaloid corticotropin releasing factor pathways. In: E.B. De Souza and C.B. Nemeroff (Eds.), Corticotropin-releasing factor: Basic and Clinical Studies of a Neuropeptide. CRC Press, New York.

Gray T.S. (1988) Autonomic neuropeptide connections of the amygdala. In: Y. Tache, J.E. Morley and M.R. Brown (Eds.), *Neuropeptides and Stress.* Salye Symposium, Symposia Hans Selye. Springer-Verlag, New York, pp. 92 – 105.

Gray T.S., Carney M.E. and Magnuson D.J. (1989) Direct projections from the central amygdaloid nucleus to the hypothalamic paraventricular nucleus; possible role in stress-induced adrenocorticotropin release. *Neuroendocrinol.* 50: 433 – 446.

Gray T.S. and Magnuson D.J. (1987) Neuropeptide neuronal efferents from the bed nucleus of the stria terminalis and central amygdaloid nucleus to the dorsal vagal complex in the rat. *J. Comp. Neurol.,* 262: 365 – 374.

Graybiel A.M. and Ragsdale C.W. (1979) Fiber connections of the basal ganglia. In: M. Cuenod, G.W. Kreutzberg, and F.E. Bloom (Eds.), *Development and Chemical Specificity of Neurons.* Elsevier, Amsterdam.

Graybiel A.M. and Ragsdale C.W.Jr. (1983) Biochemical anatomy of the striatum. In: P.C. Emson (Ed,). *Chemical Neuroanatomy,* Raven Press, New York. pp. 427 – 504.

Grebb J.A., Cancro R. (1989) Schizophrenia; clinical features. In: H.I. Kaplan and B.J. Sadock (Eds,). *Comprehensive Textbook of Psychiatry* (Vol. 1, Fifth Ed). Williams and

Wilkins, Baltimore, Maryland, pp. 757 – 777.

Groenewegen H.J. (1988) Organization of the afferent connections of the mediodorsal thalamic nucleus in the rat, related to the mediodorsal-prefrontal topography. *Neuroscience,* 24: 379 – 431.

Groenewegen H.J., Room P., Witter M.P. and Lohman A.H.M. (1982) Cortical afferents of the nucleus accumbens in the cat studied with anterograde and retrograde transport techniques. *Neuroscience,* 7: 977 – 995.

Groenewegen H.J. and Russchen F.T. (1984) Organization of the efferent projections of the nucleus accumbens to pallidal, hypothalamic and mesencephalic structures: a tracing and immunohistochemical study in the cat. *J. Comp. Neurol.,* 223: 347 – 367.

Groenewegen H.J., Vermeulen-van der Zee E., te Kortshot A. and Witter M.P. (1987) Organization of the projections from the subiculum to the ventral striatum in the rat. A study using anterograde transport of phaseolus vulgaris leucoagglutinin. *Neuroscience,* 23, 103 – 120.

Grove E.A. (1988a) Neural associations of the substantia innominata in the rat: Afferent connections. *J. Comp. Neurol.,* 277: 315 – 346.

Grove E.A. (1988b) Efferent connections of the substantia innominata in the rat. *J. Comp. Neurol.,* 277: 347 – 364.

Growdon J.H. and Corkin S. (1986) Cognitive impairments in Parkinson's disease. In: M.D. Yahr and K.J. Bergmann (Eds.), *Advances in Neurology (Vol. 45).* Raven Press, New York, pp. 383 – 392.

Haber S.N. (1987) Anatomical relationship between the basal ganglia and the basal nucleus of Meynert in human and monkey forebrain. *Proc. Natl. Acad. Sci.* 84: 1408 – 1412.

Haber S.N. and Elde R. (1981) Correlation between met-enkephalin and substance P immunoreactivity in the primate globus pallidus. *Neuroscience,* 6: 1291 – 1297.

Haber S.N., Groenewegen H.J., Grove E.A. and Nauta W.J.H. (1985) Efferent connections of the ventral pallidum: Evidence of a dual striato-pallidofugal pathway. *J. Comp. Neurol.,* 235: 322 – 335.

Haber S.N. and Nauta W.J.H. (1983) Ramifications of the globus pallidus in the rat as indicated by patterns of immunohistochemistry. *Neuroscience,* 9: 245 – 260.

Haber S.N. and Watson S.J. (1985) The comparative distribution of enkephalin, dynorphin and substance P in the human globus pallidus and basal forebrain. *Neuroscience,* 14: 1011 – 1024.

Hall E. (1972a) Some aspects of the structural organization of the amygdala. In: B.E. Eleftheriou (Ed.), *The Neurobiology of the Amygdala.* Plenum Press, New York, pp. 95 – 121.

Hall E. (1972b) The amygdala of the cat; A Golgi study. *Z. Zellorsch.,* 134: 439 – 458.

Hallanger A.E., Levey A.I., Henry J.L., Rye D.B. and Wainer B.H. (1987) The origins of cholinergic and other subcortical afferents to the thalamus in the rat. *J. Comp. Neurol.,* 262: 105 – 124.

Haracz J.L. (1985) Neural plasticity in schizophrenia. *Schizophrenia* Bull. 11: 191 – 229.

Hartmann-Von Monakow K., Akert K. and Künzle H. (1978) Projections of precentral motor cortex and other cortical areas of the frontal lobe to the subthalamic nucleus in the monkey. *Exp. Brain Res.,* 33: 395 – 403.

Hassler R. (1938) Zur Pathologie der Paralysis agitans und des postencephalitischen Parkinsonismus. *J. Psychol. U. Neur.,* 48: 387 – 476.

Hattori T. and Sugimoto T. (1983) Direct projections of the globus pallidus to the medial thalamus in the rat. *Soc. Neurosci. Abst.,* 9: 1230.

Hedreen J.C., Struble R.G., Whitehouse P.J. and Price D.L. (1984) Topography of the magnocellular basal forebrain system in human brain. *J. Neuropathol. Exp. Neurol.,* 43: 1 – 21.

Heimer L., Alheid G.F. and Zaborszky L. (1985) The basal ganglia. In: G. Paxinos (Ed.), The Rat Nervous System. Academic Press, Sydney, pp. 37 – 74.

Heimer L. and Wilson R.D. (1975) The subcortical projections of allocortex; similarities in the neural associations of the hippocampus, the piriform cortex and the neocortex. In: M. Santini (Ed.), *Golgi Centennial Symposium Proceedings.* Raven Press, New York, pp. 177 – 193.

Heimer L. (1978) The olfactory cortex and the ventral striatum. In: K.E. Livingston and O. Hornykiewicz (Eds.), *Limbic Mechanisms.* Plenum Press, New York, pp. 95 – 187.

Heimer L., Van Hoesen G.W. and Rosene D.L. (1977) The olfactory pathways and the anterior perforated substance in the primate brain. *Int. J. Neurol.,* 12: 42 – 52.

Heimer L., Zaborszky L., Zahm D.S., Alheid G.F. (1987) The ventral striatopallidothalamic projection. I. The striatopallidal link originating in striatal parts of the olfactory tubercle. *J. Comp. Neurol.,* 255: 571 – 591.

Heimer L., Zahm D.S., Churchill, L., Kalivas, P.W. and Wohltmann, C. (1990) Specificity in the projection patterns of accumbal core and shell in the rat. *Neuroscience,* (in press).

Herzog A.G. and Kemper T.L. (1980) Amygdaloid changes in aging and dementia. *Arch. Neurol.,* 37: 625 – 629.

Hill D. (1962) The schizophrenia-like psychoses of epilepsy. *Proc. Royal. Soc. B.* 55: 315 – 316.

Hill J.M. and Switzer R.C. III (1984) The regional distribution and cellular localization of iron in the rat brain. *Neuroscience,* 11: 595 – 603.

Holstege G.. Meiners L. and Tan K. (1985) Projections of the bed nucleus of the stria terminlis to the mesencephalon, pons, and medulla oblongata in the cat. *Expl. Brain Res.,* 58: 379 – 391.

Hopkins D.A. (1975) Amygalotegmental projections in rat, cat and rhesus monkey. *Neurosci. Lett.,* 1: 263 – 270.

Hopkins D.A. and Holstege G. (1978) Amygdaloid projections to the mesencephalon, pons and medulla oblongata in the cat. *Expl. Brain Res.,* 32: 529 – 547.

Hopper M.W. and Vogel F.S. (1976) The limbic system in Alzheimer's disease; a neuropathologic investigation. *Am. J. Pathology,* 85: 1 – 20.

Hornykiewicz O. (1977) Biogenic amines in the centeral nervous system. In: P.J. Viaken, Bruyn G.W., H.L. Klamans (Eds.), *Handbook of Clinical Neurology - Vol. 29,* Part III. Elsevier, Amsterdam, pp. 459 – 483.

Hornykiewicz O. and Kish S.J. (1984) Neurochemical basis of dementia in Parkinson's disease. *Can. J. Neurol. Sci. 1.* (Supplement), 101.

Horvath T.B., Siever L.J., Mohs R.C. and Davis K. (1989) Organic mental syndromes and disorders. In: H.I. Kaplan and B.J. Sadock (Eds.), *Comprehensive Textbook of Psychiatry (Vol. 1, Fifth Ed.).* Williams and Wilkins, Baltimore, MD, pp. 599 – 641.

Hreib K.K., Rosene D.L. and Moss M.B. (1988) Basal forebrain efferents to the medial dorsal thalamic nucleus in the rhesus monkey. *J. Comp. Neurol.,* 277: 365 – 390.

Hyman B.T., Damasio A.R., Van Hoesen G.W. and Barnes C.L. (1984) Alzheimer's disease; cell specific pathology isolates the hippocampal formation. *Science, (Wash. DC),* 225: 1168 – 1170.

Inagaki N., Yamatodani A., Ando-Yamamoto M., Tohyama M., Watanabe T. and Wada H. (1988) Organization of histaminergic fibers in the rat brain. *J. Comp. Neurol.,* 273: 283 – 300.

Ingvar D.H. and Franzen G. (1974) Distribution of cerebral activity in chronic schizophrenia. *Lancet,* II: 1484 – 1486.

Irle E. and Markowitsch H.J. (1986) Afferent connections of the substantia innominata basal nucleus of Meynert in carnivores and primates. *J. Hirnforsch,* 27: 343 – 367.

Jackson A. and Crossman A.R. (1983) Nucleus tegmenti pedunculopontinus efferent connections with special reference to the basal ganglia, studied in the rat by anterograde and retrograde transport of horseradish peroxidase. *Neuroscience,* 10: 725 – 765.

Jakob H. and Beckmann H. (1986) Prenatal developmental disturbances in the limbic allocortex in schizophrenics. *J. Neural Trans.,* 65: 303 – 326.

Jacobs R.W. and Butcher L.L. (1986) Pathology of the basal forebrain in Alzheimer's disease and other dementias. In: A.B. Scheibel and A.F. Wechsler (Eds.), *The Biological Substrates of Alzheimer's Disease.* Academic Press, New York, pp. 87 – 100.

Johnston J.B. (1923) Further contributions to the study of the evolution of the forebrain. *J. Comp. Neurol.,* 35: 337 – 481.

Jones E.G., Burton H., Saper C.B. and Swanson L.W. (1976) Midbrain, diencephalic and cortical relationships of the basal nucleus of Meynert and associated structures in primates. *J. Comp. Neurol.,* 167: 385 – 420.

Jones B.E. and Cuello A.C. (1989) Afferents to the basal forebrain cholinergic cell area from pontomesencephalic-catecholamine, serotonin, and acetylcholine-neurons. *Neuroscience,* 31: 37 – 61.

Javoy-Agid F. and Agid Y. (1980) Is the mesocortical dopaminergic system involved in Parkinson disease? *Neurology,* 30: 1326 – 1330.

Javoy-Agid F., Taguet H., Plaska A., Cherif-Zahar C., Raberg M. and Agid Y. (1981) Distribution of catecholamines in the ventral mesencephalon of human brain, with special reference to Parkinson's disease *J. Neurochem.,* 36: 2101 – 2105.

Jellinger K. (1985) Neuromorphological background of pathochemical studies in major psychoses. In: H. Beckmann and P. Riederer (Eds.), *Pathochemical Markers in Major Psychoses.* Springer-Verlag, New York, pp. 1 – 23.

Jourdain A., Semba K. and Fibiger H.C. (1989) Basal forebrain and mesopontine tegmental projections to the reticular thalamic nucleus: an axonal collateralization and immunohistochemical study in the rat. *Brain Res.,* 505: 55 – 65.

Jürgens U. and Ploog D. (1970) Cerebral respresentation of vocalization in the squirrel monkey. *Exp. Brain Res.,* 10: 532 – 554.

Kapp B.S., Pascoe J.P. and Bixler M.A. (1984) The amygdala; a neuroanatomical systems approach to its contribution to aversive conditioning. In: L. Squire and N. Butters (Eds.), *The Neuropsychology of Memory.* Guilford Press, New York. pp. 473 – 488.

Kelley A.E. and Domesick V.B. (1982) The distribution of the projection from the hippocampal formation to the nucleus accumbens in the rat; an anterograde and retrograde horseradish peroxidase study. *Neuroscience,* 7: 2321 – 2335.

Kelley A.E., Domesick V.B. and Nauta W.J.H. (1982) The amygdalostriatal projection in the rat; an anatomical study by anterograde and retrograde tracing methods. *Neuroscience,* 7: 615 – 630.

Kelley J., Alheid G.F., McDermott L.J., Halaris A. and Grossman S.P. (1977) Behavioral and biochemical effects of knife cuts that preferentially interrupt afferent and efferent connections of the striatum in the rat. *Pharmac. Biochem. Behav.* 6: 31 – 45.

Kevetter G.A. and Winans S.S. (1981a) Connections of the corticomedial amygdala in the golden hamster I. Efferents of the "vomeronasal amygdala". *J. Comp. neurol.,* 197: 81 – 98.

Kevetter G.A. and Winans S.S. (1981b) Connections of the corticomedial amygdala in the golden hamster. II Efferents of the "olfactory amygdala". *J. Comp. Neurol.* 197: 99 – 111.

Khachaturian H., Akil H., Brownstein M.J., Olney J.W. and Voigt K.H. (1986) Further characterization of the extra-arcuate alphamelanocyte stimulating hormone-like material in hypothalamus: Biochemical and anatomical studies. *Neuropeptides,* 7: 291 – 313.

Khachaturian H., Lewis M.E., Tsou K. and Watson S.T. (1985) β-Endorphin, α-MSH, ACTH, and related peptides. In A. Björklund and T. Hökfelt (Eds.), *Handbook of Chemical Neuroanatomy (Vol. 4, Part I);* GABA and Neuropeptides in the CNS. Elsevier, Amsterdam, pp. 216 – 272.

Kievit J. and Kuypers H.G.J.M. (1975) Basal forebrain and

hypothalamic connections to frontal and parietal cortex in the rhesus monkey. *Science,* 187: 660 – 662.

Kitai S.T. (1981) Anatomy and psysiology of the neostriatum. *Adv. Biochem. Psychopharmacol.,* 30: 1 – 21.

Kitai S.T. and Deniau J.M. (1981) Cortical inputs to the subthalamus; intracellular analysis. *Brain Res.,* 214: 411 – 415.

Kitai S.T., Kita H. (1984) Intracellular recording and labeling of globus pallidus neurons in the rat. *Soc. Neurosci. Abst.,* 10: 703.

Kodama S. (1929) Pathologisch-anatomische Untersuchen mit Bezug auf die sogennanten Basalganglien und ihre Adnexe. *Neurol. Psych. Abh. Schwiez. Arch. Neurol. Psychol.,* 8: 1 – 206.

Köhler C., Haglund L. and Swanson L.W. (1984) A diffuse αMSH-immunoreactive projection to the hippocampus and spinal cord from individual neurons in the lateral hypothalamic area and zona incerta. *J. Comp. Neurol.,* 223: 501 – 514.

Köhler C., Swanson L.W., Haglund L. and Wu J. -Y. (1985) The cytoarchitecture, histochemistry and projections of the tuberomammillary nucleus in the rat. *Neuroscience,* 16: 85 – 110.

Köhler C. and Swanson L.W. (1984) Acetylcholinesterase-containing cells in the lateral hypothalamic area are immunoreactive for alpha-melanocyte stimulating hormone (alpha-MSH) and have cortical projections in the rat. *Neurosci. Lett.,* 49: 39 – 43.

Koliatsos V.E., Martin L.J., Walker L.C., Richardson R.T., DeLong M.R. and Price D.L. (1988) Topographic, noncollateralized basal forebrain projections to amygdala, hippocampus, and anterior cingulate cortex in the rhesus monkey. *Brain Res.,* 463: 133 – 139.

Kölliker, A. (1896) Handbuch der Gewebelehre des Menschen (Vol. 2): Nervensystem. Engelmann, Leipzig.

Korczyn A.D., Inzelberg R., Treves T., Neufeld M., Reider, I. and Rabey, P.M. (1986) Dementia of Parkinson's disease. In: M.D. Yahr and K.I. Bergmann (Eds.), Advances in Neurology (Vol. 45). New York: Raven Press, pp. 399 – 402.

Kovelman J.A. and Scheibel A.B. (1984) A neurohistological correlate of schizophrenia. *Biol. Psychiatry,* 19: 1601 – 1621.

Kraepelin E. (1919) *Dementia Prœcox and paraphrenia.* In: R.M. Barclay (English Trans, reprinted 1971). Robert E. Krieger Publishing Co., Huntington, NY.

Krayniak P.F., Meibach R.C. and Siegel A. (1981) A projection from the entorhinal cortex to the nucleus accumbens in the rat. *Brain Res.,* 209: 427 – 431.

Krettek J.E. and Price J.L. (1978) Amygdaloid projections to subcortical structures within the basal forebrain and brainstem in the rat and cat. *J. Comp. Neurol.,* 178: 225 – 254.

Künzle H. (1976) Thalamic projections from the precentral motor cortex in Macaca fascicularis. *Brain Res.,* 105: 253 – 267.

Künzle H. (1978) An autoradiographic analysis of the efferent connections from premotor and adjacent prefrontal regions (areas 6 and 9) in *Macaca fascicularis. Brain Behav. Evol.,* 15: 185 – 234.

Künzle H. and Akert K. (1977) Efferent connections of cortical area 8 (frontal eye field) in Macaca fascicularis; a reinvestigation using the autoradiographic technique. *J. Comp. Neurol.,* 173: 147 – 164.

Lauer E.W. (1945) The nuclear pattern and fiber connections of certain basal telencephalic centers in the macaque. *J. Comp. Neurol.,* 183: 785 – 816.

Le Doux J.E. (1986) Sensory systems and emotion; a model of affective processing. *Integr. Psychiatry,* 4: 237 – 248.

LeDoux J.E. (1987) Emotion. In: V.B. Mountcastle, R. Plum and S.R. Geiger (Eds.), *Handbook of Physiology; section 1, The Nervous System (Vol 5).* American Physiological Society, Bethesda, MA, pp. 419 – 459.

Lee H.J., Rye D.B., Hallanger A.E., Levey A.I. and Wainer B.H. (1988) Cholinergic vs noncholinergic efferents from the mesopontine tegmentum to the extrapyramidal motor system nuclei. *J. Comp. Neurol.,* 275: 469 – 492.

Lemann W., Saper C.B. (1985) Evidence for a cortical projection to the magnocellular basal nucleus in the rat: An electron microscopic axonal transport study. *Brain Res.,* 334: 339 – 343.

Leranth C., Froscher M. (1989) Organization of the septal region in the rat brain; cholinergic-GABAergic interconnections and the termination of hippocampo-septal fibers. *J. Comp Neurol.,* 289: 304 – 314.

Leverenz J., Sumi S.M. (1984) Prevalence of Parkinson's disease in patients with Alzheimer's disease. *Neurology,* 34 (Suppl. 1) : 101.

Levey A.I., Hallanger A.E., Wainer B.H. (1987) Cholinergic nucleus basalis neurons may influence the cortex via the thalamus. *Neurosci. Lett.,* 74: 7 – 13.

Lewy F.H. (1912) Paralysis agitans. I. Pathologische Anatomie. In: M. Lewandowsky (Ed.), Handbuch der Neurologie (Vol. 3). Julius Springer, Berlin. pp. 920 – 933.

Lewy F.H. (1913) Zur pathologischen Anatomie der Paralysis agitans. *Dtsch Z. Nervenheik.,* 50: 50 – 55.

Lind R.W., Swanson L.W., Ganten D. (1985) Organization of immunoreactive cells and fibers in the rat central nervous system. *Neuroendocrinology,* 40: 2 – 24.

Lishman W.A. (1987) Organic Psychiatry: The Psychological Consequences of Cerebral Disorder (2nd Ed). Blackwell Scientific Publications, Palo Alto, U.S.A.

Luskin M.B., Price J.L. (1983) The topographic organization of associational fibers of the olfactory system in the rat, including centrifugal fibers to the olfactory bulb. *J. Comp. Neurol.,* 216: 264 – 291.

Lynd E., Klein C., Groenewegen H.J., Haber S.N. (1988) Organization of the efferent projections from the primate ventromedial striatum. *Soc. Neurosci. Abstract,* 14: 156.

Macchi G. (1951) The ontogenetic development of the olfactory telencephalon in man. *J. Comp. Neurol.,* 95: 245 – 305.

Mai J.K. and Cuello A.C. (1990) Distribution of Substance P

in the human brain. In: G. Paxinos (Es.), *The human nervous system.* Academic Press, San Diego pp. 1051 – 1094.

Mai J.K., Stephens P.H., Hope A. and Cuello A.C. (1986) Substance P in the human brain. *Neuroscience,* 17: 709 – 739.

Malamud N. (1967) Psychiatric disorder with intracranial tumors of limbic system. *Arch. Neurol.,* 17: 113 – 123.

Mann D.M.A., Tucker C.M. and Yates P.O. (1988) Alzheimer's disease; an olfactory connection? *Mechanisms Ageing Devel.,* 42: 1 – 15.

Mann D.M.A., Yates P.O. and Marcyniuk B. (1984) Alzheimer's disease; cell counts and cortical biochemistry. *Neuropath. Appl. neurobiol.,* 10: 185 – 207.

Marsden C.D., Tarsy D. and Baldessarine R.H. (1975) Spontaneous and drug-induced movement disorders in psychotic patients. In: D.F. Benson and D. Blumer (Ed.), *Psychiatric Aspects of Neurologic Disease.* Grune and Stratton, New York. pp. 219 – 266.

Martinez-Murillo R., Semenenko F. and Cuello A.C. (1988) The origin of tyrosine hydroxylase-immunoreactive fibers in the regions of the nucleus basalis magnocellularis of the rat. *Brain Res.,* 451: 227 – 236.

Martin J.B. (1984) Huntington's disease; new approaches to an old problem. *Neurol.* (Cleveland), 34: 1059 – 1072.

Mayeux R., Stern Y. (1985) Clinical heterogeneity in patients with dementia of the Alzheimer type. In: A. Fisher, I. Hanin, and C. Lachman (Eds.), *Alzheimer's and Parkinson's Disease: Advances in Behavioral Biology (Vol. 29).* Plenum Press, New York, pp. 129 – 134.

Mayeux R., Williams J.B.W., Stern Y. and Cote L. (1984) Depression and Parkinson's disease. In: R.G. Hassler and J.F. Christ (Eds.), *Advances in Neurology (Vol. 40).* Raven Press, New York, 241 – 250.

McDonald A.J. (1983) Neurons of the bed nucleus of the stria terminalis: a Golgi study in the rat. *Brain Res. Bull.* 10: 111 – 120.

McDonald A.J. (1984) Neuronal organization of the lateral and basolateral amygdaloid nuclei in the rat. *J. Comp. Neurol.,* 222: 589 – 606.

McGeer P.L., McGeer E.G., Suzuki J., Dolman C.E. and Nagai T. (1984) Aging, Alzheimer's disease, and the cholinergic system of the basal forebrain. *Neurology,* 34: 741 – 745.

McHugh, P.R. and Folstein M.F. (1975) Psychiatric syndromes of Huntington's chorea; a clinical and phenomenologic study. In: D.F. Benson and D. Blumer (Eds.), *Psychiatric Aspects of Neurologic Disease.* Grune and Stratton, New York. pp. 267 – 286.

McNeil T.F. (1988) Obstetric factors and perinatal injuries (Ch14). In: M.T. Tsuang and J.C. Simpson (Eds.), *Handbook of Schizophrenia: Nosology, Epidemiology and Genetics.* Elsevier Science Publishers, Amsterdam pp. 319 – 344.

Mehler W.R. (1980) Subcortical afferent connections of the amygdala in the monkey. *J. Comp. Neurol.,* 190: 733 – 762.

Mehler W.R. (1982) The basal ganglia-circa 1982; a review and commentary. *App. Neurophysiol.,* 44: 261 – 290.

Mehler W.R. and Nauta W.J.H. (1974) Connections of the basal ganglia and of the cerebellum. Proc. 6th Symp. Int. Soc. Res. Stereoencephalotomy, Tokyo (Part I). *Confin. Neurol.,* 36: 205 – 222.

Melander T., Staines W.A., Hökfelt T., Rokaeus A., Eckenstein F., Salvaterra P.M. and Wainer B.H. (1985) Galanin-like immunoreactivity in cholinergic neurons of the septum-basal forebrain complex projecting to the hippocampus of the rat. *Brain Res.,* 360: 130 – 138.

Mesulam M.M. and Geula C. (1988) Nucleus basalis (Ch4) and cortical cholinergic innervation in the human brain; observations based on the distribution of acetylcholinesterase and choline acetyltransferase. *J. Comp. neurol.,* 275: 216 – 240.

Mesulam M.M. and Mufson E.J. (1984) Neural inputs into the nucleus basalis of the substantia innominata (Ch4) in the rhesus monkey. *Brain,* 107: 253 – 274.

Mesulam M.M., Mufson E.J., Levey A.I. and Wainer B.H. (1983) Cholinergic innervation of cortex by the basal forebrain; cytochemistry and cortical connections of the septal area, diagonal band nuclei, nucleus basalis (substantia innominata), and hypothalamus in the rhesus monkey. *J. Comp. Neurol.,* 214: 170 – 197.

Mesulam M.M. and Van Hoesen G.W. (1978) Acetylcholinesterase-rich projections from the basal forebrain of the rhesus monkey to neocortex. *Brain Res.,* 109: 152 – 157.

Meyer G., Gonzalez-Hernandez T, Carrillo-Padilla F. and Ferres-Torres R. (1989) Aggregations of granule cells in the basal forebrain (islands of Calleja). A Golgi and cytoarchitectonic study in different mammals including man. *J. Comp. Neurol.,* 284: 405 – 478.

Meynert T. (1872) The brain of mammals. In: S. Stricker (J.J. Putnam, Trans.): *A Manual of Histology.* William Wood, New York, pp. 650 – 766.

Michel J.P., Sakamoto N., Kopp N. and Pearson J. (1986) Neurotensin immunoreactive structures in the human infant striatum, septum, amygdala, and cerebral cortex. *Brain Res.,* 397: 93 – 102.

Michel J.P, Sakamoto N. and Pearson J. (1988) Catecholaminergic anatomy of the human forebrain. In: *Progress in catecholamine research Part B: Central aspects.* New York, Alan R. Liss Inc., pp. 175 – 178.

Millhouse O.E. and Heimer L. (1984) Cell configurations in the olfactory tubercle of the rat. *J. Comp. Neurol.,* 265: 1 – 24.

Millhouse O.E. and de Olmos J. (1983) Neuronal configurations in lateral and basolateral amygdala. *Neuroscience,* 10: 1269 – 1300.

Miodonski R. (1967) Myeloarchitectonics and connections of substantia innominata in the dog brain. *Acta Biologiae Experimentalis (Warszawa),* 27: 61 – 84.

Mishkin M. (1978) Memory in monkeys severely impaired by combined but not by separate removal of amygdala and hippocampus. *Nature,* 273, 297 – 298.

Mishkin M. Malamut B. and Bachevalier J. (1984) Memories and habits; two neural systems. In: G. Lynch, J.L. McGaugh, and N.M. Weinberger (Eds.), *Neurobiology of Learning and Memory.* Guildford Press, New York, pp. 65 – 77,.

Mizuno N., Takahashi O., Satoda T. and Matsushima R. (1985) Amygdalospinal projections in the macaque monkey. *Neurosci. Lett.,* 53: 327 – 330.

Moga M.M. and Gray T.S. (1985a) Evidence for corticotropin-releasing factor, neurotensin, and somatostatin in the neural pathway from the central nucleus of the amygdala to the parabrachial nucleus. *J. Comp. Neur.,* 241: 275 – 284.

Moga M.M. and Gray T.S. (1985b) Peptidergic efferents from the intercalated nuclei of the amygdala to the parabrachial nucleus in the rat. *Neurosci. Lett.,* 61: 13 – 18.

Moga M.M., Saper C.B. and Gray T.S. (1989) Bed nucleus of the stria terminalis; cytoarchitecture, immunohistochemistry, and projection to the parabrachial nucleus in the rat. *J. Comp. Neurol.,* 283: 315 – 332.

Mogenson G.J., Ciriello J., Garland J. and Wu M. (1987) Ventral pallidum projections to mediodorsal nucleus of the thalamus; an anatomical and electrophysiological investigation in the rat. *Brain Res.,* 404: 221 – 230.

Mogenson G.J., Jones D.L. and Yim C.Y. (1980) From motivation to action; functional interface between the limbic system and the motor system. *Progr. Neurobiol.,* 14: 69 – 97.

Mogenson G.J., Swanson L.W. and Wu M. (1983) Neural projections from nucleus accumbens to globus pallidus, substantia innominata, and lateral preoptic-lateral hypothalamic area: An anatomical and electrophysiological investigation in the rat. *J. Neurosci.* 3: 189 – 202.

Mölsa P.K., Marttila R.J. and Rinne U.K. (1984) Extrapyramidal signs in Alzheimer's disease. *Neurology,* 34: 1114 – 1116.

Mufson E.J., Benoit R. and M.M. Mesulam. (1988) Immunohistochemical evidence for a possible somatostatin-containing amygdalostriatal pathway in normal and Alzheimer's disease brain. *Brain Res.,* 453: 117 – 128.

Mufson E.J., Bothwell M., Hersh L.B. and Kordower J.H. (1989) Nerve growth factor receptor immunoreactive profiles in the normal, aged human basal forebrain; colocalization with cholinergic neurons. *J. Comp. Neurol.,* 5: 196 – 217.

Müller H.F. (1985) Prefrontal cortex dysfunction as a common factor in psychosis. *Acta. Psychiatr. Scand.,* 71: 431 – 440.

Müller-Preuss P. and Jürgens U. (1976) Projections from the "cingular" vocalization area in the squirrel monkey. *Brain Res.,* 103: 29 – 43.

Nagai T., Kimura H., Maeda T., McGeer P.L., Peng F. and McGeer E.G. (1982) Cholinergic projections from the basal forebrain of rat to the amygdala. *J. Neurosci.* 2: 513 – 520.

Nakano I. and Hirano A. (1983) Neuron loss in the nucleus basalis of Meynert in parkinsonism-dementia complex of Guam. *Ann Neurol.,* 13: 87 – 91.

Nakano I. and Hirano A. (1984) Parkinson's disease; neuron loss in the nucleus basalis without concomitant Alzheimer's disease. *Ann. Neurol.,* 15: 415 – 418.

Nasrallah H.A., Fowler R.C. and Judd L.L. (1981) Schizophrenia-like illness following head injury. *Psychsomatics,* 22: 359 – 361.

Nauta W.J.H. and Domesick V.B. (1984) Afferent and efferent relationships of the basal ganglia. *Ciba Found. Symp.,* 107: 3 – 23.

Nauta W.J.H. and Mehler W.R. (1966) Projections of the lentiform nuclei in the monkey. *Brain Res.,* 1: 3 – 42.

Nauta W.J.H., Smith G.P., Faull R.L.M. and Domesick V.B. (1978) Efferent connections and nigral afferents of the nucleus accumbens septi in the rat. *Neuroscience,* 3, 385 – 401.

Newman R. and Winans S.S. (1980a) An experimental study of the ventral striatum of the golden hamster. I. Neuronal connections of the nucleus accumbens. *J. Comp. Neurol.,* 191: 167 – 192.

Newman R. and Winans S.S. (1980b) An experimental study of the ventral striatum of the golden hamster. II. Neuronal connections of the olfactory tubercle. *J. Comp. Neurol.,* 191: 193 – 212.

Nieto D. and Escobar A. (1972) Major psychoses. In: J. Minkler (Ed.), *Pathology of the Nervous System.* McGraw Hill, New York, pp. 2654 – 2665.

Novotny G.E.K. (1977) A direct ventral connection between the bed nucleus of the stria terminalis and the amygdaloid complex in the monkey (macaca fascicularis). *J. Hirnforsch.* 18: 217 – 284.

Otterson O.P. and Ben-Ari Y. (1979) Afferent connections to the amygdaloid complex of the rat and cat. I. Projections from the thalamus. *J. Comp. Neurol.,* 187: 401 – 424.

Oyanagi K., Takahashi H., Wakabayashi K. and Ikuta F. (1987) Selective involvement of large neurons in the neostriatum of Alzheimer's disease and senile dementia; a morphometric investigation. *Brain Res.,* 411: 205 – 211.

Parent A., Bouchard C. and Smith Y. (1984) The striatopallidal and striatonigral projections; two distinct fiber systems in primate. *Brain,* 85 – 390.

Parent A., Paré D., Smith Y. and Steriade M. (1988) Basal forebrain cholinergic and noncholinergic projections to the thalamus and brainstem in cats and monkeys. *J. Comp. Neurol.,* 277: 281 – 391.

Paxinos G. and Butcher L.L. Organizational principles of the brain as revealed by choline acetyltransferase and acetylcholinesterase distribution and projections. (1985) In: G. Paxinos (Ed.), *The Rat Nervous System, Vol. 1.* Academic Press, Sydney. pp. 487 – 512.

Pearce J. (1974) The extrapyramidal disorder of Alzheimer's disease. *Europ. Neurol.,* 12: 94 – 103.

Pearson R.C.A., Esiri M.M., Hiorns R.W. Wilcock G.K. and Powell T.P.S. (1985) Anatomical correlates of the distribution of the pathological changes in the neocortex in

Alzheimer disease. Proc. Natl. Sci. USA, 82: 4531 – 4534.

Penny G.R., Afsharpour S. and Kitai S.T. (1986) The glutamate decarboxylase-, leucine enkephalin-, methionine enkephalin- and substance P-immunoreactive neurons in the neostriatum of the rat and cat; evidence for partial population overlap. *Neuroscience,* 17: 1011 – 1045.

Percheron G., Yelnik J. and Francois C. (1984) A Golgi analysis of the primate globus pallidus. III. Spatial organization of the striato-pallidal complex. *J. Comp. Neurol.,* 227: 214 – 227.

Perez M.M., Trimble M.R., Murray N.M.F. and Reider I. (1985) Epileptic psychosis; an evaluation of PSE profiles. *Br. J. Psychiatry.* 146: 155 – 163.

Perry R.H., Candy J.M., Perry E.K., Thompson J. and Oakley A.E. (1984) The substantia innominata and adjacent regions in the human brain; histochemical and biochemical observations. *J. Anat.,* 134: 713 – 732.

Perry R.H., Tomlinson B.E. and Candy J.M. (1983) Cortical cholinergic deficit in mentally impaired Parkinsonian patients. *Lancet,* II: 789 – 790.

Petras J.M. (1969) Some efferent connections of the motor and somatosensory cortex of simian primates and field, canid and procyonid carnivores. *Ann. NY Acad. Sci.,* 167: 469 – 505.

Phillipson O.T. (1979) Afferent projections to the ventral tegmental area of Tsai and interfascicular nucleus: A horseradish peroxidase study in the rat. *J. Comp. Neurol.,* 187: 117 – 144.

Poletti C.E. (1986) Is the limbic system a limbic system? Studies of hippocampal efferents; their functional and clincial implications. In: B.K. Doane and K.F. Livingston (Eds.), *The Limbic System: Functional Organization and Clinical Disorders.* Raven Press, New York, pp. 79 – 94.

Price D.L., Whitehouse P.J., Struble R.G., Coyle J.T., Clark A.W., De Long, M.R., Cork, L.C. and Hedreen, J.C. (1982) Altzheimer's disease and Down's syndrome. *Ann. NY Acad. Sci.,* 396: 145 – 164.

Price J.L. (1990) The olfactory system. In: Paxinos G. (Ed.), *The human nervous system.* Academic Press, San Diego, (in press).

Price J.L. and Amaral D.G. (1981) An autoradiographic study of the projections of the central nucleus of the monkey amygdala. *J. Neurosci.,* 11: 1242 – 1259.

Price J.L., Russchen F.T. and Amaral D.G. (1987) The limbic region. II. The amygdaloid complex. In: A. Bjrklund, T. Hkfelt and L.W. Swanson (Eds.), *Handbook of Chemical Neuroanatomy (Vol 5).* Elsevier Science Publishers, Amsterdam. pp. 279 – 388.

Price J.L. and Slotnick B.M. (1983) Dual olfactory representation in the rat thalamus; an anatomical and electrophysiological study. *J. Comp. Neurol.,* 215: 63 – 77.

Price J.L. and Stern R. (1983) Individual cells in the nucleus basalis-diagonal band complex have restricted axonal projections to the cerebral cortex in the rat. *Brain Res.,* 269: 352 – 356.

Ragsdale C.W. Jr. and Graybiel A.M. (1988) Fibers from the basolateral nucleus of the amygdala selectively innervate striosomes in the caudate nucleus of the cat. *J. Comp Neurol.,* 269: 506 – 522.

Ramon Y Cajal S. (1955) Studies on the Cerebral Cortex. Lloyd-Luke (Medical Books) Ltd, London.

Randrup A. and Munkvad I. (1974) Pharmacology and physiology of sterotyped behavior. *J. Psychiat. Res.,* 11:1 – 10.

Reichert K.B. (1859-1861) Der Bau des Menschlichen Gehirns durch Abbildung mit erlauterndem Texte, 2 Vols. Engelmann. Leipzig.

Reil J.C. (1809) Untersuchungen über den Bau des grossen Gehirns im Menschen. *Arch. Psysiol.* (Halle), 9: 136 – 208.

Richardson R.T., Mitchell S.J., Baker F.H. and DeLong M.R. (1988) Responses of nucleus basalis of Meynert neurons in behaving monkeys. In: C.D. Woody, D.L. Alkon, and J.L. McGaugh (Eds.), *Cellular Mechanisms of Conditioning and Behavioral Plasticity.* Plenum Publishing, New York, pp. 161 – 173.

Riederer P. and Jellinger K. (1983) Morphologie und Patholbiochemie der Parkinson-Krnakheit. In: Gnshirt M. (Ed.), Pathophysiologie, Klinik und Therapie des Parkinsonismus, Ed Roche, Basal pp. 31 – 50.

Rinne J.O., Rummukainen J., Paljarvi L. and Rinne U.K. (1989) Dementia in Parkinson's disease is related to neuronal loss in the medial substantia nigra. *Ann. Neurol.,* 26, 47 – 50

Rinvik E., Grofov I., Hammond C., Fger J. and Deniau J.M. (1979) A Study of the afferent connections to the subthalamic nucleus in the monkey and the cat using the HRP technique. *Adv. Neurol.,* 24: 53 – 70.

Robins A.H. (1976) Depression in patients with parkinsonism. *Br. J. Psychiatry,* 128: 141 – 145.

Rolls E.T., Sanghera M.K. and Roper-Hall A. (1979) The latency of activation of neurones in the lateral hypothalamus and substantia innominata during feeding in the monkey. *Brain Res.,* 164: 121 – 135.

Romansky K.V., Usunoff K.G., Ivanov, D.P. and Galabov G.P. (1979) Corticosubthalamic projection in the cat; an electron microscopic study. *Brain Res.,* 163: 319 – 322.

Room P., Russchen F.T., Groenewegen H.J. and Lohman A.H.M. (1985) Efferent connections of the prelimbic (area 32) and the infralimbic (area 25) cortices: An anterograde tracing study in the cat. *J. Comp. Neurol.,* 242: 40 – 55.

Rosene D.L. and Van Hoesen G.W. (1977) Hippocampal efferents reach widespread areas of cerebral cortex and amygdala in the rhesus monkey. *Science,* (NY), 198: 315 – 317.

Rossor M.N. (1981) Parkinson's disease and Alzheimer's disease as disorders of the isodendritic core. *Br. Med. J. Clin. Res.,* 283: 1588 – 1590.

Rossor M., Svendsen C., Hent S., Montjoy C., Roth M. and Iversen L. (1982) The substantia innominata in Alzheimer's disease: A histochemical and biochemical study of cholinergic marker enzymes. *Neurosci. Lett.,* 28: 217 – 222.

Ruberg M., Ploska A. and Javoy-Agid F. (1982) Muscarinic binding and choline acetyl-transferase activity in Parkinsonian subjects with reference to dementia. *Brain Res.,* 232: 129 – 139.

Russchen F.T. (1986) Cortical and subcortical afferents of the amygdaloid complex. In: Schwarz R. and Ben-Ari Y. (Eds.), *Excitatory amino acids and epilepsy.* Plenum Press, New York, pp. 35 – 52.

Russchen F.T., Amaral D.G. and Price J.L. (1985a) The afferent connections of the substantia innominata in the monkey, *Macaca Fascicularis. J. Comp. Neurol.,* 242: 1 – 27.

Russchen F.T., Amaral D.G. and Price J.L. (1987) The afferent input to the magnocellular division of the mediodorsal thalamic nucleus in the monkey, Macaca fascinularis. *J. Comp. Neurol.,* 256: 175 – 210.

Russchen F.T., Bakst I., Amaral D.G. and Price J.L. (1985b) The amygdalostriatal projections in the monkey. An anterograde tracing study. *Brain Res.,* 329: 241 – 257.

Russchen F.T. and Price J.L. (1984) Amygdalostriatal projections in the rat. Topographical organization and fiber morphology shown using the lectin PHA-L as an anterograde tracer. *Neurosci. Lett.,* 47: 15 – 22.

Rye D.B., Saper C.B., Lee H.J. and Wainer B.H. (1987) Pedunculopontine tegmental nucleus of the rat: cytoarchitecture, cytochemistry, and some extrapyramidal connections of the mesopontine tegmentum. *J. Comp. Neurol.,* 259: 483 – 528.

Rye D.B., Wainer B.H., Mesulam M.M., Mufson E.J. and Saper C.B. (1984) Cortical projections arising from the basal forebrain: A study of cholinergic and non-cholinergic components employing combined retrograde tracing and immunohistochemical localizations of choline acetyltransferase. *Neuroscience,* 13: 627 – 643.

Sakai S.T. (1988) Corticonigral projections from area 6 in the raccoon. *Exp. Brain Res.,* 73: 498 – 504.

Sakamoto N., Pearson J. and Reisberg B. (1988) The human subcommissural basal forebrain. *Soc. Neurosci. Abstr.,* 14: 719.

Sandrew B.B., Edwards D.L., Poletti C.E. and Foote W.E. (1986) Amygdalo-spinal projections in the cat. *Brain Res.,* 35 – 239.

Saper C.B. (1984) Organization of cerebral cortical afferent systems in the rat. II. Magnocellular basal nucleus. *J. Comp. Neurol.* 222: 313 – 342.

Saper C.B. (1987) Diffuse cortical projection systems: anatomical organization and role in cortical function. In: V.B. Mountcastle, R. Plum. and S.R. Geiger (Eds.), *Handbook of Psysiology; The Nervous System (Vol 5).* American Physiological Society, Bethesda, MA. pp. 169 – 210.

Saper C.B. (1990) The cholonergic system. In: G. Paxinos (Ed.), *The human nervous system.* Academic Press, San Diego, pp. 483 – 582.

Saper C.B. and Chelimsky T.C. (1984) A cytoarchitectonic and histochemical study of nucleus basalis and associated cell groups in the normal human brain. *Neuroscience,* 13: 1023 – 1037.

Saper C.B., Wainer B.H. and German D.C. (1987) Axonal and transneuronal transport in the transmission of neurological disease; potential role in system degenerations. *Neuroscience,* 23: 389 – 398.

Schneider G.E. (1979) Is it really better to have your brain lesion early? A revision of the "Kennard Principle". *Neuropsychologia,* 17: 557 – 583.

Schwaber J.S., Kapp B.S., Higgins G.A. and Rapp P.R. (1982) Amygdaloid and basal forebrain direct connections with the nucleus of the solitary tract and the dorsal motor nucleus of the vagus. *J. Neurosci.,* 2: 1424 – 1438.

Schwaber J.S., Rogers W.T., Satoh K. and Fibiger H.C. (1987) Distribution and organization of cholinergic neurons in the rat forebrain demonstrated by computer-aided data acquisition and three-dimensional reconstruction. *J. Comp. Neurol.,* 263: 309 – 325.

Scoville W.B. and Milner B. (1957) Loss of recent memory after bilateral hippocampal lesions. *J. Neurol. Neurosurg. Psychiat.,* 20: 11 – 21.

Selemon L.D. and Goldman-Rakic P.S. (1985) Longitudinal topography and interdigitation of corticastriatal projections in the rhesus monkey. *J. Neurosci.,* 5: 776 – 794.

Semba K., Reiner P.B., McGeer E.G. and Fibiger H.C. (1988) Brainstem afferents to the magnocellular basal forebrain studied by axonal transport, immunohistochemistry, and electrophysiology in the rat. *J. Comp. Neurol.,* 267: 433 – 453.

Slater E. and Bear G. (1963) The schizophrenia like psychoses of epilepsy. *Br. J. Psychiat.,* 109: 95 – 150.

Smith Y., Parent A. (1986) Differential connections of caudate nucleus and putamen in the squirrel monkey *(Saimiri sciureus). Neuroscience,* 18: 347 – 371.

Sofroniew M.V., Campbell P.E., Cuello A.C. and Eckenstein F. (1985) Central cholinergic neurons visualized by immunohistochemical detection of choline acetyltransferase. In: G. Paxinos (Ed.), *The Rat Nervous System (Vol 1).* Academic Press, Sydney, pp. 471 – 485.

Spatz H. (1922) Uber den Eisennachweis im Gehirn, besonders in Zentren des extrapyramidal-motorischen Systems. *Z. Ges. Neurol. Psychiat.,* 77: 261 – 390.

Squire L.R. (1987) Memory; neural organization and behavior. In: V.B. Mountcastle, F. Plum, and S.R. Geiger (Eds.), *Handbook of Physiology (Section 1): The Nervous System (Vol. 5, Part 1).* Amereican Physiological Society, Bethesda, MD, pp. 295 – 371.

Sripanidkulchai K., Sripanidkulchai B. and Wyss J.M. (1984) The cortical projection of the basolateral amygdaloid nucleus in the rat: A retrograde fluorescent dye study. *J. Comp. Neurol.,* 229: 418 – 431.

Staines W.A. and Fibiger H.C. (1984) Collateral projections of neurons of the rat globus pallidus to the striatum and substantia nigra. *Exp. Brain. Res.*, 56: 217 – 220.

Steinbusch H.W.M., Sauren Y., Groenewegen H., Watanabe T. and Mulder A.H. (1986) Histaminergic projections from the premammillary and posterior hypothalamic region to the caudate-putamen complex in the rat. *Brain Res.*, 368: 389 – 393.

Stephan H. (1975) Allocortex. In: *Handbuch der Mikrokospishen Anatomie des Menschen (Vol, IV/9).* Springer-Verlag, Berlin.

Steriade M., Parent A., Pare D. and Smith Y. (1987) Cholinergic and non-cholinergic neurons of cat basal forebrain project to reticular and mediodorsal thalamic nuclei. *Brain Res.*, 408: 372 – 376.

Stevens J.R. (1982) Neuropathology of schizophrenia. *Arch. Gen. Psychiat.*, 39: 1131 – 1139.

Stevens J.R. (1983) Pathophysiology of schizophrenia. *Clin. Neuropharm.*, 6: 77 – 90.

Stevens J.R. (1986) Epilepsy and psychosis; neuropathological studies of six cases. In: M.R. Trimble and T. Bolwig (Eds.), *Aspects of Epilepsy and Psychiatry.* John Wiley and Sons, pp. 117 – 145.

Stevens J.R. (1989) The search for an anatomical basis of schizophrenia; review and update. In: Mueller (Ed.), *Neurology and Psychiatry: A Meeting of Minds.* Karger, Basel, New York, pp.64 – 87.

Stevens J.R. (1991) Psychosis and the Temporal Lobe. In D. Smith, D. Treiman and M. Trimble (Eds.), *Advances in Neurology,* Vol. 55, Raven Press, New York.

Sugimoto T. and Mizuno N. (1987) Neurotensin in projection neurons of the striatum and nucleus accumbens, with reference to coexistence with enkephalin and GABA; an immunohistochemical study in the cat. *J. Comp. Neurol.*, 257: 383 – 395.

Swanson L.W. (1982) Projections of the ventral tegmental area and adjacent regions: A combined fluorescent tracer and immunofluorescence study in the rat. *Brain Res. Bull.*, 9:321 – 353.

Swanson L.W. (1987) The hypothalamus. In: A. Björklund, T. Hökfelt, and L.W. Swanson (Eds.), *Handbook of Chemical Neuroanatomy (Vol. 5):* Integrated Systems of the CNS (Part 1). Elsevier Science Publishers, Amsterdam, pp. 1 – 124.

Swanson, L.W. and Cowan, W.M. (1975) A note on the connections and development of the nucleus accumbens. *Brain Res.*, 92: 324 – 330.

Swanson L.W. and Köhler C. (1986) Anatomical evidence for direct projections from entorhinal area to the entire cortical mantle in the rat. *J. Neurosci.*, 6: 3010 – 3023.

Swanson L.W., Köhler C. and Björklund A. (1987) The limbic region. I. The septohippocampal system. In: A. Björklund, T. Hökfelt, and L.W. Swanson (Eds.), *Handbook of Chemical Neuroanatomy (Vol 5);* Integrated Systems of the CNS. Elsevier Science Publisher, Amsterdam, pp. 125 – 277.

Switzer R.C., Hill J. and Heimer L. (1982) The globus pallidus and its rostro-ventral extension into the olfactory tubercle of the rat: a cyto- and chemoarchitectural study. *Neuroscience,* 7: 1891 – 1904.

Tagliavini F. and Pilleri G. (1983) Neuronal counts in basal nucleus of Meynert in Alzheimer's disease and in simple senile dementia. *Lancet, I:* 469 – 470.

Tagliavini F., Pilleri G., Bouras C. and Constantinidis J. (1984) The basal nucleus of Meynert in idiopathic Parkinson's disease. *Acta, Neurologica Scandinavia,* 69: 20 – 28.

Takada M., Ng G. and Hattori T. (1986) Single pallidal neurons project both to the striatum and thalamus in the rat. *Neurosci. Lett.*, 69: 217 – 220.

Torrey E.F. and Peterson M.R. (1974) Schizophrenia and the limbic system. *Lancet, II:* 942 – 946.

Trimble M.R. (1981) *Neuropsychiatry.* John Wiley and Sons, Chichester.

Trimble M.R. and Bolwig T.G. (Eds.), (1986) *Aspects of Epilepsy and Psychiatry.* John Wiley and Sons, New York.

Turner B.H. (1981) The cortical sequence and terminal distribution of sensory related afferents to the amygdaloid complex of the rat and monkey. In: Y. Ben-Ari (Ed.), *The Amygdaloid Complex (INSERM Symposium No. 20).* Elsevier Biomedial Press, Amsterdam, pp. 51 – 76.

Turner B.H., Gupta K.C. and Mishkin M. (1978) The locus and cytoarchitecture of the projection areas of the olfactory bulb in Macaca mulatta. *J. Comp. Neurol.*, 177: 381 – 396.

Ulfig N. (1989) Altered lipofuscin pigmentation in the basal nucleus (Meynert) in Parkinson's disease. *Neurosci. Res.*, 6: 456 – 462.

Ulfig N. (1989) Configuration of the magnocellular nuclei in the basal forebrain of the human adult. *Acta Anatomica,* 134: 100 – 105.

Ulfig N., Braak E., Ohm T.G. and Pool C.W. (1990) Vasopressinergic neurons in the magnocellular nuclei of the human basal forebrain. (In press.)

Umegaki K., Shiosaka S., Kawai Y., Shinoda K., Yagura A., Shibasaki T., Ling N. and Tohyama M. (1983) The distribution of alpha-melanocyte stimulating hormone [alpha MSH] in the central nervous system of the rat: An immunohistochemical study. I. Forebrain and upper brainstem. *Cell Molec. Biol.*, 29: 377 – 386.

Van Hoesen G.W. (1981) The differential distribution, diversity and sprouting of cortical projections to the amygdala in the Rhesus monkey. In: Y. Ben-Ari (Ed.), *The Amygdaloid Complex. INSERM Symposium No. 20.* Elsevier Biomedical Press, Amsterdam, pp. 77 – 104.

Van Hoesen G.W. (1985) Neural system of the nonhuman primate forebrain implicated in memory. *Am. NY. Acad. Sci.*, 444, 97 – 112.

Van Hoesen G.W. and Damasio A.R. (1987) Neural correlates of cognitive impairment in Alzheimer's disease. In: V.B. Mountcastle, F. Plum, and S.R. Geiger (Eds.), *Handbook of Physiology, Section 1: The Nervous System* (Vol 5, Ch 22). American Physiological Society, Bethesda, MA, pp.

871 – 898.

Van Hoesen G.W., Yeterian E.H. and Lavizzo-Mourey R. (1981) Widespread corticostriate projections from temporal cortex of rhesus monkey. *J. Comp. Neurol.*, 199, 205 – 219.

Van Hoesen G.W., Mesulam M. -M. and Haaxma R. (1976) Temporel cortical projections to the olfactory tubercle in the rhesus monkey. *Brain Res.*, 109: 375 – 381.

Van Praag H.M. (1981) Socio-biological psychiatry. *Comp. Psychiatry,* 22: 441 – 450.

Van Rossen J.M. (1966) The significance of dopamine receptor blockade for the mechanism of action of neuroleptic drugs. *Arch. Int. Pharmacodyn Ther.*, 160: 492 – 494.

Veening J.G., Swanson L.W. and Sawchenko P.E. (1984) The organization of projections from the central nucleus of the amygdala to brainstem sites involved in central autonomic regulation; a combined retrograde transport-immunohistochemical study. *Brain Res.*, 303: 337 – 357.

Vincent S.R., McIntosh C.H.S., Buchan A.M.J. and Brown J.C. (1985) Central somatostatin systems revealed with monoclonal antibodies. *J. Comp. Neur.*, 238: 169 – 186.

Vogt C. and Vogt O. (1952) Altérations anatomiques de la schizophrenie et d'autres psychoses dites fonctionnelles. In: Rosenberg and Sellier (Eds.), *Proceedings of the First International Congress on Neuropathology (Vol 1).* Toronto, 515 – 532.

Von Buttlar-Brentano K. (1952) Pathohistologische Feststellungen am Basalkern Schizophrener. *J. Nerv. Ment. Dis.*, 116: 646 – 653.

Von Buttlar-Brentano K. (1955) Das Parkinsonsyndrom in Lichte der Lebensgeschichtlichen Veranderungen des Nucleus Basalis. *J. Hirnforsch.*, 2: 55 – 76.

Von Economo C. and Koskinas G.N. (1925) *Die Cytoarchitektonik der Hirnrinde des Erwachsenen Menschen.* Springer Verlag, Berlin.

Walker L.C., Kitt C.A., DeLong M.R. and Price D.L. (1985) Noncollateral projections of basal forebrain neurons to frontal and parietal neocortex in primates. *Brain Res. Bull.* 15: 307 – 314.

Walker L.C., Price D.L. and Young W.S. (1989) GABAergic neurons in the primate basal forebrain magnocellular complex. *Brain Res.*, 499: 188 – 192.

Warburton J.W. (1967) Depressive symptoms in Parkinson patient referred for thalamotomy. *J. Neurosurg. Psychiatry,* 30: 368 – 370.

Watanabe T., Taguchi Y., Shiosako S., Tanaka J., Kubota H., Terano Y., Tohyama M. and Wada H. (1984) Distribution of the histaminergic neuron system in the central nervous system of rats: A fluorescent immunohistochemical analysis with histidine decarboxybase as a marker. *Brain Res.*, 295: 3 – 25.

Weinberger D.R. (1986) The pathogenesis of schizophrenia: a neurodevelopmental theory. In: H.A. Nasrallah and D.R. Weinberger (Eds.), *Handbook of Schizophrenia I: The Neurology of Schizophrenia.* Elsevier Science Publishers B.V., Amsterdam, 397 – 406.

Weinberger D.R. and Berman K.F. (1988) Speculation on the meaning of cerebral metabolic hypofrontality in schizophrenia. *Schizophrenia Bull.*, 14: 157 – 168.

Whitehouse P.J., Hedreen J.C., White C.L. and Price J.L. (1983) Basal forebrain neurons in the dementia of Parkinson disease. *Ann. Neurol.*, 13: 243 – 248.

Whitehouse P.J., Price D.L., Clark A.W., Coyle J.T. and DeLong M.R. (1981) Alzheimer disease; evidence for selective loss of cholinergic neurons in the nucleus basalis. *Ann. Neurol.*, 10: 122 – 126.

Wilcock G.K., Esiri M.M., Bowen D.M. and Smith C.C.T. (1983) The nucleus basalis in Alzheimer's disease; cell counts and cortical biochemistry. *Neuropathol. Appl. Neurobiol.*, 9: 175 – 179.

Woodhams P.L., Roberts G.W., Polak J.M. and Crow T.J. (1983) Distribution of neuropeptides in the limbic system: The bed nucleus of the stria terminalis. *Neuroscience,* 8: 677 – 703.

Woolf N.J. and Butcher L.L. (1982) Cholinergic projections to the basolateral amygdala: A combined Evans Blue and acetylcholinesterase analysis. *Brain Res. Bull.*, 8: 751 – 763.

Woolf N.J., Eckenstein F., Butcher L.L. (1984) Cholinergic systems in the rat brain. I. Projections to the limbic telencephalon. *Brain Res. Bull.*, 13: 751 – 784.

Wyss J.M. and Sripanidkulchai K. (1984) Topography of the mesencephalic and pontine projections from the cingulate cortex in the rat. *Brain Res.*, 293: 1 – 15.

Yasui Y., Itoh K. and Mizuno N. (1987) Direct projections from the caudal spinal trigeminal nucleus to the striatum in the cat. *Brain Res.*, 408: 334 – 338.

Yoshimura M. (1988) Pathological basis for dementia in elderly patients with idiopathic Parkinson's disease. *Eur. Neurol.*, 28: 29 – 35.

Young W.S. III, Alheid G.F. and Heimer L. (1984) The ventral pallidal projection to the mediodorsal thalamus; a study with fluorescent retrograde tracers and immunohistofluorescence. *J. Neurosci.*, 4: 1626 – 1638.

Zaborszky L. (1989) Afferent connections of the forebrain cholinergic projection neurons, with special reference to monoaminergic and peptidergic fibers. In: M. Frotscher and U. Misgeld (Eds.), Central Cholinergic Synaptic Transmission. Birkhauser, Basel. pp. 12 – 32.

Zaborszky L., Alheid G.F., Beinfeld M.L., Eiden L.E., Heimer L. and Palkovits M. (1985) Cholecystokinin innervation of the ventral striatum; a morphological and radioimmunological study. *Neuroscience,* 14: 427 – 453.

Zaborszky L., Carlsen J., Brashear H.R. and Heimer L. (1986) Cholinergic and GABAergic afferents to the olfactory bulb in the rat with special emphasis on the projection neurons in the nucleus of the horizontal limb of the diagonal band. *J. Comp. Neurol.*, 243: 488 – 509.

Zaborszky L. and Cullinan W.E. (1989) Hypothalamic axons terminate of forebrain cholinergic neurons; an ultrastructural double-labeling study using PHA-L tracing and ChAT immunocytochemistry. *Brain Res.,* 479: 177 – 184.

Zaborszky L., Leranth C. and Heimer L. (1984) Ultrastructural evidence of amygdalofugal axons terminating on cholinergic cells of the rostral forebrain. *Neurosci. Lett.,* 52: 219 – 225.

Zaborszky L., Luine V.N., Cullinan W.E. and Heimer L. (1990) Direct catecholaminergic-cholinergic interactions in the basal forebrain: morphological and biochemical studies. (Submitted for publication.)

Zahm D.S. (1989) The ventral striatopallidal parts of the basal ganglia in the rat. II. Compartmentation of ventral pallidal efferents. *Neuroscience,* 30: 33 – 50.

Zahm, D.S. (1990) The ditribution of neurotensin immunoreactive neurons in relation to dorsal and ventral striatal infrastructure in rat; clochicine and haloperidol administration. *Synapse,* in review.

Zahm D.S. and Heimer L. (1987) The ventral striatopallidothalamic projection. III. Striatal cells of the olfactory tubercle establish direct synaptic contact with ventral pallidal cells projecting to mediodorsal thalamus. *Brain Res.,* 404: 327 – 331.

Zahm, D.S. and Johnson, S.N. (1989) Asymmetrical distribution of neurotensin immunoreactivity in the basal ganglia of the rat following unilateral injections of 6-hydroxydopamine into the ventral tegmental area of Tsai. *Brain Res.,* 483: 301 – 311.

Zahm D.S., Zaborszky L., Alones V.E. and Heimer L. (1985) Evidence for the coexistence of glutamate decarboxylase and metenkephalin immunoreactivities in axon terminals of rat ventral pallidum. *Brain Res.,* 325: 317 – 321.

Zahm D.S., Zaborszky L., Alheid G.F. and Heimer L. (1987) The ventral striatopallidothalamic projection. II. The ventral pallidothalamic link. *J. Comp. Neurol.,* 255: 592 – 605.

Zola-Morgan S., Squire L.R. and Amaral D.G. (1986) Human amnesia and the medial temporal region: Enduring memory impairment following a bilateral lesion limited to field CA1 of the hippocampus. *J. Neurosci.* 6: 2950 – 2967.

G. Holstege (Ed.)
Progress in Brain Research, Vol. 87

CHAPTER 8

Contributions of the amygdalar complex to behavior in macaque monkeys

Elisabeth A. Murray

Laboratory of Neuropsychology, National Institute of Mental Health, Bethesda, MD 20892, U.S.A.

Introduction

Although the amygdalar complex has long been considered to contribute to emotional and motivational processes, an amygdalar contribution to cognition is less widely accepted.* Many investigators believe that the amygdala tags sensory events with the affective (or internal) state of the organism (see Kesner and DiMattia, 1987). Thus, the amygdala would allow an organism to operate on stored information concerning whether a previously-experienced environmental stimulus was "good", "important", "bad", etc. It would also color events and give them a distinctive quality in memory. In this view, the amygdala acts primarily as a telencephalic modulator, promoting appropriate behavior that may affect actions either consciously or unconsciously. Alternatively, the amygdala may be viewed as an active part of the sensory processing system, as one of several structures involved in the storage of sensory (and perhaps motor) events. In this view the amygdala would be in a position to relate specific information concerning either affective states or nonaffective environmental stimuli.

In this chapter I will argue for the second view set forth in the preceding paragraph. Neurobehavioral investigations in monkeys support the idea that the amygdala may play a critical role not only in emotional behavior, by associating environmental stimuli with affective states, but also in cognitive behaviors without obvious affective components, by associating sensory stimuli that arise from different sensory modalities.

First, I will briefly summarize the major anatomical relations of the amygdala, in order to discuss how these connections may support behavior. Then I will examine ways in which the amygdalar complex may contribute to behavior. Results from a few recent behavioral studies, conducted as part of a larger program investigating the neural basis for learning and memory, will be presented to illustrate major points.

Anatomical relations of the amygdalar complex

The amygdalar complex is a telencephalic structure consisting of several separate nuclei that can be identified on the basis of cytoarchitectonic criteria, anatomical relations, and histochemical markers (Johnston, 1923; Crosby and Humphrey, 1941; Price, 1981; de Olmos et al., 1985; Amaral, 1987). Two major nuclear groups are evident: 1) the basolateral group, comprised of the lateral nucleus, the lateral basal nucleus, the medial basal nucleus, and the accessory basal nucleus; and 2) the centromedial group, comprised of the central nucleus, the cortical nucleus, and the medial nucleus (see Fig. 1).

* Most modern textbooks on cognition do not even consider the topic of emotion; consequently, there is considerable disarray surrounding the issue of whether emotion contributes to cognition, and if so, how it manifests itself.

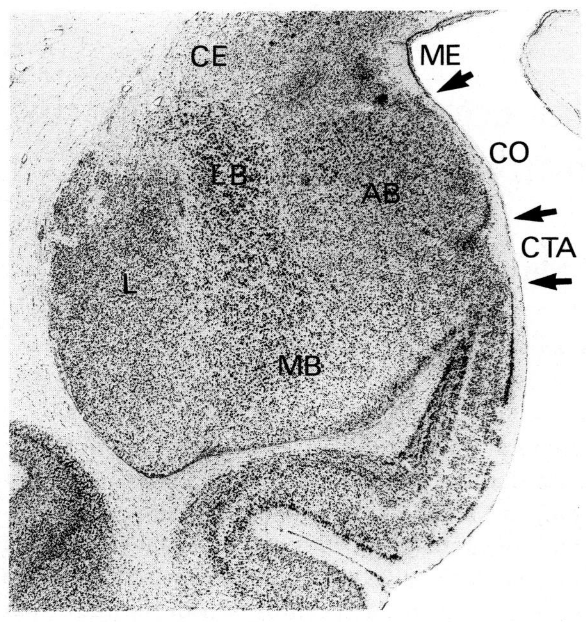

Fig. 1. Photomicrograph of a Nissl-stained coronal section through the amygdalar complex in a rhesus monkey. Nuclear designations are based on the work of Crosby and Humphrey (1941). Abbreviations: AB, accessory basal nucleus; CO, cortical nucleus; CE, central nucleus; CTA, cortical transition area; L, lateral nucleus; LB, lateral basal nucleus; ME, medial nucleus; MB, medial basal nucleus.

The anatomical relations of the amygdalar complex can be divided into four major groups. Major projection systems connect the amygdala with the cortex, the medial and midline thalamus, other parts of the basal forebrain, and the hypothalamus and brainstem. These connections are summarized in Fig. 2. Except where otherwise indicated, the discussion is restricted to investigations involving nonhuman primates.

Cortical relations

Briefly, the amygdala receives projections from modality-specific neocortical areas serving all the sensory systems (with the exception of olfaction, which is not represented at the neocortical level, but influences the amygdala more directly). These areas include the inferior temporal cortex for vision (Herzog and Van Hoesen, 1976; Aggleton et al., 1980; Turner et al., 1980; Van Hoesen, 1981; Iwai and Yukie, 1987), the posterior two-thirds of the insular cortex for touch (Aggleton et al., 1980; Turner et al., 1980; Mufson et al., 1981; Friedman et al., 1986), the superior temporal gyrus for audition (Herzog and Van Hoesen, 1976; Aggleton et al., 1980; Turner et al., 1980; Van Hoesen, 1981; Amaral et al., 1983), and the frontal operculum

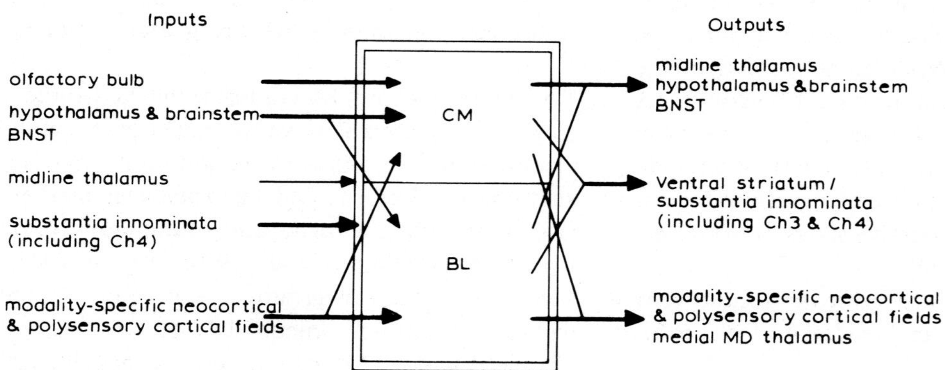

Fig. 2. Schematic diagram of the major inputs and outputs of the amygdalar complex. Thick arrows denote relatively heavy projections and thin arrows denote relatively light projections. Note that the basolateral group of the amygdala projects densely into the centromedial group of the amygdala (Aggleton, 1985). Thus sensory information from cortical fields, although directed primarily to the basolateral group, is in a position to influence the centromedial group as well.

and anterior insular cortex for gustation (Turner et al., 1980; Mufson et al., 1981). In addition, the amygdala receives projections from many polysensory cortical regions, some of which are neocortical and others of which are either periallocortical or mesolimbic. These areas include the temporal polar cortex (TG), the perirhinal cortex (areas 35 and 36), the entorhinal cortex (area 28), cortex in the depths of the superior temporal sulcus, orbital frontal cortex (areas 12 and 13), and anterior cingulate cortex (area 24) (Turner et al., 1980; Herzog and Van Hoesen, 1976, 1981; Pandya et al., 1981; Iwai and Yukie, 1987).

One of the most striking aspects of amygdalar connectivity is that the neocortical areas receiving amygdalofugal projections are much more numerous and widespread than those giving rise to amygdalopetal projections. For example, of the neocortical fields that are modality-specific for vision, only the most ventral and rostral of these (areas TEO and TE) contain neurons that project to the amygdala, whereas these same two areas and many more, including prestriate areas and the striate cortex itself, receive projections from the amygdala, particularly from cells in the lateral basal nucleus (Tigges et al., 1982; Amaral and Price, 1984; Iwai and Yukie, 1987). A similar arrangement has been observed for amygdalar relations with somatosensory cortical fields as well (Amaral and Price, 1984; Friedman et al., 1986). Indeed, this marked asymmetry in amygdalocortical and cortico-amygdalar relations may provide an important key to understanding amygdalar function. This issue will be discussed further in the section on amygdalar contributions to learning and memory.

Amygdalofugal projections to polysensory cortex terminate in entorhinal and perirhinal cortex, area TG, and medial (areas 24, 25, and 32) and orbital (areas 12, 13, and 14) prefrontal cortex (Amaral and Price, 1984; Iwai and Yukie, 1987; Moran et al., 1987; Saunders and Rosene, 1988).

Thalamic relations

The most prominent amygdalothalamic projection, arising primarily from the basolateral group, terminates in the magnocellular portion of the mediodorsal nucleus (MDmc) (Nauta, 1961; Porrino et al., 1981; Aggleton and Mishkin, 1984; Russchen et al., 1987). The amygdala may also influence MDmc indirectly via relays in the basal forebrain (see Hreib et al., 1988). Additional amygdalothalamic projections, arising primarily in the centromedial group, terminate in the midline thalamic nuclei (Price and Amaral, 1981; Aggleton and Mishkin, 1984). Although MD does not appear to project to the amygdala, the paraventricular nucleus of the thalamus and the midline central nuclear complex do (Mehler, 1980).

Connections with the basal forebrain

The basolateral group of the amygdala gives rise to a dense projection to the nucleus accumbens and olfactory tubercle, structures comprising the bulk of the ventral striatum (Russchen et al., 1985b; Aggleton et al., 1987). The basolateral group, together with the centromedial, gives rise to a projection to the substantia innominata that encompasses cholinergic cell groups Ch3 and Ch4 (Russchen et al., 1985a; Aggleton et al., 1987). Both the ventral striatum and substantia innominata have been implicated in reward mechanisms (Rolls et al., 1979; Rolls, 1984; Taylor and Robbins, 1986; White, 1989), and it is likely that the amygdala interacts with these structures in learning about rewarding events (Everitt et al., 1989).

Many cells within the Ch4 group, as well as some noncholinergic cells of the substantia innominata, project to the amygdala (Mesulam et al., 1983; Aggleton et al., 1987; Kordower et al., 1989). Other basal forebrain regions appear to supply little input to the amygdala.

Hypothalamic and brainstem connections

The amygdalar projections to the hypothalamus terminate primarily in the lateral hypothalamic area, with additional terminations in the supramammillary area and paramammillary nucleus. Brainstem projections appear to arise solely from the central nucleus of the amygdala. In the midbrain, projections to the central grey and in the region of the substantia nigra and peripeduncular nucleus predominate. In addition, the central nucleus projects heavily to the parabrachial region of the pons and to the dorsal motor nucleus of the vagus and nucleus of the solitary tract, regions related to autonomic function (Price and Amaral, 1984). Another major amygdalar projection terminates in the bed nucleus of the stria terminalis (BNST). The BNST has been considered, on cytoarchitectonic, connectional, and immunohistochemical grounds, an extension of the central and medial amygdalar nuclei (Holstege et al., 1985; Alheid and Heimer, 1988). As such, it affords an additional route for amygdalo-hypothalamic influences (Price and Amaral, 1984).

Projections from the hypothalamus to the amygdala arise primarily from the ventromedial nucleus and lateral hypothalamic area and terminate principally, though by no means exclusively, in the centromedial group of the amygdala (Jones et al., 1976; Mehler, 1980; Amaral et al., 1982). In addition, the peripeduncular nucleus and parabrachial region send a heavy projection to the amygdala (Jones et al., 1976; Mehler, 1980). Results based on HRP histochemistry also suggest that the nucleus of the solitary tract and paravagal cell groups project to the amygdala, but because these areas often contain endogenously pigmented cells, this finding must be accepted with caution (Mehler, 1980). A report based on both anterograde and retrograde tracing techniques employed in the rat (Ricardo and Koh, 1978), however, has also described a projection from the nucleus of the solitary tract to the central nucleus of the amygdala, thus supporting the evidence for this projection in the monkey.

Amygdalar contributions to emotional and social behavior

The behavioral effects of amygdalar removal include both the readily observable changes in emotional and social behavior, many of which comprise the Klüver-Bucy syndrome, as well as more formal observations afforded by training on cognitive problem-solving tasks.

Klüver and Bucy (1939) noted the possible significance of the temporal lobes for emotional behavior when they described a set of behaviors, now known as the Klüver-Bucy syndrome, that followed bilateral temporal lobectomy in monkeys. The syndrome is comprised of a number of bizarre and striking behaviors such as psychic blindness (the inability of animals to "recognize" stimuli), apparent lack of fear, hypermetamorphosis (the excessive tendency to grasp for and reach for objects, and to attend to objects in the environment), coprophagia, increased orality, and hypoemotionality. These same symptoms have more recently been found by Weiskrantz (1956) to follow aspiration lesions of the amygdala, and by Aggleton and Passingham (1981) to follow radio-frequency lesions of the amygdala, findings which strongly suggest that the critical damage responsible for this syndrome is restricted to the amygdalar complex itself.

The alteration in emotional behavior that follows amygdalar removal is remarkable; when confronted with a variety of stimulus objects, amygdalectomized monkeys display a paucity of i) aggressive behaviors (e.g., lunging, mouth threats, flattened ears), ii) submissive behaviors (e.g., grimacing, lip smacking) and iii) conflict behaviors (e.g., yawning, piloerection) relative to controls (Aggleton and Passingham, 1981).

The consensus interpretation of these data is that bilateral amygdala removal disrupts the ability of environmental stimuli to influence emotional behavior (see Aggleton and Mishkin, 1986). Two lines of evidence support this idea. First, removal of one or more sensory systems or damage to sensory-limbic pathways result in a hypoemotionality like that observed after bilateral amygdalectomy (Downer, 1961; Doty et al., 1973; Horel and Misantone, 1974; Horel et al., 1975). In the course of a study on routes of interhemispheric transfer of visual discrimination problems, Downer (1961) came upon an amazing demonstration of this phenomenon. Some of his monkeys had received sagittal sections of the optic chiasm, corpus callosum and anterior commissure in order to restrict the visual input to one hemisphere. Further, one of these animals had, in addition, received a unilateral temporal pole resection. Downer observed that when visual input was restricted to the hemisphere with the temporal pole removal the monkey appeared placid and displayed apparently indiscriminate visual behavior. This finding was confirmed in a second animal with the same pattern of chiasm and forebrain commissure sections, but with unilateral amygdalar removal instead of temporal pole removal. When visual input was restricted to the hemisphere with the amygdala removal, this monkey, too, displayed many of the aberrant behaviors described by Klüver and Bucy. Interestingly, the placid emotional behavior was elicited only in response to inputs from the visual sensory system; touching the animal would elicit a strong affective reaction that matched the animal's typical preoperative response. Thus, the bizarre behaviors were evident only in response to stimuli in the sensory modality disconnected from the amygdala. A second reason for thinking that the amygdala mediates the influence of environmental stimuli on emotional behavior is that the amygdala itself is not necessary for the expression of emotional behavior: electrical stimulation of the hypothalamus in amygdalectomized cats can evoke fear and aggressive attack (Fernandez de Molina and Hunsperger, 1962; Egger and Flynn, 1967), and electrical stimulation of the midbrain in precollicular decerebrate cats can elicit integrated patterns of somatic and autonomic changes characteristic of defense reactions (Bard and Macht, 1958; see Bandler et al., this volume, for review).

Although little formal work has addressed the role of the amygdala in primate social behavior, adult rhesus monkeys that have sustained amygdalar removals have been reported to display unusual social behaviors and lowered dominance rankings in group situations. These alterations are somewhat complex, and appear to interact with the amount of time that the social relations were in force prior to surgery and the preoperative social status of the monkey (Rosvold et al., 1954; Thompson et al., 1977).

Amygdalar contributions to learning and memory

More formal observations on the effects of amygdalar removal on behavior have been found in the course of studies examining the contributions of the medial temporal lobe limbic structures, the amygdalar complex and hippocampal formation, to memory. Ablation studies in monkeys have focussed on the neural structures critical for storing information about what particular sensory events have been experienced (recognition memory), and what particular sensory events occurred together (associative memory).

Recognition memory

Monkey's recognition memory was assessed using delayed nonmatching-to-sample, a test of visual memory for objects. In this task, which is shown schematically in Fig. 3, each trial is composed of two parts: sample presentation and choice test. For the sample presentation the monkey is shown a single object overlying the central well of a three-well test tray. The monkey displaces this object in order to obtain the food reward hidden underneath it. Ten seconds later, on the choice test, the monkey is shown the sample plus a new object, now overlying the lateral wells of the test tray. The monkey must learn to displace the novel object in order to obtain another food reward. Following a 30-s intertrial interval, this procedure is repeated, and so on, until 20 such trials, comprising a test session, have been completed. With trial-unique objects, monkeys learn this task very rapidly — in just 100 – 150 trials. In 1978, Mishkin directly examined the contribution of the amygdala and hippocampus to recognition memory in monkeys. Following training on the basic task, each monkey received bilateral removal of the amygdala, the hippocampus, or both structures combined. In this study and the others that I will describe in this chapter, the amygdalar removals included not only the amygdalar complex itself, but also approximately the anterior half of the entorhinal cortex. In addition, the hippocampal removals included not only the hippocampal formation but also approximately the posterior half of the entorhinal cortex and the parahippocampal gyrus as well. Following surgery the monkeys were given a two-week rest period and were then retrained on the basic task (i.e., on delayed nonmatching-to-sample with 10-s delays). Once the animals reattained criterion, they were given a performance test in which their memory was taxed in two ways — first by increasing the delays between sample presentation and choice test from 10 s to 30, 60, and 120 s and, second, by requiring the monkeys to remember a list of 3, 5, or 10 objects. For this list-length testing the samples are shown one at a time, separated by 20 s, and then the choice tests are given, one at a time, separated by 20 s.

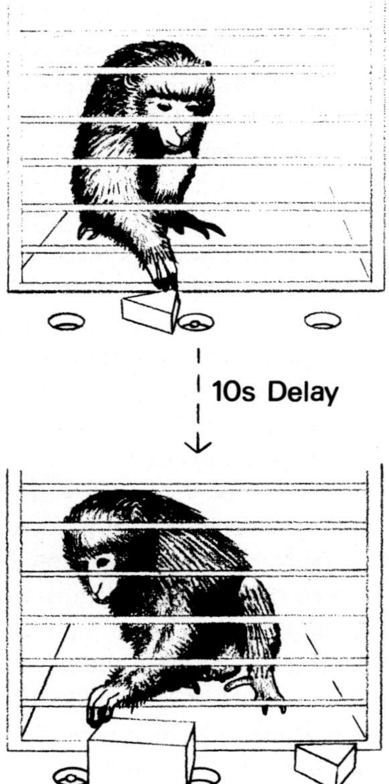

Fig. 3. Schematic diagram of a rhesus monkey performing a single trial of the delayed nonmatching-to-sample task. First the monkey is shown a sample object covering the central well of a three-well test tray, which it displaces to obtain the half peanut hidden underneath. Following a 10-s delay, the monkey is confronted with the same object plus a novel one. The animal must learn to displace the novel (or nonmatching) object in order to obtain another half peanut. In the recognition memory study described here, new pairs of objects were used on every trial and the intertrial interval was 30 s.

The results of this study in object recognition memory indicated that whereas amygdalar removal alone and hippocampal removal alone had only a mild effect on recognition, the combined removal of these two structures had a profound effect. When tested with delays of 60 s or longer, monkeys with the combined amygdalar and hippocampal removals scored at near chance levels whereas the controls scored better than 90% correct responses. At the time these data were published, Mishkin (1978) suggested that perhaps it was this combined damage to the amygdala and hippocampus that was responsible for the global anterograde amnesia seen in the patient H.M.* This was certainly a very exciting possibility, but there were still alternative interpretations of the data. For example, one possibility was that the severe memory impairment was due not to combined damage to the amygdala and hippocampus but to inadvertent damage to the inferior temporal cortex or the white matter underlying this cortex, tissue known to be important for visual perception and memory. To test this possibility, we decided to evaluate recognition memory in monkeys in another sensory modality. In the somatic sensory system, the insular cortex is the last in a series of interconnected cortical fields that relays information to the medial temporal lobe (Friedman et al., 1986). Because it is highly unlikely that the insular cortex or its underlying white matter would be

* In 1953, the patient H.M. underwent a bilateral medial temporal lobe resection for relief of intractable epileptic seizures. H.M.'s operation, which resulted in a global amnesia that remains severe even today, closely approximates the combined amygdalar and hippocampal removal in the monkeys described here.

compromised during the combined removal of the amygdala and hippocampus, we trained monkeys on a tactile version of delayed nonmatching-to-sample. Several modifications of the visual task were undertaken in order to help the animals learn the new, tactile version of the task. First, the monkeys were trained with a small set of 40 tactually-discriminable objects that were mounted on corks. The corks fit snugly into the wells of the test tray, thereby forcing the monkeys to grasp and lift the objects in order to displace them. In addition, small light-emitting diodes (LEDs) were recessed in front of each well in order to help orient the animals in the dark. Illuminated LEDs marked the locations of occupied foodwells; accordingly, on the sample presentation, the central LED was lit, but not the side ones, and on the choice test, the side LEDs were lit, but not the central one. Each animal's behavior was monitored via an infrared-sensitive camera connected to a video monitor. In this study the animals were first trained on visual delayed nonmatching-to-sample. Then they were taken through a light-dimming phase of training until they would work in complete darkness. Once this had been achieved, they were given a performance test in which the delays between sample presentation and choice test were increased. For this tactile version of the task, the monkeys compared the objects (manually) on well over 50% of the choice tests, so it was clear that the animals were indeed choosing on the basis of touch.

After training, the animals received either bilateral amygdalar removal, bilateral hippocampal removal, or the combination of these two removals. As in the earlier study in vision, the animals were allowed to relearn the task following surgery, and were then given a performance test, which in this case employed delay but not list conditions. The effects of the lesions in tactile recognition were generally similar to those obtained in visual recognition (Murray and Mishkin, 1984). Monkeys with hippocampal removals actually performed slightly better than they had preoperatively, whereas monkeys with amygdalar removals were moderately impaired. Monkeys with combined amygdalar and hippocampal removals were severely impaired; their scores dropped to near chance levels of performance with delays of 60 s or longer.

Two conclusions can be drawn from this study. First, it appeared that the interpretation of the earlier experiment, that combined damage to the amygdala and hippocampus is required to produce a severe impairment in recognitions was correct. Second, the results suggested that the memory deficit that follows combined amygdalar and hippocampal removal in monkeys is at least bimodal. Thus, the experiments described above, together with other studies not discussed here (Saunders et al., 1984; Murray and Mishkin, 1986), point toward the contribution of both the amygdala and hippocampus to recognition memory in monkeys. This latter statement is meant to imply not that the structures are contributing in the same way — certainly there are a number of lines of evidence suggesting that these structures play different roles in memory — but only that each structure can carry on the process fairly efficiently in the absence of the other.

These findings are consistent with the idea that the amygdalar complex, by virtue of its receipt of sensory inputs from modality-specific neocortical areas as well as from polysensory cortical areas, is an active participant in the storage of information. It has been suggested that there are actually two parallel cortico-limbo-thalamo-cortical circuits that participate in recognition memory: one circuit involving the amygdala and mediodorsal nucleus of the thalamus, and the other, the hippocampus and anterior nuclear complex of the thalamus (Mishkin, 1982). This proposal is based on behavioral experiments similar to those discussed previously, but which are beyond the scope of this paper. Nevertheless, it is worth noting that both the amygdala and the medial thalamic structure to which it projects contribute to recognition memory in monkeys, and, furthermore, that a limited set of structures outside the amygdalar system also contribute to recognition memory.

Associative memory

Associative memory is the ability to link sensory events with other sensory events, motor acts, or affective states.* Although the amygdala and hippocampus appear to be contributing roughly equally to recognition memory, recent experiments have indicated that these structures may be making independent and selective contributions to associative memory.

There is an extensive literature indicating that the amygdala is important for learning about food reward, presumably because the amygdala contributes to the rapid association of stimuli with primary reinforcement (Spiegler and Mishkin, 1981; Gaffan and Harrison, 1987; Gaffan et al., 1988). As discussed in detail elsewhere (Gaffan et al., 1989; Murray, 1990), food reward usually encompasses a constellation of features (e.g. taste, appearance, intrinsic reward value), and associations made with food reward may therefore involve either its affective or nonaffective qualities, or both.

Some recent work carried out by Gaffan and Murray (1990) will be used to illustrate the contribution of the amygdala to stimulus-reward association. In this experiment, monkeys learned visual discriminations for food reward in a learning set paradigm. Each daily session consisted of five new discrimination problems presented serially. For each problem, the monkey was shown two 2-dimensional stimuli simultaneously on a color monitor and was required to touch one as a response. The same two stimuli were shown on the next trial, and so on, for 20 trials. A response to one (the positive) of these two stimuli was always rewarded whereas a response to the other was never rewarded, and the monkey learned, through trial and error, to choose the positive stimulus. The left-right position of the positive stimulus was randomized to ensure that the monkey linked stimulus quality, and not stimulus position, with reward. When baseline performance was determined, the monkeys received either bilateral amygdalar removals or bilateral lesions of the medial portion of the medial dorsal nucleus (MD) of the thalamus. The results, illustrated in Fig. 4, show that the bilaterally symmetrical removals produced significant and equally severe deficits in discrimination learning for food reward.

Because the amygdalar complex projects directly to the medial portion of MD, the behavioral results suggested the possibility that the amygdala and medial MD might comprise a single, tightly linked functional system for stimulus-reward association. To test this possibility, in a separate group of monkeys we disconnected the amygdala from medial MD. The disconnection was achieved by removing medial MD in one hemisphere in one stage, and the amygdala in the other hemisphere in a second stage, a procedure that effectively

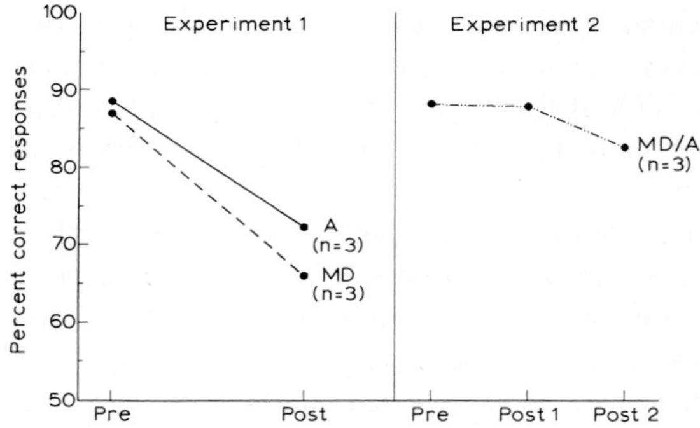

Fig. 4. Discrimination learning for food reward. In experiment 1, monkeys received bilaterally symmetrical lesions of either the amygdala (A) or medial portion of the medial dorsal nucleus of the thalamus (MD). In experiment 2, a separate group of monkeys received disconnection of the amygdala from the medial thalamus (MD/A). Abbreviations: Pre, mean score for the last five sessions (25 discrimination problems) given preoperatively; Post, mean score for the last five sessions (25 problems) given postoperatively.

* A theoretical distinction has been made (see Mishkin and Petri, 1984) between associations that are presumably based on stored neural representations (e.g. sensory-sensory, sensory-motor, sensory-affective, etc.), and associations that are presumably based on selective reinforcement of one among many responses (stimulus-response). These two kinds of associations may be distinguished by their neural basis as well; medial temporal lobe damage severely disrupts the ability of monkeys to learn the former kind of association but not the latter. This discussion will be restricted to the neural substrates for the limbic-dependent associations.

removes amygdalar interaction with medial MD. The scores of monkeys in the disconnection group are also shown in Fig. 4. After the first stage of surgery the monkeys performed as well as they had preoperatively. Following the second operation, however, there was a relatively mild but statistically significant decrement in performance. So the answer to the question as to whether these two structures constitute a single functional system essential for stimulus-reward association is "no". Although there was a significant, measurable effect of the asymmetrical or crossed lesion, the behavioral effect was not nearly so great as that following the bilaterally symmetrical removals. One possible explanation for this finding is that there are some remaining contralateral projections of amygdala to MD that might sustain the behavior. This possibility seems unlikely, however, because such contralateral projections are sparse (Aggleton and Mishkin, 1984), and might be expected to cross in the massa intermedia, which was transected. Alternatively, amygdalar interaction with the ventral striatal or hypothalamic regions, portions of which are implicated in reward learning (Mora et al., 1976; Fukuda et al., 1986; Robbins et al., 1989), may be important for stimulus-reward association. Regardless, the neural substrate supporting stimulus-reward associations must involve more than the single functional system (amygdala and MD) suggested above.

Another behavioral task that has provided us with some information about amygdalar contributions to associative memory is a crossmodal version of delayed nonmatching-to-sample (Murray and Mishkin, 1985). Monkeys that had already been trained on the visual and tactile versions of delayed nonmatching-to-sample described earlier in the section on "Recognition memory" were confronted with a tactile-to-visual crossmodal version of this task. A schematic diagram of the task is shown in Fig. 5. The monkeys were given a sample presentation in the dark, in which only tactile cues were available, followed by a choice test in the light, in which only visual cues were available. (The monkeys were forced to make a visual choice because the first object touched was scored as the animal's response). Although the structure of the trial on this crossmodal version of delayed nonmatching-to-sample was just the same as on the recognition tests, it is important to note that the task has been converted from one requiring short-term sensory memory to one requiring, in addition, long-term associative memory. That is, on a choice test in the traditional recognition tasks, the monkey simply experiences the sample once again; now, on a choice test in the crossmodal version of the task, the monkey must actually bring together both tactile and visual information from the individual objects in order to choose correctly. These tactile-visual associations have presumably been learned either through the long course of training with these objects, or perhaps through the monkeys' experiences prior to entering the laboratory. Thus, the crossmodal task has two memory components: a short-term sensory memory component, because the monkey must remember the sample object for 10 s, and, also, a long-term associative memory component, because the monkey must link the tactile and visual qualities of the object. As it turned out (see Fig. 6), animals with amygdalar removals performed extremely poorly on the crossmodal task for the

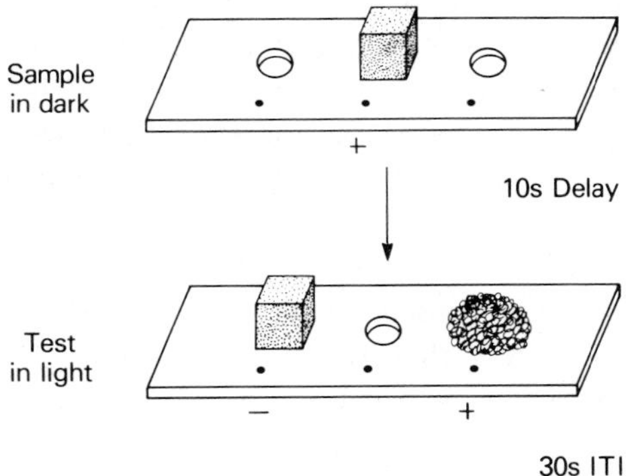

Fig. 5. Schematic diagram of a trial in the crossmodal (tactual-to-visual) delayed nonmatching-to-sample task. A new pair of objects is used on every trial within a session for a total of 20 trials, and these same objects are paired again for use the next day (session). Abbreviations: ITI, intertrial interval; s, seconds.

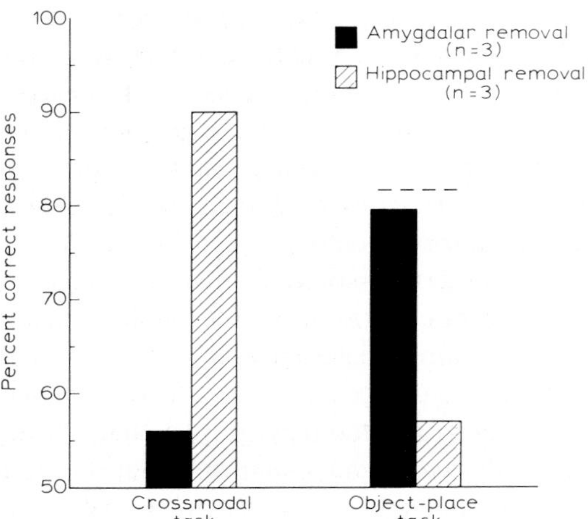

Fig. 6. Effects of amygdalar removal alone and hippocampal removal alone on two different associative memory tasks. The crossmodal task (left side of figure) was administered postoperatively only. The height of the bars indicates the mean postoperative level of performance for each operated group based on a total of 500 trials per monkey. The object-place task (right side of figure) was given both pre- and postoperatively. The dashed line indicates the mean preoperative level of performance for all the monkeys in this study, based on 600 trials per animal, whereas the height of the bars indicates the mean postoperative level of performance for each group of monkeys, based on 1200 trials per monkey.

duration of training, whereas operated control monkeys with hippocampal removals performed quite well. Importantly, the same amygdalectomized monkeys were able to perform well on the intramodal versions of this task employing the same apparatus, the same objects, and the same delay conditions; hence, perception and short-term sensory memory were intact. The poor performance of the amygdalectomized monkeys on the crossmodal task must therefore reflect impairment in long-term (crossmodal) associative memory. These data suggest that the amygdala may be critical for linking, in memory, sensory stimuli from different sensory modalities.

Because the amygdala is traditionally considered to contribute to emotional and social behavior, it is important to consider, at least briefly, how the amygdala could be critical for such apparently disparate behaviors as crossmodal sensory-sensory associations on the one hand, and emotional and social behavior on the other. Perhaps the amygdala processes information about affective states in the same way it processes information from the neocortex about the traditional senses. If so, then associations involving both i) cortically-processed information derived from two or more sensory modalities, and ii) cortically-processed sensory information and cortically- or subcortically-processed affective states, can be thought of as "crossmodal" associations. That is, perhaps just as a tactile sensory input may elicit a stored visual representation of an object, an environmental stimulus — say a stick or a net — may elicit an associated emotional state. In this view, the amygdala might act as a switch or relay whereby a sensory stimulus might evoke, via cortico-amygdalar pathways projecting to the hypothalamus and brainstem, an appropriate emotional response. Similarly, sensory information derived from one modality might elicit, via cortico-amygdalo-cortical projections, a stimulus representation stored in a neocortical area serving another modality. In this way, given a sensory event, the amygdala may be critical for recalling either an associated affective state, a stored stimulus representation in another sensory modality, or both.

It is instructive to contrast the results of the crossmodal experiment with the results of another recently published study (Parkinson et al., 1988). In this latter study, monkeys were trained to associate objects and their locations. In this task, which is shown schematically in Fig. 7, there were two trial types — one called "object and place" and one called "place only". During the sample presentation for each trial type the monkey displaced two different objects overlying two of three wells. A few seconds later, on the choice test, the monkeys were shown two identical objects and could obtain a food reward by displacing the object that covered the same well that it had at sample presentation. In the object-place trial type, both the objects at the choice test covered previously occupied wells, so the animal actually

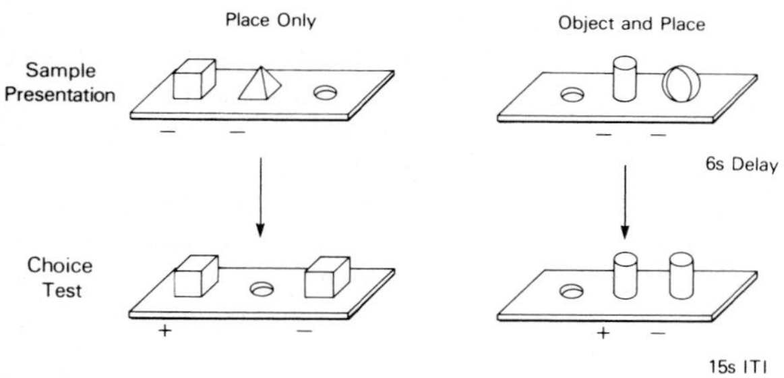

Fig. 7. Schematic diagram of the two trial types in the object-place association task. Each trial type appears equally often in the 24-trial session, and new pairs of objects are used on every trial. Abbreviations as in Fig. 5.

had to remember both object quality and place information in order to choose correctly. In the place-only trial type, by contrast, only one of the objects available for choice was in a previously occupied location, so place information was sufficient to guide choice behavior. As it turned out, there was no interaction of lesion and trial type. Consequently, the histogram shown in Fig. 6 simply combines the data from these two trial types. Monkeys with hippocampal removals were severely impaired on this task; they dropped from the 80% correct responses obtained preoperatively to approximately 50 – 60% correct responses. Furthermore, they were unable to improve their scores even over a long postoperative course of training. Monkeys with amygdalar removals, by contrast, scored close to their preoperative level of performance almost immediately. As in the crossmodal task, both operated groups of monkeys performed well on tests of visual object recognition. Thus, the results of this experiment are the converse of those obtained in the crossmodal experiment. The hippocampus, but not the amygdala, is critical for remembering places and for associating sensory stimuli with places.

These results are of interest for at least two reasons. First, this is the only task that has been given to monkeys to my knowledge that has shown a dissociation of this type, that is, a hippocampal but not an amygdalar contribution to memory. Second, this is a fairly difficult task — probably as difficult as the crossmodal task, based on the number of trials that it takes animals to learn — yet the monkeys with amygdalar removals perform quite well. This rules out the possibility that the impairment of the monkeys with amygdalar removals on the crossmodal task was due specifically to task difficulty or to some global change in motivational or emotional state.

Additional anatomical considerations

Because much of the work concerning the behavioral effects of amygdalar removal is based on lesions like those described here, which include both the amygdala and subjacent cortex, further experiments will have to address whether some of the effects ascribed to the amygdalar complex might instead be due to removal of the underlying cortex.

The speculation concerning the functions of specific projection systems is not meant to be an exhaustive exploration of the possibilities. Although I have suggested that the projection from the amygdala to the neocortex may mediate the process of associative recall, this projection may have other functions that do not exclude the present one. For example, it has been suggested that one of the effects of learning is to "tune" the sensory apparatus to promote the processing of significant stimuli (see Weinberger, 1984). Perhaps this process is achieved via the widespread amygdalar projection to the neocortex. Further, an unexplored topic that may be related to the "tuning" idea is whether the amygdala mediates influences of autonomic/affective centers on sensory processing.

Resolution of these questions will help clarify the precise contribution of amygdalar complex to behavior.

Conclusions

The amygdalar complex is anatomically related both to cortical processing areas devoted to all the traditional sensory modalities, such as vision, touch, audition, etc., as well as to cortical and subcortical processing systems known to be related to the quasi-modality of emotion. Thus the amygdala is in a position to process information about both affective and nonaffective sensory events. Behavioral studies suggest that the amygdala is critical for crossmodal associations; this may include the association of sensory stimuli derived from different sensory modalities, as in the crossmodal task, as well as stimulus-affect and stimulus-reward associations. The hippocampus, the medial temporal lobe neighbor of the amygdala, may be necessary for some aspects of spatial memory, including object-place associations. The amygdala and hippocampus thus appear to make independent and selective contributions to associative memory.

Acknowledgements

I gratefully acknowledge the valuable contributions of Mortimer Mishkin, who helped develop and support this work. I thank both Mortimer Mishkin and John Aggleton for their numerous helpful comments on an earlier version of this manuscript, David Gaffan for fruitful discussions of some of the ideas set forth in this chapter, and Judy Morgan and Dragana Ivkovich for help with the illustrations. Some of this work has been supported by NATO grant number 0184/87 for International Collaboration in Research (E.A.M. and D. Gaffan).

References

Aggleton, J.P. (1985) A description of intra-amygdaloid connections in old world monkeys. *Exp. Brain Res.,* 57: 390 – 399.

Aggleton, J.P., Burton, M.J. and Passingham, R.E. (1980) Cortical and subcortical afferents to the amygdala of the rhesus monkey (*Macaca mulatta*). *Brain Res.,* 190: 347 – 368.

Aggleton, J.P., Friedman, D.P. and Mishkin, M. (1987) A comparison between the connections of the amygdala and hippocampus with the basal forebrain in the macaque. *Exp. Brain Res.,* 67: 556 – 568.

Aggleton, J.P. and Mishkin, M. (1984) Projections of the amygdala to the thalamus in the cynomolgus monkey. *J. Comp. Neurol.,* 222: 56 – 68.

Aggleton, J.P. and Mishkin, M. (1986) The amygdala: sensory gateway to the emotions. In: R. Plutchik and H. Kellerman (Eds.), *Emotion: theory, research, and experience,* vol. 3, Academic Press, Orlando, pp. 281 – 299.

Aggleton, J.P. and Passingham, R.E. (1981) Syndrome produced by lesions of the amygdala in monkeys (*Macaca mulatta*). *J. Comp. Physiol. Psychol.,* 95: 961 – 977.

Alheid, G.F. and Heimer, L. (1988) New perspectives in basal forebrain organization of special relevance for neuropsychiatric disorders: the striatopallidal, amygdaloid, and corticopetal components of substantia innominata. *Neuroscience,* 27: 1 – 39.

Amaral, D.G. (1987) Memory: anatomical organization of candidate brain regions. In: V.B. Mountcastle, F. Plum and S.R. Geiger (Eds.), *Handbook of Physiology, Section 1, The Nervous System,* vol. 5., American Physiological Association, Bethesda, MD, pp. 211 – 294.

Amaral, D.G., Insausti, R. and Cowan, W.M. (1983) Evidence for a direct projection from the superior temporal gyrus to the entorhinal cortex in the monkey. *Brain Res.,* 275: 263 – 277.

Amaral, D.G. and Price, J.L. (1984) Amygdalo-cortical projections in the monkey (*Macaca fascicularis*). *J. Comp. Neurol.,* 230: 465 – 496.

Amaral, D.G., Veazey, R.B. and Cowan, W.M. (1982) Some observations on hypothalamo-amygdaloid connections in the monkey. *Brain Res.,* 252: 13 – 27.

Bandler, R., Carrive, P. and Zhang, S.P. (1991) Integration of somatic and automomic reactions within the midbrain periaqueductal grey: Viscerotopic somatopic and functional organization. In: G. Holstege (Ed.), *Progress in Brain Research Vol. 87,* Elsevier, Amsterdam, pp. 269 – 305.

Bard, P. and Macht, M.B. (1958) The behavior of chronically decerebrated cats. In: *Neurological Basis of Behavior,* Ciba Foundation Symposium, Churchill Ltd., London, pp. 55 – 75.

Crosby, E.C. and Humphrey, T. (1941) Studies of the vertebrate telencephalon. *J. Comp. Neurol.,* 74: 309 – 352.

de Olmos, J., Alheid, G.F. and Beltramino, C.A. (1985) Amygdala. In: G. Paxinos (Ed.), *The rat nervous system,* vol. 1. Academic Press, Sydney, pp. 223 – 334.

Doty, R.W., Negrao, N. and Yamaga, K. (1973) The unilateral engram. *Acta Neurobiologiae Experimentalis,* 33: 711 – 728.

Downer, J.L. (1961) Changes in visual gnostic functions and emotional behaviour following unilateral temporal pole damage in the "split brain" monkey. *Nature,* 191: 50 – 51.

Egger, M.D. and Flynn, J.P. (1967) Further studies on the effect of amygdaloid stimulation and ablation on hypothalamically elicited attack behavior in cats. In: W.R. Adey and T. Tokizane (Eds.), *Progress in Brain Research, vol. 27,* Elsevier, Amsterdam, pp. 165 – 182.

Everitt, B.J., Cador, M. and Robbins, T.W. (1989) Interactions between the amygdala and ventral striatum in stimulus-reward association: studies using a second-order schedule of sexual reinforcement. *Neuroscience,* 30: 63 – 75.

Fernandez de Molina, A. and Hunsperger, R.W. (1962) Organization of the subcortical system governing defense and flight reactions in the cat. *J. Physiol.,* 160: 200 – 213.

Friedman, D.P., Murray, E.A., O'Neill, J.B. and Mishkin, M. (1986) Cortical connections of the somatosensory fields in the lateral sulcus of macaques: evidence for a corticolimbic pathway for touch. *J. Comp. Neurol.,* 252: 323 – 347.

Fukuda, M., Ono, T., Nishino, H. and Nakamura, K. (1986) Neuronal responses in monkey lateral hypothalamus during operant feeding behavior. *Brain Res. Bull.,* 17: 879 – 884.

Gaffan, D. and Harrison, S. (1987) Amygdalectomy and disconnection in visual learning for auditory secondary reinforcement by monkeys. *J. Neurosci.,* 7: 2285 – 2292.

Gaffan, E.A., Gaffan, D. and Harrison, S. (1988) Disconnection of the amygdala from visual association cortex impairs reward-association learning in monkeys. *J. Neurosci.,* 8: 3144 – 3150.

Gaffan, D., Gaffan, E.A. and Harrison, S. (1989) Visual-visual associative learning and reward-association learning in monkeys: the role of the amygdala. *J. Neurosci.,* 9: 558 – 564.

Gaffan, D.G. and Murray, E.A. (1990) Amygdalar interaction with the medial dorsal nucleus of the thalamus and the ventromedial prefrontal cortex in stimulus-reward associative learning in the monkey. *J. Neurosci.,* 10: 3479 – 3493.

Herzog, A.G. and Van Hoesen, G.W. (1976) Temporal neocortical afferent connections to the amygdala in the rhesus monkey. *Brain Res.,* 115: 57 – 69.

Holstege, G., Meiners, L. and Tan, K. (1985) Projections of the bed nucleus of the stria terminalis to the mesencephalon, pons, and medulla oblongata in the cat. *Exp. Brain Res.,* 58: 379 – 391.

Horel, J.A. and Misantone, L.J. (1974) The Klüver-Bucy syndrome produced by partial isolation of the temporal lobe. *Exp. Neurol.,* 42: 101 – 112.

Horel, J.A., Keating, E.G. and Misantone, L.J. (1975) Partial Klüver-Bucy syndrome produced by destroying temporal neocortex or amygdala. *Brain Res.,* 94: 347 – 359.

Hreib, K.K., Rosene, D.L. and Moss, M.B. (1988) Basal forebrain efferents to the medial dorsal thalamic nucleus in the rhesus monkey. *J. Comp. Neurol.,* 277: 365 – 390.

Iwai, E. and Yukie, M. (1987) Amygdalofugal and amygdalopetal connections with modality-specific visual cortical areas in macaques (*Macaca fuscata, M. mulatta, and M. fascicularis*). *J. Comp. Neurol.,* 261: 362 – 387.

Johnston, J.B. (1923) Further contributions to the study of the evolution of the forebrain. *J. Comp. Neurol.,* 36: 143 – 192.

Jones, E.G., Burton, H., Saper, C.B. and Swanson, L.W. (1976) Midbrain, diencephalic and cortical relationships of the basal nucleus of Meynert and associated structures in primates. *J. Comp. Neurol.,* 167: 385 – 419.

Kesner, R.P. and DiMattia, B.V. (1987) Neurobiology of an attribute model of memory. In: A.N. Epstein and A.R. Morrison (Eds.), *Progress in Psychobiology and Physiological Psychology,* vol. 12, Academic Press, Orlando, pp. 207 – 277.

Klüver, H. and Bucy, P.C. (1939) Preliminary analysis of functions of the temporal lobes in monkeys. *Archives Neurol. Psychiat.,* 42: 979 – 1000.

Kordower, J.H., Bartus, R.T., Marciano, F.F. and Gash, D.M. (1989) Telencephalic cholinergic system of the New World monkey (*Cebus apella*): morphological and cytoarchitectonic assessment and analysis of the projection to the amygdala. *J. Comp. Neurol.,* 279: 528 – 545.

Mehler, W.R. (1980) Subcortical afferent connections of the amygdala in the monkey. *J. Comp. Neurol.,* 190: 733 – 762.

Mesulam, M.-M., Mufson, E.J., Levey, A.I. and Wainer, B.H. (1983) Cholinergic innervation of the cortex by the basal forebrain: cytochemistry and cortical connections of the septal area, diagonal band nuclei, nucleus basalis (substantia innominata), and hypothalamus in the rhesus monkey. *J. Comp. Neurol.,* 214: 170 – 197.

Mishkin, M. (1978) Memory in monkeys severly impaired by combined but not by separate removal of amygdala and hippocampus. *Nature,* 273: 297 – 298.

Mishkin, M. (1982) A memory system in the monkey. *Phil. Trans. R. Soc. Lond. B.,* 298: 85 – 95.

Mishkin, M. and Petri, H.L. (1984) Memories and habits: some implications for the analysis of learning and retention. In: L.R. Squire and N. Butters (Eds.), *Neuropsychology of Memory,* Guilford Press, New York, pp. 287 – 296.

Mora, F., Rolls, E.T. and Burton, M.J. (1976) Modulation during learning of the responses of neurons in the lateral hypothalamus to the sight of food. *Exp. Neurol.,* 53: 508 – 519.

Moran, M.A., Mufson, E.J. and Mesulam, M.-M. (1987) Neural inputs into the temporopolar cortex of the rhesus monkey. *J. Comp. Neurol.,* 256: 88 – 103.

Mufson, E.J., Mesulam, M.-M. and Pandya, D.N. (1981) Insular interconnections with the amygdala in the rhesus monkey. *Neuroscience,* 6: 1231 – 1248.

Murray, E.A. (1990) Representational memory in nonhuman primates. In: D.S. Olton and R.P. Kesner (Eds.), *Neurobiology of Comparative Cognition,* Erlbaum, pp. 127 – 155.

Murray, E.A. and Mishkin, M. (1984) Severe tactual as well as visual memory deficits follow combined removal of the amygdala and hippocampus in monkeys. *J. Neuroscience,* 4: 2565 – 2580.

Murray, E.A. and Mishkin, M. (1985) Amygdalectomy impairs crossmodal association in monkeys. *Science,* 228: 604 – 606.

Murray, E.A. and Mishkin, M. (1986) Visual recognition in monkeys following rhinal cortical ablations combined with either amygdalectomy or hippocampectomy. *J. Neuroscience,* 6: 1991 – 2003.

Nauta, W.J.H. (1961) Fibre degeneration following lesions of the amygdaloid complex in the monkey. *J. Anat.,* 95: 515 – 530.

Pandya, D.N., Van Hoesen, G.W. and Mesulam, M.-M. (1981) Efferent connections of the cingulate gyrus in the rhesus monkey. *Exp. Brain Res.,* 42: 319 – 330.

Parkinson, J.K., Murray, E.A. and Mishkin, M. (1988) A selective mnemonic role for the hippocampus in monkeys: memory for the location of objects. *J. Neuroscience,* 8: 4159 – 4167.

Porrino, L.P., Crane, A.M. and Goldman-Rakic, P.S. (1981) Direct and indirect pathways from the amygdala to the frontal lobe in rhesus monkeys. *J. Comp. Neurol.,* 198: 121 – 136.

Price, J.L. (1981) Toward a consistent terminology for the amygdaloid complex. In: Y. Ben-Ari (Ed.), *The amygdaloid complex.* Elsevier/North-Holland Biomedical Press, Amsterdam, pp. 13 – 18.

Price, J.L. and Amaral, D.G. (1981) An autoradiographic study of the projections of the central nucleus of the monkey amygdala. *J. Neurosci.,* 11: 1242 – 1259.

Ricardo, J.A. and Koh, E.T. (1978) Anatomical evidence of direct projections from the nucleus of the solitary tract to the hypothalamus, amygdala, and other forebrain structures in the rat. *Brain Res.,* 153: 1 – 26.

Robbins, T.W., Cador, M., Taylor, J.R. and Everitt, B.J. (1989) Limbic-striatal interactions in reward-related processes. *Neuroscience and Biobehavioral Reviews,* 13: 155 – 162.

Rolls, E.T. (1984) Responses of neurons in different regions of the striatum of the behaving monkey. In: J.S. McKenzie, R.E. Kemm and L.N. Wilcox (Eds.) *The basal ganglia: structure and function,* Plenum, New York, pp. 467 – 493.

Rolls, E.T., Sanghera, M.K. and Roper-Hall, A. (1979) The latency of activation of neurones in the lateral hypothalamus and substantia innominata during feeding in the monkey. *Brain Res.,* 164: 121 – 135.

Rosvold, H.E., Mirsky, A.F. and Pribram, K. (1954) Influence of amygdalectomy on social behavior in monkeys. *J. Comp. Physiol. Psychol.,* 47: 173 – 178.

Russchen, F.T., Amaral, D.G. and Price, J.L. (1985a) The afferent connections of the substantia innominata in the monkey *Macaca fascicularis. J. Comp. Neurol.,* 242: 1 – 27.

Russchen, F.T., Amaral, D.G. and Price, J.L. (1987) The afferent input to the magnocellular division of the mediodorsal thalamic nucleus in the monkey, *Macaca fascicularis. J. Comp. Neurol.,* 256: 175 – 210.

Russchen, F.T., Bakst, I. Amaral, D.G. and Price, J.L. (1985b) The amygdalostriatal projections in the monkey. An anterograde tracing study. *Brain Res.,* 329: 241 – 257.

Saunders, R.C., Murray, E.A. and Mishkin, M. (1984) Further evidence that amygdala and hippocampus contribute equally to recognition memory. *Neuropsychologia,* 22: 785 – 796.

Saunders, R.C. and Rosene, D.L. (1988) A comparison of the efferents of the amygdala and the hippocampal formation in the rhesus monkey: I. Convergence in the entorhinal, prorhinal, and perirhinal cortices. *J. Comp. Neurol.,* 271: 153 – 184.

Spiegler, B.J. and Mishkin, M. (1981) Evidence for the sequential participation of inferior temporal cortex and amygdala in the acquisition of stimulus-reward associations. *Behav. Brain Res.,* 3: 303 – 317.

Taylor, J.R. and Robbins, T.W. (1986) 6-Hydroxydopamine lesions of the nucleus accumbens, but not of the caudate nucleus, attenuate enhanced responding with reward-related stimuli produced by intra-accumbens d-amphetamine. *Psychopharmacology,* 90: 390 – 397.

Thompson, C.I., Bergland, R.M. and Towfighi, J.T. (1977) Social and nonsocial behaviors of adult rhesus monkeys after amygdalectomy in infancy or adulthood. *J. Comp. Physiol. Psychol.,* 91: 533 – 548.

Tigges, J., Tigges, M., Cross, N.A., McBride, R.L., Letbetter, W.D. and Anschel, S. (1982) Subcortical structures projecting to visual cortical areas in squirrel monkey. *J. Comp. Neurol.,* 209: 29 – 40.

Turner, B.H., Mishkin, M. and Knapp, M. (1980) Organization of amygdalopetal projections from modality-specific cortical association areas in the monkey. *J. Comp. Neurol.,* 191: 515 – 543.

Van Hoesen, G.W. (1981) The differential distribution, diversity and sprouting of cortical projections to the amygdala in the rhesus monkey. In: Y. Ben-Ari (Ed.), *The amygdaloid complex.* Elsevier/North-Holland Biomedical Press, Amsterdam, pp. 77 – 90.

Weinberger, N.M. (1984) The neurophysiology of learning: A view from the sensory side. In: L.R. Squire and N. Butters (Eds.), *Neuropsychology of Memory,* Guilford Press, New York, pp. 489 – 503.

Weiskrantz, L. (1956) Behavioral changes associated with ablation of the amygdaloid complex in monkeys. *J. Comp. Physiol. Psychol.,* 49: 381 – 391.

White, N.M. (1989) A functional hypothesis concerning the striatal matrix and patches: mediation of S-R memory and reward. *Life Sciences,* 45: 1943 – 1957.

G. Holstege (Ed.)
Progress in Brain Research, Vol. 87

CHAPTER 9

Biochemical switching in hypothalamic circuits mediating responses to stress

L.W. Swanson*

Howard Hughes Medical Institute, The Salk Institute for Biological Studies, La Jolla, CA 92037, U.S.A.

Introduction

Over the last half-century, the generally held view has emerged that the hypothalamus plays a particularly important role in coordinating the endocrine, autonomic, and behavioral responses that assure survival of the individual (homeostasis) as well as survival of the species (reproduction). And since stress (or a stressor) is usually regarded as any condition or factor that disturbs the dynamic equilibrium (homeostasis) of the body, it has seemed reasonable to assume that hypothalamic circuitry mediates a number of the adaptive responses initiated by such factors.

Unfortunately, our understanding of the basic organizing principles of hypothalamic circuitry lags far behind that of the major sensory and motor systems of the CNS, although considerable progress has been made in the last 15 years with the application of neuroanatomical methods based on axonal transport and histochemistry. The purpose of this review is to outline one view of the general organization of hypothalamic circuitry, as well as evidence that information flow through this circuitry may be influenced by changes in the ratios of neuropeptides released by individual links in this circuitry.

* *Present address:* Hedco Neurosciences Building MC 2520, University of Southern California, Los Angeles, CA 90089-2520, U.S.A.

Organization of the hypothalamus

As reviewed in detail elsewhere (Swanson, 1986, 1987), the hypothalamus contains three longitudinal zones, each of which displays relatively distinct morphological and functional characteristics, at least to a first level of approximation (Fig. 1). The periventricular zone is a narrow band of generally small, bipolar neurons that lies adjacent to the third ventricle and subserves two cardinal functions. First, the vast majority of neuroendocrine motoneurons associated with the pituitary gland lie within or near the periventricular zone. Furthermore, separate pools of these motoneurons associated with control of the anterior pituitary (the parvicellular neurosecretory system) are arranged in rostral-caudal order. Thus, gonadotropin-releasing hormone (GnRH) neurons are scattered in and around periventricular tissue surrounding the rostral end of the third ventricle; somatostatin (SS) neurons that inhibit growth hormone release are centered in the anterior periventricular nucleus; corticotropin-releasing hormone (CRH) and thyrotropin-releasing hormone (TRH) cells lie within the paraventricular nucleus (PVH, see below); and dopamine (DA) cells (which inhibit prolactin release), along with growth hormone-releasing hormone (GRH) cells are concentrated caudally in the arcuate nucleus. And second, two cell groups associated with the periventricular zone are essential for the generation of fundamental

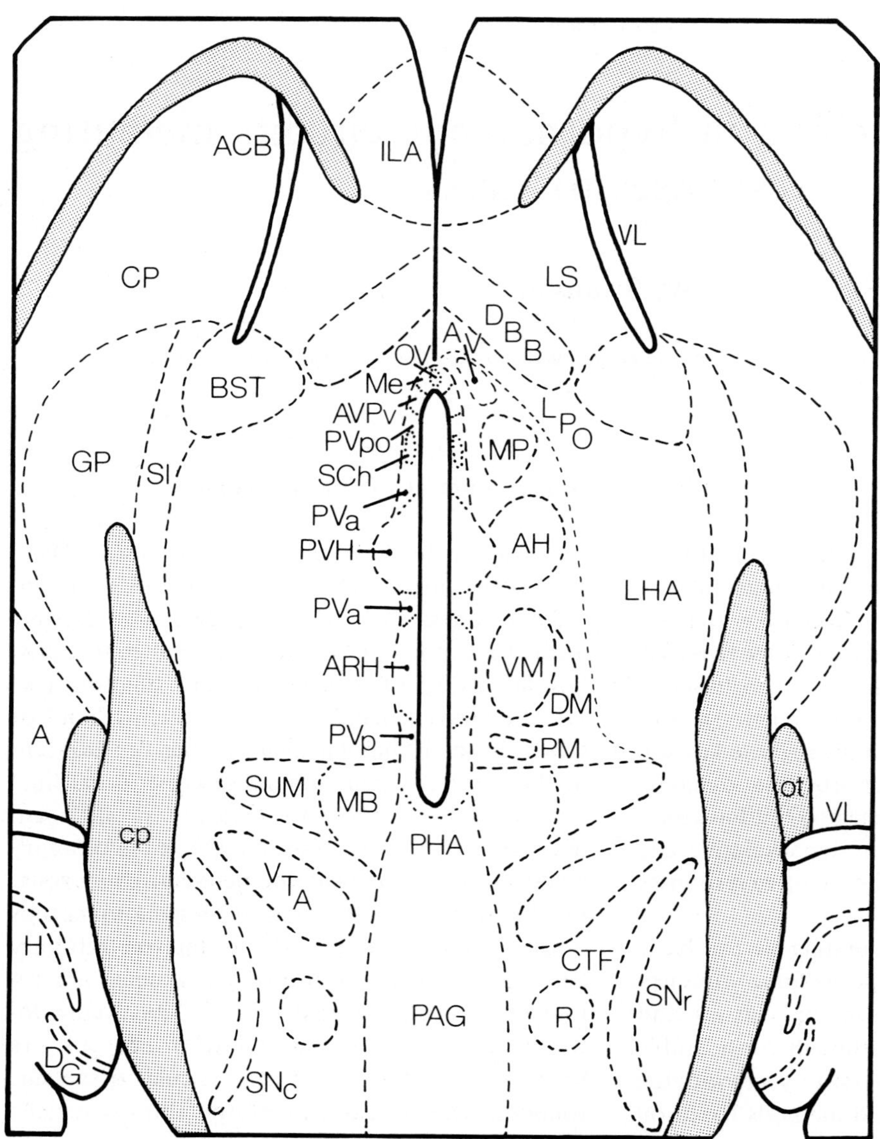

Fig. 1. A schematic horizontal view of the rat brain to show the major cell groups in and around the hypothalamus. *Abbreviations:* A, amygdala; ACB, nucleus accumbens; AH, anterior hypothalamic nucleus; ARH, arcuate nucleus; AV, anteroventral preoptic nucleus; AVPv, anteroventral periventricular nucleus; BST, bed nuclei of the stria terminalis; CP, caudoputamen; CTF, central tegmental field; DBB, nucleus of the diagonal band; DG, dentate gyrus; DM, dorsomedial nucleus; GP, globus pallidus; H, hippocampus; ILA, infralimbic area; LHA, lateral hypothalamic area; LPO, lateral preoptic area; LS, lateral septal nucleus; MB, mammillary body; Me, median preoptic nucleus; MP, medial preoptic nucleus; OV, vascular organ of the lamina terminalis; PAG, periaqueductal gray; PHA, posterior hypothalamic area; PM, premammillary nucleus; PV_a, anterior periventricular nucleus; PV_p, posterior periventricular nucleus; PV_{po}, preoptic periventricular nucleus; PVH, paraventricular nucleus; R, red nucleus; SCh, suprachiasmatic nucleus; SI, substantia innominata (ventral pallidum); $SN_{c,r}$, compact and reticular parts of the substantia nigra; SUM, supramammillary nucleus; VL, lateral ventricle; VM, ventromedial nucleus, hypothalamus; VTA, ventral tegmental area; cp, cerebral peduncle; ot, optic tract. (From Swanson, 1987).

biological rhythms. The suprachiasmatic nucleus is an endogenous circadian rhythm generator, and the anteroventral periventricular nucleus rostral to it plays a critical role in generating the estrous cycle.

The medial zone of the hypothalamus lies just lateral to the periventricular zone, and can be thought of as a series of relatively well-defined nuclei embedded within a rather diffuse matrix of generally medium-sized neurons. From rostral to caudal, the major well-defined cell groups include the medial preoptic nucleus, the anterior hypothalamic nucleus, the dorsomedial and ventromedial nuclei, the premammillary nucleus, and the mammillary complex. LeGros Clark (1938) first pointed out that these nuclei conveniently serve to divide the hypothalamus as a whole into four rostrocaudal levels: preoptic, anterior, tuberal, and mammillary. Although the connections of the medial zone are very complex, they appear as a whole to receive their major specific inputs from various components of the limbic region of the telencephalon, and to distribute this information to the periventricular zone on the one hand, and to the medial forebrain bundle on the other.

The lateral zone is a heterogeneous, poorly differentiated region that is often regarded as a rostral continuation of the brainstem reticular formation. The typical multipolar neurons in this zone are relatively large, with long dendrites that course among, and are contacted by, fibers of the medial forebrain bundle, the most complex fiber system in the brain. The axons of lateral zone neurons project to the periventricular and medial zones of the hypothalamus, as well as throughout the rostral and caudal extent of the medial forebrain bundle. The latter set of projections are very extensive and ''diffuse'', and innervate the entire cerebral cortical mantle and limbic parts of the subcortical telencephalon rostrally, as well as extensive parts of the reticular core and spinal cord, including autonomic nuclei, caudally. In the broadest functional sense, the lateral zone appears to play an important role in modulating the behavioral state (e.g., attention and arousal) of the animal, as well as the output of the autonomic nervous system.

In summary, the one feature that distinguishes the hypothalamus from the rest of the CNS is the periventricular zone, which directly controls the output of the pituitary gland. Taken as a whole, the lateral zone functions in a much less specific way, appearing to modulate the general behavioral state of the animal and the autonomic nervous system. The medial zone appears to relay information from limbic parts of the telencephalon to both the neuroendocrine system and to the medial forebrain system.

The PVH and its circuitry

The PVH in the rat is a cytoarchitectonically well-defined region in the rostrodorsal part of the periventricular zone that contains on the order of 10^4 neurons in about 0.5 mm^2 of tissue (Swanson and Sawchenko, 1983). The nucleus is of particular interest because it has provided a unique model for examining the hypothalamic coordination of endocrine, autonomic, and behavioral responses. Thus, direct axonal projections from the PVH reach the posterior pituitary (Scharrer and Scharrer, 1940), the neurohemal zone of the median eminence (Vandesande et al., 1977), and reticular and autonomic parts of the brainstem and spinal cord (Saper et al., 1976) (Fig. 2). Subsequent neuroanatomical work based on immunohistochemical and multiple retrograde tracer techniques has established that projections to the posterior pituitary, neurohemal zone of the median eminence, as well as brainstem and spinal cord arise from essentially separate populations of neurons that are topographically segregated within the PVH, and that each of these three compartments can be further subdivided (for reviews see Swanson, 1987; Swanson et al., 1987).

Figure 3A is a schematic view of the basic organization of cell groups in the caudal half of the PVH, although it must be emphasized that the physical segregation of cell types is not complete; a small number of neurons of a particular type are

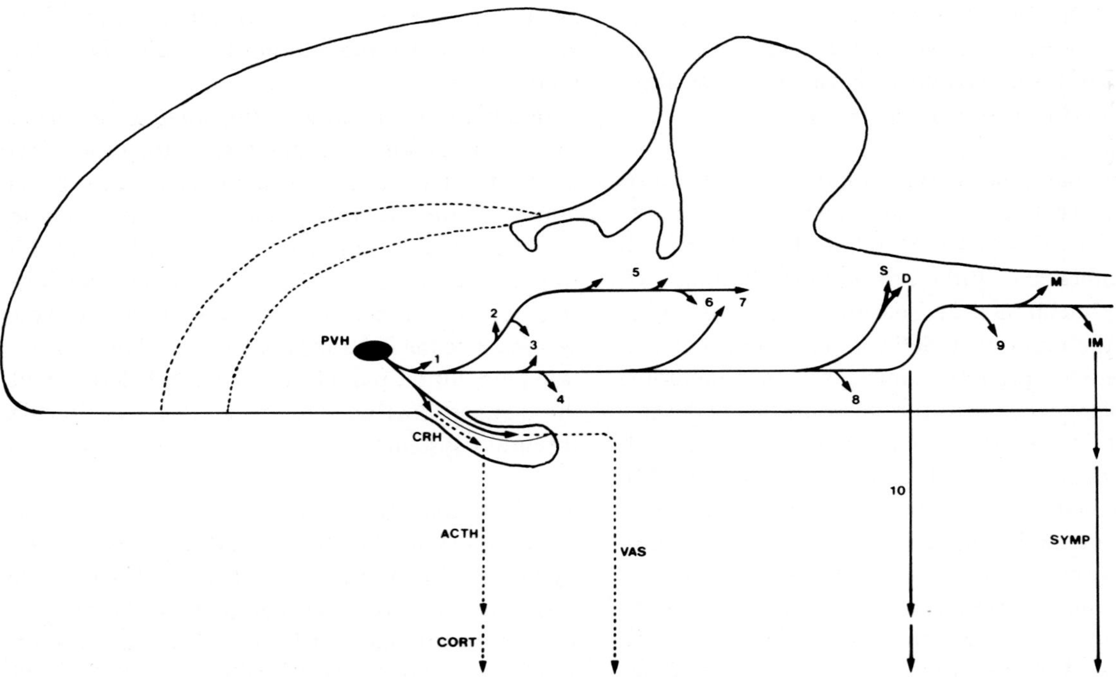

Fig. 2. Another schematic horizontal view of the rat brain to illustrate the major efferent projections of the PVH. *Abbreviations:* ACTH, adrenocorticotropic hormone; CORT, corticosterone; D, dorsal motor nucleus of the vagus; IM, intermediolateral column; M, marginal zone; S, nucleus of the solitary tract; SYMP, postganglionic sympathetic neurons; VAS, vasopressin; 1, lateral hypothalamic area; 2, posterior hypothalamic area; 3, mesencephalic reticular formation; 4, ventral tegmental area; 5, periaqueductal gray; 6, pedunculopontine nucleus; 7, locus coeruleus and parabrachial nucleus; 8, ventrolateral medulla; 9, spinal central gray; 10, vagus nerve.

typically found scattered in adjacent parts of the nucleus. As this figure makes clear, the magnocellular neurosecretory division contains separate pools of neurons that synthesize oxytocin or vasopressin and project to the posterior pituitary. The parvicellular neurosecretory division is quite complex; virtually all of the CRH and TRH delivered to the neurohemal zone of the median eminence arises from separate groups of neurons in this division of the PVH (see Ceccatelli et al., 1989), which thus constitutes the final common pathway for the central control of ACTH and thyroid-stimulating hormone (TSH) release from the anterior pituitary. In addition, this division harbors the dorsal region of the neuroendocrine SS cell group that is centered in the anterior periventricular nucleus, as well as a small number of what are probably neuroendocrine DA (Kawano and Daikoko, 1987) and GRH (Sawchenko et al., 1985a) cells, the majority of which are found in the arcuate nucleus. Thus, at least some neurons in the parvicellular division of the PVH synthesize five of the six classical hypophysiotrophic factors (GnRH is not produced in the PVH).

Finally, the mediocellular division with descending projections (the "descending" division) can be parcellated into at least three parts (Swanson and Kuypers, 1980), although a great deal remains to be learned about its topographical organization. Nevertheless, it has been clear for some time (Swanson and Kuypers, 1980) that the dorsal part preferentially innervates the spinal cord (and particularly the preganglionic sympathetic column), whereas the ventral subdivision provides substantial inputs to both parasympathetic (especially the dorsal vagal complex) and sympathetic cell groups,

	Posterior Pituitary (M)		Median Eminence/ Anterior Pituitary (P)					Descending (D) Symp 7, PS/Symp 8/9
	1	2	3	4	5	6a	6b	7 8/9
•		VAS	VAS					VAS
	OXY							OXY
•	CRH		CRH					CRH
				TRH				TRH
					SS			SS
						GRH		
•		DA					DA	DA
•		ANG	ANG					ANG
	CCK		CCK					
			NT					NT
			ENK					ENK
•	DYN	DYN	(DYN)					DYN
		GAL						
	7B2	7B2						
			GABA					

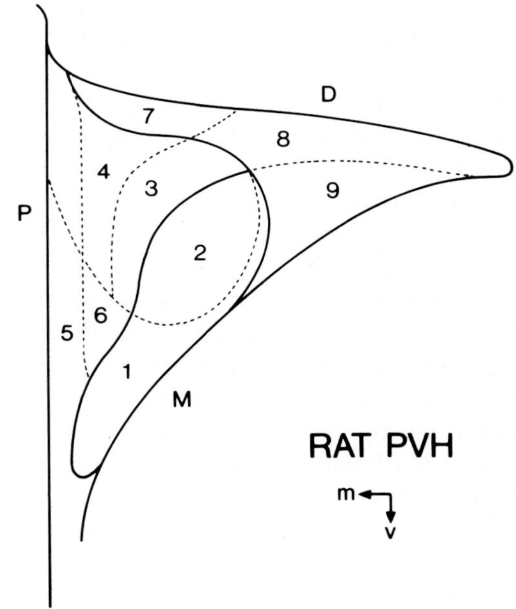

Fig. 3. The drawing on the right is a schematic representation of the major components of the posterior half of the rat PVH (D, descending division; M, magnocellular neurosecretory division; P, parvicellular neurosecretory division). The numbers within subdivisions of the PVH refer to cell types that appear to contain the neuroactive substances listed in the chart on the left. *Abbreviations* in chart (not used in text): ANG, angiotensin; CCK, cholecystokinin; DA, dopamine; DYN, dynorphin; ENK, enkephalin; GAL, galanin; NT, neurotensin; OXY, oxytocin; PS/Symp, to parasympathetic and sympathetic systems; VAS, vasopressin. References to the information in this figure can be found in Swanson et al., 1986, 1987; Sawchenko and Levin, 1989; Swanson and Simmons, 1989; and in the text.

and recent evidence indicates (Strack et al., 1989) that neurons projecting to organ-specific groups of sympathetic preganglionic neurons are also topographically organized.

Taken together, the evidence just reviewed suggests that the PVH may be viewed essentially as a motor nuclear complex, with separate divisions related to control of the posterior pituitary, the anterior pituitary, and the autonomic nervous system and reticular core.

Afferent control of the PVH

Having defined the projections of the PVH in terms of three functionally and anatomically distinct compartments, the question naturally arises as to mechanisms involved in coordinating appropriate responses initiated by these projections. At least three possible mechanisms are obvious: specific neural afferents that innervate more than one cell type, interneurons, and recurrent collaterals. To date, there is no convincing evidence for interneurons in the PVH, and the results of intracellular filling studies indicate that only descending neurons give rise to recurrent collaterals, which may end preferentially in the mediocellular, "descending" compartment itself (see Rho and Swanson, 1989).

It seems likely, therefore, that coordinated responses from different cell types in the PVH are affected primarily by neural afferents. Unfortunately, neuroanatomical work has shown that, perhaps not surprisingly, the afferent control of the PVH is exceedingly complex, consisting of inputs from literally dozens of different cell groups, most of which appear to innervate more than one compartment.

Before considering general features of the afferent control of the PVH, it is worth pointing out that intracellular filling experiments indicate that the dendrites of neurons in one of the major compartments tend to stay within the boundaries of that compartment, although their distal processes often end in immediately adjacent parts of neighboring compartments or just outside the lateral border of the nucleus itself (Rho and Swanson, 1989). Nevertheless, the evidence suggests that a neural pathway giving rise to a clear terminal field in a particular compartment almost certainly innervates neurons in that compartment.

It is not necessary for our purposes here to review all known afferents to various components of the PVH (see Swanson, 1987 and below). Instead, we shall focus on inputs to parvicellular CRH neurons that project to the neurohemal zone of the median eminence (Fig. 4), and thus presumably relay information from stressors that leads to ACTH and glucocorticoid secretion. At least for descriptive purposes, major known inputs to the "CRH" part of the PVH (the dorsal medial parvicellular division, PVHmpd) can be divided into four broad classes. The first consists of a complex series of ascending projections from the dorsal vagal complex, ventrolateral medulla, and parabrachial nucleus that appear to relay visceral sensory information from the vagus and glossopharyngeal nerves. The highly differentiated pathways from the medulla have been shown to contain at least epinephrine, norepinephrine, neuropeptide Y, galanin, somatostatin, and activin (see Sawchenko and Swanson, 1982; Sawchenko et al., 1985b; Levin et al., 1987; Cunningham and Sawchenko, 1988, 1990; Sawchenko et al., 1988a,b).

The second broad class of afferents arises in the subfornical organ, a circumventricular nucleus that lacks a blood-brain barrier, and is particularly involved in mediating the central effects of circulating angiotensin II on water balance. Interestingly, the direct projection from the subfornical organ reaches all parts of the PVH, including

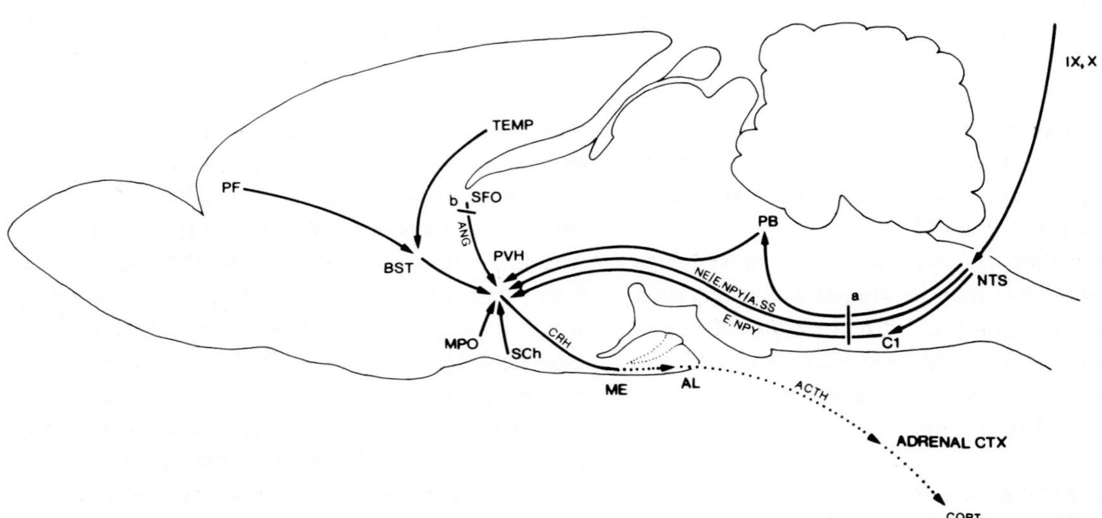

Fig. 4. A summary of the major known inputs to the PVHmpd in the rat. *Abbreviations*: A, activin; AL, anterior lobe (pituitary); ACTH, adrenocorticotropic hormone; ANG, angiotensin; BST, bed nuclei of the stria terminalis; C_1, adrenergic cell group in ventrolateral medulla; CORT, corticosterone; E, epinephrine; ME, neurohemal zone of median eminence; MPO, medial preoptic nucleus; NE, norepinephrine; NPY, neuropeptide Y; NTS, nucleus of the solitary tract; PB, parabrachial nucleus; PF, medial prefrontal cortex; SCh, suprachiasmatic nucleus; SFO, subfornical organ; SS, somatostatin; TEMP, medial temporal lobe (amygdala and hippocampal formation); IX, glossopharyngeal nerve; X, vagus nerve; a & b, sites of knife cuts discussed in text.

the PVHmpd, and appears at least in part to use angiotensin as a neurotransmitter (Lind et al., 1985a). Thus, the subfornical organ is in a position to mediate direct humoral chemosensory-neuroendocrine reflexes at the level of the PVH (and supraoptic nucleus), as well as other autonomic and behavioral responses to hypovolemia (see Swanson and Lind, 1986).

The third class of afferents arises in the telencephalon, and is presumably concerned with cognitive influences on CRH/ACTH/glucocorticoid secretion. As reviewed elsewhere (Swanson, 1987), the only established dense projection from the telencephalon to virtually all parts of the PVH arises in the bed nuclei of the stria terminalis (BST), a ventral component of the septal region. The most likely functional significance of this projection is suggested by the fact that the BST receives massive inputs from ventral parts of the hippocampal formation and the amygdala, as well as from medial parts of the prefrontal cortex. Since these three regions in turn all receive inputs from the isocortex, the anatomical evidence suggests that the BST acts as a "funnel" for isocortical influences on ACTH release after relays through other parts of the limbic region.

And finally, many different cell groups in the hypothalamus itself project to the PVHmpd. This issue was first addressed with retrograde transport methods and the anterograde autoradiographic technique (Sawchenko and Swanson, 1983). Since then, we have begun to reexamine hypothalamic projections with the method based on the anterograde transport of PHA-L (Gerfen and Sawchenko, 1984), which is a more powerful approach than the autoradiographic method because terminal boutons can be identified unequivocally. Table I summarizes the relative distribution of PHA-L-labeled fibers with terminal boutons from various hypothalamic regions, based on our published and unpublished results.

While the functional significance of most of these hypothalamic inputs remains obscure, at the very least they provide a substrate for the potential relay of a broad array of limbic and reticular information to the PVH, including CRH parvicellular neurosecretory cells in the PVHmpd.

Coexpression of neuroactive substances in PVH neurons

In the preceding sections what might be viewed as the classical morphological and connectional features of the hypothalamus, and of the PVH in particular, have been reviewed. We shall now venture into an aspect of functional neuroanatomy that may someday revolutionize thinking about the flow of information through neural circuitry.

A convenient starting point for this discussion is provided by the demonstration that individual neurons may contain more than one neuroactive substance (see Burnstock, 1976; Chan-Palay et al., 1978; Hökfelt et al., 1978). This fundamental observation has since been confirmed for many types of neurons (see Hökfelt et al., 1986), and indeed it does not seem unreasonable to suggest that the expression of multiple "transmitters' may be a feature common to a majority of neurons.

Nowhere in the brain does the multiple expression of neuroactive substances appear more pervasive and obvious than in the PVH. As summarized in Fig. 2, a set of over a dozen neuropeptide genes is expressed in the PVH, along with certain other nonpeptidergic compounds, including dopamine and GABA (Meister et al., 1988). Two features of the information summarized in Fig. 2 deserve particular attention. First, the evidence suggests that a particular cell type, such as the parvicellular neurosecretory CRH population in the PVHmpd, may, under appropriate physiological conditions, express at least eight different neuroactive substances. And second, many neuroactive substances are expressed across two or more cell types within the PVH. In the extreme case, vasopressin, CRH, dopamine, angiotensin, and dynorphin appear to be contained within all three major cell types in the PVH.

This evidence, which is based on the application of immunohistochemical and in situ hybridization techniques, suggests that the PVH provides an excellent model for examining the functional

TABLE I

Possible hypothalamic inputs to PVH/SO observed with the PHA-L method

*Reference**	*Source of Projection*	SO	PVH								
			am	*pmm*	*pml*	*ap*	*mpd*	*mpv*	*dp*	*lp*	*pv*
(1) and u.o.	substantia innominata †	+	+	+	+	+	+	++	++	++	+++
u.o., RS198	lateral preoptic area	+	+	+	–	++	+	+	+	+	+
u.o., RBS 118	parastrial n.	+++	+++	+++	+++	+++	++	++++	++++	++++	+++
u.o., RBS 55	anterodorsal preoptic n.	++	+++	++	++	+++	++	++	++	++	+++
u.o., RBS 54	anteroventral preoptic n.	–	++	++	++	++	++	++	++	+++	++
u.o., RBS 92	anteroventral periventricular n.	–	+++	+++	++	++++	++	++	++++	++	++++
u.o., A 48	preoptic suprachiasmatic n.	+	+++	++	+	+++	++	+++	+++	+	++++
(2)	suprachiasmatic n.	–	+	+	+	++	+	++	+	+	+
u.o., A 34	dorsal to SCh	+	+	+	+	+++	+	++	+++	+	++
u.o., A 53	retrochiasmatic a.	+	+	+	+	+++	++	+	+	+	++
u.o., RBS 21	medial preoptic n., central	–	++	+	+	++++	+	++	+++	+	+++
u.o., RBS 83	medial preoptic n., medial	+	+++	++	+	++++	+	++	+++	++	+++++
u.o., RBS 135	medial preoptic n., lateral	–	+	++	–	++++	++	+	++	+	+++
u.o., RBS 204	anterior hypothalamic n., anterior	+	++	++	–	++	+	++	++	++	++
u.o., RBS 81	ventromedial n., dorsomedial	–	–	–	+	++	++	+	+	+	+
u.o., RBS 73	arcuate n.	–	+	+	–	++	+	+	+	+	+++

* References: (1) Swanson et al., 1984; (2) Watts et al., 1987; u.o.: unpublished observations along with experiment number. † The substantia innominata is usually regarded as part of the telencephalon, but shares a number of features in common with the lateral preoptic area. *Abbreviations*: PVH, paraventricular n.; SCh, suprachiasmatic n.; SO, supraoptic n.; a, area; n., nucleus; parts of PVH (see Swanson et al., 1986): am, anterior magnocellular; mpd, dorsal medial parvicellular; mpv, ventral medial parvicellular; pml, lateral (vasopressinergic) posterior magnocellular; pmm, medial (oxytocinergic) posterior magnocellular; pv, periventricular.

significance of multiple neurotransmitter expression in central neurons, as well as their possible differential regulation.

Differential regulation of neuropeptide genes in the PVHmpd: Adrenal steroids

The possibility that the ratio of multiple neurotransmitters can vary substantially within a particular cell type was first clearly established in cultures of developing sympathetic ganglion cells, and later during the in vivo development of the cholinergic sympathetic innervation of particular sweat glands (for reviews see Patterson, 1978; Landis, 1988). Furthermore, the sympathetic system was also exploited to demonstrate that neural activity appears to change the ratio of substance P and catecholamines in ganglion cells (Kessler and Black, 1982; Black et al., 1987).

We shall now review evidence that similar effects occur within the CNS, specifically within the PVH, and consider their possible functional significance. Following the characterization of CRH by Vale and his colleagues in 1981, and the production of specific antisera to the 41-amino acid peptide, it became clear that removal of glucocorticoid negative feedback (by adrenalectomy) led to a dramatic increase in CRH levels in the PVHmpd after 3 – 7 days (Bugnon et al., 1983; Merchenthaler et al., 1983; Paull and Gibbs, 1983; Swanson et al., 1983; Tramu et al., 1983).

This evidence clearly demonstrated that adrenalectomy profoundly alters CRH levels in the PVHmpd, and subsequent work indicates that the change is due in part at least to a depressive effect of glucocorticoids on CRH peptide and mRNA levels in neurons of the PVHmpd (Agnati et al., 1985; Young et al., 1986; Cintra et al., 1987; Kóvacs and Mezey, 1987; Sawchenko, 1987a; Swanson and Simmons, 1989). That physiologically relevant levels of circulating glucocorticoids may alter CRH mRNA levels in the PVHmpd has recently been demonstrated with in situ hybridization methods. By perfusing normal, unstressed rats at different times of the day-night cycle, clear declines in CRH mRNA levels were shown to follow the characteristic diurnal surge of corticosterone (Fig. 5; Watts and Swanson, 1989).

Of greater interest was the finding that adrenalectomy also leads to a massive increase in vasopressin (Tramu et al., 1983; Kiss et al., 1984a; Sawchenko et al., 1984a) and angiotensin (Lind et al., 1985a,b) levels in CRH cells of the PVHmpd.

The response of vasopressin has been examined most carefully, and the evidence suggests that a direct depressive effect of corticosterone on vasopressin mRNA levels is also involved (see Wolfson et al., 1985, and references just cited for CRH); in sharp contrast, however, corticosterone does not appear to influence angiotensin mRNA levels in the PVHmpd (Swanson and Simmons, 1989).

Although low levels of vasopressin (Vandesande et al., 1977) and angiotensin (see Lind et al., 1985a,b) can be detected in terminals of the neurohemal zone of the median eminence in normal animals, the peptides are below the level of detectability in cell bodies of PVHmpd neurons, even following colchicine treatment, unless animals are adrenalectomized. This is in sharp contrast to CRH levels in the same neurons, and in view of the immunohistochemical and in situ evidence cited above, indicates strongly that the vasopressin gene in PVHmpd neurons is much more sensitive to the depressive effects of glucocorticoids than the CRH gene. The possible functional significance of this observation will be considered below.

Multiple immunohistochemical staining methods have been used to show that CRH neurons in the PVHmpd may also contain enkephalin (Hökfelt et al., 1983), neurotensin (Sawchenko et al., 1984b), and cholecystokinin (Kiss et al., 1984b). The evidence to date suggests that cholecystokinin immunoreactivity in the PVHmpd increases following adrenalectomy (Mezey et al., 1986; but see Swanson and Simmons, 1989), whereas levels of enkephalin and neurotensin do not change significantly (see Sawchenko, 1987b). Taken as a whole, this evidence is of interest because CRH, vasopressin, angiotensin, and cholecystokinin all appear to act at the level of the anterior pituitary corticotrope to release ACTH, whereas neurotensin and enkephalin do not share this activity. Thus, glucocorticoids appear to regulate negatively a set of neuropeptides in PVHmpd neurons that in turn regulate ACTH secretion, but do not influence other neuropeptides in the same cells that do not influence directly ACTH secretion.

Differential regulation of neuropeptide genes across cell types in the PVH: Steroid hormones

As mentioned above, several neuropeptides are expressed in all three major compartments of the PVH. It has been of interest, therefore, to determine whether the effects of adrenal steroids on neuropeptides in CRH neurons of the PVHmpd are the same or different in other parts of the PVH. The major conclusions of this work (see Swanson and Simmons, 1989) are the following: 1) While corticosterone depresses CRH mRNA levels in PVHmpd neurons, it increases CRH mRNA levels in magnocellular (oxytocinergic) neurosecretory neurons, and in neurons with descending projections. 2) Whereas corticosterone exerts a profound inhibitory influence on vasopressin mRNA levels in the PVHmpd, it has no measurable influence on these mRNA levels in magnocellular neurosecretory neurons, or in PVH neurons with descending projections.

As summarized in Table II, this evidence suggests that in the PVH corticosterone can have op-

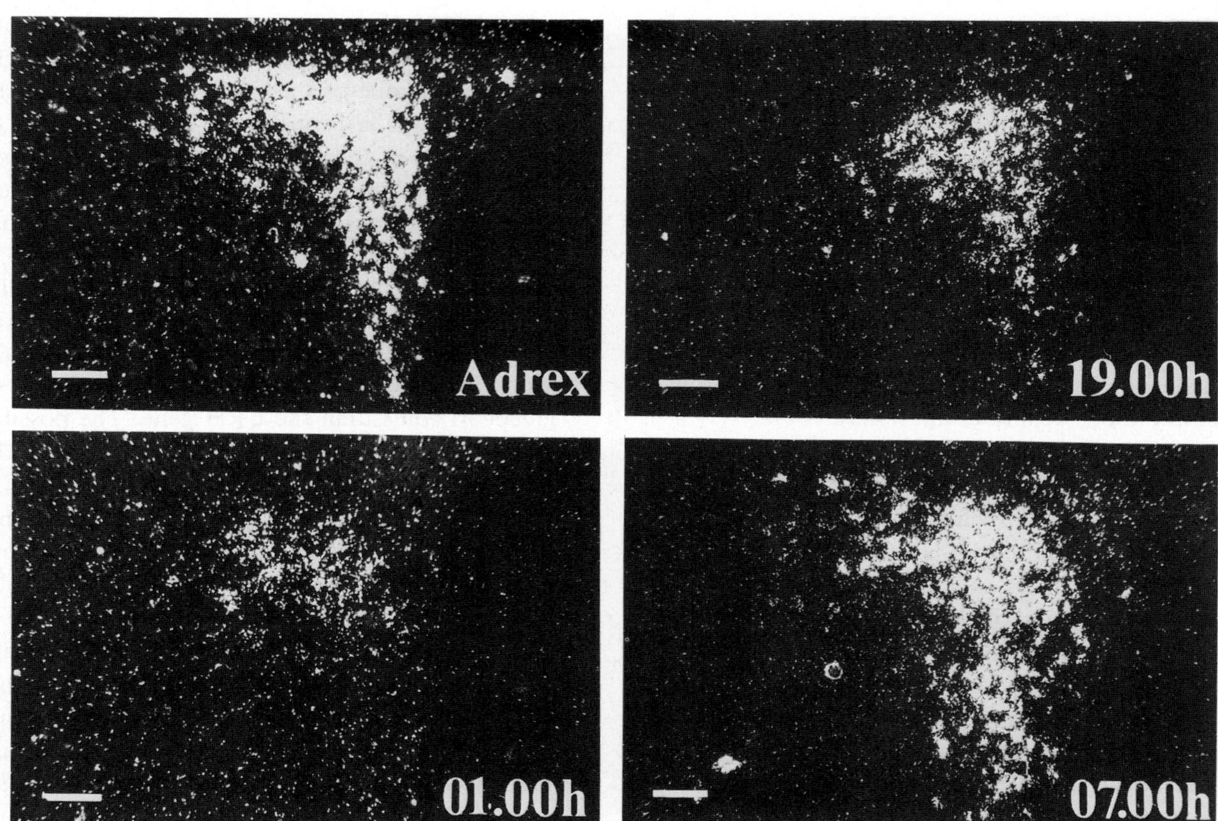

Fig. 5. Darkfield photomicrographs showing *in situ* hybridization for CRH mRNA in the PVH (left side of the brain) of female rats perfused at different times of the day-night cycle, as compared to an adrenalectomized (Adrex) animal. Scale bars = 100 μm. (From Watts and Swanson, 1989).

TABLE II

Effects of corticosterone on neuropeptide mRNA levels in different neuron cell types of the rat PVH

	Parvicellular Neuroendocrine	Magnocellular Neuroendocrine	Mediocellular Descending
CRH	↓	↑	↑
VAS	↓	–	–

posite effects on CRH mRNA levels in different cell types, and that the hormone can have the same effect on a pair of neuropeptide genes in one cell type (depression of CRH and vasopressin mRNA in the PVHmpd), and different effects on the same pair in different cell types. The most obvious explanation for these findings is that the expression of particular neuropeptide genes in the PVH is regulated by combinations of multiple transcription factors, since all three major cell types appear to express the glucocorticoid (and mineralocorticoid) receptor (Swanson and Simmons, 1989). The identity of other relevant transcription factors remains to be determined, although they may include certain proto-oncogenes (Sagar et al., 1988) and members of the POU-domain family (He et al., 1989).

Other steroid hormones may also influence neuropeptide levels in the PVH, although this problem remains to be examined in detail. However, it does seem likely that aldosterone and testosterone (Baldino and Davis, 1986; Sawchenko, 1987a,c) do not influence CRH and vasopressin levels in the PVH. On the other hand, immunohistochemical studies indicate that, in magnocellular neurons, estrogen increases levels of angiotensin, galanin, and dynorphin (but not vasopressin) in vasopressinergic cells, and increases levels of oxytocin but decreases levels of CRH and cholecystokinin in oxytocinergic cells (Sawchenko and Levin, 1989). It is not clear whether these are direct effects of estrogen on magnocellular neurosecretory neurons, since they do not appear to express the estrogen receptor (see Simerly et al., 1990), although estrogen does appear to increase oxytocin mRNA levels in this cell type (Miller et al., 1989), perhaps by an indirect (neural) mechanism.

Differential regulation of neuropeptide levels in the PVHmpd: Neural influences

It is thus clear that steroid hormones can alter dramatically the ratio of neuropeptides in particular cell types in the PVH. There is also evidence to suggest that substances released from neural inputs to the PVH may also change neuropeptide levels in the nucleus. Mezey et al. (1984) first reported that systemic injections of a phenylethanolamine N-methyl transferase (PNMT) inhibitor, which among other things decreased epinephrine levels in the PVH, led to an increase in CRH levels in the PVHmpd. However, it has since been shown that chemical (Alonso et al., 1986) or surgical (Sawchenko, 1988) interruption of ascending brainstem catecholamine inputs to the PVH (see Fig. 4) leads to a decrease in PVHmpd CRH levels, as well as an increase in neurotensin levels in the same cell group (Kawakami et al., 1984). Interestingly, experiments using in situ hybridization indicate that such brainstem lesions do not change levels of mRNA for CRH, vasopressin, angiotensin, cholecystokinin, or enkephalin, or for the glucocorticoid or mineralocorticoid receptor (Swanson and Simmons, 1989).

The results of these experiments indicate that both hormonal and neural inputs can change the ratios of neuropeptides in specific PVH cell types, although the mechanisms underlying these changes may be quite different (Sawchenko, 1988; Swanson and Simmons, 1989).

Functional implications

The evidence reviewed here suggests that the PVH is a particularly useful model for beginning to understand the structure and chemistry of hypothalamic circuitry that coordinates endocrine, autonomic, and behavioral responses to a wide variety of stressors. General principles governing the PVH regulation of neuroendocrine and autonomic responses are clear: the nucleus contains several classes of neuroendocrine motoneurons, as well as a separate pool of neurons that projects directly to autonomic and reticular centers in the brainstem and spinal cord. The role of the PVH in behavior is less clear, although it now seems likely that ascending catecholamine/peptidergic inputs from the medulla stimulate ingestive behaviors that require a certain minimal level of glucocorticoids to be effective, along with an intact descending projection to the reticular core (see Weiss and Leibowitz, 1985; Roland et al., 1986).

The parvicellular neurosecretory CRH neuron in the PVHmpd has also emerged as an intriguing model of a multifunctional neuronal cell type with a motor output that may depend on the functional status of the animal as well as on the pattern of action potentials travelling down its axon. As illustrated schematically in Fig. 6, the morphology of these neurons is rather simple. The cell body is typically bipolar and gives rise to two dendrites, each of which branches once or twice, has a sparse complement of spines, and tends to be aligned parallel to the dendrites of similar neurons (Rho and Swanson, 1989). It is well established that the axon of these cells arches laterally around the fornix before ending in the neurohemal zone of the median eminence, but it is also clear that it may give rise to terminal boutons, particularly in the region just lateral to the PVH itself (Rho and Swanson, 1987). It is likely therefore that the axons of these cells establish intrahypothalamic synapses as well as releasing substances from terminals in the median eminence.

There is no doubt that substances released at the level of the median eminence enter the hypophyseal portal system and exert endocrine influences on the secretion of hormones from the anterior pituitary (see Plotsky and Sawchenko, 1987). It also seems likely, however, that substances released into the extracellular fluid of the median eminence exert paracrine influences on other types of nerve terminals within the median eminence. Perhaps the best example of this in the present context is the reported action of CRH to inhibit the secretion of GnRH at the level of the median eminence (Gambacciani et al., 1986).

The evidence suggests, therefore, that the axon of a parvicellular neuroendocrine CRH neuron

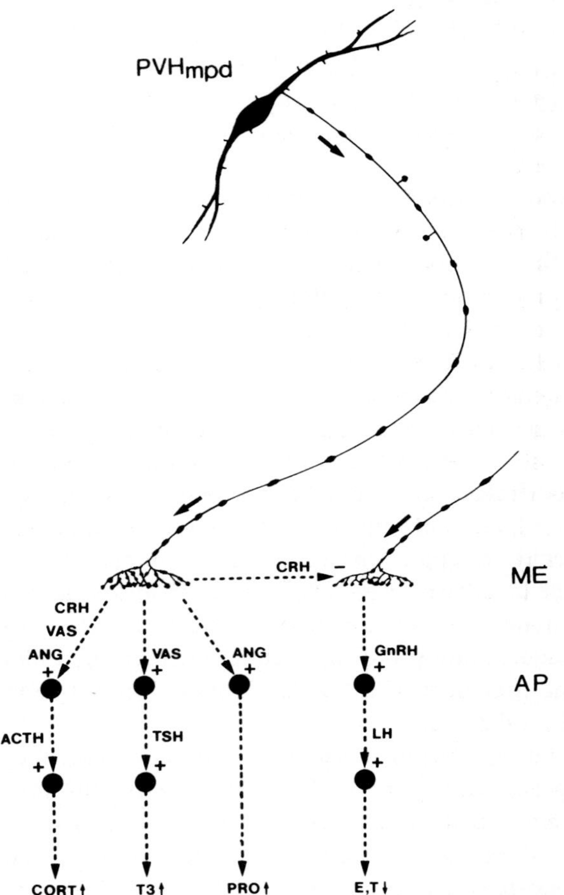

Fig. 6. An idealized CRH neuron in the PVHmpd. As discussed in the text, such neurons appear to be in a position to exert intrahypothalamic synaptic influences from axonal terminal boutons, paracrine influences at the level of the median eminence (ME), and endocrine influences at the level of the anterior pituitary (AP). It is important to point out that at this time it seems reasonable to assume that all of the neuroactive substances expressed in such a neuron are released from all of its axon terminals (see Eccles, 1986). *Abbreviations*: ACTH, adrenocorticotropic hormone; ANG, angiotensin; CORT, corticosterone; E, estrogen; GnRH, gonadotropin releasing hormone; LH, luteinizing hormone; PRO, prolactin; T, testosterone; TSH, thyroid stimulating hormone; T3, triiodothyronine; VAS, vasopressin.

may exert synaptic influences within the hypothalamus, paracrine effects at the level of the median eminence (e.g., to help lower gonadal steroid levels during stress in the rat), and endocrine effects at the level of the anterior pituitary. The functional significance of this arrangement comes into sharper focus when the multitude of neuroactive substances elaborated by this cell type is taken into account, and when the fact that the ratios of these substances can vary markedly is considered.

As indicated in Fig. 6, one consequence of multiple peptide release in the median eminence is that these substances could influence the release of hormones from several different cell types in the anterior pituitary. Thus, CRH and vasopressin (as well as angiotensin and cholecystokinin) act synergistically to release ACTH (and β-endorphin) from corticotropes (see Lind et al., 1985b; Mezey et al., 1986; Plotsky and Sawchenko, 1987); vasopressin stimulates TSH release (Lumpkin et al., 1987), and angiotensin stimulates prolactin release (Schramme and Denef, 1984). Parvicellular CRH neurons may also indirectly increase the secretion of prolactin by way of a paracrine effect of enkephalin at the level of the median eminence. Enkephalin may act at this level to decrease the release of dopamine (which inhibits prolactin secretion) from terminals arising in the arcuate nucleus (see Deyo et al., 1979).

The fact that adrenal steroids and neural inputs may change the ratio of neuroactive substances released by PVHmpd CRH neurons adds a layer of complexity to the scheme illustrated in Fig. 6, and suggests that the same pattern of electrical activity in their axons may produce different motor effects at different times, a form of biochemical switching in what may be assumed for the sake of the present argument to be an anatomically fixed component of a neural circuit (Swanson, 1983). The functional implications predicted by this hypothesis are illustrated in Fig. 7. Under chronically low circulating levels of corticosterone, the CRH and vasopressin genes are released from steroid inhibition, and large quantities of the two hormones are

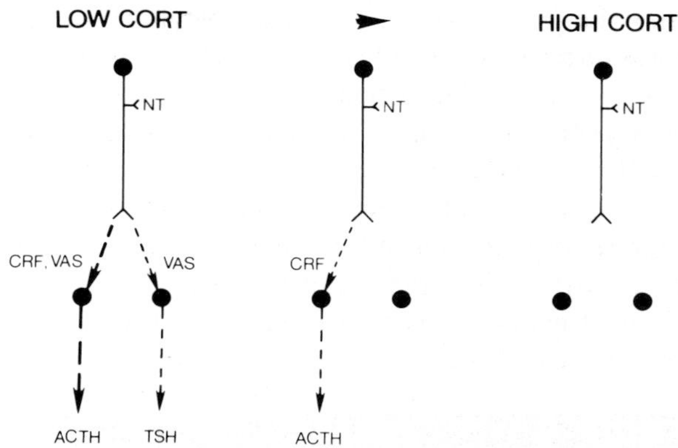

Fig. 7. Different chronic levels of circulating corticosterone (CORT) appear to change the ratio of corticotropin releasing hormone (CRF) and vasopressin (VAS), but not neurotensin (NT), released from the axon terminals of neurons in the PVHmpd (upper row of dots). This drawing illustrates the possible functional significance of these altered neuropeptide ratios on the secretion of hormones from cells in the anterior pituitary (lower row of dots). This model presumes that CRF, VAS, and NT are released from all terminals of the axon, but that different postsynaptic cell types have different complements of receptors for these three neuropeptides. *Abbreviations*: ACTH, adrenocorticotropic hormone; TSH, thyroid stimulating hormone.

synthesized and reach the anterior pituitary, where maximal secretion of ACTH is effected, and vasopressin stimulates TSH secretion as well. If circulating steroid levels remain at low-to-moderate levels, vasopressin mRNA levels are severely depressed, and CRH mRNA levels remain high; thus, ACTH will still be secreted, but little vasopressin from CRH cells will be available for TSH secretion. Finally, chronically elevated corticosterone levels drastically reduce CRH and vasopressin levels in PVHmpd neurons, thus resulting in little ACTH or TSH secretion by PVHmpd neurons. In summary, the endocrine status of the animal may determine the mixture of anterior pituitary hormones secreted in response to the same neural stimuli applied to PVHmpd CRH neurons.

In contrast, since neurotensin levels in these neurons do not appear to be influenced by corticosterone, responses elicited by this neuropeptide may not be influenced by the endocrine status of the animal. One possible role of neurotensin in this neuron may be as a neurotransmitter at the intrahypothalamic synapses formed by the axons of PVHmpd CRH neurons just outside the lateral border of the PVH. This is suggested by the large number of neurotensin binding sites in this region (see Moyse et al., 1988, and Fig. 8).

One final point about the multiple expression of neuroactive substances is worth emphasizing. In the discussion thus far we have referred to the typical PVHmpd CRH neuron, and the influence of various factors on the neuropeptide content of such a neuron. It is obvious, however, that we are dealing with a population of cells, and the question naturally arises as to how this population is defined; and even more specifically, how uniform are the characteristics of this cell type? This is a general problem in neuroanatomy, but is particularly vexing in this instance for two reasons. First, the neurotransmitter content of these neurons is quite different under different physiological conditions; and second, as described elsewhere (e.g., Lind et al. 1984; Sawchenko et al., 1984b; Swanson et al., 1987), different cells within this population clearly display different ratios of neuropeptides. Therefore, the population of cells does not contain a uniform ratio of neuroactive substances at a particular time, and these ratios in individual cells may respond quite differently to a particular physiological challenge.

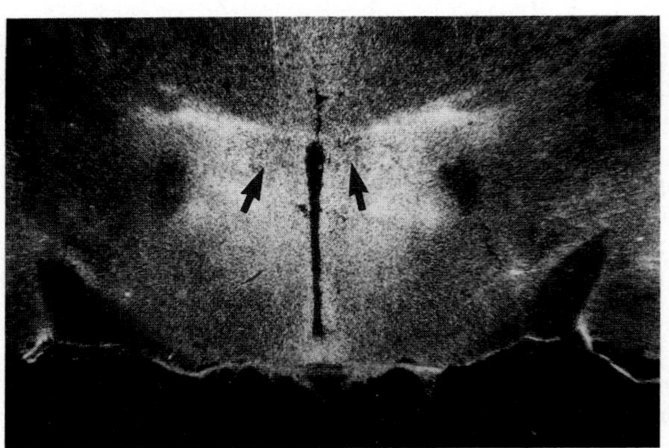

Fig. 8. This darkfield photomicrograph shows the distribution of ^{125}I-neurotensin binding to a frontal section through the level of the PVH (arrows) in the rat. X 15. (Kindly provided by Dr. A. Beaudet).

These points are well illustrated in the data presented in Tables III and IV (R.W. Lind and L.W. Swanson, previously unpublished observations). To maximize CRH, vasopressin, and angiotensin immunostaining, 5 adult rats were

TABLE III

Extent of CRH, vasopressin, and angiotensin immunocolocalization in neurons of the dorsal medial parvicellular part of the rat paraventricular nucleus (N = 5)

	$\bar{X}$ (± SEM)	% Total	Range
Total cells	2831 (± 340)	(100%)	2202 – 4097
Triply labeled	695 (± 124)	25 (± 4)%	489 – 1118
CRF/VAS labeled	154 (± 86)	5 (± 3)%	16 – 495
CRF/ANG labeled	194 (± 49)	7 (± 2)%	66 – 354
VAS/ANG labeled	242 (± 93)	8 (± 3)%	51 – 597
CRF only labeling	820 (± 149)	29 (± 5)%	633 – 1414
ANG only labeling	455 (± 49)	16 (± 2%)	311 – 576
VAS only labeling	271 (± 76)	10 (± 3)%	109 – 522

4 week ADX, 24 h colchicine; 1-in-5 series, 15 μm sections; nuclei counted, corrected (Abercrombie); VAS mAb + ANG polyclonal-elute-CRF polyclonal.

TABLE IV

Relative density (% absorbance) of immunohistochemical staining in 13 different, triply-labeled PVHmpd neurons after adrenalectomy and colchicine treatment

Cell no.	*CRF*	*VAS*	*AII*
1.	30	67	33
2.	32	63	32
3.	45	65	50
4.	54	88	49
5.	31	69	65
6.	31	52	59
7.	36	48	57
8.	71	76	54
9.	68	42	59
10.	78	61	50
11.	43	39	38
12.	58	54	44
13.	60	58	46
Range	16-100	29-99	29-100

adrenalectomized and 4 weeks later an injection of colchicine was made into the lateral ventricle; 24 h later they were perfused, and a 1-in-5 series of 15 μm thick frontal sections through the PVH was stained simultaneously with a monoclonal antibody to vasopressin and a polyclonal antibody to angiotensin, photographed, the antibodies eluted, and the sections restained with an antiserum to CRH and rephotographed (for methods see Sawchenko et al., 1984a and Lind et al., 1985b; for representative photomicrographs of this material see Fig. 8 in Swanson et al., 1986). All CRH, vasopressin, and angiotensin immunostained neurons with a clear nucleus in the PVHmpd were counted and the results are presented in Table III. On the average, the PVHmpd contained about 2,800 immunostained neurons, only 25% of which were triply-labeled. The remaining cells contained combinations of any two peptides, or any of the three peptides alone. It is possible, of course, that all cells contain at least a small amount of each peptide, often below the level of detectability of the immunohistochemical method employed in this study. Nevertheless, this evidence clearly indicates that different neurons in the PVHmpd contain vastly different ratios of the peptides. It is also worth mentioning that we could detect no obvious, reproducible pattern in the location of triply, doubly, or singly labeled neurons in the PVHmpd.

More direct evidence for different ratios of the 3 peptides in individual neurons of the PVHmpd was obtained by carrying out densitometric measurements of immunohistochemical staining intensity in photomicrographs of the material just described (for method see Swanson and Simmons, 1989). As shown in Table IV, the staining intensity for each of the 3 peptides varied widely in the population of 13 neurons sampled, suggesting that each neuron contained a different ratio of neuropeptides. For a variety of technical reasons (e.g., section thickness and associated problems with antibody penetration), it is not valid to compare directly staining intensities for a particular antibody between cells. However, comparisons of different antibody staining intensities within an individual cell do appear to be valid because the peptides are (at this level of analysis) distributed uniformly throughout the cytoplasm.

Taken together, the evidence thus suggests that while the ratios of neuropeptides in particular PVHmpd neurons may vary widely, definite trends and shifts in these ratios are evident in the population of cells as a whole, under normal and experimental conditions.

Conclusion

Clear alterations in the ratios of multiple neuroactive substances due to hormonal and/or neural influences have been established in the sympathetic system and in the PVH. And while the functional significance of these particular changes remain to be established with certainty, it is tempting to suggest that the underlying phenomenon represents the substrate for biochemical switching of information flow in what could be anatomically fixed

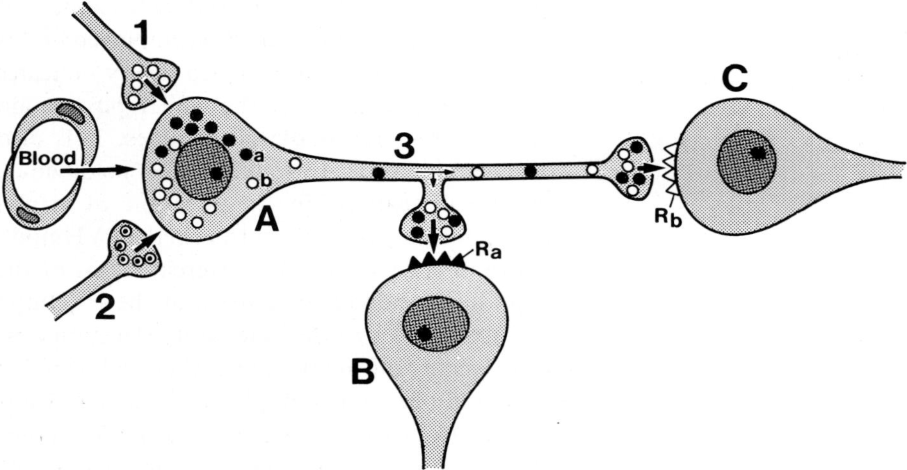

Fig. 9. Biochemical switching in a neuroanatomically fixed circuit may be implemented by changes in the ratio of neuropeptides a and b within a particular neuron (A), if the neuron innervates two different cell types (B, C), each of which expresses receptors (Ra, Rb) for one neuropeptide or the other. The a/b ratio may be altered by substances released from neural inputs 1 and 2, or by steroid hormones entering from nearby capillaries. (From Swanson, 1983).

circuitry, and that it could represent a strategy used in many other parts of the brain.

The biochemical switching hypothesis generates a number of hypotheses, some of which are evident in Fig. 9. First, the ability of a neuron to synthesize and release multiple neuroactive substances (all of which are probably released at each axon terminal) implies that the neuron could innervate multiple cell types defined by their complement of postsynaptic receptors. Thus, a cell innervated by one axon collateral may express receptors for only one neuroactive substance, while a different collateral may synapse with a cell expressing receptors for a different neuroactive substance. Second, significantly altered ratios of neuroactive substances may bias the efficacy of synaptic transmission through the synapses associated with the different collaterals just mentioned. Third, if neuropeptides are involved, the functional consequences of altered ratios must have a relatively long time-course, since the peptides must be synthesized in the cell body, and transported down the axon to its various terminal fields. Fourth, the time-course of these effects will vary at different terminals of an axon in proportion to the distance of the terminal from the cell body (due to axonal transport time of neuropeptides). And fifth, changes in the ratios of multiple neuroactive substances within individual neurons may be effected by neural and/or hormonal signals.

References

Agnati, L.F., Fuxe, K., Yu, Z.-Y., Härfstrand, A., Okret, S., Wikström, A.-C., Goldstein, M., Zoli, M., Vale, W. and Gustafsson, J.-Å. (1985) Morphometrical analysis of the distribution of corticotrophin releasing factor, glucocorticoid receptor and phenylethanolamine-*N*-methyltransferaseimmunoreactive structures in the paraventricular hypothalamic nucleus of the rat. *Neurosci. Lett.,* 54: 147–154.

Alonso, G., Szafarczyk, A. and Assenmacher, I. (1986) Immunoreactivity of hypothalamoneurohypophysial neurons with secrete corticotropin-releasing hormone (CRH) and vasopressin (Vp): Immunocytochemical evidence for a correlation with their functional state in colchicine-treated rats. *Exp. Brain Res.,* 61: 497–505.

Baldino Jr., F. and Davis, L.G. (1986) Glucocorticoid regulation of vasopressin messenger RNA. In *In Situ Hybridization in Brain, G.R. Uhl (Ed.), Plenum Press, New York, pp. 97–116.*

Black, I.B., Adler, J.E., Dreyfus, C.F., Friedman, W.F., LaGamma, E.F. and Roach, A.H. (1987) Biochemistry of information storage in the nervous system. *Science,* 236: 1263 – 1268.

Bugnon, C., Fellman, D. and Gouget, A. (1983) Changes in corticoliberin and vasopressin-like immunoreactivities in the zona externa of the median eminence in adrenalectomized rats. Immunocytochemical study. *Neurosci. Lett.,* 37: 43 – 49.

Burnstock, G. (1976) Do some nerve cells release more than one transmitter? *Neurosci.,* 1: 239 – 248.

Ceccatelli, S., Eriksson, M. and Hökfelt, T. (1989) Distribution and coexistence of corticotropin-releasing factor-, neurotensin-, enkephalin-, cholecystokinin-, galanin- and vasoactive intestinal polypeptide/peptide histidine isoleucine-like peptides in the parvocellular part of the paraventricular nucleus. *Neuroendocrinol.,* 49: 309 – 323.

Chan-Palay, V., Jonsson, G. and Palay, S.L. (1978) Serotonin and substance P coexist in neurons of the rat's central nervous system. *Proc. Natl. Acad. Sci., U.S.A.,* 75: 1582 – 1586.

Cintra, A., Fuxe, K., Härfstrand, A., Agnati, L.F., Wikström, A.-C., Okret, S., Vale, W. and Gustafsson, J.-Å. (1987) Presence of glucocorticoid receptor immunoreactivity in corticotropin releasing factor and in growth hormone releasing factor immunoreactive neurons of the rat di- and telencephalon. *Neurosci. Lett.,* 77: 25 – 30.

Clark, W.E.L. (1938) Morphological aspects of the hypothalamus. In: W.E.L. Clark, J. Beattie, G. Riddoch and N.M. Dott (Eds.), *The Hypothalamus. Morphological, Functional, Clinical and Surgical Aspects.* Oliver and Boyd, Edinburgh, pp. 2 – 68.

Cunningham Jr., E.T. and Sawchenko, P.E. (1988) Anatomical specificity of noradrenergic inputs to the paraventricular and supraoptic nuclei of the rat hypothalamus. *J. Comp. Neurol.,* 274: 60 – 76.

Cunningham Jr., E.T. and Sawchenko, P.E. (1990) Anatomical organization of adrenergic inputs to the paraventricular and supraoptic nuclei of the rat hypothalamus. *J. Comp. Neurol.,* (in press).

Deyo, S.N., Swift, R.M. and Miller, R.J. (1979) Morphine and endorphins modulate dopamine turnover in rat median eminence. *Proc. Natl. Acad. Sci., U.S.A.,* 76: 3006 – 3009.

Eccles J.C. (1986) Chemical transmission and Dale's principle. *Prog. Brain Res.,* 68, 3 – 13.

Gambacciani, M., Yen, S.S.C. and Rasmussen, D.D. (1986) GnRH release from the mediobasal hypothalamus: in vitro inhibition by corticotropin-releasing factor. *Neuroendocrinol.,* 43: 533 – 536.

Gerfen, C.R. and Sawchenko, P.E. (1984) An anterograde neuroanatomical tracing method that shows the detailed morphology of neurons, their axons and terminals: Immunohistochemical localization of an axonally transported plant lectin, *Phaseolus vulgaris* leucoagglutinin (PHA-L). *Brain Res.,* 290: 219 – 238.

He, X., Treacy, M.N., Simmons, D.M. Ingraham, H.A., Swanson, L.W. and Rosenfeld, M.G. (1989) Expression of a large family of POU-domain regulatory genes in mammalian brain development. *Nature,* 340: 35 – 42.

Hökfelt, T., Fahrenkrug, J., Tatemoto, K., Mutt, V., Werner, S., Hulting, A.-L., Terenius, L. and Chang, K.J. (1983) The PHI (PHI-27)/corticotropin-releasing factor/enkephalin immunoreactive hypothalamic neuron: Possible morphological basis for integrated control of prolactin, corticotropin, and growth hormone secretion. *Proc. Natl. Acad. Sci., U.S.A.* 80: 895 – 898.

Hökfelt, T., Holets, V.R., Staines, W., Meister, J., Melander, T., Schalling, M., Schultzberg, M., Freedman, J., Björklund, H., Olson, L., Lindh, B., Elfvin, L.-G., Lundberg, J.M., Lindgren, J.Å., Samuelsson, B., Pernow, B., Terenius, L., Post, C., Everitt, B. and Goldstein, M. (1986) Coexistence of neuronal messengers – an overview. *Prog. Brain Res.,* 68: 33 – 70.

Hökfelt, T., Ljungdahl, A., Steinbusch, H., Verhofstad, A., Nilsson, G., Brodin, E., Pernow, B., and Goldstein, M. (1978) Immunohistochemical evidence of substance P-like immunoreactivity in some 5-hydroxytryptamine-containing neurons in the rat central nervous system. *Neurosci.,* 3: 517 – 538.

Kawakami, K., Fukiu, K., Oomura, H., Nakajima, T., Yanaihara, T. and Ibata, Y. (1984) Influence of ascending noradrenergic fibers on the neurotensin-like immunoreactive neurons in the rat paraventricular nucleus. *Neurosci. Lett.,* 44: 149 – 154.

Kawano, H. and Daikoku, S. (1987) Functional topography of the rat hypothalamic dopamine neurons systems: Retrograde tracing and immunohistochemical study. *J. Comp. Neurol.,* 265: 242 – 253.

Kessler, J.A. and Black, I.B. (1982) Regulation of substance P in adult rat sympathetic ganglia. *Brain Res.,* 234: 182 – 187.

Kiss, J.Z., Mezey, É. and Skirboll, L. (1984a) Corticotropin-releasing factor-immunoreactive neurons of the paraventricular nucleus become vasopressin-positive after adrenalectomy. *Proc. Natl. Acad. Sci., U.S.A.,* 81: 1854 – 1858.

Kiss, J.Z., Williams, T.H. and Palkovits, M. (1984b) Distribution and projections of cholecystokinin-immunoreactive neurons in the hypothalamic paraventricular nucleus of rat. *J. Comp. Neurol.,* 227: 173 – 181.

Kóvacs, K.J. and Mezey, É. (1987) Dexamethasone inhibits corticotropin-releasing factor gene expression in the rat paraventricular nucleus. *Neuroendocrinol.,* 46: 365 – 368.

Landis, S.C. (1988) Neurotransmitter plasticity in sympathetic neurons and its regulation by environmental factors *in vitro* and *in vivo*. In: A. Björklund, T. Hökfelt, and C. Owman (Eds.), *Handbook of Chemical Neuroanatomy, Vol. 6: The Peripheral Nervous System.* Elsevier, Amsterdam, pp. 65 – 116.

Levin, M.C., Sawchenko, P.E., Howe, P.R.C., Polak, J. and Bloom, S.R. (1987) The organization of galanin-immunoreactive inputs to the paraventricular nucleus with special reference to their relationship to catecholaminergic afferents. *J. Comp. Neurol.,* 261: 562 – 583.

Lind, R.W., Swanson, L.W. and Sawchenko, P.E. (1985a) Anatomical evidence that neural circuits related to the subfornical organ contain angiotensin II. *Brain Res. Bull.,* 15: 79 – 82.

Lind, R.W., Swanson, L.W., Bruhn, T.O. and Ganten, D. (1985b) The distribution of angiotensin II-immunoreactive cells and fibers in the paraventriculo-hypophysial system of the rat. *Brain Res.,* 338: 81 – 89.

Lind, R.W., Swanson, L.W., Chin, D.A., Bruhn, T.O. and Ganten, D. (1984) Angiotensin II: An immunohistochemical study of its distribution in the paraventriculo-hypophysial system and its co-localization with vasopressin and CRF in parvocellular neurons. *Soc. Neurosci. Abstr.,* 10: 88.

Lumpkin, M.D., Samson, W.K. and McCann, S.M. (1987) Arginine vasopressin as a thyrotropin-releasing hormone. *Science,* 235: 1070 – 1073.

Meister, B., Hökfelt, T., Geffard, M. and Oertel, W. (1988) Glutamic acid decarboxylase- and γ-aminobutyric acid-like immunoreactivities in corticotropin-releasing factor-containing parvocellular neurons of the hypothalamic paraventricular nucleus. *Neuroendocrinol.,* 48: 516 – 526.

Merchenthaler, I., Vigh, S., Petrusz, P. and Schally, A.V. (1983) The paraventriculo-infundibular corticotropin releasing factor (CRF) pathway as revealed by immunocytochemistry in long-term hypophysectomized or adrenalectomized rats. *Regul. Pept.,* 5: 295 – 305.

Mezey, É., Kiss, J.Z., Skirboll, L.R., Goldstein, M. and Axelrod, J. (1984) Increase of corticotropin-releasing factor staining in rat paraventricular nucleus neurones by depletion of hypothalamic adrenaline. *Science,* 310: 140 – 141.

Mezey, É., Reisine, T.D., Skirboll, L., Beinfeld, M. and Kiss, J.Z. (1986) Role of cholecystokinin in corticotropin release: Coexistence with vasopressin and corticotropin-releasing factor in cells of the rat hypothalamic paraventricular nucleus. *Proc. Natl. Acad. Sci., U.S.A.,* 83: 3510 – 3512.

Miller, F.D., Oximek, G., Milner, R.J. and Bloom, F.E. (1989) Regulation of neuronal oxytocin mRNA by ovarian steroids in the mature and developing hypothalamus. *Proc. Natl. Acad. Sci., U.S.A.,* 86: 2468 – 2472.

Moyse, E., Miller, M.M., Rostène, W. and Beaudet, A. (1988) Effects of ovariectomy and estradeiol replacement on the binding of ^{125}I-neurotensin in rat suprachiasmatic nucleus. *Neuroendocrinol.,* 48: 53 – 60.

Patterson, P.H. (1978) Environmental determination of autonomic neurotransmitter functions. *Ann. Rev. Neurosci.,* 1: 1 – 17.

Paull, W.K. and Gibbs, F.P. (1983) The corticoptrin releasing factor (CRF) neurosecretory system in intact, adrenalectomized, and adrenalectomized-dexamethasone treated rats. *Histochem.,* 78: 303 – 316.

Plotsky, P.M. and Sawchenko, P.E. (1987) Hypophysial-portal plasma levels, median eminence content, and immunohistochemical staining of corticotropin-releasing factor, arginine vasopressin, and oxytocine after pharmacological adrenalectomy. *Endocrinol.,* 120: 1361 – 1369.

Rho, J.-H. and Swanson, L.W. (1987) Neuroendocrine CRF motoneurons: Intrahypothalamic axon terminals shown with a new retrograde-lucifer-immuno method. *Brain Res.,* 436: 143 – 147.

Rho, J.-H. and Swanson, L.W. (1989) A morphometric analysis of functionally defined subpopulations of neurons in the paraventricular nucleus of the rat with observations on the effects of colchicine. *J. Neurosci.,* 9: 1375 – 1388.

Roland, C.R., Bhakthavatsalam, P. and Leibowitz, S.F. (1986) Interaction between corticosterone and α2-noradrenergic system of the paraventricular nucleus in relation to feeding behavior. *Neuroendocrinol.,* 42: 296 – 305.

Sagar, S.M., Sharp, F.R. and Curran, T. (1988) Expression of c-fos protein in brain: Metabolic mapping at the cellular level. *Science,* 240: 1328 – 1331.

Saper, C.B., Loewy, A.D., Swanson, L.W. and Cowan, W.M. (1976) Direct hypothalamo-autonomic connections. *Brain Res.,* 117: 305 – 312.

Sawchenko, P.E. (1987a) Evidence for a local site of action for glucocorticoids in inhibiting CRF and vasopressin expression in the paraventricular nucleus. *Brain Res.,* 403: 213 – 224.

Sawchenko, P.E. (1987b) Evidence for differential regulation of corticotropin-releasing factor and vasopressin immunoreactivities in parvocellular neurosecretory and autonomic-related projections of the paraventricular nucleus. *Brain Res.,* 437: 253 – 263.

Sawchenko, P.E. (1987c) Adrenalectomy-induced enhancement of CRF and vasopressin immunoreactivity in parvocellular neurosecretory neurons: Autonomic, peptide, and steroid specificity. *J. Neurosci.,* 7: 1093 – 1106.

Sawchenko, P.E. (1988) The effects of catecholamine-depleting medullary knife cuts on CRF-and vasopressin-immunoreactivity in the hypothalamus of normal and steroid-manipulated rats. *Neuroendocrinol.,* 48: 459 – 470.

Sawchenko, P.E., Benoit, R. and Brown, M.R. (1988a) Somatostatin 28-immunoreactive inputs to the paraventricular and supraoptic nuclei: Principal origin from non-aminergic neurons in the nucleus of the solitary tract. *J. Chem. Neuroanat.,* 1: 81 – 94.

Sawchenko, P.E., Plotsky, P.M., Pfeiffer, S.W., Cunningham Jr., E.T., Vaughan, J., Rivier, J. and Vale, W. (1988b) Inhibin β in central neural pathways involved in the control of oxytocin secretion. *Nature,* 334: 615 – 617.

Sawchenko, P.E. and Levin, M.C. (1989) Neuropeptide co-expressin in the magnocellular neurosecretory system of the female rat: Evidence for differential modulation by estrogen. *J. Comp. Neurol.,* (in press).

Sawchenko, P.E. and Swanson, L.W. (1982) The organization of noradrenergic pathways from the brainstem to the paraventricular and supraoptic nuclei in the rat. *Brain Res. Rev.,* 4: 275 – 325.

Sawchenko, P.E. and Swanson, L.W. (1983) The organization of forebrain afferents to the paraventricular and supraoptic nuclei of the rat. *J. Comp. Neurol.*, 218: 121 – 144.

Sawchenko, P.E., Swanson, L.W., Rivier, J. and Vale, W.W. (1985a) The distribution of growth hormone-releasing factor (GRF) immunoreactivity in the central nervous system of the rat: An immunohistochemical study using antisera directed against rat hypothalamic GRF. *J. Comp. Neurol.*, 237: 100 – 115.

Sawchenko, P.E., Swanson, L.W., Grzanna, R., Howe, P.R.C., Polak, J.M. and Bloom, S.R. (1985b) Colocalization of neuropeptide Y-immunoreactivity in brainstem catecholaminergic neurons that project to the paraventricular nucleus of the hypothalamus. *J. Comp. Neurol.*, 241: 138 – 153.

Sawchenko, P.E., Swanson, L.W. and Vale, W.W. (1984a) Coexpression of corticotropin-releasing factor and vasopressin immunoreactivity in parvocellular neurosecretory neurons of the adrenalectomized rat. *Proc. Natl. Acad. Sci., U.S.A.*, 81: 1883 – 1887.

Sawchenko, P.E., Swanson, L.W. and Vale, W.W. (1984b) Corticotropin-releasing factor: Coexpression within distinct subsets of oxytocin-, vasopressin-, and neurotensin-immunoreactive neurons in the hypothalamus of the male rat. *J. Neurosci.*, 4: 1118 – 1129.

Scharrer, E. and Scharrer, B. (1940) Secretory cells within the hypothalamus. *Proc. Assoc. Res. Nervous Mental Dis.*, 20: 170 – 194.

Schramme, C. and Denef, C. (1984) Stimulation of spontaneous and dopamine-inhibited prolactin release from anterior pituitary reaggregate cell cultures by angiotensin peptides. *Life Sci.*, 34: 1651 – 1658.

Simerly, R.B., Chang, C., Muramatsu, M. and Swanson, L.W. (1990) The distribution of androgen and estrogen receptor mRNA-containing cells in the rat brain: An *in situ* hybridization study. *J. Comp. Neurol.*, (in press).

Strack, A.M., Sawyer, W.B., Hughes, J.H., Platt, K.B. and Loewy, A.D. (1989) A general pattern of CNS innervation of the sympathetic outflow demonstrated by transneuronal pseudorabies viral infections. *Brain Res.*, 491: 145 – 162.

Swanson, L.W. (1983) Neuropeptides. New vistas on synaptic transmission. *TINS*, 6: 294 – 295.

Swanson, L.W. (1986) Organization of mammalian neuroendocrine system. In: F.E. Bloom (Ed.), *Handbook of Physiology, The Nervous System, IV*. Waverly Press, Baltimore, pp. 317 – 363.

Swanson, L.W. (1987) The hypothalamus. In: A. Björklund, T. Hökfelt, and L.W. Swanson (Eds.), *Handbook of Chemical Neuroanatomy, Vol. 5: Integrated Systems of the CNS, Part I*. Elsevier, Amsterdam, pp. 1 – 125.

Swanson, L.W. and Kuypers, H.G.J.M. (1980) The paraventricular nucleus of the hypothalamus: Cytoarchitectonic subdivisions and organization of projections to the pituitary, dorsal vagal complex, and spinal cord as demonstrated by retrograde fluorescence double-labeling methods. *J. Comp. Neurol.*, 194: 555 – 570.

Swanson, L.W. and Lind, R.W. (1986) Neural projections subserving the initiation of a specific motivated behavior in the rat: New projections from the subfornical organ. *Brain Res.*, 379: 399 – 403.

Swanson, L.W., Mogenson, G.J., Gerfen, C.R. and Robinson, P. (1984) Evidence for a projection from the lateral preoptic area and substantia innominata to the mesencephalic locomotor region in the rat. *Brain Res.*, 295: 161 – 178.

Swanson, L.W. and Sawchenko, P.E. (1983) Hypothalamic integration: Organization of the paraventricular and supraoptic nuclei. *Ann. Rev. Neurosci.*, 6: 275 – 325.

Swanson, L.W., Sawchenko, P.E. and Lind, R.W. (1986) Regulation of multiple peptides in CRF parvocellular neurosecretory neurons: Implications for the stress response. *Prog. Brain Res.*, 68: 169 – 190.

Swanson, L.W., Sawchenko, P.E., Lind, R.W. and Rho, J.-H. (1987) The CRH motoneuron: Differential peptide regulation in neurons with possible synaptic, paracrine, and endocrine outputs. *Ann. N.Y. Acad. Sci.*, 512: 12 – 23.

Swanson, L.W., Sawchenko, P.E., Rivier, J. and Vale, W.W. (1983) Organization of ovine corticotropin-releasing factor immunoreactive cells and fibers in the rat brain: An immunohistochemical study. *Neuroendocrinol.*, 36: 165 – 186.

Swanson, L.W. and Simmons, D.M. (1989) Differential steroid hormone and neural influences on peptide mRNA levels in CRH cells of the paraventricular nucleus: A hybridization histochemical study in the rat. *J. Comp. Neurol.*, 285: 413 – 435.

Tramu, G., Croix, C. and Pillez, A. (1983) Ability of the CRF immunoreactive neurons of the paraventricular nucleus to produce a vasopressin-like material. *Neuroendocrinol.*, 37: 467 – 469.

Vale, W., Spiess, J., Rivier, C. and Rivier, J. (1981) Characterization of a 41-residue ovine hypothalamic peptide that stimulates secretion of corticotropin and β-endorphin. *Science*, 213: 1394 – 1397.

Vandesande, F., Dierickx, K. and De Mey, J. (1977) The origin of the vasopressinergic and oxytocinergic fibres of the external region of the median eminence of the rat hypophysis. *Cell Tiss. Res.*, 180: 443 – 452.

Watts, A.G. and Swanson, L.W. (1989) Diurnal variations in the content of preprocorticotropin-releasing hormone messengre ribonucleic acids in the hypothalamic paraventricular nucleus of rats of both sexes as measured by *in situ* hybridization. *Endocrinol.*, 125: 1734 – 1738.

Watts, A.G. Swanson, L.W. and Sanchez-Watts, G. (1987) Efferent projections of the suprachiasmatic nucleus: I. Studies using anterograde transport of *Phaseolus vulgaris* leucoagglutinin in the rat. *J. Comp. Neurol.*, 258: 204 – 229.

Weiss, G.F. and Leibowitz, S.F. (1985) Efferent projections from the paraventricular nucleus mediating α2-noradrenergic feeding. *Brain Res.*, 347: 225 – 238.

Wolfson, B., Manning, R.W., Davis, L.G., Arentzen, R. and Baldino Jr., F. (1985) Co-localization of corticotropin releasing factor and vasopressin mRNA in neurones after adrenalectomy. *Nature (Lond.)*, 315: 59 – 61.

Young III, W.S., Mezey, É. and Siegel, R.E. (1986) Quantitative *in situ* hybridization histochemistry reveals increased levels of corticotropin-releasing factor mRNA after adrenalectomy in rats. *Neurosci. Lett.*, 70: 198 – 203.

G. Holstege (Ed.)
Progress in Brain Research, Vol. 87

CHAPTER 10

The prefrontal cortex and its relation to behavior

Joaquin M. Fuster

Department of Psychiatry and Brain Research Institute, School of Medicine, University of California at Los Angeles, CA 90024, U.S.A.

Introduction

It is now well established that the prefrontal cortex plays an important role in the organization of behavior and, therefore, the order and timing of behavioral acts. There is mounting evidence that the essence of that role is what I have called the mediation of cross-temporal contingencies (Fuster 1985), that is, the integration of behavior in accord with sensory information that is temporally separate from the action itself. Accordingly, the prefrontal cortex would be that part of the neocortex that allows the organism to reconcile sensations and acts that are mutually contingent but temporally separate from each other. This view puts the prefrontal cortex at the top of neural structures involved in sensory-motor integration and in charge of bridging temporal gaps in the perception-action cycle. That is the cybernetic cycle of influences from sensory receptors to motor effectors, to the environment, and back to sensory receptors, that governs orderly behavior. I have postulated that the prefrontal cortex mediates those temporal gaps by critically supporting at least two cognitive functions that make that temporal bridging possible and, consequently, the temporal organization of behavior possible: (1) a temporally "retrospective" function of short-term memory for sensory information, and (2) a temporally "prospective" function of preparatory motor set. Both these functions appear represented in the dorsolateral prefrontal cortex of the primate. In this paper, I briefly summarize some electrophysiological evidence for these propositions. In particular, my focus will be on single-unit activity from the prefrontal cortex of monkeys performing a class of behavioral tasks that epitomize cross-temporal integration: delay tasks.

Prefrontal cortex and the mediation of cross-temporal contingencies

The logic of delay tasks is the logic of cross-temporal contingencies. It can be summarized in two statements: "If now this, then later that; if earlier that, then now this". Figure 1 illustrates examples of the most commonly used delay tasks. All these tasks require, on every trial, the performance of a discrete behavioral act in accord with a discrete item of sensory information that has been received in the recent past. All of them are impaired by lesions of dorsolateral prefrontal cortex. Such impairments are a clear indication of the involvement of the dorsolateral prefrontal cortex in cross-temporal integration.

The first electrical indication of that prefrontal role was obtained by Walter and his colleagues in the human (Walter et al., 1964): a slow surface-negative potential which can be recorded from the frontal region in the interval of time, imposed by the investigator, between a stimulus and a motor act contingent on it. Those investigators called it the "contingent negative variation" (CNV). In the early 1970's, single-unit recordings from prefron-

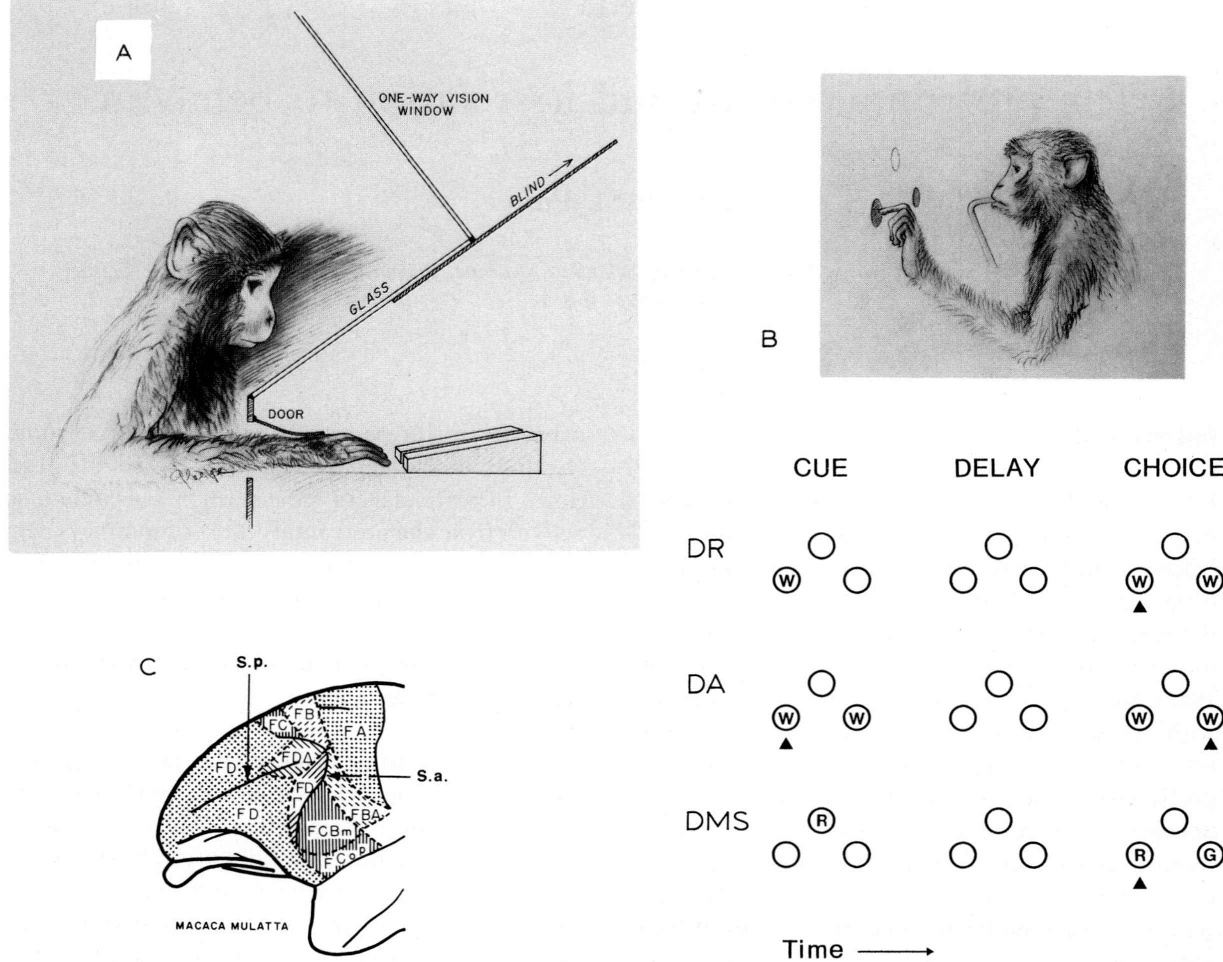

Fig. 1. Schematic diagram of delay tasks. (A) Typical direct-method delayed-response task. A trial begins with placement of a food morsel under one of the two identical objects in full view of the animal; the opaque screen (blind) is then lowered. After a delay of a few seconds or minutes, the screen is raised and the animal offered the choice of one object. If the choice is correct (object with concealed food), the animal retrieves the food as reward; an incorrect choice terminates the trial without reward. The position of the bait is changed at random from one trial to the next. (B) Diagram of test situation for indirect-method, automated, delay tasks. The subject faces a panel with three stimulus-response buttons. Below is the sequence of events for three different tasks (W, white light; G, green light; R, red light); triangles mark site of correct response, which is rewarded with fruit juice. DR: Indirect-method delayed response. The cue is the brief illumination of one of the lower buttons; after the delay, the two lower buttons are lit for choice; correct response is pressing the button lit before the delay. DA: Delayed alternation. The subject must press one of the two lower buttons when they appear simultaneously lit between delays; the correct button alternates between right and left. DMS: Delayed matching to sample. The sample (cue) is the brief colored illumination of the top button. After the delay, two colors appear simultaneously in the lower buttons; correct response is pressing the button with the sample color; the sample color and its position in the lower buttons are changed randomly from trial to trial. (C) Cytoarchitectonic map of the frontal cortex of the rhesus monkey according to von Bonin and Bailey. Prefrontal cortex is labeled FD. Animals with prefrontal lesions show deficits in performance of the four tasks illustrated above. The magnitude of the deficit depends on the location and extent of the lesion.

tal areas in monkeys performing delay tasks provided the first indications at the neuronal level of the involvement of the prefrontal cortex in cross-temporal contingencies (Fuster, 1973). One of the most striking findings was that of neurons that fired continuously and at high levels during the period of delay that in those tasks is interposed between a sensory cue and the motor response contingent on it (Fig. 2). Sustained inhibition was also encountered, although less commonly (Fig. 3). Both the sustained activation and the sustained inhibition of the delay period were shown to depend on the presence of a relationship of mutual contingency between the events that preceded and those that succeeded that period. For example, that sustained activation or inhibition disappeared in mock trials, when the animal was deprived of the information that determined the response at the end of the delay (Fig. 3).

Those early data clearly suggested the cross-temporal integrative role of prefrontal neurons. I attributed those kinds of activity to the involvement of those neurons in a form of transient or short-term memory. Such a memory involvement was subsequently made more evident by data from our lab and from others. Also later, it became clear that prefrontal cells do not only engage in short-term memory but in a second temporally in-

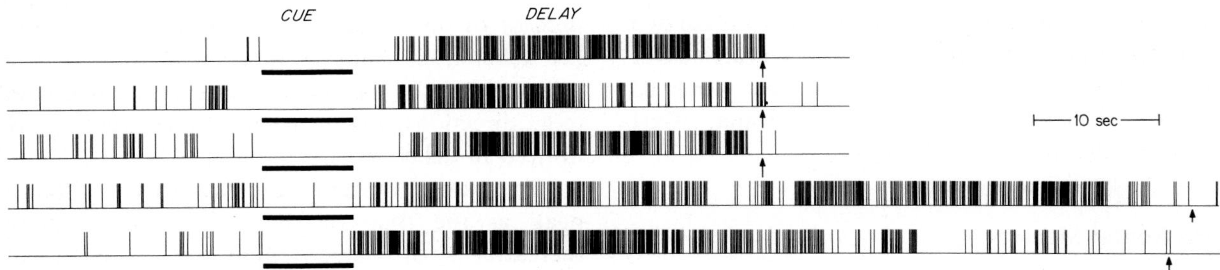

Fig. 2. Discharge of a prefrontal unit during five trials of a delayed-response task (direct method). A horizontal bar marks the cue period and an arrow the end of each trial. Note the activation of the cell during the delay (30 s in the upper three trials, 60 sec in the lower two).

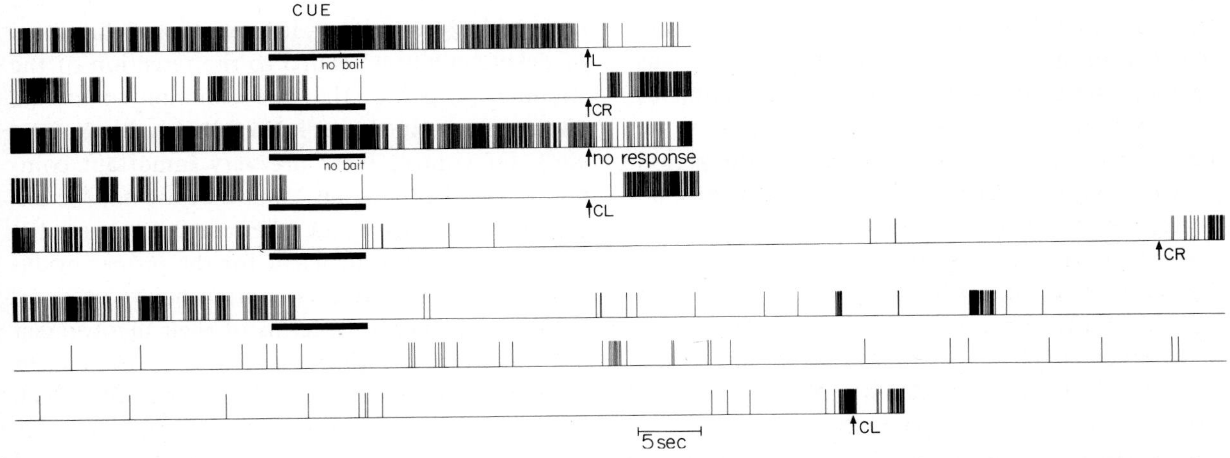

Fig. 3. Discharge of a prefrontal unit during six trials of a delayed-response task (direct method). On the first and third trial, the cue (bait under one object, as in Fig. 1A) is not given. In those two mock trials, with absence of cross-temporal contingency, the unit fails to show the normal inhibition during the delay that, in the last trial, is nearly 4-min long. (*Abbreviations*: C, correct response; R, right; L, left).

tegrative function that I have postulated to be essential for the mediation of cross-temporal contingencies of behavior, that is, preparatory motor set. Both the memory role and the motor-set role of prefrontal neurons were essentially ascertained by observation that in some units delay activity was coupled to the stimulus, while in others it was coupled to the motor response: Stimulus-coupling was observed for considerable time after the stimulus, while response-coupling was observed well in advance of the response. In the next two sections I briefly describe the evidence obtained in our laboratory and elsewhere for those two prefrontal processes of cross-temporal integration, that is, short-term or working memory and preparatory motor set. My work on both these two aspects of prefrontal function has been carried out in collaboration with Gary Alexander, Richard Bauer, John Jervey, Javier Quintana, Carl Rosenkilde, and Javier Yajeya.

Prefrontal Memory

By selectively cooling the dorsolateral convexity of the prefrontal cortex, we were able to demonstrate a reversible impairment of delay-task performance (Bauer and Fuster, 1976). That impairment had two outstanding features: (1) It was equally severe whether or not the cue to be remembered was spatially defined; (2) It increased in magnitude as a function of the delay (Fig. 4). In other words, the deficit became greater as the length of the period between cue and choice was increased. This second feature of the cryogenic prefrontal deficit was fully consistent with the assumption that the function impaired was one with a temporal decay. Of course, short-term memory is one such function.

Another characteristic of the prefrontal delay-task deficit is its supramodality. Not only does it occur whether the cue is spatially defined or not, but whether it is visual, auditory, or somesthetic. This supramodality of the deficit was first demonstrated in the human (Lewinsohn et al., 1972). Our recent cooling data from monkeys do not only suggest that the deficit applies to visual short-term memory but to haptic short-term memory as well. Furthermore, these data also suggest that the deficit is not only supramodal but cross-modal (i.e., it occurs in delay tasks requiring transfer across time from vision to touch, or vice versa).

During the delay, that is, during the retention period of delay tasks, many dorsolateral prefrontal units are coupled to the stimulus just presented. That coupling to the sensory stimulus after it has disappeared from the environment can be taken, of course, as an indication of those units' involvement in retention of the stimulus. The coupling has two different forms or manifestations: (1) gradual descent of discharge as the delay progresses; and (2) differential stimulus-dependent firing of the unit in terms of the two or more alternative cues (e.g., directions, colors or patterns) conventionally utilized in delay tasks.

The gradual descent of delay activity after a peak at the time of the cue or immediately thereafter is, of course, reminiscent of mnemonic decay. It is exemplified by the types C and D of my original classification (Fig. 5). However, in the absence of differential stimulus-dependent delay firing, the argument for cellular memory, simply on the basis of firing trend, is only suggestive and not conclusive. At most, it suggests that that form of delay activity is related to the retention of the stimulus properties that are common to all the alternate cues in the task (like shape, brightness, etc.). Of course, these are very important components of the "engram", but they are not the only ones that determine the correctness of the choice; they are insufficient for the proper bridging of the cross-temporal contingency.

More convincing, in terms of their involvement in memory, is the differential stimulus-dependent discharge of prefrontal cells during the delay. Such units have been demonstrated in spatial delay tasks, such as delayed response (Fig. 6) and delayed alternation, as well as in nonspatial delay tasks, such as delayed matching (Niki, 1974; Niki and Watanabe, 1976; Rosenkilde et al., 1981;

Fuster et al., 1982; Kojima and Golman-Rakic, 1984; Quintanta et al., 1988; Funahashi et al., 1989). Even in such cells, however, the argument for memory may be inconclusive, especially in spatial tasks. For in these tasks the direction of the correct response can be predicted by the animal either from the cue or from the direction of the previous response. As a result, unit activity related to memory cannot be easily distinguished from unit activity related to the motor response. This is especially true in units, such as the one in Fig. 6, in which both factors seem to play a role, in other words, units in which delay-activity is to some degree coupled to both the cue just presented and

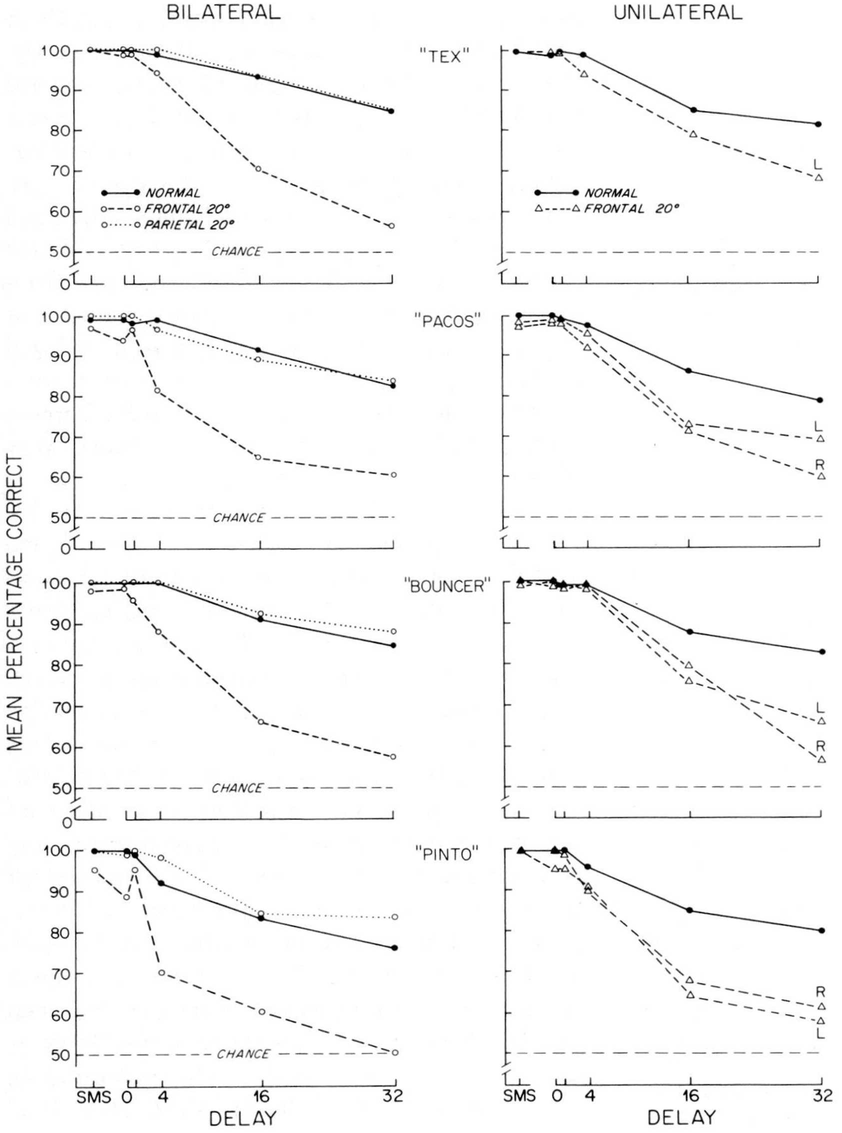

Fig. 4. Performance of four monkeys in delayed matching-to-sample (DMS: Fig. 2, B) at normal cortical temperature and under cooling of dorsolateral prefrontal or posterior parietal cortex. (SMS, simultaneous matching-to-sample; delay in seconds.) Note increasing prefrontal deficit as a function of delay.

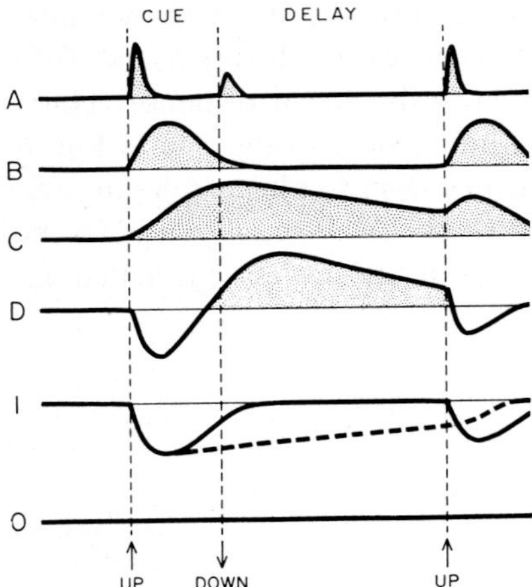

Fig. 5. Types of units in prefrontal cortex of the monkey during delayed-response testing. Heavy line represent deviations of firing from inter-trial base line. Arrows mark displacements of opaque screen between animal and test objects (Fig. 1A).

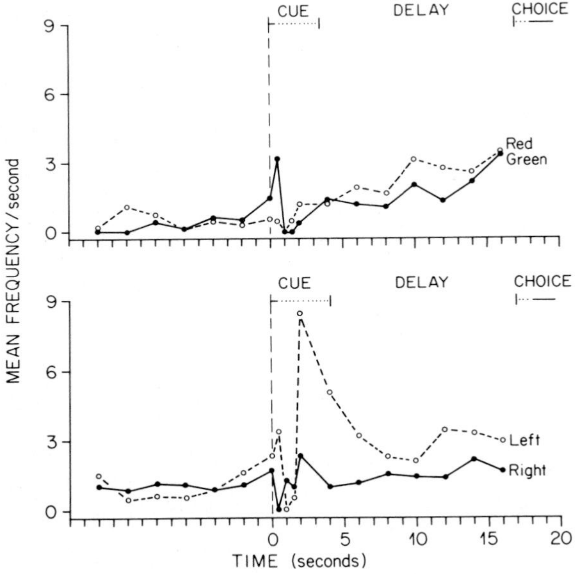

Fig. 6. Firing frequency of a prefrontal unit during testing in delayed matching-to-sample with colors (upper graph) and delayed response (lower graph). (In these tests (see Fig. 1B) the cue was terminated by the animal's pressing of a button; hence the variability of cue duration.) Note, during cue and delay periods, differential firing in delayed response and accelerating firing in color-matching trials.

the impending response. In any event, the phenomenon of sensory-coupling (i.e. memory-coupling) can be, and has been, demonstrated in tasks with spatial dissociation between cue and response.

It is of course debatable whether the sustained, cue-dependent, activation of some prefrontal neurons during the delay reflects the involvement of those neurons in the cell assemblies that Hebb postulated to be the essence of short-term memory. A reasonable case can be made for this, provided that a cell assembly is not construed simply as a cluster of neurons but as a network, as I have attempted to do elsewhere (Fuster 1989): a network that extends well beyond the prefrontal cortex and includes other sectors of association cortex. Which sector will be involved, in addition to the prefrontal cortex, will depend on the sensory character of the cue. If the cue is visual, as it is in visual delayed matching, the inferotemporal cortex will be involved (Fuster and Jervey, 1982; Fuster, 1990), where neurons evidently take part in the retention of very specific visual information. If the cue is somesthetic, the posterior parietal cortex will be involved (Koch and Fuster, 1989), where some neurons seem to take part in retention of haptic information. In any case, those are cortical areas that interact functionally with the prefrontal cortex (Fuster et al., 1985, Quintana et al., in press). The important point I wish to make here is that the prefrontal cortex is part of all neuronal networks that mediate the kind of cross-temporal contingencies that delay tasks contain; those other areas are also part of those networks inasmuch as the sensory information that needs to be transferred across time is, so to speak, within their specialty.

In conclusion, it seems indisputable that the neurons of the prefrontal cortex are very much engaged in a form or aspect of memory that can best be characterized as short-term and context-dependent memory. It is short-term inasmuch as the action is to occur in the short-term. It is context-dependent in that it depends on the context of the action itself. Whatever the content of that memory, it is memory primarily and perhaps exclusively in the service of behavioral action.

Prefrontal Set

In addition to the retrospective, mnemonic, aspects of prefrontal function, its prospective, future-related, aspects have also been documented in the neuropsychological literature (Fuster, 1989). In the human, dorsolateral prefrontal lesions are associated with well-known difficulties in planning; they can be exposed by such formal tests as the Tower of London, which is a test of the ability to organize motor action in the short-term (Shallice, 1982). It seems, therefore, that we are dealing with the failure of a function that is temporally symmetrical to the short-term memory function we have just discussed, though not by any means independent from it. Ingvar (1984) dubbed it "the memory of the future".

Just as there is electrophysiological evidence of the involvement of dorsolateral prefrontal neurons in short-term memory, there is evidence of their involvement in short-term preparation for movement or motor set. In delay tasks, such as delayed response, delayed matching and the like, motor-set cells behave in a manner directly opposite to that of the memory cells we have seen. Whereas memory cells seem to be looking backwards, to the cue, motor-set cells seem to be looking forward, to the impending motor response. Thus, we observe units that instead of gradually diminishing their firing between cue and response, they accelerate it. In any event, units that show accelerating discharge during the delay are probably a special case of a general category of units that have been shown to do so while the monkey prepares for movement in a variety of tasks, including delay tasks (Kubota et al., 1974; Sakai, 1974; Niki and Watanabe, 1976; Fuster et al., 1982; Boch and Goldberg, 1989). A unit may accelerate its discharge regardless of which cue the monkey has been given or which response he is about the execute, provided that a motor act is in the making (Fig. 7). More direct evidence of involvement in specific-response set can be found in units that show a different rate of discharge depending on the particular motor response that the monkey is preparing. This evidence can best be obtained by use of behavioral tasks in which the cue is spatially dissociated from the response.

Lately, with Quintana, we have been investigating the cellular phenomena associated with preparatory motor set in the dorsolateral prefrontal cortex. For that, we are using a number of delay tasks in which cue and response are spatially dissociated. These include, for example, delayed matching to sample and delayed conditional discrimination. In one such task, for example, the cue consists of a color always displayed in the same position of the field; the color determines the direction of the response, left or right, at the end of the delay. By use of reversible, cryogenic, lesions we are gathering further evidence that the integrative functions of the prefrontal cortex are important for performance of these tasks (Quintana and Fuster, 1988).

The most important microelectrode findings from these latest studies can be summarized as follows: Units that fire differentially at the time of the motor response (i.e., with different firing frequence on right than on left response) commonly show selective response-coupling well in advance of the response itself. In fact, response-coupling may already appear at the time of the cue, if that cue defines and determines the direction of the forthcoming response. In other words a prefrontal cell may reveal its tuning to a particular response direction already upon appearance of the sensory cue that symbolizes that direction; thus, the discharge of the cell, in accord with the color of the cue, "predicts" by several seconds the motor response of the animal. Furthermore, in the course of the delay, direction-selective cells show progressively greater discharge as their "preferred response" approaches, whether that response is to the right or to the left.

In conclusion, during the delay between cue and response, a substantial proportion of dorsolateral prefrontal units show motor-coupling in anticipa-

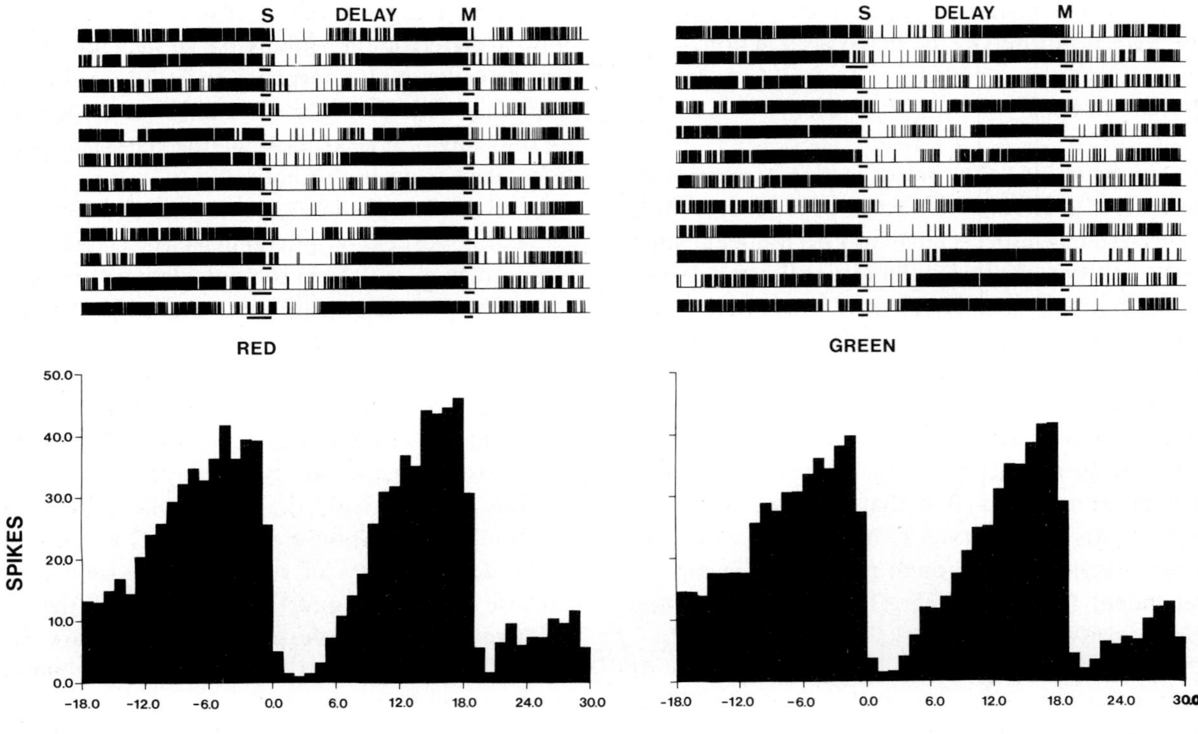

Fig. 7. Rasters and frequency histograms from a prefrontal unit during delayed matching-to-sample (red or green). Samples (S) and match (M) periods are marked by horizontal lines under the records. The unit accelerates its firing before the sample (which the animal is supposed to terminate by pressing a button) and during the 18-s delays.

tion of movement. Their discharge tends to increase as the time for expected movement approaches, whereas, as we have seen, the opposite is true for sensory-coupled cells, whose discharge tends to diminish during the same period. It is reasonable to infer that sensory-coupled cells are somehow involved in the retention of sensory information, while motor-coupled cells engage in preparation of the response that is consonant with that information according to the rules of the task.

Functional Interactions

Thus, it appears that two general types of neurons in dorsolateral prefrontal cortex participate in the two complementary processes of (1) holding sensory information and (2) preparation for motor action in accord with that information. It is not yet possible to determine the mechanisms by which the information is transferred across time and incorporated into the appropriate action. That transfer may at least in part occur locally within dorsolateral cortex. It should be noted that, during the delay, units with descelerating activity have been found there in close proximity of units with accelerating activity (Fuster et al., 1982). Therefore, it is not inconceivable that information is relayed more or less directly from the former to the latter cells within small cortical confines, perhaps within functional modules or columns of prefrontal cortex.

It seems also likely, however, that those transactions take place within and between widely distributed neuronal networks, of which the prefrontal cortex, along with other cortical areas, is a part. In order to understand this kind of interactions it is useful to look at the larger picture of cortical involvement in the perception-action cycle (Neisser, 1976; Arbib, 1981; Fuster, 1989). As mentioned above, this cycle is defined by the circular pattern of cybernetic influences running from the environment through sensory systems, through motor systems, and back to the environment, that supports and regulates any orderly sequence of behavior. There is an extensive array of well-substantiated cortical and subcortical connections underlying that cycle of influences (Fig. 8).

Two general points need to be made here. The first is that the prefrontal cortex, together with polysensory association areas of posterior cortex with which it is well connected, constitutes the highest level of the sensory and motor hierarchies of cortical structures involved in the perception-action cycle. The prefrontal cortex, through its connections with those other cortical areas, closes at the top the ring of neural structures involved in sensory-motor integration. One implication of its supraordinate position, which I have attempted to defend with physiological evidence, is that the prefrontal cortex, especially its dorsolateral portion, is in charge of closing via those connections the temporal gaps within the cycle. The dorsolateral prefrontal cortex is needed to integrate sensory input with later action, in other words, to close the cross-temporal contingencies within the cycle. In order to accomplish this, the prefrontal cortex probably interacts with other associative areas and with subcortical structures that are part of motor systems. Reciprocal interactions with these cortical and subcortical structures may, perhaps through some form of neural reverberation, support the short-term memory and motor-set functions of the prefrontal cortex that I postulate are needed for cross-temporal integration.

The second point that I want to make to close this discussion is that at least part of the output of prefrontal cortex that flows back upon sensory

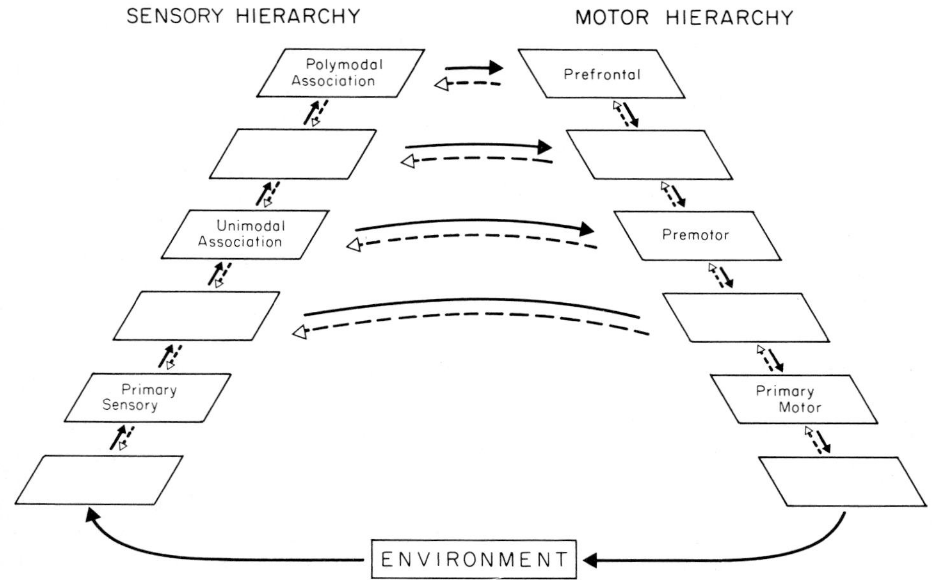

Fig. 8. Scheme of connectivity between cortical regions that are part of the sensory and motor hierarchies of information processing and are involved in the perception-action cycle. Blank boxes represent intermediate stages of cortical or subcortical processing within or between labeled regions. Note that connections are bidirectional. The basic scheme, as represented here (and especially well substantiated in visual and somesthetic systems), is consistent with a large body of anatomical and functional data (for details, see Fuster 1989).

areas may well serve the role of corollary discharge. In this context, corollary discharge is another cybernetic function that serves cross-temporal integration and the perception-action cycle. As Teuber proposed (1972), the corollary discharge of the prefrontal cortex is some kind of output that this cortex sends to sensory structures concomitantly with action. It is supposed to prepare these structures for the anticipated effects of the action. Thus, whereas above we have dealt with motor set deriving from recent sensory information, here we are dealing with the converse, that is, sensory set deriving from recent action. In any event, the physiological evidence for corollary discharge is less compelling and the physiological mechanisms no less obscure than for motor set. At present, it seems appropriate to consider corollary discharge as at least another hypothetical mechanism, in addition to those of short-term memory and motor set, by which the prefrontal cortex ensures the integration of behavior in the temporal domain.

Summary

The prefrontal cortex is critical for temporal organization of behavior. It mediates cross-temporal sensory-motor contingencies, integrating motor action (including speech) with recent sensory information. It performs this role through cooperation of two cognitive functions represented in its dorsolateral areas: short-term memory (STM) and preparatory set. Supporting data have been obtained from monkeys performing delay tasks, which epitomize the principle of cross-temporal contingency. In a given trial, the animal performs an act contingent on a sensory cue given a few seconds or minutes earlier. During the delay between cue and response, cells in dorsolateral prefrontal cortex show sustained activation. Two cell categories can be identified in tasks in which cue and response are spatially separate. Cells of the first participate in STM: Their activation tends to diminish as the delay progresses; in some, the activation level depends on the particular cue received. Similar cells are found elsewhere in cortex. Cells of the second category seem to take part in preparation of motor response: Their activation tends to increase in anticipation of it and may be attuned to the particular movement the cue calls for. This cell type is rare outside of frontal cortex. The temporally integrative function of the prefrontal cortex is probably based on local interactions between "memory" and "motor-set" cells, as well as on neural associations between prefrontal cortex and posterior cortical areas.

References

Arbib, M.A. (1981) Perceptual structures and distributed motor control. In: V.B. Brooks (Ed.), Handbook of Physiology; Nervous System, Vol. II *Am. Physiol. Soc.*, Bethesda, pp. 1448 – 1480.

Bauer, R.H. and Fuster, J.M. (1976) Delayed-matching and delayed-response deficit from cooling dorsolateral prefrontal cortex in monkeys. *J. Comp. Physiol. Psychol.*, 90: 293 – 302.

Boch, R.A. and Goldberg, M.E. (1989) Participation of prefrontal neurons in the preparation of visually guided eye movements in the rhesus monkey. *J. Neurophysiol.*, 61: 1064 – 1084.

Funahashi, S., Bruce, C.J. and Goldman-Rakic, P.S. (1988) Memory fields: directional tuning of delay activity in the dorsolateral prefrontal cortex of rhesus monkey. *Soc. Neurosci. Abstr.*, 14: 860.

Fuster, J.M. (1973) Unit activity in prefrontal cortex during delayed-response performance: Neuronal correlates of transient memory. *J. Neurophysiol.*, 36: 61 – 78.

Fuster, J.M. (1985) The prefrontal cortex, mediator of cross-temporal contingencies. *Human Neurobiol.*, 4: 169 – 179.

Fuster, J.M. (1989) *The Prefrontal Cortex* (2nd Edition). Raven Press, New York.

Fuster, J.M. (1990) Inferotemporal units in selective visual attention and short-term memory. *J. Neurophysiol.*, 64: 681 – 697.

Fuster, J.M., Bauer, R.H. and Jervey, J.P. (1982) Cellular discharge in the dorsolateral prefrontal cortex of the monkey in cognitive tasks. *Exp. Neurol.*, 77: 679 – 694.

Fuster, J.M., Bauer, R.H. and Jervey, J.P. (1985) Functional interactions between inferotemporal and prefrontal cortex in a cognitive task. *Brain Res.*, 330: 299 – 307.

Fuster, J.M. and Jervey, J.P. (1982) Neuronal firing in the inferotemporal cortex of the monkey in a visual memory task. *J. Neurosci.*, 2: 361 – 375.

Ingvar, D.H. (1985) *"Memory of the future"*: An essay on the temporal organization of conscious awareness. *Human*

Neurobiol., 4: 127 – 136.

Koch, K. and Fuster, J.M. (1989) Unit activity in monkey parietal cortex related to haptic perception and temporary memory. *Exp. Brain Res.,* 76: 292 – 306.

Kojima, S. and Goldman-Rakic, P.S. (1984) Functional analysis of spatially discriminative neurons in prefrontal cortex of rhesus monkeys. *Brain Res.,* 291: 229 – 240.

Kubota, K., Iwamoto, T. and Suzuki, H. (1974) Visuokinetic activities of primate prefrontal neurons during delayed-response performance. *J. Neurophysiol.,* 37: 1197 – 1212.

Lewinsohn, P., Zieler, R., Libet, J., Eyeberg, S. and Nielson, G. (1972) Short-term memory – a comparison between frontal and nonfrontal right- and left-hemisphere brain-damaged patients. *J. Comp. Physiol. Psychol.,* 81: 248 – 255.

Neisser, U. (1976) Cognition and Reality: Principles and Implications of Cognitive Psychology. Freeman, San Francisco.

Niki, H. (1974) Differential activity of prefrontal units during right and left delayed response trials. *Brain Res.,* 70: 346 – 349.

Niki, H. and Watanabe, M. (1976) Prefrontal unit activity and delayed response: relation to cue location versus direction of response. *Brain Res.,* 105: 79 – 88.

Quintana, J. and Fuster, J.M. (1988) Effects of cooling parietal or prefrontal cortex on spatial and nonspatial visuo-motor tasks. *Soc. Neurosci. Abstr.,* 14: 160.

Quintana, J., Fuster, J.M. and Yajeya, J. (1991) Effects of cooling parietal cortex on prefrontal units in delay tasks. *Brain Res.,* (in press).

Quintana, J., Yajeya, J. and Fuster, J.M. (1988) Prefrontal representation of stimulus attributes during delay tasks. I. Unit activity in cross-temporal integration of sensory and sensory-motor information. *Brain Res.,* 474: 211 – 222.

Rosenkilde, C.E., Bauer, R.H. and Fuster, J.M. (1981) Single cell activity in ventral prefrontal cortex on behaving monkeys. *Brain Res.,* 209: 375 – 394.

Sakai, M. (1974) Prefrontal unit activity during visually guided lever pressing reaction in the monkey. *Brain Res.,* 81: 297 – 309.

Shallice, T. (1982) Specific impairments of planning. Philos. *Trans. R. Soc. Lond.* (Biol.), 298: 199 – 209.

Walter, W., Cooper, R., Aldridge, V., McCallum, W. and Winter, A. (1964) Contingent negative variation: an electric sign of sensori-motor association and expectancy in the human brain. *Nature,* 203: 380 – 384.

G. Holstege (Ed.)
Progress in Brain Research, Vol. 87

CHAPTER 11

Neural mechanisms underlying corticospinal and rubrospinal control of limb movements

Paul D. Cheney[1], Eberhard E. Fetz[2] and Klaus Mewes[1]

[1] *Department of Physiology and Ralph L. Smith Research Center, University of Kansas Medical Center, Kansas City, KS 66103 and* [2] *Department of Physiology and Biophysics, University of Washington, Seattle, WA, 98195, U.S.A.*

Introduction

Commands for movements of the limbs are transmitted from the brain to the spinal cord through descending systems. Some neurons of these systems contact motoneurons directly and will be referred to as premotor neurons. The anatomical organization, synaptic effects and discharge properties of premotor neurons are of central importance to understanding how the brain controls movement. This paper reviews our current understanding of the organization and functional properties of descending systems and recent advances that have come from single unit recording in awake monkeys using new techniques that reveal the synaptic connections of single premotor neurons with motoneurons of agonist and antagonist muscles. Emphasis will be placed on the role of descending systems in the control of limb movements, although it is recognized that locomotion and other motor behaviors involving axial, head and/or facial muscles may involve similar principles. Emphasis will also be on motor control in primates although relevant data from the cat and other species will be included where no primate data is available.

Identification of descending systems controlling limb movements

In the history of work on motor function of the CNS, a variety of techniques have been used to identify brain structures projecting to motoneurons. Fritsch and Hitzig (1870) first evoked muscle contractions by applying electrical stimulation to the motor area of cerebral cortex in the dog. Recording movements evoked by gross electrical stimulation of the brain surface was followed by more elaborate techniques such as measurement of the actual forces produced in isolated muscles by focal surface stimulation of the cortex (Chang et al., 1947). The historical progression toward using more refined and sensitive methods to detect cortical output ultimately led in the 1960's to recording synaptic potentials evoked in motoneurons from electrical stimulation of the cerebral cortex or subcortical structures (Phillips and Porter, 1977). Most recently, considerable progress has been made in developing microstimulation techniques for more refined and discrete activation of descending neurons (Asanuma and Sakata, 1967). This effort has culminated with methods capable of detecting the excitatory and inhibitory effects of single neurons on muscle activity in the awake animal during task performance (Fetz et al., 1976; Cheney, 1980; Fetz and Cheney, 1980; Buys et al., 1986).

Paralleling these electrophysiological developments, anatomical studies became increasingly more refined and sensitive. Degeneration methods provided the first clear evidence concerning the origin of various spinally projecting neurons

(Brodal, 1981). However, the application of various neuroanatomical tracers such as horseradish peroxidase (HRP) has yielded enormous progress in understanding the origin and organization of descending systems.

Holstege (this volume, Chapter 14) has divided spinal cord projecting descending systems into two categories: somatic and limbic. This subdivision recognizes not only the traditional somatic descending systems but also substantial recent evidence for another group of descending systems which arise from limbic structures (Holstege, 1987). Traditional descending systems include the corticospinal, rubrospinal, reticulospinal, vestibulospinal, tectospinal and interstitiospinal systems (Fig. 1). These systems are known to: 1) exert powerful, relatively direct excitatory and inhibitory synaptic effects on motoneurons, 2) exhibit somatotopic organization (except the reticulospinal system), and 3) be highly modulated in relation to the kinematic features of movement. Limbic descending systems arise from locus coeruleus, raphe nuclei, and hypothalamic nuclei. These neurons are also labelled by spinal cord injections of the retrograde tracer HRP. Similarly the spinal terminations of these neurons can be labelled by the anterograde tracer ^{3}H-leucine (Holstege, this volume). Like the somatic descending systems, the limbic systems also terminate among motoneurons but are believed to influence motoneuron excitability in a more tonic fashion related to behavioral state and/or to exert some trophic influence over motoneurons and spinal cord circuitry. This paper will focus on the somatic descending systems involved in the control of muscle contraction and movement parameters.

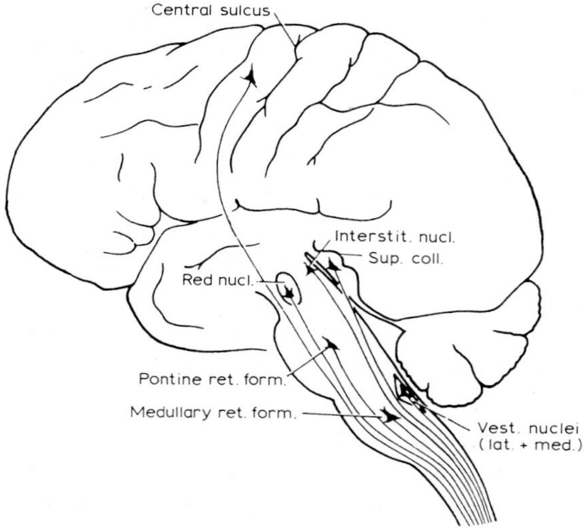

Fig. 1. Origin of brain descending systems containing neurons that contact spinal motoneurons. (Modified from Brodal, 1981)

It is clear that not all descending systems are equipotent in their access to motoneuron pools of the limb when viewed along a continuum extending from most distal to proximal and finally to most axial. This was recognized very early in mapping studies of motor cortex, which revealed that distal muscles, although much smaller in mass than more proximal and axial muscles, were represented by a much larger area of cortex. The classic studies of Lawrence and Kuypers (1968a,b) also showed that deficits from lesions of the pyramidal tract (corticospinal) and rubrospinal system are most severe and lasting for movements of the distal extremity whereas deficits from lesions of the reticulospinal and vestibulospinal systems are most severe for movements involving proximal and axial muscles. Based on these findings and the different anatomical locations of these tracts in the spinal cord, Lawrence and Kuypers divided descending systems into a dorso-lateral component, which included the corticospinal and rubrospinal systems, and a ventro-medial component which included the reticulospinal and vestibulospinal systems. One of the basic findings of their studies was that lesions of the corticospinal system resulted in permanent loss of relatively independent finger movements (RIFMs) and severe distal weakness; however, the monkey could maintain an upright posture, run and climb the side of the cage with little or no difficulty. Deficits from corticospinal lesions were less severe if the rubrospinal system was intact. Similarly, deficits from rubrospinal system lesions were virtually unnoticeable if the corticospinal system was intact. In contrast, lesions of the ventro-medial system rendered the monkey immobile and unable to maintain an upright posture.

In this respect, such lesions were much more disabling than those of the dorso-lateral system.

This lesion work and other anatomical and electrophysiological studies emphasize the importance of the dorso-lateral descending systems in the control of distal musculature and the mediolateral systems in the control of proximal and axial muscles. Consequently, studies on descending control of limb movements, appropriately, have focussed on the corticospinal and rubrospinal tracts. However, it should be noted that the reticulospinal and vestibulospinal systems also make synaptic linkages with motoneurons of distal limb muscles (see later section of this paper) and their involvement in limb movements should not be overlooked.

Categories of limb movements

The limbs participate in a wide range of movements which can be classified in terms of the various control problems they present to the neural apparatus. The following factors may all be of significance in determining underlying neural mechanisms and shaping the relevant motor program (Cheney, 1985):

1. Movement speed: slow (ramp) versus ballistic (Delong and Strick, 1974).
2. The number of joints involved: simple (1 joint) versus compound (coordination of two or more joints).
3. The type of feedback guidance: somesthetic, vestibular, auditory, visual or some combination of these.
4. Movement complexity: for instance the number of discrete steps in a movement sequence (Roland et al., 1980) and whether movement targets are remembered or visible.
5. The mechanism by which the movement is stopped: self terminated or externally terminated.
6. Accuracy constraints.
7. Muscle groups involved: 1) distal versus proximal/axial, 2) flexors versus extensors, and 3) fast versus slow muscles (Preston et al., 1967; Burke et al., 1970).
8. The degree of learning and mental concentration required, ranging from the most automatic or stereotyped (e.g., respiration and locomotion) to the least automatic such as playing the piano (Phillips and Porter, 1977).

Of all these factors, the subdivision of movements on a continuous scale from most automatic to least automatic seems particularly useful. This distinction was first proposed by Hughlings Jackson (as cited in Phillips and Porter, 1977) and seems to be a key factor in determining the involvement of various descending systems in movement. For example, lesions of the corticospinal system in monkeys interfere with the use of the hand for skilled movements such as removing a food morsel from a narrow well but the same monkeys show no obvious deficit in using the hand for more automatic locomotor movements such as running or climbing the side of the cage (Tower, 1940). In evolution, the forebrain has come to occupy a position of supreme importance for executing the least automatic, most skilled movements. Accordingly, the severity of deficits in skilled movements following lesions of the pyramidal system increases with the size of the forebrain (Phillips and Porter, 1977).

Synaptic linkage from descending premotor neurons to spinal motoneurons

The synaptic linkage between neurons of descending systems and alpha motoneurons has been investigated using: 1) intracellular recording of EPSPs and IPSPs evoked by stimulation of descending systems (Table I), and 2) facilitation or suppression of the muscle spindle Ia monosynaptic reflexes after stimulation of a descending system (Table I; Preston et al., 1967; Asanuma and Sakata, 1967). Intracellular recordings provide precise timing and magnitude information about EPSPs and IPSPs associated with different descending systems. However, because impaling individual motoneurons is technically difficult, only limited intracellular data is available on the distribution of premotor EPSPs and IPSPs to dif-

TABLE I
Summary of results from studies of synaptic effects from premotor descending systems on motoneurons

Primate	Forearm digits F	E	Wrist F	E	Elbow F	E	Shoulder F	E	Hindlimb digits F	E	Ankle F	E	Knee F	E	Hip F	E	Neck	Axial	Facial
Corticospinal																			
Intracellular	+m	+m	+m/−	+m/−	+m/−	−/+m			+m	+m	+m/−	+m/−	+m/−	+m/−		+m			
Ia conditioning	+m	+m	+m/−	+m/−	−/+	+/−					+m/−	+m	+m/−	−d	+m/−	−d			
Spike trig. ave.	+/−	+/−	+/−	+/−															
Rubrospinal																			
Intracellular									+m		+m	+m/− (fdl) −d/+ (gsol)							
Spike trig. ave	+/−	++/−	+/−	++/−															
Reticulospinal*																			
Intracellular											+m/−	+m/−	+m	+m					
Vestibulospinal*																			
Intracellular										0		+m		+m					
Cat	**Forearm digits F**	**E**	**Wrist F**	**E**	**Elbow F**	**E**	**Shoulder F**	**E**	**Hindlimb digits F**	**E**	**Ankle F**	**E**	**Knee F**	**E**	**Hip F**	**E**	**Neck**	**Axial**	**Facial**
Corticospinal																			
Intracellular	+d	−/+d	+d/−t	+d/−t	+d/−t	+d/−t −d,t	+d	−/+d									+d, −d		
Ia conditioning	+	+	+/−	+/−	+/−	−slow +/− (fast)					+d	−d (slow) +/− (fast)	+d	−d	+d/−	−d			
Rubrospinal																			
Intracellular			+d/−		d/−t	+d/−t			−	+d/−	+d/−	−sol +mg −/+fdl +−pl	+d/−	+d/−	+d/−	+d/−			+m
Reticulospinal																			
Intracellular	+m 38%	+m/− 38%	+m/− 38%	+m/− 38%	+m/− 78%	+m/− 50%			+m/− 50%	+m/− 70%	+m/− 86%	m/− 85%	+m/− 60%	−d/+ 50%		+m/−d 60%	+m 85% −m 68%		+m 72% −m −d
Vestibulospinal																			
Intracellular	+p/−p	+p/−p	+p/−p	+p/−p	+p/−p	+p/−p			−p	+m	−d	+m +p	−d	+m +p		+m +p	+m −m		+m −m

m = monosynaptic, d = disynaptic, t = trisynaptic, p = polysynaptic, + = excitatory, − = inhibitory, +/− = mixed with predominant effect listed first, % = % of motoneurons receiving effects. Methods used to examine synaptic effects on motoneurons include intracellular recording, Ia reflex conditioning and spike triggered averaging of EMG activity (SpTA). Excitatory and inhibitory components of mixed effects are probably generated by different premotor neurons. All inhibitory effects probably have a minimal disynaptic linkage. Data from Alstermark and Sasaki (1985), Alstermark et al. (1985), Baev (1971), Burke et al. (1970), Clough et al. (1968), Grillner et al. (1971), Hongo et al. (1969), Illert et al. (1976a,b), Illert and Wiedemann (1984), Jankowska et al. (1975), Landgren et al. (1962a,b), Peterson et al. (1978, 1979), Peterson (1979), Phillips and Porter (1964), Preston (1961), Preston et al. (1967), Shapovalov (1972), Shapovalov et al. (1971, 1973), Wilson et al. (1970), Wilson and Yoshida (1969), Yu et al. (1972). SpTA data from Cheney et al. (1988), Fetz and Cheney (1980), and Kaser and Cheney (1985).

ferent motoneuron pools. Monosynaptic reflex testing also provides relatively precise timing information on synaptic events. However, unlike intracellular recording, which yields detailed information about synaptic input to a single motoneuron, monosynaptic reflex testing provides a measure of the net effect of the stimulated premotor neurons on an entire population of motoneurons, for example motoneurons of a specific muscle.

Table I summarizes results from existing studies of the distribution of synaptic effects from premotor descending systems to motoneurons of different muscles in cats and primates – the two most widely studied species. The data was derived from both intracellular and monosynaptic reflex testing experiments. For comparison, data derived from recent work using the technique of spike-triggered averaging of EMG activity in awake monkeys is included. This new approach to examining the correlational linkages from single premotor cells to motoneurons will be considered in detail in later sections. Despite the critical role of descending systems in the control of limb movements, quantitative detail about the synaptic connections of these systems is relatively sketchy, especially in primates. Nevertheless, some generalizations concerning the synaptic effects of descending systems on motoneurons have emerged:

1. In primates, all descending systems make monosynaptic connections with at least some motoneurons. The proportion of motoneurons receiving monosynaptic corticospinal or rubrospinal input is 100% for the most distal muscles and diminishes for more proximal muscles. (Clough et al., 1968; Phillips and Porter, 1977). The magnitudes of corticospinal EPSPs vary in a parallel manner for motoneurons of distal and proximal muscles. Conversely, the incidence of monosynaptic input to motoneurons of proximal and axial muscles is greater for the ventro-medial descending systems than dorso-lateral systems.
2. In the cat, the dorso-lateral descending systems have a minimum disynaptic linkage to motoneurons, although some monosynaptic connections to muscles of the digits have been reported (Enberg, 1963; McCurdy et al., 1984). In the rat, about half of distal forelimb and hindlimb motoneurons receive monosynaptic input from the corticospinal system (Elger et al., 1977; Janzen et al., 1977). These connections may be related to the greater development of independent digits in the rat than in the cat and the rat's greater skill in their use.
3. The fast or slow nature of a muscle, and perhaps individual motor units within a muscle seems to be an important factor determining the synaptic action of the rubrospinal and corticospinal systems (Burke et al., 1970; Preston et al., 1967). Fast, phasic muscles such as the medial gastrocnemius are facilitated from cortex, whereas slow postural muscles such as soleus are predominantly inhibited. Within the gastrocneumius muscle, fast and slow motor units are also distinguished by the corticospinal and rubrospinal systems with fast units receiving facilitation and slow ones inhibition (Burke et al., 1970).
4. Information on unitary EPSPs from neurons of descending systems has been limited and fragmentary. Asanuma and Rosen (1972) reported an individual corticospinal EPSP of 100 μV. This experiment is technically much more difficult than the detection of individual EPSPs in motoneurons from muscle afferents partly because the identity of the premotor neuron's target muscles is uncertain. More systematic information on the magnitude and distribution of individual EPSPs and IPSPs, analogous to that which exists for spindle afferent postsynaptic potentials would clearly be of interest. The synaptic effects of individual corticospinal neurons on single motor units have been detected with cross-correlation techniques (Mantel and Lemon, 1987; Fortier et al., 1989).
5. As is clear from Table I, large gaps exist in our knowledge of input to motoneurons from

descending systems, particularly in the primate. For example, only corticospinal input has been investigated for forelimb muscles in the primate. In view of the large number of monkeys required for intracellular experiments, it seems unlikely that significant new studies can be expected. However, while not providing the same level of quantitative information about synaptic effects, spike-triggered averaging of EMG activity does yield detailed information about the sign, magnitude and distribution of synaptic effects on motoneurons and in conjunction with response properties of the same cells, provides a powerful approach toward achieving a more complete knowledge of premotor descending control of different muscles.

Spike-triggered averaging of EMG activity: Method for identifying the output properties of single premotor neurons

Rationale and procedure

The introduction of recording from single neurons in awake animals by Jasper et al. (1958) and its application to issues related to the cortical control of movement by Evarts (1966) has brought about great progress in understanding the functional role of descending systems. However, this approach has always been limited by the lack of information about the axonal projections of individual neurons. Ideally, the discharge of a particular premotor neuron should be interpreted in relation to its synaptic effects on motoneurons of its target muscles. With the introduction of spike-triggered averaging of EMG activity in awake animals, it has become possible to examine for the first time, not only the movement related discharge of single premotor neurons, but also the organization of their output effects on the activity of agonist and antagonist motoneurons.

To identify, in awake monkeys, cortical premotor cells with a functional linkage to motoneurons, Fetz and Cheney (1980) developed the method of spike-triggered averaging of rectified EMG activity. The rationale for this method is as follows. Premotor neurons with a direct excitatory synaptic linkage to motoneurons will produce individual EPSPs at a fixed latency following discharge of the premotor cell. The magnitude of these EPSPs will be too small to reliably discharge the motoneuron with each occurrence. Nevertheless, the EPSPs will depolarize the membrane, bringing the motoneuron closer to firing threshold and transiently increasing its firing probability. EMG activity is the sum of the spike trains of a population of motor units within a muscle. Since the neuromuscular junction normally has a high safety factor characterized by a one-to-one relationship between motoneuron and muscle fiber action potentials, motor unit spike trains provide an accurate reflection of the firing of spinal motoneurons. Therefore, the synaptic effect of a single premotor cell on motoneuron firing probability can be detected by averaging the EMG activity associated with many premotor cell spikes. These events are illustrated in Fig. 2 for the effects of a single muscle spindle Ia afferent on the firing probability of a target motoneuron and average EMG activity of the corresponding muscle.

Further details of the spike-triggered averaging procedure are illustrated in Fig. 3. In this case, the discharge of a single cortical neuron was recorded in relation to the extension phase of a ramp-and-hold wrist movement. EMG activity was full-wave rectified and the 30 ms segments extending from 5 ms before the trigger spike to 25 ms after the spike were digitized at 4 KHz and averaged. The EMG associated with each of the first five spikes in the record is shown (perispike EMG) along with the cumulative average of these EMG segments. Note that the prominent waveforms occurring about 10 ms after the first cortical spike are largely lost after the EMG segments associated with the first five spikes are averaged. However, an average of 2,000 spike events shows a clear peak beginning at a latency of 6 ms. Such a transient increase in average EMG activity is referred to as postspike facilitation (PSpF) and is interpreted as evidence of an underlying synaptic linkage between the trig-

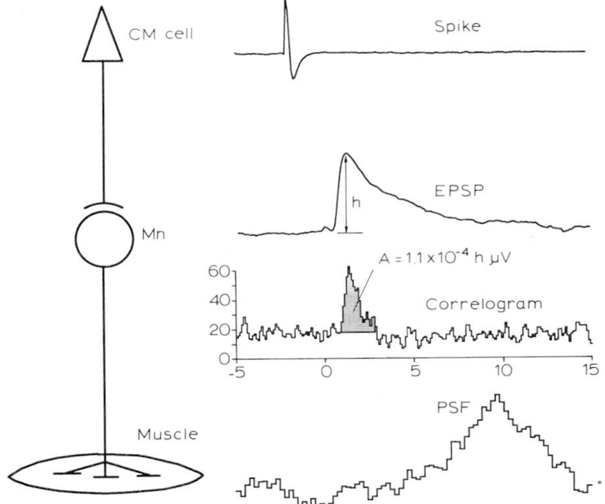

Fig. 2. Events mediating the postspike effects of a premotoneuronal cell connected monosynaptically to motoneurons. Spike discharges are followed by unitary EPSPs and an increase in motor unit firing probability reflecting the derivative of the EPSP. PSpF in the corresponding average of rectified EMG activity is delayed by conduction time from the spinal cord to the muscle. The area of the correlogram peak was found to be proportional to the height of the EPSP. The time course of PSpF is greater than the correlogram peak for a single motor unit because: 1) PSpF is the sum of facilitation in several motor units with different conduction velocities, and 2) the duration of the motor unit potential waveform contributes to PSpF. Data shown is for a muscle spindle Ia afferent (Cope et al., 1987). Figure from Fetz et al. (1989)

ger neuron and motoneurons. Cortical neurons yielding PSpF are referred to as corticomotoneuronal or CM cells; red nucleus neurons yielding PSpF are referred to as rubromotoneuronal or RM cells.

The strength of the spike-triggered averaging method is that it can be applied in awake animals enabling the identification of cells that are causally involved in producing muscle activity. The response properties of these motor output neurons can then be investigated during specific motor tasks. The response properties of these neurons are particularly important in understanding the contribution of descending systems to movement. Thus, the spike-triggered averaging method enables parallel investigation of the synaptic organization of premotor cells with motoneurons and investigation of relations between cell discharge and specific kinematic parameters of movement.

Spike-triggered averaging of rectified EMG activity is capable of revealing a cell's correlational linkages with motoneurons. However, compared to spike-triggered averages of intracellularly recorded synaptic potentials, it provides less precise information about the timing of synaptic events and, hence, the number of synapses in the linkage. Moreover, although postspike effects can be quantified to provide some measure of the relative strength of an underlying synaptic effect, the magnitudes of PSpF must be interpreted with caution. For example, PSpF from a premotor neuron that facilitated a small fraction of recorded motor units strongly might be similar in magnitude to PSpF from a neuron that facilitated a large fraction of the recorded motor units weakly. Cross correlating premotor cell discharge with single motor units avoids these ambiguities and provides a more exact and interpretable measure of the strength of a synaptic effect. However, recording isolated motor units is more difficult, and the probability of finding an effect may be low if the motor unit field of a premotor neuron is small.

Reliability and reproducibility of postspike effects

Identifying features in spike-triggered averages can sometimes be difficult, and a variety of approaches have been used to assess their reliability. A conceptually simple but statistically rigorous approach would be to compile several consecutive averages (five or more) all with the same number of trigger events (Kasser and Cheney, 1985). The effects in these averages could then be tested statistically by comparing them to averages computed under the same conditions but with random triggers (Fig. 4). Although this might be ideal from a statistical viewpoint, it requires an extensive amount of redundant data, which cannot always

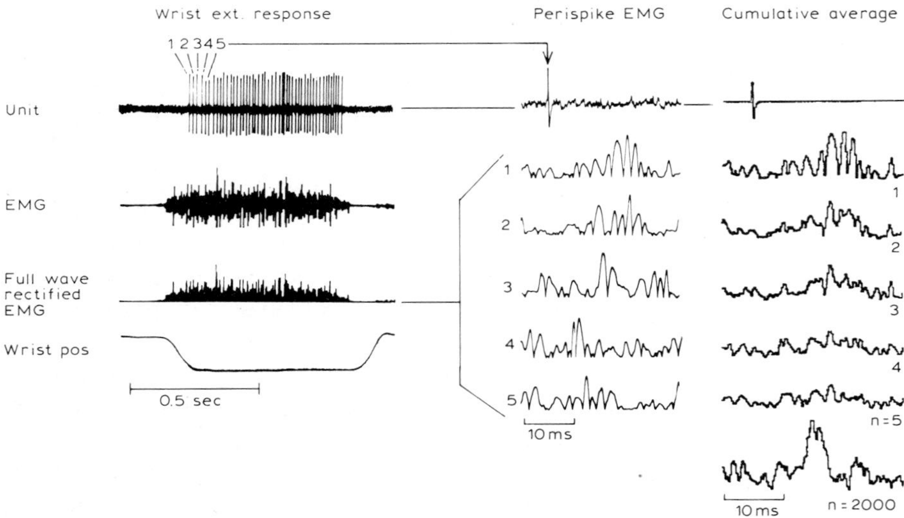

Fig. 3. Spike-triggered averaging procedure used to detect postspike effects from single premotor neurons. Spikes associated with movement are used to trigger averages of rectified EMG activity. The response at the left illustrates the discharge of a cortical cell and normal and rectified EMG activity of one agonist muscle associated with wrist extension. Thirty millisecond segments of EMG activity associated with each premotor cell spike are averaged. The cumulative average of EMG segments associated with the first five cell spikes are shown in the column at the right. Although no clear effects are present after five sweeps, the average of 2000 events shows a clear, transient postspike facilitation. (From Fetz and Cheney, 1980)

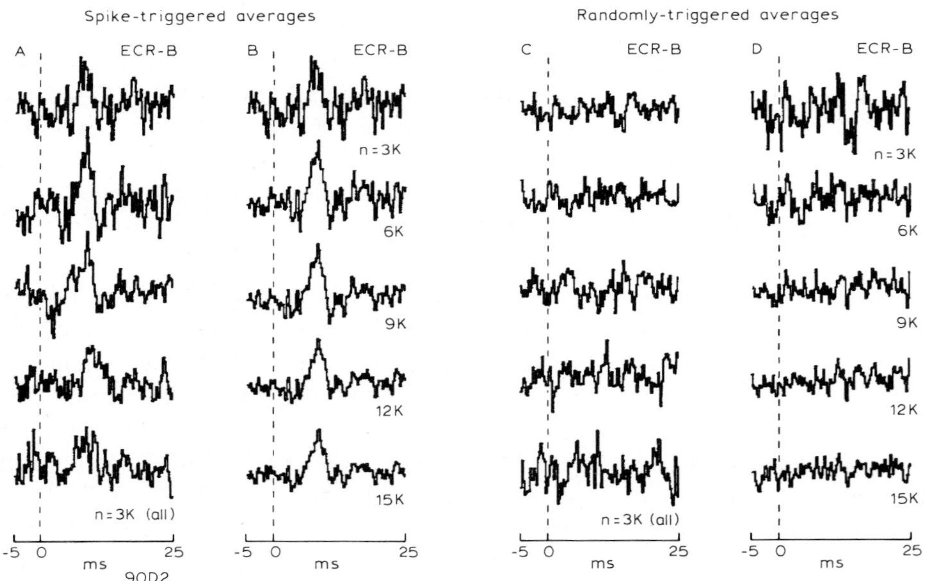

Fig. 4. CM cell spike-triggered averages and randomly-triggered averages of the same agonist muscle. Columns A and C show five consecutive averages of 3000 trigger events. Columns B and D show the cumulative averages of the records in A and C. Note the presence of clear PSpF in each 3K spike-triggered average and the absence of a clear effect in the randomly-triggered average. Also note the continuous improvement in signal-to-noise ratio with increasing numbers of trigger events. (From Kasser and Cheney, 1985)

be obtained during actual recording. Furthermore, this procedure seriously limits recording time available to complete a diverse protocol of tests. As a compromise, a similar but abbreviated approach to analysis of significance can be applied. The reproducibility of an effect must be demonstrated by showing that: 1) it appears in at least two consecutive averages of 2000 trigger events or more, or, more commonly, 2) that the signal to noise ratio of an effect improves as more sweeps are averaged (Botteron and Cheney, 1989). Statistical significance of facilitated or suppressed segments of a particular average is assessed by *t*-test comparisons with points in the baseline segment preceding the trigger spike (Fetz and Cheney, 1980; Kasser and Cheney, 1985). The onset and termination of an effect is measured as the point where the smoothed envelope of an effect crosses a line representing one or two standard deviations of the baseline points (Fig. 5). All averages are based on at least 2000 trigger events, although the number of trigger events is usually much higher.

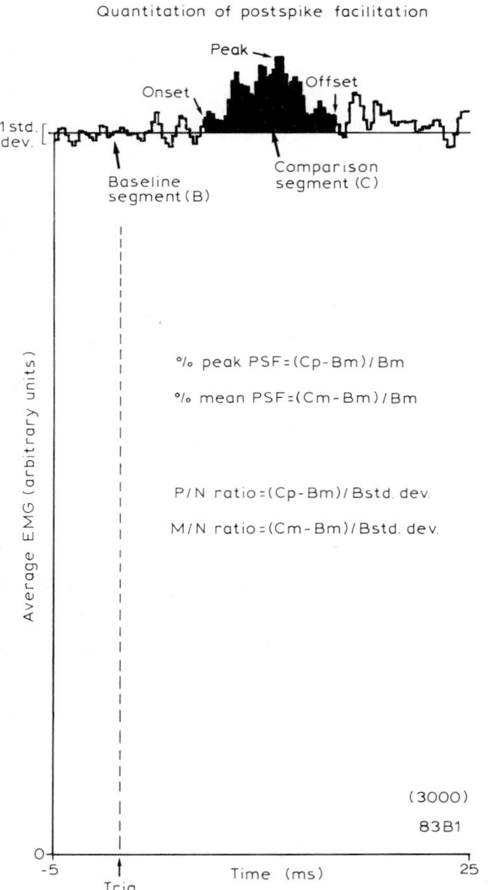

Fig. 5. Methods of quantifying postspike and poststimulus effects. The change from baseline of the facilitated or suppressed segment may be expressed as a percent of baseline or as a signal-to-noise ratio. In both cases, magnitude may be measured as either a peak or mean value. Bm = baseline mean, Cp = peak value, Cm = mean value in C segment. A related approach to quantifying postspike effects is to calculate a ratio of the peak effect to base line (referred to as k value) or the mean effect to base line (referred to as k′) (Mantel and Lemon, 1987)

Quantifying postspike effects

Postspike effects in averages of rectified EMG activity can be quantified by two different methods (Fig. 5). One measure expresses the increase or decrease in average EMG activity as a percent of baseline; the other expresses the increase or decrease as a signal-to-noise ratio. In both cases, facilitation and suppression can be measured as a peak or a mean of the facilitated or suppressed points. Signal-to-noise measures have the advantage of being independent of baseline level making comparisons of the strength of effects under widely varying conditions possible (Cheney and Mewes, 1985). Postspike effects in averages of EMG activity seem to obey the principle that applies generally to signal averaging: signal-to-noise ratio increases in proportion to the square root of the number of sweeps or trigger events. This has been directly validated for both PSpF and PSpS. For example, in Fig. 4, the peak-to-noise ratio of PSpF at 12,000 trigger events is double that at 3000 trigger events. Quantitative comparisons using signal-to-noise ratio measures must be normalized to a standard number of trigger events using the proportionality between magnitude and square root of the number of trigger events.

Detection of inhibitory effects with spike-triggered averaging of EMG activity

The utility of the spike-triggered averaging technique extends beyond the detection of excitatory synaptic effects. Cheney et al. (1982) and Kasser and Cheney (1985) first showed that postspike suppression (PSpS) of antagonist muscles from CM cells is detectable with spike-triggered averaging of rectified EMG activity. Fig. 6 is an example of PSpS from a cortical cell whose discharge increased during wrist flexion. Spike-triggered averages show clear facilitation of multiple agonist muscles (extensors) and reciprocal suppression of the antagonists. FCR was strongly suppressed at a latency slightly longer than the PSpF of the extensors. Additional flexors showed weaker but clear PSpS. The average magnitude of PSpS is about half that of PSpF and the onset latency of PSpS is about 3 ms longer than that of PSpF. These findings are consistent with involvement of interneurons in mediation of PSpS. Kasser and Cheney (1985) concluded that PSpS is probably mediated by collaterals of CM cells to Ia inhibitory interneurons, since corticospinal input to these interneurons is well established (Jankowska and Tanaka, 1974; Jankowska et al., 1976). CM cell collaterals to other cortical cells with direct inhibitory synapses on motoneurons is unlikely because monosynaptic IPSPs from motor cortex have never been reported. Therefore, detection of effects with spike-triggered averaging of EMG activity is not limited to monosynaptic linkages but

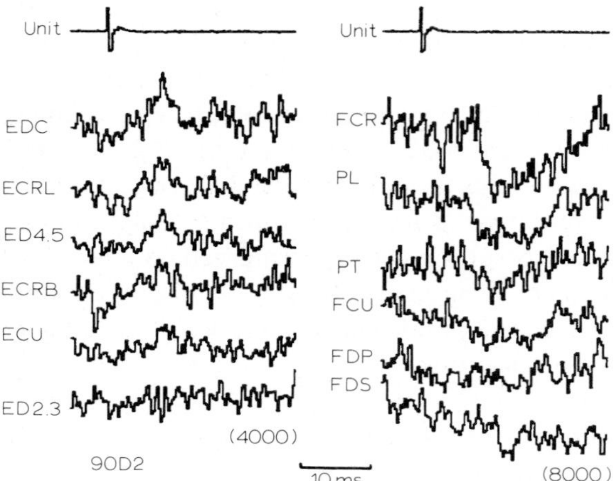

Fig. 6. Spike-triggered averages for a reciprocally organized CM cell. This cell produced clear PSpF in multiple extensor muscles and clear PSpS in multiple flexor muscles. (Kasser and Cheney, unpublished)

also includes less direct linkages. Additional non-obligatory synapses, however, will weaken the strength of the primary correlation peak and will broaden its time course (Fetz and Cheney, 1980). Consequently, the clearest effects will generally be those mediated by monosynaptic linkages. Comparison of PSpF with reciprocal PSpS confirms this view (Kasser and Cheney, 1985).

The fact that disynaptic inhibitory linkages are detectable with spike-triggered averaging raises the question of detectability of disynaptic excitatory events. Preliminary studies of postspike effects from cells in motor thalamus of the monkey show some cases of clear, reproducible PSpF (Fig. 7, from unpublished work of Mewes and Cheney). Since cells of motor thalamus are known to project monosynaptically to pyramidal tract cells, the minimum synaptic linkage to motoneurons is disynaptic (Amassian and Weiner, 1966; Araki and Endo, 1976; Purpura et al., 1964). Therefore, disynaptic excitatory linkages are also clearly detectable with spike-triggered averaging of EMG activity. Sensitivity capable of revealing non-monosynaptic linkages is an asset in so far as it enables identification of cells, such as those in motor thalamus, that provide input to premotor neurons of descending systems and ultimately have powerful effects on muscle activity. The relations of these cells to movement and to the discharge of premotor neurons to which they project can then be investigated knowing that the cells are causally involved in the movement. The contribution of disynaptic linkages to PSpF from CM and RM cells must also be considered possible.

Interpretation of cross correlograms in relation to underlying EPSPs

Postspike effects are generated only from EPSPs that cause the motoneuron to fire or IPSPs that prevent motoneuron firing. It should be noted that spike-triggered averaging of EMG activity requires that both the trigger neuron and muscle are simultaneously active. In this case, the postsynaptic potentials from the trigger cell will be superimposed on motoneuron membrane trajectories associated with repetitive firing in which voltage threshold for spike initiation is approached as a

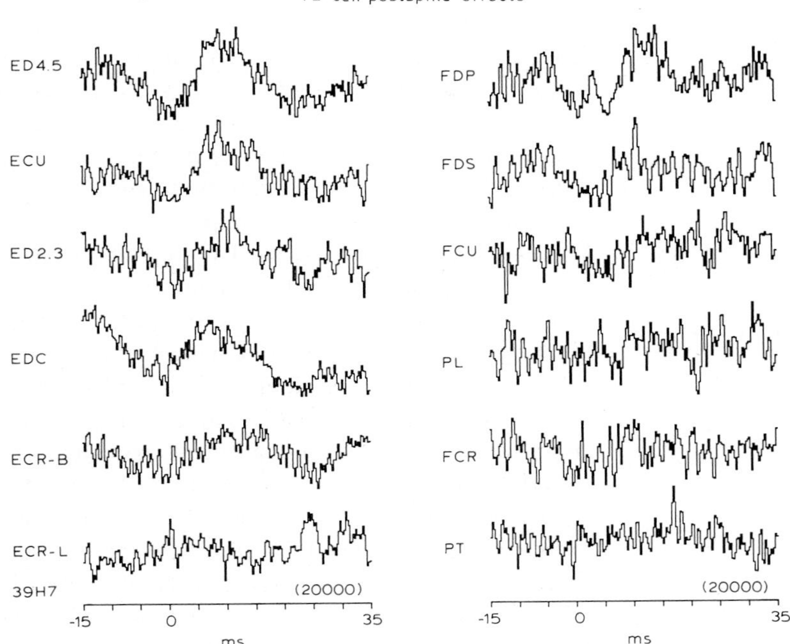

Fig. 7. Postspike facilitation of multiple extensor muscles from a cell in motor thalamus of a monkey. Minimum linkage for these effects is disynaptic. Number of trigger events in parentheses. (Mewes and Cheney, unpublished)

ramp trajectory (Fig. 8). Only EPSPs that depolarize the motoneuron to threshold or IPSPs that prevent its depolarization to threshold will contribute to postspike effects observed in averages of EMG activity. Since the motoneuron membrane potential moves toward threshold during the rising phase of an EPSP, the increased firing probability of a motoneuron is associated primarily with the rise of the EPSP. The advanced occurrence of these spikes in the correlogram peak leaves a subsequent trough, that is, a period of reduced firing probability. Consequently, the changes in firing probability of a motoneuron associated with the EPSP reflect primarily the derivative of the EPSP rather than the EPSP itself (Fetz and Cheney, 1980). The trough will be shallower than the peak because the interval from which spikes are drawn is longer than the rising phase of the EPSP. These predictions were directly confirmed in cat motoneurons: the increase in motoneuron firing probability following electrical stimulation of Ia afferents in the peripheral nerve coincided with the rising phase of the compound EPSP (Fetz and Gustafsson, 1983). The mean half-width of correlogram peaks (0.65 ms) agreed closely with the mean half width of the EPSP derivatives (0.55 ms) but not with the mean half width of the EPSPs (4.31 ms). Large EPSPs always produced correlogram peaks that best matched their derivatives, whereas small EPSPs in the presence of synaptic noise often produced correlogram peaks that were wider than their derivatives. The duration of correlogram peaks for single motor units from CM cells spikes (Mantel and Lemon, 1987) and microstimuli applied in the vicinity of CM cells (Palmer and Fetz, 1985b) also had durations consistent with the derivative of the CM -EPSP rather than the EPSP itself.

More recently, Cope et al. (1987) examined the shapes of correlogram peaks produced by the smaller amplitude, fast rising unitary EPSPs evoked from single Ia afferent fibers. Again, the dura-

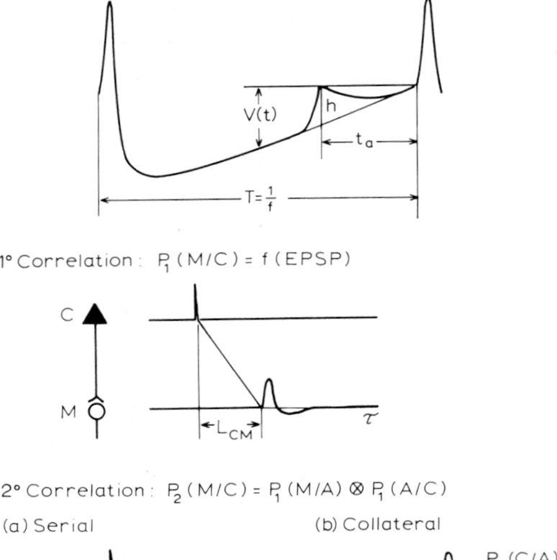

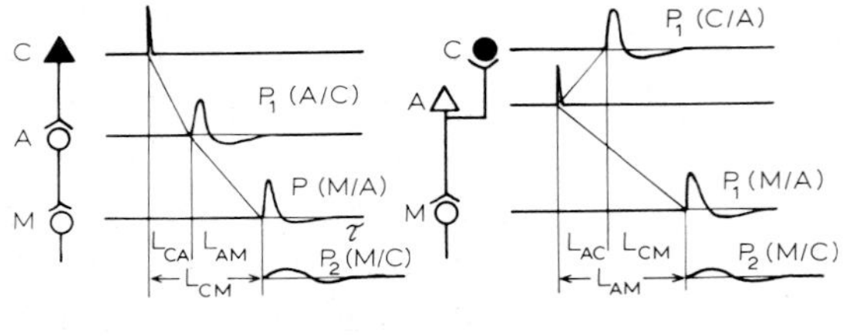

Fig. 8. Relation between synaptic connections and cross-correlogram features. *Top*: schematic representation of EPSP superimposed on membrane potential of a repetitively firing motoneuron; t_a = time during which EPSP may trigger a motoneuron action potential. *Bottom*: neural connections which could yield PSpF. Monosynaptic connection produces primary correlation; disynaptic links produce secondary correlations that is the convolution of underlying primary correlations (From Fetz and Cheney, 1980)

tion of the correlogram peak could be accounted for largely by a component proportional to the derivative of the EPSP (Fig. 2). The correlogram peak area was best correlated with EPSP amplitude. In SpTAs of multiunit EMG activity, the onset of PSpF is delayed from the onset of the motoneuron correlogram peak due to conduction time to the muscle. PSpF is also much broader than the motor unit correlogram peak because of contributions from the motor unit potentials themselves (about 4 ms) and contributions resulting from the summation of potentials from multiple facilitated motor units with different conduction times to the periphery.

IPSPs produced primary correlogram troughs followed by compensatory peaks (Fetz and Gustafsson, 1983). Again, this is consistent with the ramp trajectory of membrane potential toward threshold in a repetitively firing motoneuron. The IPSP delays the occurrence of spikes, forming a correlogram trough followed by a compensatory peak. These delayed spikes will tend to collect at a later point forming the compensatory peak. Unlike correlogram peaks associated with EPSPs, correlogram troughs associated with IPSPs were wider than the IPSP derivatives and did not correspond to any linear combination of the shape of the IPSPs or its derivative. Another significant difference between EPSPs and IPSPs is the increase in magnitude of the IPSP near threshold; this means that IPSPs having the same amplitude as EPSPs when measured at rest actually have a three-fold greater effect when the motoneuron is firing.

Contribution of discharge synchrony to postspike effects

A question raised frequently concerning the interpretation of spike-triggered averages is the degree to which postspike effects may be mediated by other cells that are synchronized with the trigger cell. For example, a cell lacking axonal connections with motoneurons could, nevertheless, show PSpF if its discharge was sufficiently synchronized with a true premotor cell. Synchrony might result from collateral synaptic input (Fig. 8b) or from shared input from the same afferent axons. PSpFs resulting from synchrony with a true premotor cell arising from axon collaterals or common synaptic input constitute second and third order correlations respectively (Fetz and Cheney, 1980). Such higher order correlations are the convolution of the individual primary correlations in the circuit. In the case of collateral synaptic input to a non-premotor cell (C in Fig. 8b), the primary correlations are between cell C and A (the actual premotor cell) and between A and the motoneuron

(M). Common synaptic input to A and C (not illustrated) would involve primary correlations between C and the afferent input cell, from the afferent input cell to a true premotor cell (A), and finally from the premotor cell to the motoneuron. In each case, the increase in probability of firing of the motoneuron associated with the spikes of the non-premotor cell is the product of the primary correlations in the circuit. PSpF resulting from such indirect neuronal circuits should be weaker and broader than that from monosynaptic linkages.

Smith and Fetz (1989) recently quantified the contribution of synchrony between neighboring cortical neurons, including CM cells, to PSpF. Thirty-five percent of 217 cortical cell pairs exhibited correlogram peaks that straddled the origin, consistent with common synaptic input. Fifteen cell pairs with common synaptic input were combinations of a non-CM with a CM cell. Despite the presence of a clear correlogram peak between the CM cell and non-CM cell, none of the 15 non-CM cells showed significant postspike effects. This demonstrates that synchrony of discharge arising from common synaptic input is insufficient to mediate PSpF from a cell lacking axonal connections with motoneurons.

For CM cells facilitating the same muscles, the contribution of synchrony to PSpF was evaluated by computing spike-triggered averages from cells after eliminating the synchronized spikes as triggers (Fig. 9). The records in the left column were all compiled with the spikes of Cell A as the trigger. Record (a) shows the distribution of spikes from cell B relative to spikes of Cell A aligned at zero time (cross-correlogram of A on B). The solid line is the correlogram after eliminating the triggers that were synchronized with spikes of Cell B; the dotted line shows the correlogram peak of synchronized spikes without any spike selection. After eliminating synchronized spikes, PSpF from each cell was observed in the same muscles and was in all respects similar to the control averages computed from all the cell's spikes (compare b and c). The contribution of synchronized spikes is revealed by subtracting the SpTAs obtained from non-synchronized spikes from the corresponding control SpTA (b from c). The difference between control and selected SpTAs is essentially flat (f). Records in the column under Cell B show the correlogram of cell B on A before and after eliminating synchronized spikes and the corresponding control PSpF and spike selected PSpF. Again, synchrony made virtually no contribution to PSpF. As a further test of the contribution of synchrony, the cross-correlogram containing the synchronized spikes was convolved with the PSpF of the CM cell (records d and e for cell A). The peak in the convolution was much smaller than the peak of the PSpF and had a time course matching the broad shoulders of the PSpF but lacking the sharply defined center peak of the PSpF.

Some important conclusions can be drawn from these findings. First, the contribution of one CM cell to the PSpF of a synchronized CM cell seems to be negligible and not a major concern in using spike-triggered averaging of EMG activity to identify CM cells or the distribution of their effects to motoneurons of different muscles. Second, the contribution that synchrony does make is largely to the broad, gradually changing shoulders of the PSpF rather than to the primary PSpF peak itself. This may account for the early onset of some PSpFs.

The modest contribution of synchrony to PSpF may seem to contradict evidence of clear PSpF from cells in motor thalamus (Fig. 7) and clear PSpS of antagonist muscles (Fig. 6), both of which must be mediated by a minimum disynaptic linkage. However, the strength of synapses in indirect linkages and the number of interneurons are important factors in determining whether significant features in correlations will be detected. Stimulus-triggered averages from thalamic cells may reveal effects mediated by synaptic linkages through motor cortex, and through red nucleus, via potent connections of interpositus axons. Nevertheless, it remains clear that the characteristics of most PSpFs are consistent with mediation by a monosynaptic linkage. The later components of PSpF, however, might receive a contribution from disynaptic linkages.

Spike-triggered averages of unrectified EMG activity

Normally EMG activity is rectified before averaging to avoid possible cancellation of negative and positive components of motor unit potentials and to eliminate any ambiguity between excitatory and inhibitory events. However, Botteron and Cheney (1989) recently showed that postspike effects are also clearly detectable in averages of unrectified EMG activity. Of 110 muscles showing PSpFs in averages of rectified EMG activity, 49 (45%) also showed clear postspike effects in corresponding averages of

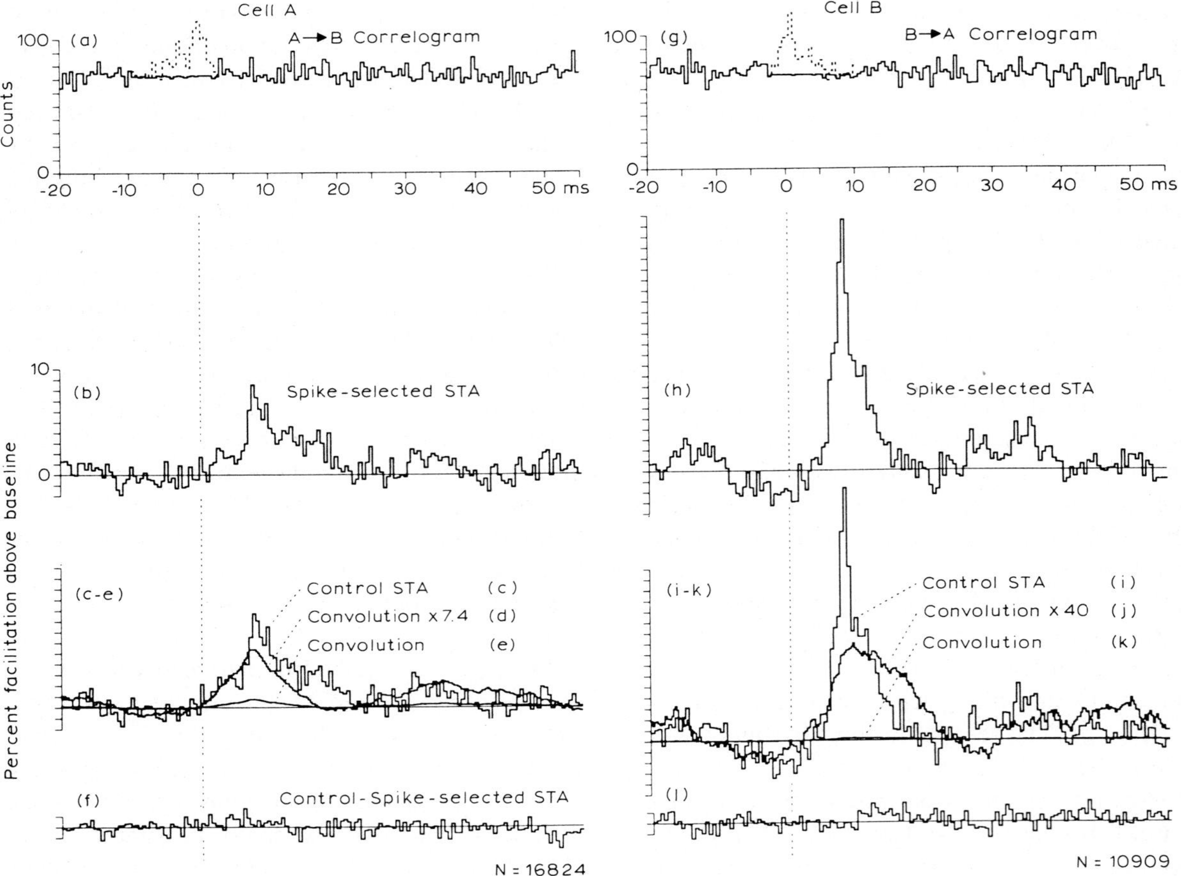

Fig. 9. Contribution of spike synchrony to PSpF. Analysis for a pair of simultaneously recorded CM cells. Effect of synchrony was evaluated by two methods. First, by eliminating the synchronized spikes as trigger events and comparing spike selected and control spike-triggered averages. Second, by convolving the cross-correlogram of cell B using A as the reference with the spike selected spike-triggered average from cell A. Same analysis was performed for Cell A using B as a reference. (a,g): cross-correlograms of Cell B with A as a reference (left) and Cell A with B as a reference (right). Dotted lines are correlograms including all spikes; solid lines are correlograms with synchronized spikes excluded. Spike selected averages (b, h) match control averages (c, i) indicating little or no contribution of synchronized spikes to PSpF. (f,l): control spike-triggered average minus spike selected average. Convolution represents the component of spike-triggered average expected from synchronized spikes of the other cell. The convolution peak corresponds with the broad component of the PSpF and has an early onset latency. The magnitude of the convolution peaks were 1/7 and 1/40 the magnitude of the broad component corresponding PSpFs. (From Smith and Fetz, 1989)

unrectified EMG activity. Remarkably, clear postspike effects in unrectified EMGs were also found in association with 50% of the cases of CM cell suppression of muscle activity (Fig. 10). The waveform that emerges from the unrectified EMG in association with PSpF is the average of the waveforms of all the facilitated motor unit potentials displaced in time according to their onset latency. Similarly, the waveform in the average of unrectified EMG activity associated with PSpS is the inverse of the suppressed motor unit potentials. Although effects in unrectified EMGs are some times clearer than in averages of rectified EMGs, cancellation of effects by summation of the positive and negative components of different motor unit potentials was confirmed as a serious problem leading, in some cases, to complete loss of

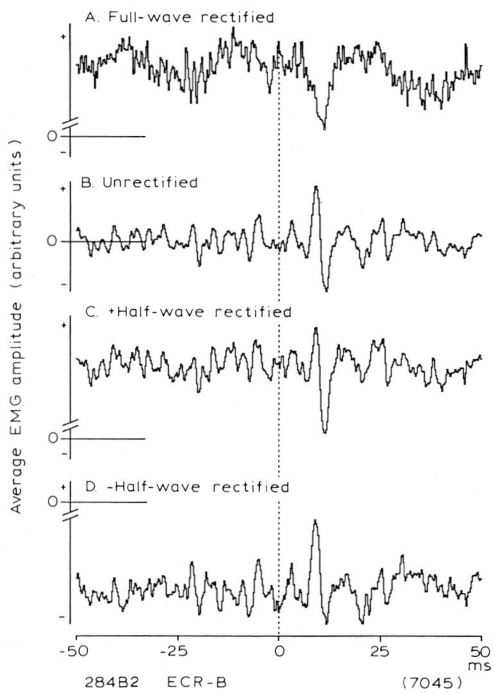

Fig. 10. Effect in unrectified EMG associated with PSpS. Waveforms of opposite polarity in half-wave rectified EMGs are not overlapping and cancellation does not occur. Waveforms in unrectified averages are the inverse of the suppressed motor unit potentials. (Botteron and Cheney, 1989)

effects. Nevertheless, averages of unrectified EMGs were useful in clarifying the nature of some postspike effects that were classified as complex based on latencies that were too short to be consistent with underlying anatomical connections. Effects in averages of unrectified EMGs had appropriate latencies and these cells could then be confidently classified as premotor cells.

Cross-correlations between premotor neurons and single motor units

Spike-triggered averaging of multinunit EMG activity with indwelling multistranded stainless steel wires benefits from broad sampling of the motor units within a muscle. This might enhance the probability of detecting postspike effects in cases of a restricted distribution of synapses from a premotor cell within a motoneuron pool. In addition, averaging the EMG signal itself prolongs the PSpF and enhances detection because the individual facilitated motor unit potentials usually straddle many sampling points. However, while this may account for some of the success of the method, it also introduces complications that render quantifying effects more difficult. Furthermore, PSpF in averages of EMG activity provides no information about the extent of facilitation of individual motor units within the muscle. These limitations can be addressed by computing cross-correlograms between the discharges of single premotor neurons and individual motor units within a muscle. Using this approach, Mantel and Lemon (1987) found clear peaks in the cross-correlograms of single CM cells and individual motor units in a target muscle. Fig. 11 is an example of a CM cell that produced clear PSpF in an average of surface EMG from abductor pollicis brevis (record A). Cross-correlations revealed that the cell also facilitated all three of the single motor units recorded with the same CM cell. The cross-correlogram peaks for individual motor units are weaker and narrower (mean half-width = 1.9 ms) than the PSpF of surface EMG. Of 31 motor units tested with 11 CM cells, 27 showed significant facilitation. Similar proportions of facilitated motor units were found by Fortier et al. (1989). These results suggest a relatively broad distribution of terminals to different motoneurons within the motoneuron pool. This conclusion is further supported by the findings of Palmer and Fetz (1985b) who cross-correlated single motor unit activity with single intracortical microstimuli (S-ICMS). As many as 8 single motor units from an individual facilitated forearm muscle were tested for effects from S-ICMS at 23 cortical output sites. Overall, 95% (99 of 104) of motor units tested were facilitated by low intensity S-ICMS, again suggesting a broad distribution of terminals from CM cells to different motoneurons within a pool.

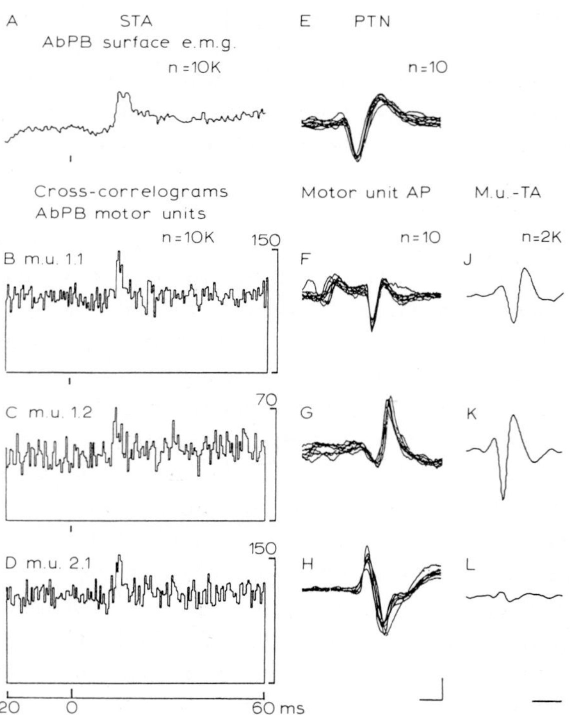

Fig. 11. Cross-correlograms of three single motor units in Abductor pollicis brevis (AbPB) triggered from a CM cell. (A). Spike-triggered average of rectified EMG activity. (B, C and D): Cross correlation functions for three AbPB motor units with reference to the discharge of a CM cell at zero time. (E). Spike waveform of the CM cell. (F, G and H): spike waveforms of the three motor units. (J, K and L): average spike waveforms of the three motor units. (From Mantel and Lemon, 1987)

Characteristics of PSpF and PSpS from single premotor neurons

Spike-triggered averaging of EMG activity has been used to analyze the output effects of single corticospinal and rubrospinal neurons on wrist and digit muscles in the monkey (Cheney et al., 1988; Fetz and Cheney, 1980; Lemon and Muir, 1983; Lemon et al., 1986; Mewes and Cheney, 1986). The sign and distribution of synaptic effects on motoneurons of agonist and antagonist muscles have been investigated under similar conditions for both CM and RM cells. Agonist muscles are defined as those which are coactivated with the cell during voluntary movement. To activate CM cells that are normally silent during the antagonist phase of movement, Kasser and Cheney (1983) developed a double barrelled microelectrode suitable for combined recording and glutamate iontophoresis in the awake monkey. Discharge during the antagonist phase of movement was evoked with glutamate. Spikes were then gated during either flexion or extension and used as triggers for compiling averages of the corresponding muscles. RM cells always showed a sustained background discharge throughout the alternating wrist movement cycle. Consequently, the output effects of these cells on antagonist muscles could be tested without using glutamate iontophoresis.

The characteristics of PSpF and PSpS studied with the same methods and under the same behavioral conditions are detailed in Table II. As expected, the latency of RM postspike effects are shorter than those of CM cell effects by about one millisecond. Since the conduction velocities of CM and RM cells are similar (Landgren et al., 1962a,b; Shapovalov et al., 1971; Shapovalov, 1973), this difference can be attributed to the shorter conduction distance to motoneurons for RM cells. It is also worth noting that for both CM and RM cells, the latency of PSpS is about 3 ms longer than the latency of PSpF. As discussed above, this suggests mediation of suppression by non-monosynaptic pathways. Disynaptic inhibition from Ia afferents to antagonist motoneurons has a latency that is

TABLE II

Characteristics of postspike effects from CM and RM cells

Postspike effects	CM	RM
Onset latency		
PSpF	6.3 ± 1.6	5.9 ± 1.9
PSpS	10.1 ± 2.8	9.3 ± 3.0
Peak magnitude (% of baseline)		
PSpF	7.0 ± 6.6	4.1 ± 2.0
PSpS	4.1 ± 2.4	4.0 ± 2.3
Number muscles with PSpF/cell	3.0	3.0
Number muscles with PSpS/cell	1.3	2.1

CM cell data from Kasser and Cheney (1985); RM cell data from work of Mewes and Cheney.

about one millisecond longer than excitation (Jankowska and Roberts, 1972). The three millisecond latency difference between PSpF and PSpS, therefore, seems somewhat long and remains unexplained. Nevertheless, it is known that corticospinal and rubrospinal neurons terminate on Ia inhibitory interneurons, and this seems to be a likely pathway for PSpS.

CM and RM cells facilitated not one but an average of three muscles of the five to six coactivated forearm agonists tested. The distribution of PSpS was more restricted for both CM and RM cells; this may be related to the fact that PSpS is weaker and more difficult to detect (Table II). It should be noted that three facilitated muscles per CM or RM cell holds for cells related to alternating wrist movements involving simple coactivation of forearm wrist and digit muscles. Cells related to more discrete tasks, such as precision grip between the thumb and index finger, show more restricted muscle fields (Lemon et al., 1986).

Functional output patterns of PSpF and PSpS from single premotor neurons

The output effects of CM and RM cells on motoneurons of agonist and antagonist muscles are organized in functionally meaningful patterns. Three fundamental categories of output effects on agonist and antagonist muscles can be identified – pure facilitation, reciprocal and cofacilitation (Fig. 12; Data compiled from: Kasser and Cheney, 1985; Smith and Fetz, unpublished work; Mewes and Cheney, unpublished work). Pure facilitation cells facilitated agonist muscles but had no detectable effect on the antagonists. Just over half of the CM cells and 39% of the RM cells were of this type. Reciprocal cells facilitated the agonists and simultaneously suppressed the antagonists. Thirty percent of CM cells and 27% of RM cells were of this type. Cofacilitation cells were common in the RM cell population (18%) but only a few examples were identified in CM cell recordings.

The reciprocal and cofacilitation cell types are particularly noteworthy because they represent clear examples of ways in which descending systems are functionally organized for specific types of movements. Reciprocally organized cells are well suited for mediating the reciprocal pattern of extensor and flexor muscle activation associated

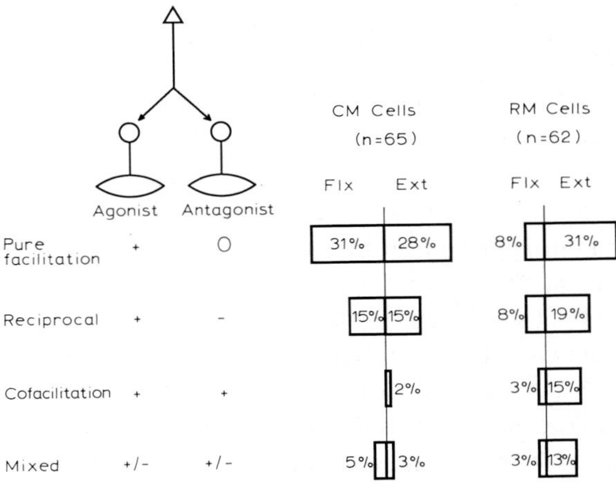

Fig. 12. Projection patterns of CM and RM cell output types to flexor and extensor muscles. Pure facilitation cells facilitated agonist muscles and had no effect on antagonists; reciprocal cells facilitated agonists and reciprocally suppressed the antagonists; cofacilitation cells simultaneously facilitated both flexor and extensor muscles; and mixed cells facilitated some agonists and suppressed others. Note that RM cells preferentially facilitate extensor muscles but CM cells are equally divided between those that facilitate extensors and flexors. (From Fetz et al., 1989)

with alternating movements. Similarly, the cofacilitation pattern is well suited for responses such as power grip that involve coactivation of forearm flexors and extensors to stabilize the wrist. Cofacilitation cells may also help bring motoneurons to threshold, independent of the direction of movement. Some additional minor categories of cells produced: 1) mixed effects, that is, facilitation and suppression in different synergist muscles, 2) pure suppression of antagonist muscles with no effects on agonists, and 3) inverse effects – facilitation of antagonists coupled, in some cases, with suppression of agonists.

In addition to these functional patterns of CM and RM cell output organization, other preferences in the distribution of PSpF and PSpS were observed. Most striking was the preferential facilitation of extensor muscles by RM cells (Fig. 12). Whereas CM cells were equally divided between those that facilitated either flexor or extensor muscles, 78% of RM cells facilitated extensors either exclusively or predominantly. This strong preference in favor of facilitation of extensors was also present in the microstimulation data. Even at sites where individual cells facilitated flexor muscles, stimulation predominantly facilitated extensor muscles (Mewes et al., 1987).

Although the number of CM cells facilitating flexor and extensor muscles was not different, the magnitude of PSpF in extensors was greater than that in flexors, and a similar tendency existed for RM cells (Cheney et al., 1988).

Beyond these preferences, individual CM and RM cells did not show a strong bias favoring facilitation of a specific muscle or combination of muscles. No particular muscle or combination of muscles was facilitated with any greater probability than others, although a weak tendency for stronger and more frequent facilitation of EDC was evident.

Modules of output organization in descending systems

Maps of topographic representation

Premotor neurons of most descending systems are not arranged randomly but rather show ordered representation of the peripheral muscular apparatus at two different levels. On a large scale, premotor neurons are arranged in an orderly fashion such that neurons controlling adjacent body parts occupy contiguous areas of the cortical or brainstem region. The existence of such a topographic organization for motor cortex has been known since the earliest stimulation experiments. More recently, movements evoked by applying electrical stimuli to the surface of motor cortex have been mapped in detail for a variety of species including humans and these general maps are well known (Phillips and Porter, 1977). A broad orderly representation of the contralateral musculature exists in motor cortex of all primate species. The basic pattern of organization is one in which the foot is represented most medially in the precentral gyrus followed laterally by more proximal muscles of the leg, the trunk, arm, hand and, most laterally, the representation of the face and tongue. An important feature of such maps is the disproportionately large representation devoted to muscles used in skilled movements of the face and hands compared to that devoted to control of large proximal muscles used in postural control and locomotion. Kwan et al. (1978) presented a variation of this motor map based on movement relations of arm neurons and microstimulation findings in the monkey. They concluded that muscles of the arm are represented in a radial pattern in the cortex with hand muscles at the center, wrist muscles in a band encircling the hand representation, elbow muscles next and finally shoulder muscles in the most peripheral band. Clear topographic organization has also been established for the rubrospinal and vestibulospinal systems, but as yet, none has been established for the reticulospinal system (Brodal, 1981).

The maps of motor representation derived from these studies have been very useful in understanding the coarse features of descending system organization; but how much variability exists in the maps from one subject to the another? Topographic maps provide only a general picture of the organization. Detailed features of the organization will vary across subjects and to an even greater extent across species. For example, from the topographic maps of red nucleus it is only possible to conclude that the arm representation is located dorso medially and the leg representation ventolaterally. Further details may vary and must be established on an individual basis. Similarly, in motor cortex the relative location of representation for major body parts, for example, the hand, is consistent across subjects but the relative locations from which specific movements of the hand and digits can be elicited with electrical stimulation of cortex will vary in different subjects. The amount of cortical area from which a particular movement can be evoked with intracortical microstimulation may also vary in different subjects. Such variations may reflect the history of the subject's use of that movement. Nudo and Merzenich (unpublished data) showed that the area of motor cortex in monkeys from which movements of the hand and digits could be evoked with microstimulation enlarged after several days of performing a skilled movement of the hand. Therefore, the details of cortical motor maps show plasticity and may become remodelled adaptively as a function of use.

Columnar organization in motor cortex?

As Phillips and Porter (1977) pointed out, the most elemental unit of output organization from motor cortex is the single spinal cord-projecting premotor neuron – the CM cell. However, do these neurons form higher order functional aggregates in which all cells of the aggregate share common features? In motor cortex, a further consideration is whether the common features extend across cortical lamina to form columns. Although evidence for columnar organization in primary sensory cortical areas is very clear, comparable evidence for columns in motor cortex is lacking. There can be no doubt that the basic architecture of motor cortex is radial in its orientation. The thalamocortical and association fibers supplying afferent inputs to motor cortex are radially oriented as are the apical dendrites of pyramidal tract neurons themselves (Phillips and Porter, 1977). Asanuma and Rosen (1972) presented evidence for a columnar organization of input-output modules in motor cortex. In experiments combining microstimulation and unit recording in tranquilized monkeys, they found that sites evoking the same movement, for example, abduction of the thumb, tended to be aligned as columns within the cortex. Moreover, the sensory receptive fields of neurons in a column typically included the joint or skin region moved by stimulation at that site. Based on these results, a columnar organization of tightly organized input-output processing modules was proposed. However, Lemon and Porter (1976) failed to find evidence of a precise segregation of sensory inputs to cortical cells of a single output zone in awake monkeys, meticulously trained to allow passive manipulation of the limbs. Of 18 pairs of neighboring neurons (within 500 μm of each other), 11 pairs showed closely related afferent input zones but the remainder had widely disparate sensory inputs. Existing evidence concerning the columnar organization of motor output zones is also complicated by the fact the "columns" thus far studied have been largely in the bank of the precentral gyrus making vertical penetration through the full length of a single column difficult. Furthermore, conclusions about the size and distribution of motor cortical columns have been based on relatively few observations. Also, evoked movements rather than a more sensitive measure of muscle activation, such as EMG activity, has been used to identify motor output effects. It seems clear that much additional work is needed to place columnar organization in motor cortex on a firm footing.

Functional aggregates of CM and RM cells

Although strong evidence for columnar organization of cells in motor cortex is lacking, evidence favoring the existence of functional aggregates or assemblies of CM cells in lamina V of motor cortex is compelling. Large injections of HRP in the spinal cord have shown that corticospinal neurons are not uniformly distributed in lamina V of motor cortex but rather are organized as aggregates or clusters consisting of 4 – 20 cells occupying a 0.5 – 1.0 mm diameter area (Coulter et al., 1976; Jones and Wise, 1977; Murray and Coulter, 1981). Clustering of corticospinal neurons has also been suggested based on antidromic activation of pyramidal tract neurons (Humphrey and Rietz, 1976; Kwan et al., 1978). Fig. 13 illustrates corticospinal cell clustering from an experiment in which all or nearly all the corticospinal neurons were labelled with HRP (Jones and Wise, 1977). This reconstruction shows the distribution of corticospinal neurons both in sagittal sections and viewing the surface of the cortex as a flattened sheet. Aggregation of corticospinal neurons in area 4 and adjacent cortical areas is clear from sagittal sections. Reconstruction of the distribution of these neurons across the entire territory of area 4 and SI viewed as a flattened sheet shows that the corticospinal cell aggregates tend to form strips oriented medio-laterally. Individual strips give off

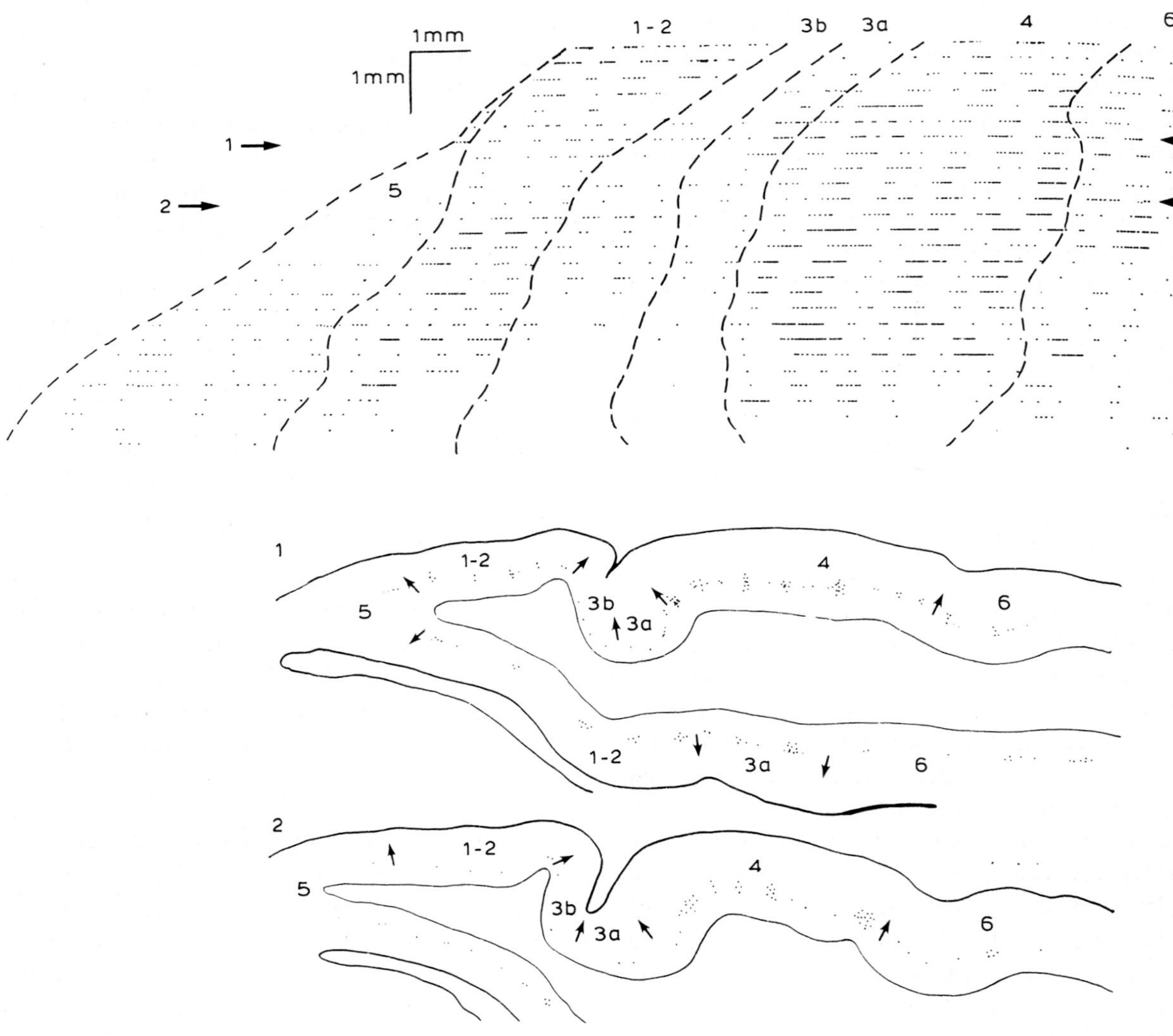

Fig. 13. Distribution of HRP labelled corticospinal neurons in cerebral cortex of monkey. Distribution is shown for cross sections and for the flattened cortex. Arrows indicate levels of cross sections. Note that corticospinal neurons occur as clusters and that the clusters tend to form medio-laterally oriented strips. (From Jones and Wise, 1977)

branches that merge with adjacent strips.

Although the functional significance of the strips is unknown, clusters of corticospinal cells may represent fundamental modules of output from motor cortex. If these clusters are to be viewed as unit modules of output organization, it must be shown that the cells of a cluster share common functional properties. What may be the common functional property of neurons belonging to a cluster? Recent evidence comparing the postspike and poststimulus effects obtained at CM cell sites suggests that the common property shared by neighboring CM cells (probably cells of the same cluster) is the distribution of output terminations to motoneurons. Cheney and Fetz (1985) found that the pattern of poststimulus facilitation across a set of six extensor or flexor muscles closely matched the pattern of postspike facilitation obtained from a single CM cell recorded at the same site. Stimuli were applied through the microelectrode at the recording sites of CM cells under the same behavioral conditions that were used to compute spike-triggered averages (Fig. 14). To avoid spread of effects by temporal summation, stimuli were delivered at a rate of 15 Hz or less. Because this intracranial microstimulation method reveals the effects of a single stimulus, it is referred to as stimulus-triggered averaging or S-ICMS. The results from one CM cell site are illustrated in Fig. 15. In this example, FCU was the only muscle facilitated by the CM cell. Stimulus-triggered averages at 8, 10 and 20 μA revealed poststimulus facilitation (PStF) restricted to FCU, strengthening the conclusion that PSpF was mediated by the recorded CM cell. Although exhibiting a similar distribution, PStF was much greater in magnitude than PSpF. In Fig. 15, the magnitude of effects in FCU at 8 μA appear similar to that of PSpF. However, PStF is actually much greater in magnitude because it was obtained with only 500 trigger pulses compared to 10,000 spikes for PSpF. Because the signal-to-noise ratio increases as the square root of the number of trigger events, the PStF at 8 μA is actually about five times greater than PSpF. Whereas PSpF reflects the output effects of a single cell, PStF reflects the output ef-

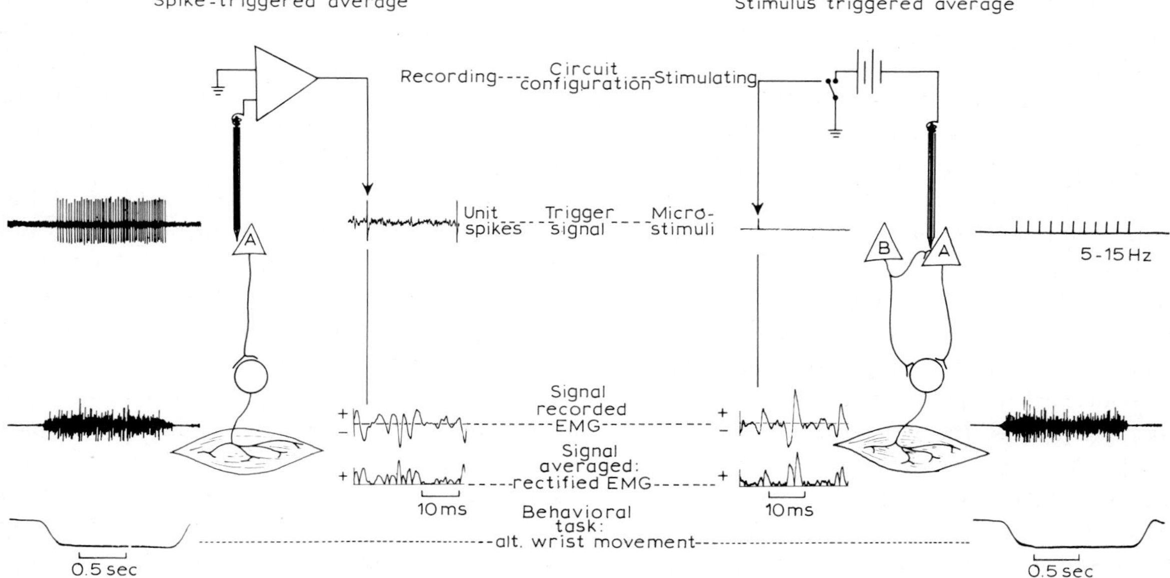

Fig. 14. Comparison of spike and stimulus-triggered averaging methods. For stimulus-triggered averaging, microstimuli are applied at a low rate (15 Hz or less) and under the same behavioral conditions used for computing the spike-triggered averages. (From Cheney and Fetz, 1985)

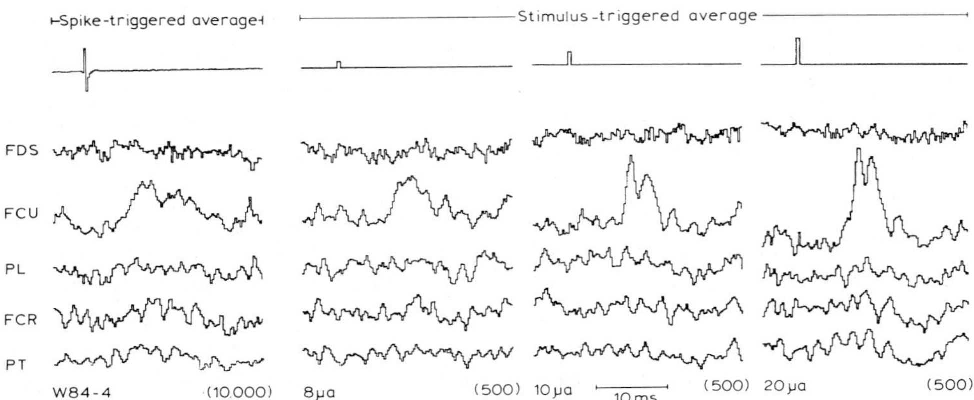

Fig. 15. Postspike facilitation (PSpF) of an individual flexor muscle (FCU) from a CM cell. Poststimulus facilitation (PStF) from microstimuli applied to the recording site during wrist flexion. Note that the pattern of PStF matches the pattern of PSpF but is greater in magnitude. Number of trigger events in parentheses. (From Cheney and Fetz, 1985)

fects of the population of cells excited by the stimulus. The strength of poststimulus effects at 5 – 10 μA was generally 2 – 20 times greater than postspike effects confirming the involvement of many CM cells. The fact that PStF involved many CM cells but had the same basic profile across synergist muscles as PSpF from the single CM cell at the same site indicates that neighboring cells activated by the stimulus have similar patterns of synaptic connections with motoneurons.

The similarity in target muscle fields of neighboring CM cells was confirmed by computing spike-triggered averages from cells located within the same track and separated by 0.6 mm or less. Results for a pair of simultaneously recorded cells are illustrated in Fig. 16. Both CM cells facilitate ECU and ED4,5 most strongly. Weaker PSpF is present in EDC and ECR and the weakest effect was in ED2,3. Stimulation at 10 μA produced a pattern of PStF closely matching the pattern of PSpF, except that the magnitude of PStF was much greater than that of PSpF. Eight pairs of neighboring cells were tested and all showed a high degree of similarity in their muscle fields. Therefore, just as neighboring sensory neurons in various parts of primary sensory cortex share common receptive fields, CM cells in lamina V of motor cortex share common muscle fields.

If the muscle fields of neighboring CM cells are similar, a related issue is whether their discharge patterns in relation to active movement are also similar. In sensory cortex, the response properties of cells in the same column are usually similar; for example, all the cells might be rapidly adapting or slowly adapting; in the visual system, orientation of an effective light stimulus might be the same for all cells of a column. In motor cortex, the details of functional properties are not necessarily similar for neighboring CM cells that presumably belong to the same cluster. Functional similarity does not seem to extend beyond the fact that neighboring CM cells are related to movements of the same joint. For example, Fig. 16 shows that both of the CM cells of this simultaneously recorded pair were coactivated with wrist extension but the pattern of discharge was dissimilar. One cell of the pair had a pure tonic pattern of discharge in relation to ramp-and-hold wrist movement while the other had a clear phasic-tonic pattern. The significance of this difference is strengthened by the fact that the qualitative pattern of discharge seems to be a rather robust feature of CM cell discharge. For example, Cheney and Fetz (1985) found that the pattern for a particular cell was the same under both isometric and auxotonic (same torque but with wrist movement) conditions. The discharge of

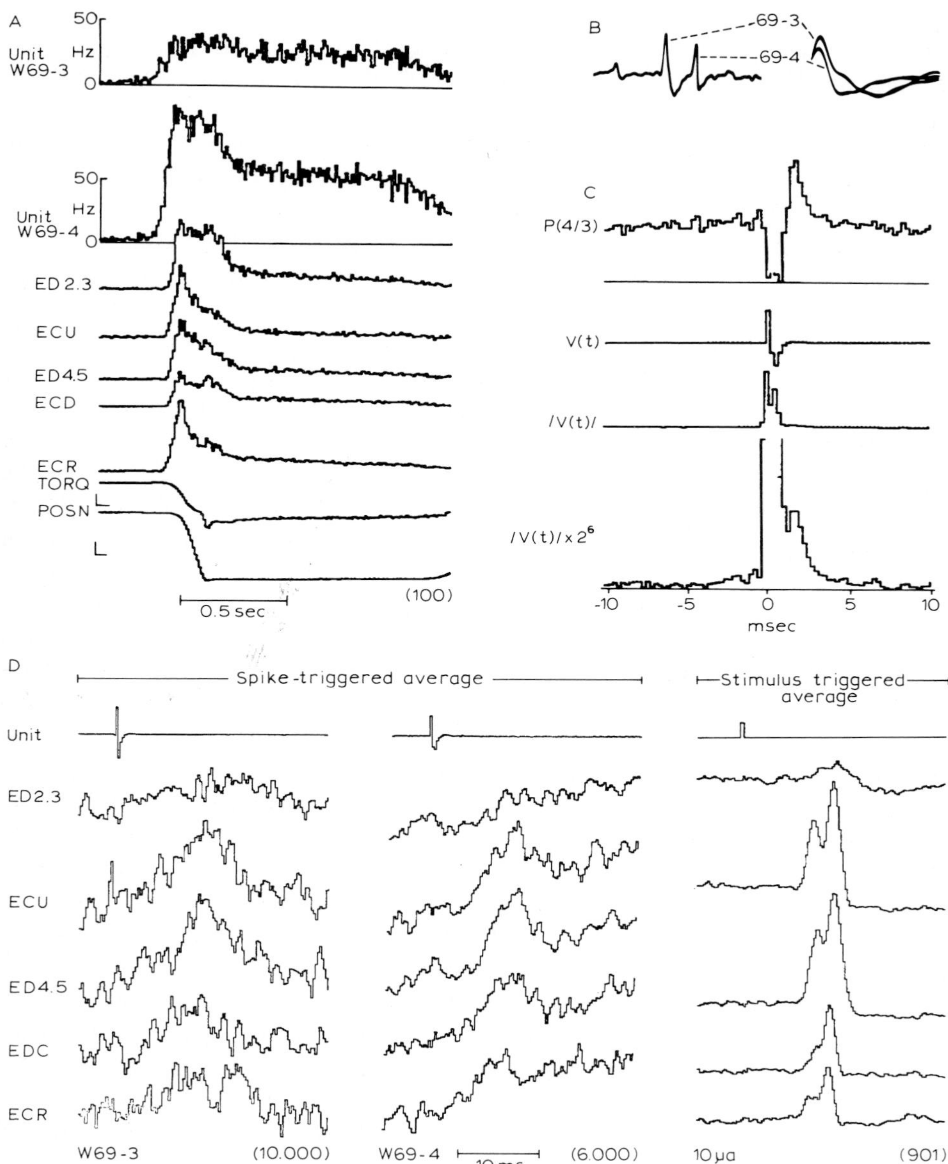

Fig. 16. Active movement relations and output effects for a pair of neighboring CM cells simultaneously recorded through the same microelectrode. (A). Discharge pattern of the two CM cells during ramp and hold wrist extension. (B). Spike waveforms of each CM cell. (C). Cross-correlogram (P4/3) of cell W69-4 with reference to the spike discharge of W69-3 at zero time. Correlogram is zero for period when spikes occur simultaneously and discrimination of separate waveforms fails. V(t) and channel below it are averages of the unrectified and rectified spike recordings respectively triggered from the spikes of cell W69-3. Lower channel is rectified average expanded. Both the correlogram and the average of rectified spike activity show peaks at about 2 ms suggesting that cell W69-4 received excitatory collateral synaptic input from cell W69-3. (D). Spike-triggered averages from each CM cell and a 10 μA stimulus-triggered average computed at the same cortical site. Note the high degree of similarity in the pattern of PSpF from each cell and the pattern of PStF. In additional tests, synchronized spikes in (C) were eliminated as triggers and a similar pattern of PSpF was observed from each cell. (Modified from Cheney and Fetz, 1985)

motor cortex cells recorded at the same site may also be related to opposite directions of movement at a joint. However, examples of neighboring CM cells with opposing target muscles have not been found.

Fig. 17 illustrates the output organization postulated by Cheney and Fetz (1985) for motor cortex. The basic module of output is a cluster of CM cells in layer V. The feature shared in common by each cell of a cluster is the muscle field. The similarity in synaptic output from different CM cells of a cluster seems to extend beyond the cell's simple muscle field. The fact that the relative magnitude of PSpF across different target muscles is similar for different cells in a cluster suggests not only that the target muscles are the same but also that the relative strength of synaptic input to target motoneuron pools is also similar. The muscle fields of different clusters involve different muscles; some facilitate a single motoneuron pool (A) but most facilitate different combinations of synergist motoneuron pools (for example, B and F). The most common output patterns for CM cells are pure facilitation, in which the cell has no effect on antagonist muscles (clusters A and C), and reciprocal, in which the cells of a cluster not only facilitate agonist muscles but simultaneously suppress antagonists, probably through spinal inhibitory interneurons (B and E).

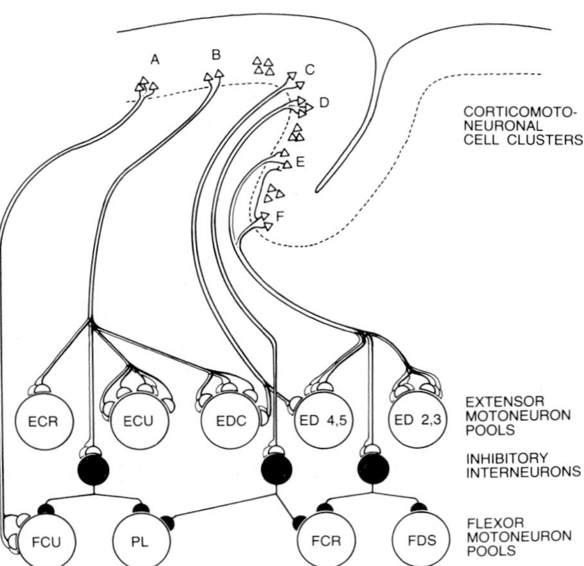

Fig. 17. Model of motor cortex output organization based on findings from spike and stimulus-triggered averaging. CM cells occur as clusters or aggregates in which each cell of the aggregate has a similar pattern of terminations with motoneurons. (From Cheney and Fetz, 1985)

Mewes et al. (1987) studied rubrospinal output organization using the same approach of comparing the pattern of poststimulus effects with the pattern of postspike effects. Although clustering of magnocellular red nucleus cells is not clear anatomically, at most RM cell sites stimulus-triggered averaging yielded results similar to those for CM cell sites (Fig. 18). However, overall the match between the pattern of PSpF and PStF at RM cell sites was less consistent than at CM cell sites. Flexor RM cell sites yielded the poorest match because stimulation always produced the strongest facilitation in extensor muscles. These results suggest that the output from red nucleus consists of functional modules in which neighboring RM cells have similar patterns of synaptic connections with motoneurons. However, the number of cells in a module (output zone) is smaller than in motor cortex and the modules show more overlap and/or less muscle field homogeneity. Greater stimulation of axons of passage might also be a factor contributing to a larger number of mismatches between the profile of PSpF and PStF across muscles at RM cell sites than at CM cell sites. The existence of actual clusters of RM cells separated by space lacking RM cells seems doubtful. However, the basic principle of organization presented here could apply just as well to neighboring cells and does not depend on the existence of actual anatomical cell clusters separated by boundary regions lacking neurons.

Discharge patterns of premotor descending neurons in relation to wrist movements

The discharge patterns of CM and RM cells in relation to a standard ramp and hold trajectory of wrist torque fall into specific categories as il-

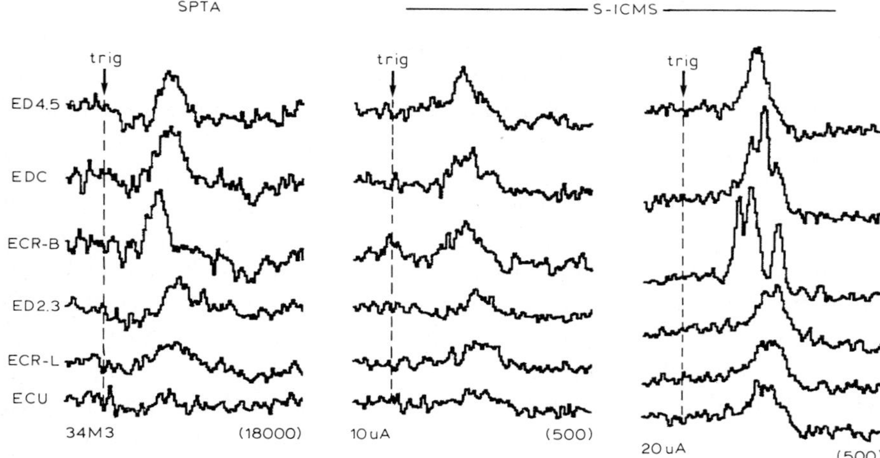

Fig. 18. Spike and stimulus-triggered averages from an RM cell site. Note the similarity between the pattern of PSpF and PStF. (Mewes and Cheney, unpublished observations)

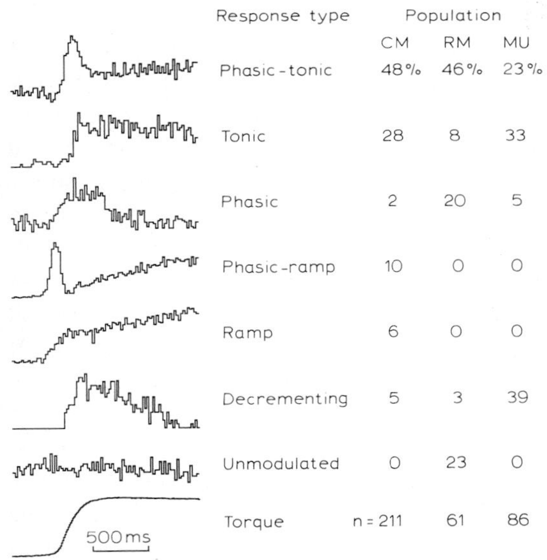

Response type	Population CM	RM	MU
Phasic-tonic	48%	46%	23%
Tonic	28	8	33
Phasic	2	20	5
Phasic-ramp	10	0	0
Ramp	6	0	0
Decrementing	5	3	39
Unmodulated	0	23	0
Torque	n = 211	61	86

Fig. 19. Response patterns of CM cells, RM cells and motor units in relation to ramp-and-hold wrist movements against moderate loads. Table gives percent of each response type in each population. (From Fetz et al., 1989.)

lustrated in Fig. 19. For comparison, the patterns exhibited by single motor units are also shown (Palmer and Fetz, 1985a). The most common pattern of discharge for premotor cells was phasic-tonic; about half of all CM and RM cells were of this type. The CM population contained a large fraction of pure tonic cells but few pure phasic cells, whereas the RM population contained a large fraction of pure phasic cells but few pure tonic cells. This is consistent with the observations of others emphasizing the phasic nature of red nucleus discharge and its involvement with the phasic aspects of movement (Ghez and Kubota, 1977; Ghez and Vicaro, 1978; Gibson et al., 1985a,b; Kohlerman et al., 1982). Nevertheless, the presence of a tonic component of discharge for most RM cells is clear (Cheney and Mewes, 1986; Cheney et al., 1988). Surprisingly, a significant fraction (23%) of the RM cell population showed no modulation of discharge in relation to wrist movements despite the presence of strong PSpF of forearm muscles directly involved in the task. These cells show gradual increases in background firing rate associated with the transition from a resting state to task performance. This activity would raise the background level of motoneuronal excitability without actually contributing to the modulation of muscle activity that generates a particular movement. It is possible that these cells might be clearly modulated in relation to some other task involving the forearm muscles. However, some unmodulated RM cells remained unmodulated when tested in relation to a much different task involving a visually guided arm movement terminating in precision grip of a food morsel. Therefore, under normal conditions, a significant fraction of the RM cell population seems to be unmodulated in relation to specific movement parameters.

Like CM cells, the majority of motor units were either phasic-tonic or tonic (Fig. 19). However, unlike either CM or RM cells, a large fraction of motor units showed a gradually decrementing discharge during the hold phase of the task when wrist torque was either constant or decreasing at a slower rate than cell discharge.

Encoding of specific movement parameters by premotor descending neurons

Identification of homogeneous premotor cell populations

One of the challenges facing neuroscientists studying the properties of brain descending systems is understanding the significance of the discharge of single neurons in functional terms. For example, what aspect of motor output or movement is encoded in the discharge of single premotor descending neurons and what do these neurons contribute to the movement? These types of questions were first directly addressed by Evarts (1968) in a study of pyramidal tract neuron discharge in relation to wrist movements against different external loads. Based on the finding that the discharge of pyramidal tract neurons preceded the onset of movement and that firing rate was graded in relation to the external load against which the monkey worked, Evarts proposed that these neurons initiate the movement and encode the force of movement. Since Evarts' original work, some reports have confirmed encoding of static force by motor cortex cells while others have emphasized that motor cortex cells are better related to movement kinematics (direction, velocity) rather than movement dynamics (force, rate of change of force, torque) (Schmidt et al., 1975; Georgopoulos et al., 1983). However, it must be recognized that motor cortex contains a wide variety of cell types with different inputs and different target structures. Different categories of neurons may encode different types of information and it becomes essential to identify the target structures of recorded neurons.

Clear delineation in an awake animal of the movement parameters encoded in premotor cell output requires demonstration that a particular cell influences motoneurons and is causally involved in the movement. The presence of PSpF in spike-triggered averages of rectified EMG activity provides confirmation of a cell's linkage to motoneurons independent of its discharge pattern. Identifying premotor neurons in this way has provided some definitive answers to questions concerning parameters of movement encoded in the discharge from motor cortex and red nucleus.

Encoding of static torque

Over a large range, the tonic activity of both CM and RM cells is linearly related to the static wrist torque to which the cell's target muscles contribute. An example of a torque-encoding RM cell is illustrated in Fig. 20. Spike-triggered averages show that this RM cell is reciprocally organized and facilitates multiple extensor muscles while suppressing multiple flexor muscles. The relation between tonic firing rate and static torque for this cell is linear with a slope of 139 Hz/Nm (Fig. 21A). Of 61 RM cells studied in relation to static torque, 54% showed a load dependent tonic discharge compared to 99% (209 of 211 tested) of CM cells. The slope of the relationship between firing rate and static torque is referred to as the rate-torque slope and provides a measure of the sensitivity with which the cell encodes wrist torque. Representative relationships for the CM and RM cells and motor units are represented in Fig. 22. Although both CM and RM cells encode the torque of movement, the mean rate-torque slope for CM cells was 3 – 4 times that of RM cells (Table III). CM cells, therefore, encode static torque with greater resolution than RM cells. Another consistent finding, evident from the plots in Fig. 22, is that the rate-torque slopes of cells facilitating extensor muscles

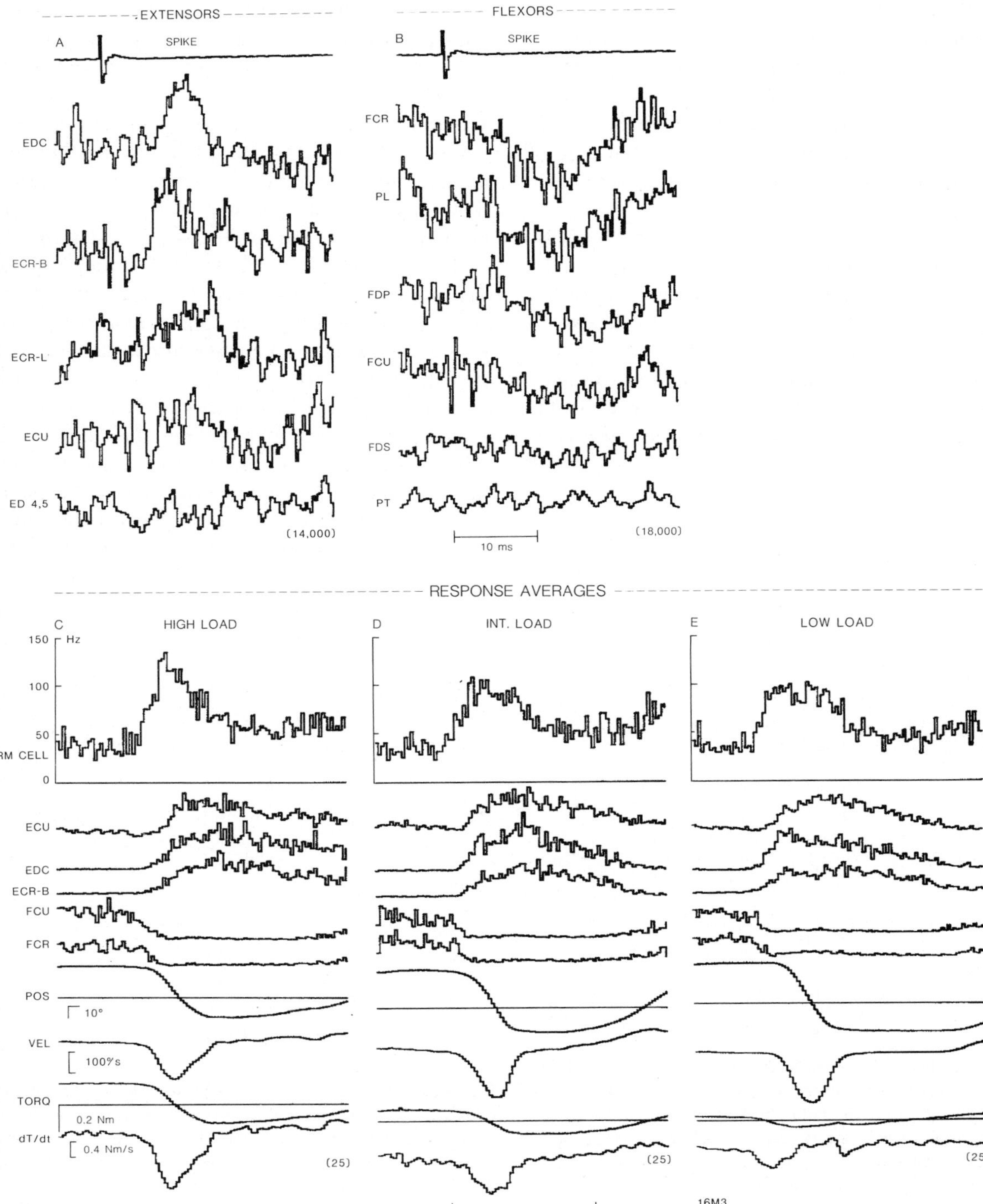

Fig. 20. Responses of an RM cell in relation to three different external load levels. Spike-triggered averages (top) show that the cell was reciprocally organized and facilitated extensor muscles while suppressing flexor muscles. (From Cheney et al., 1988)

are greater than those of cells facilitating flexor muscles. This difference was present in both the CM and RM cell data but its explanation is unclear. It does not appear to result from a peripheral factor, such as a greater mechanical advantage of flexor muscles compared to extensors because a similar difference was not present in the data for motor units recorded under the same conditions.

Encoding of static torque by CM and RM cells has also been confirmed under isometric conditions where wrist torque can be clearly and unambiguously dissociated from position. In all cases, rate-torque relationships determined under isometric conditions were similar to those for auxotonic conditions in which movements away from a zero position were opposed by a spring-like load (Cheney and Fetz, 1980; Cheney and Mewes, 1986). In conclusion, encoding of static force is a consistent property of nearly all CM and RM cells with a tonic discharge in relation to movement.

Relation to phasic parameters of movement

Many CM and RM cells exhibit a clear phasic component of discharge at movement onset, either alone or in combination with a tonic component. The phasic component of discharge is measured as the peak or mean discharge rate associated with the phasic burst minus the tonic discharge rate occurring during the static hold phase of the task. In general, correlations between discharge rate and movement velocity or rate of torque change are more mixed and variable across cells than relations to static torque. This could be due in part to greater difficulty in accurately measuring the relevant variables and examining an adequate range of the parameter of interest, but it is also clear that premotor cells simply show more variability in the extent and nature of encoding of phasic features of

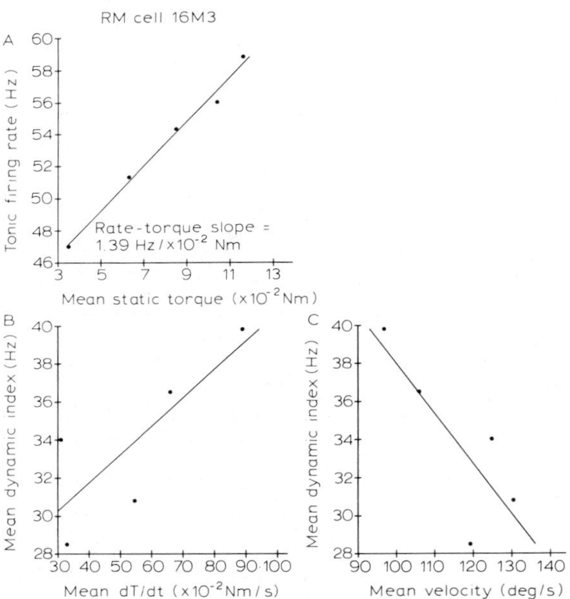

Fig. 21. Relations between discharge rate and movement parameters for the cell illustrated in Fig. 20. (A). Tonic firing rate measured during the hold phase of the task (0.25 – 0.5 s after the peak of movement) versus static torque. (B and C). Plots of the cell's phasic activity measured as dynamic index against movement velocity and mean dT/dt. Dynamic index was calculated by subtracting tonic activity from the phasic discharge during movement. (From Cheney et al., 1988)

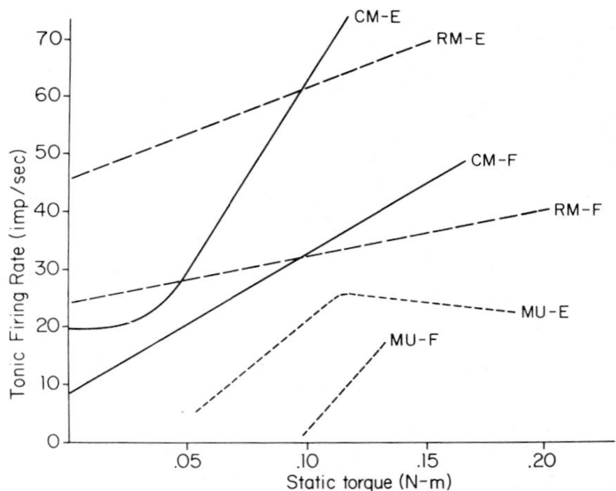

Fig. 22. Relationships between firing rate and static torque for typical CM cells, RM cells and motor units. Extensor and flexor units are plotted separately. Note that the mean rate-torque slopes for the CM cells are greater than for the RM cells. Supraspinal premotor cells are active at the lowest force levels, while motor units are recruited at increasing forces. (From Fetz et al., 1989)

TABLE III

Functional properties of CM and RM cells

Discharge properties for active movement	CM	RM
Onset relative to target muscle	− 54 ms *(− 71, − 63,	− 89 ms + 5, + 101)
Tonic component of activity		
% of tonic cells with relation to static torque	100%	100%
Rate-torque slope		
Extension	480 Hz/Nm (140 − 800)	159 Hz/Nm (39 − 342)
Flexion	250 Hz/Nm (60 − 500)	61 Hz/Nm (28 − 99)
Phasic component of activity		
Number cells tested	16	32
Relation to dT/dt	50%	34%
Relation to velocity	?	31%
Unrelated	50%	34%

* Mean onset times for phasic-tonic, phasic-ramp, tonic, and ramp CM cells respectively.
CM cell data from Cheney and Fetz (1980); RM cell data from work of Mewes and Cheney.

movement than the static features of movement. Evarts (1968) concluded that just as the tonic discharge of PTNs was related to static force, so the phasic discharge of many PTNs was related to the rate of change of force. Other studies since have confirmed this relation for motor cortex cells (Smith et al., 1975) and for red nucleus cells (Ghez and Vicaro, 1978). Cheney and Fetz (1980) reported that the phasic discharge of about half of CM cells was related to the rate of change of torque (dT/dt) and that the phasic discharge was the same for similar torque trajectories under both auxotonic or isometric conditions, confirming that the key parameter encoded was dT/dt not velocity. However, CM cell relations to velocity have not been specifically investigated.

Ghez and Vicaro (1978) emphasized the phasic nature of discharge of magnocellular red nucleus neurons in the cat studied in relation to a forelimb isometric task and concluded that the discharge encoded the rate of change of force. More recently, Gibson et al. (1985a,b) and Houk et al. (1988) found that the discharge of many magnocellular red nucleus neurons in the monkey was highly correlated with movement velocity. Cheney and Mewes (1986; also see Cheney et al., 1988) found that the phasic discharge of about a third of RM cells was best related to movement velocity. Correlation coefficients were greater for velocity than dT/dt and the phasic component of discharge was diminished under isometric conditions. However, the phasic discharge of another third of RM cells was best related to dT/dt and the remaining third were not significantly correlated with either velocity or dT/dt (Table III).

Fig. 21 shows plots of phasic activity measured as dynamic index for the RM cell illustrated in Fig. 20. Dynamic index was calculated by subtracting the tonic discharge rate measured during the hold period of the task from the mean firing rate of the phasic component of discharge. The magnitude of the phasic discharge of this cell was positively correlated with the rate of torque change in the extension direction − the direction of the cell's target muscles. Because this monkey's movements slowed somewhat as external load and dT/dt increased, velocity and dT/dt were inversely related. Consequently, the cell's phasic discharge was also inversely related to movement velocity in the extension direction. A primary relation to dT/dt was further confirmed under isometric conditions, for which movement velocity was zero.

Significant correlations with specific movement parameters can be established for RM cells suggesting encoding of these parameters by the central motor program. However, the varied nature of the best parameter − velocity in some cases, dT/dt in others and neither in still others − coupled with a large trial by trial variability raise the question of whether any of these parameters can actually be said to be encoded by RM cell discharge. Certainly any one cell makes a relatively small contribution to torque and the sum of a population of cells is likely to show a much better correlation than individual cells. Nevertheless, if velocity or dT/dt were the actual primary parameter encoded by the motor program, tighter, more uniform correlations might be expected. It is possible that some other motor parameter, such as average EMG activity in the cell's target muscles, might correlate better with the movement related phasic modulation of premotor cells.

Encoding of movement vectors by populations of motor cortex cells

Humphrey et al. (1970) first showed that correlations between cortical cell discharge rate and force or rate of change of force can be improved by considering coding in a population of cells rather than any individual cell. Clearly, all movements involve thousands of premotor cells and, although the precision with which any given cell specifies a parameter of movement may show substantial variance, the sum total of the entire population of premotor neurons involved in the movement specifies key parameters with little variance. More recently, Georgopoulos and colleagues examined the encoding of arm movement direction by populations of motor cortex neurons (Georgopoulos et al., 1983). Monkeys were trained to move a handle to each of eight targets in two dimensional space. The discharge of motor cortex neurons in relation to each direction was measured and plotted as shown in Fig. 23 for one neuron. This neuron, like most others in motor cortex, shows broad tuning of discharge with movement direction but with a best direction, for which discharge is greatest, in this case for movements at 135 degrees. A cell's directional tuning curve represents its contribution to movement in different directions of two dimensional space. The contribution of a cell to movement in a particular direction can be plotted as a vector whose length is the change in cell discharge rate for that movement direction and whose direction is the cell's preferred movement direction. The movement vectors for 241 motor cortex neurons recorded in relation to movement in eight different directions (same task as Fig. 23) are illustrated in Fig. 24. The vectorial sum of the whole population is illustrated by the dotted line. Note the high degree of congruence between the direction of the vectorial sum of the population and the actual movement direction indicated by the arrows in the center of the figure. This data demonstrates how functions exhibited by a neuronal population can match a parameter such as movement direction.

It should be pointed out that the rationale

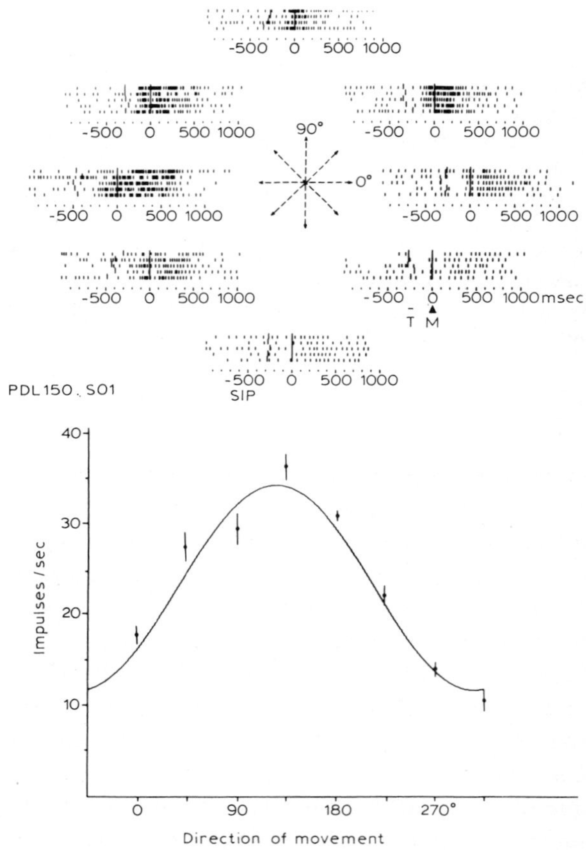

Fig. 23. Discharge of a motor cortex cell in relation to eight different directions of arm movement in a two dimensional plane. Movement started from a center point surrounded by the targets. *Top:* dot rasters of trials. *Bottom:* average rate throughout movement as a function of movement direction. This cell is typical of many motor cortex cells in showing broad tuning around a single best direction. (From Georgopoulos et al., 1983)

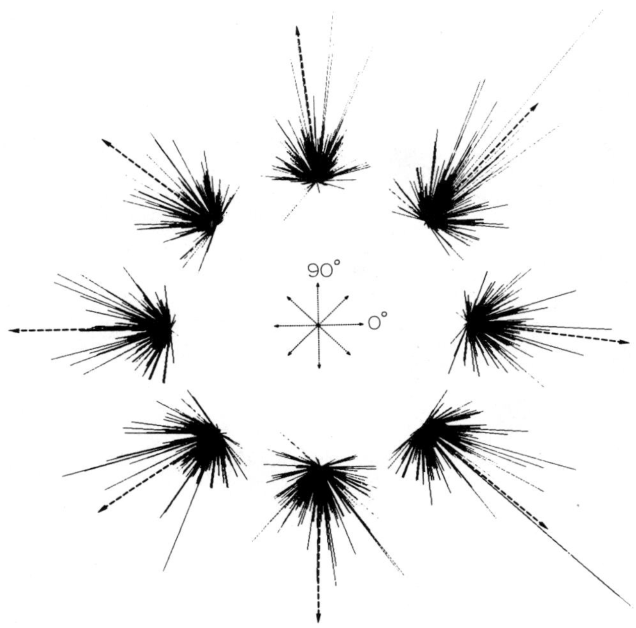

Fig. 24. Representation of the directional tuning of motor cortex cells recorded in experiments such as illustrated in Fig. 23. Discharge of each cell for each movement direction is plotted as a vector whose length is equal to the discharge rate for movements to the target in that direction and whose orientation indicates the direction for which the cell's discharge was strongest. The vector contributions of each cell to the movement were summed to yield a population vector (broken arrow). Note the high degree of conformity between the population vector and the direction of the actual movement. (From Georgopoulos et al., 1983)

underlying calculation of neuronal population vectors differs fundamentally from the approach of Humphrey et al. (1970) in that, for vector calculation, the aim of examining a population of neurons is not to reduce unwanted variability. Rather the broad directional tuning of any particular cell is a consistent property stemming from a similar broad tuning of the cell's target muscles. It is only by considering the net contribution of a population of such broadly tuned cells involved in a particular movement that the direction of movement is unambiguously matched. This type of analysis might also be applied to other movement parameters, such as force direction, with similar results (Georgopoulos et al., 1983). Kalaska et al. (1989) recently confirmed this suggestion. They applied vectorial analysis to a population of motor cortex neurons using the same task for which the data in Figs. 23 and 24 were collected but with the addition of external loads to assist or oppose movement toward each of the targets. Fig. 25 summarizes the neuronal discharge vectors for all cells recorded in the absence of external loads (A) and with external loads (B). In A, the position of each cluster of vectors relative to the center point represents the direction of movement for that cluster; in B the position of the cluster relative to the center point represents the direction the external load pulled the pendulum away from the center starting point. External loads that pulled the pendulum in each of the 8 target directions were applied for active movements in each direction. The movement direction vectors (A) are calculated and plotted in the same way as in Fig. 24. In (B), the activity of each cell is represented by a vector oriented along the axis of its preferred movement direction measured in the control block (A). The length of the vector in (B) was determined by the

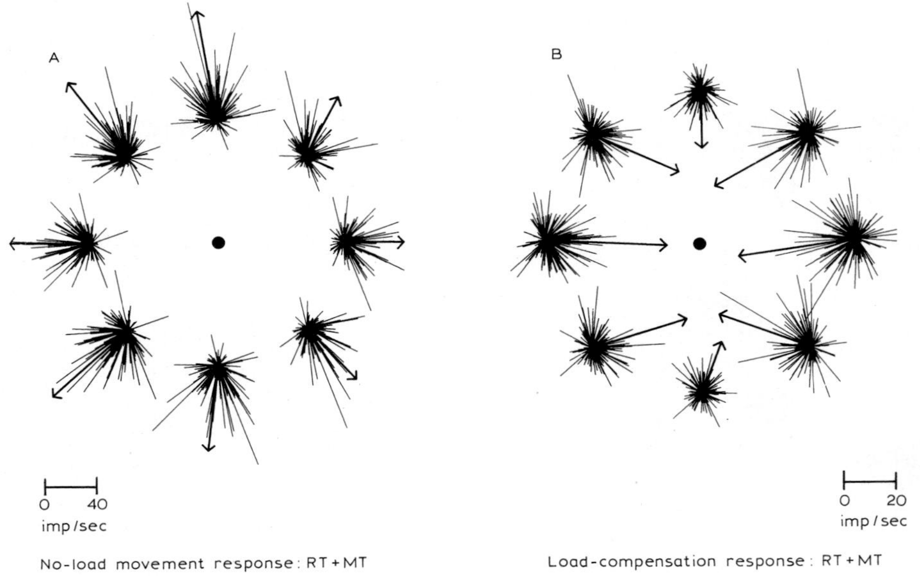

Fig. 25. Vectors representing the discharge of motor cortex neurons in relation to movement direction and load direction. Monkeys moved a handle to target positions surrounding a centrally located starting position (center filled circle). In (A) the position of each cluster of vectors relative to the center point represents the direction of movement for that cluster; in (B) the position of the cluster relative to the center point represents the direction the external load pulled the pendulum away from the center starting point. External loads that pulled the pendulum in each of the target directions were then applied for each of the 8 directions of active movement. For any movement direction, external load could reduce the magnitude of the movement vector to near zero (for loads assisting movement) or substantially increase it (for loads opposing movement). See text for further description. (From Kalaska et al., 1989)

load related change in activity of the cell, relative to the activity during the control block. Increases in discharge rate relative to the rate for the same movement direction during the control block were represented as vectors pointing towards the cell's preferred movement direction; decreases in discharge rate caused by the load were represented as vectors pointing opposite the cell's preferred movement direction. Each vector cluster represents the change in discharge of the sample population caused by one direction of load. Note that for each outwardly oriented load direction, the vector sum of the motor cortex population discharge (heavy arrows) is oriented inward, appropriate to compensate for the externally applied load. In other words, loads opposing movement in a particular direction strongly activated cells for which that was the preferred movement direction, whereas loads assisting movement in that direction greatly reduced cell activity. Most cells (95%) showed significant variations in tonic discharge associated with external loads. However, some cells showed clear modulation with movement direction, but were not influenced by loads, confirming earlier work of Thach (1978). Most of the cells were probably pyramidal neurons in layer V based on their large spike amplitudes and location at intermediate cortical depths. Preliminary findings reported by Kalaska, as part of the same study, suggest that the majority of cells in more superficial layers of motor cortex encode movement direction; that is, these cells are insensitive to external load. For example, microstimulation threshold was negatively correlated with an index of cell sensitivity to load. Based on these early findings, it is tempting to speculate that a transformation from representation of kinematics (intended direction and velocity of movement) to dynamics (joint torques required to produce the intended movement) occurs within motor cortex. In any case, the discharge of most motor cortex cells sampled from deep layers in this task was dependent on the load against which the monkey worked and the force generated by the agonist muscles. These findings are consistent with previous studies showing that motor cortex cells, and particularly CM cells, encode force or torque parameters of movement (Evarts, 1968; Cheney and Fetz, 1980).

Georgopoulos et al. (1984) found that the preferred movement direction of motor cortex cells tends to be columnarly organized in a way that may correlate with the cluster organization of CM cells described in an earlier section. CM cells probably exhibit preferred movement directions reflecting the cell's weighted facilitation of a particular combination of target muscles (Georgopoulos, 1988). The discharge of cells in more superficial layers of the same cortical column might also exhibit similar preferred movement directions but with a primary relation to movement direction rather than muscle activation parameters.

Task specific discharge of descending premotor neurons

By their facilitation of target muscles, individual CM and RM cells can be considered to represent muscle fields, in some cases individual muscles but more frequently combinations of muscles. The activity of motoneurons is rigidly coupled to the activity of the muscle fibers they innervate, and is predictable based on the principle of orderly recruitment. One can ask whether the functional activity of premotor cells is similarly linked to the activity of their target muscles? As discussed in previous sections, consistent coactivation of premotor cells with their target muscles is commonly observed; however, dissociation of premotor cell discharge and target muscle activity has been demonstrated under a variety of conditions, emphasizing the task specific nature of the discharge of some premotor neurons. Dissociation in this case is defined as coactivation under some conditions but absence of coactivation or reciprocal activation under other conditions, despite the presence of clear postspike effects in the cell's target muscles. Conditions under which dissociation has been observed for CM cells include: 1) power grip (Cheney et al., 1985), 2) precision grip (Muir and Lemon, 1983), 3) ballistic movements (Cheney and Fetz, 1980). Fig. 26 compares the discharge of a CM cell under two different task conditions, both of which were associated with strong consistent coactivation of the cell's target muscles (Cheney et al., 1985). One task was alternating wrist movement, which required reciprocal activation of wrist flexor and extensor muscles. The second was a power grip task, which involved squeezing a pair of nylon bars and required coactivation of wrist flexors and extensors to stabilize the wrist. Fig. 26 shows that the cell's activity was strongly engaged for wrist extension – the direction of its target muscles. However, during power grip cell activity was actually reduced despite equally strong activation of the cell's target muscles. Task specificity such as this might be understood in terms of the cell's output effects on muscle activity. The spike-triggered averages (top) show that this cell facilitated multiple wrist extensors and suppressed a wrist flexor. These effects were confirmed in stimulus-triggered averages computed at the same site. The functional uncoupling of the activity of this CM cell and its target muscles may be related to the fact that the cell reciprocally suppressed the flexor muscles. Because this suppression would interfere with the cocontraction of flexors and extensors needed for power grip, the central motor program for cocontraction may exclude reciprocally organized cells.

A similar dissociation was reported by Muir and Lemon (1983) for CM cells facilitating intrinsic hand muscles. They found that CM cells were preferentially active in relation to precision grip, but were relatively inactive during power grip despite the fact that power grip involved greater

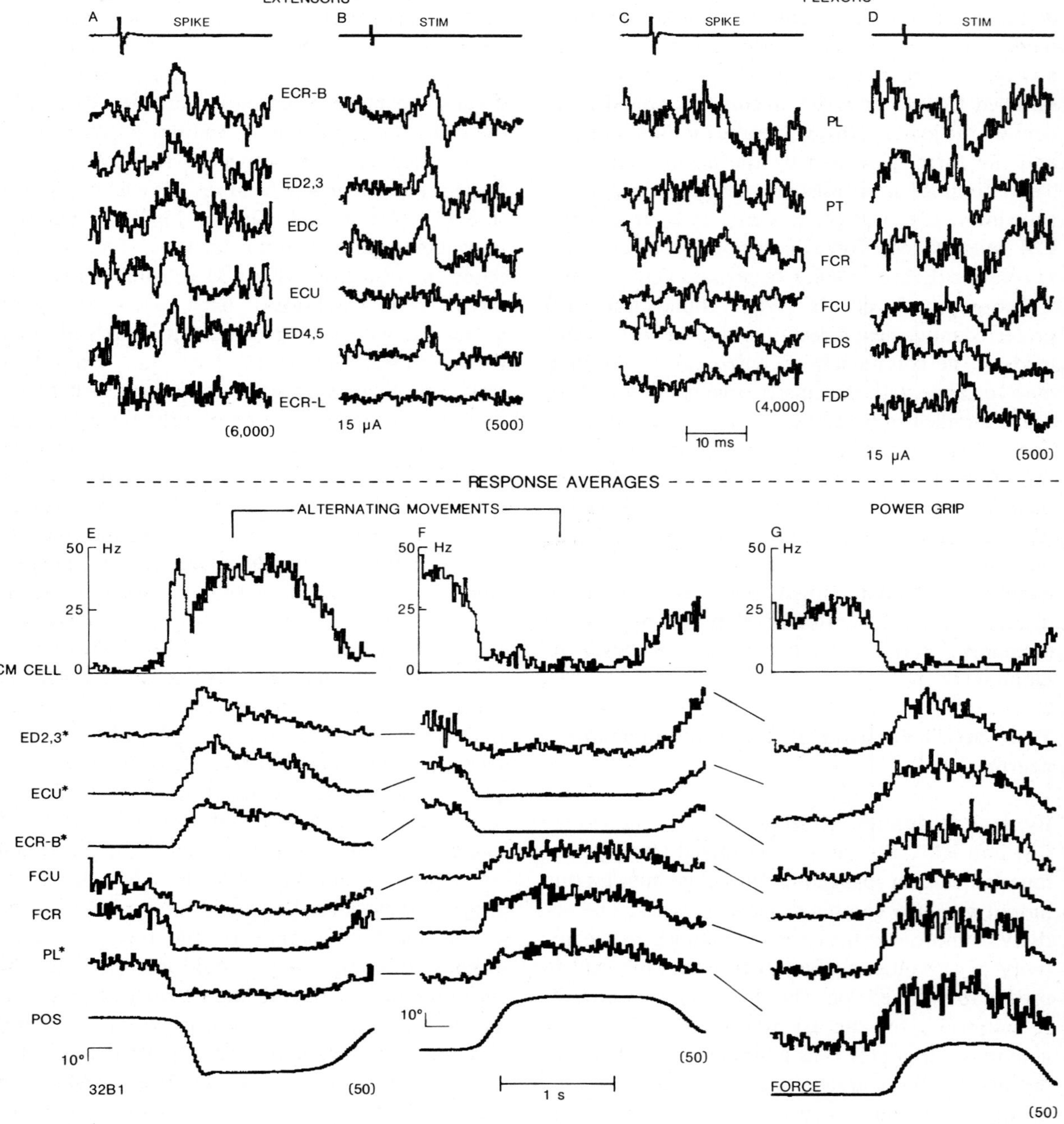

Fig. 26. Active movement discharge of a CM cell during alternating wrist movements and power grip. Spike-triggered averages show that this is a reciprocally organized cell which facilitated extensors and suppressed a flexor-PL. These effects were confirmed in stimulus-triggered averages computed at the same cortical site. Note that cell discharge shuts off during power grip despite strong activation of the cell's target muscles. (From Cheney et al., 1985)

activation of the cell's target muscles (Fig. 27).

Still another example of functional uncoupling of the activity of a premotor cell and its target muscles was reported by Cheney and Fetz (1980). CM cells were highly active during accurate, controlled wrist movements to 10 degree targets but nearly inactive during ballistic, uncontrolled movements that more strongly activated the cell's target muscles.

In all these instances, a muscle representation can be identified for each cell. PSpFs computed under different task conditions might differ somewhat in absolute magnitude and occasionally a muscle would show PSpF in one task but not the other. Nevertheless, the clearest PSpFs typically were present in both task conditions and the relative magnitude of PSpF was usually similar. Therefore, over short periods of time the muscle field seems relatively fixed, reflecting "hard wired" neural connections. Functional activation of the premotor cell, on the other hand, is subject to much greater short term flexibility. Cell activation shows a task specificity that, in some cases, may be related to the functional role of the cell's suppressed target muscles, but in other cases, seems to depend on factors beyond simple circuitry, such as the accuracy of a movement or its position along a scale from least to most automatic.

Relative contribution of CM and RM cells to movement

Much of the functional organization of different descending systems is revealed in the response properties and correlational linkages of their individual premotor neurons. However, comparisons of the relative contribution of different descending systems to movement requires that the effects of individual neurons on muscle activity be synthesized as an estimate of the population effect. Quantitative information about the magnitude of synaptic effects from single premotor neurons and the distribution of these effects, coupled with knowledge of the number of neurons converging on a typical motoneuron, enables estimates of the contribution of each descending system to movement. The relative contribution of particular systems may differ for different categories of movement and for movements at different joints. For example, it is likely that reticulospinal and vestibulospinal neurons make a greater contribution to movements at proximal joints during locomotion than the corticospinal and rubrospinal

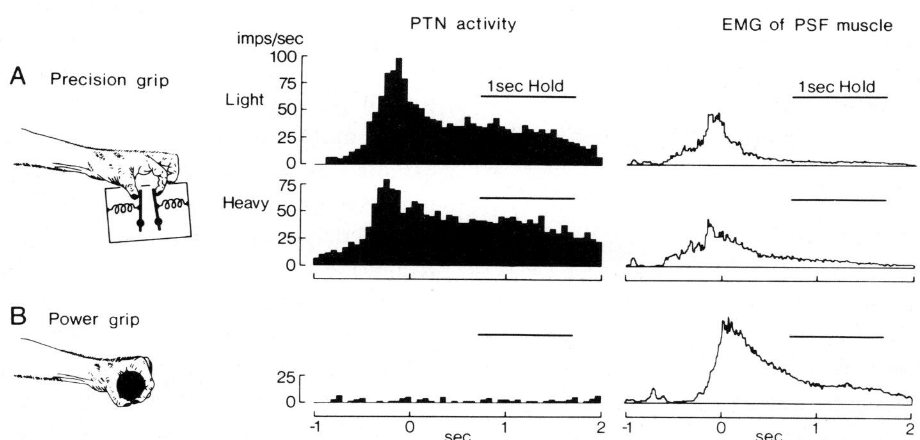

Fig. 27. Active movement discharge of a CM cell during precision grip and power grip. EMG activity of the cell's target muscle is also shown. Note that the cell discharges intensely for precision grip but is unrelated to power grip despite stronger activation of its target muscles. (From Muir and Lemon, 1983)

systems. On the other hand, skilled movements of the hand rely more heavily on the corticospinal and rubrospinal systems. Sufficient quantitative information now exists on the synaptic effects and firing patterns of individual CM and RM cells during wrist movements to begin to estimate their relative contribution to motoneuron activity.

Fetz et al. (1989) estimated the net contribution of corticospinal and rubrospinal colonies to motoneuron firing rate during the hold period of a ramp-and-hold movement. The static component of movement was chosen to avoid the complications associated with the many unknown variables that come into play during transitions between flexion to extension. The contribution of CM and RM cell populations to the firing of an average target motoneuron was estimated from:

1. The increment in firing of a motoneuron associated with a premotoneuronal EPSP of a particular amplitude. Cope et al. (1987) found that the unitary EPSPs from single muscle spindle Ia afferents produced above chance discharge of target motoneurons that was proportional to EPSP amplitude (Fig. 2). Although derived from muscle spindle Ia afferent data, this relation may also hold for other inputs to the motoneuron.
2. The number of CM or RM cells converging on a single motoneuron, that is, the size of the CM or RM colony.
3. The firing rates of CM and RM cells during the hold phase of the task.

These factors can be expressed by the following relationship:

(1) $df_m \cong 0.0001{*}h{*}n{*}f$

where df_m is the increment in motoneuron firing rate, 0.0001 is the constant that provides the transformation from EPSP amplitude to motoneuron firing (a 100 μV EPSP evokes 1 spike for every 100 occurrences), h is the mean amplitude of the EPSP for a particular input, n is the number of neurons converging onto the motoneuron and f is the mean firing rate of the presynaptic neurons. The number of CM or RM cells converging on a single motoneuron is difficult to estimate as is the size of the individual EPSPs from these neurons. However, the product of h and n is the maximal EPSP which has been measured in anesthetized preparations. Measurements of the maximal CM-EPSP range from 1 to 3 mv (Clough et al., 1968; Phillips and Porter, 1977; Shapovalov et al., 1971; Fritz et al., 1985). Shapovalov found that RM-EPSPs in macaque monkeys averaged 0.6 mv. Using an intermediate magnitude of 2 mv for CM cells in expression (1) above and a measured extensor CM cell mean firing rate of about 62 Hz for holding against an intermediate extension load of 0.1 Nm (Fig. 22) yields a motoneuron firing rate increment of 12.4 Hz attributable to the CM input. Similarly, a maximal RM-EPSP of 0.6 and a measured mean extensor RM cell firing rate of 60 Hz at 0.1 Nm yields a motoneuron firing rate increment of 3.6 Hz. The sum of these is 16 Hz which is about 75% of the mean firing rate of extensor motor units at 0.1 Nm. The contribution of the CM system is about three times greater than that of the RM system.

Conclusion

The technique of spike-triggered averaging of EMG activity in awake monkeys is yielding new information at the level of individual premotor neurons concerning the sign, strength and distribution of synaptic effects from descending systems to spinal motoneurons. This data complements and extends that derived from intracellular and monosynaptic reflex conditioning studies in anesthetized animals. More importantly, the technique can be applied in awake animals, enabling not only identification of motor output cells within the brain but also correlations between a cell's synaptic influences and its functional relations to movement. Spike-triggered averaging of EMG activity has provided new insights concerning the organization and function of the rubrospinal and corticospinal systems in primates and future applications of the method can be expected to further elucidate the role of different premotor neurons in movement.

Acknowledgements

We thank colleagues whose efforts contributed to this paper, particularly Gail Widener, Wade Smith and Rick Kasser. We also thank Drs Apostolos Georgopoulos and John Kalaska for their helpful comments on the manuscript. This work was supported by NIH grant 25646, NSF grant BMS 8216608 and BRSGSO7RR05373 to P. Cheney and NIH grants NS12542 and RR00166 to E. Fetz.

Abbreviations

CM – corticomotoneuronal
CNS – central nervous system
dT/dt – rate of change of torque
EMG – electromyogram
EPSP – excitatory postsynaptic potential
HRP – horseradish peroxidase
IPSP – inhibitory postsynaptic potential
PSpF – postspike facilitation
PSpS – postspike suppression
PStF – poststimulus facilitation
PStS – poststimulus suppression
PTN – pyramidal tract neuron
RIFMs – relatively independent finger movements
RM – rubromotoneuronal
S-ICMS – single pulse intra-cranial microstimulation
SpTA – spike triggered average
StTA – stimulus triggered average

Muscles:

ED 2,3 – extensor digitorum two and three
ED 4,5 – extensor digitorum four and five
EDC – extensor digitorum communis
ECU – extensor carpi ulnaris
ECR-B – extensor carpi radialis brevis
ECR-L – extensor carpi radialis longus
FDS – flexor digitorum sublimis
FDP – flexor digitorum profundus
FCU – flexor carpi ulnaris
PL – palmaris longus
FCR – flexor carpi radialis
PT – pronator teres

References

Alstermark, B. and Sasaki, S. (1985) Integration in descending motor pathways' controlling the forelimb in the cat. 13. Cortico-spinal effects in shoulder, elbow, wrist and digit motorneurons. *Exp. Brain Res., 59:* 353 – 364.

Alstermark, B., Pinter, M.J. and Sasaki, S. (1985) Pyramidal effects in dorsal neck motoneurones of the cat. *J. Physiol.,* 363: 287 – 302.

Amassian, V.E. and Weiner, H. (1966) Monosynaptic and polysynaptic activation of pyramidal tract neurons by thalamic stimulation. In: D.P. Purpura and M.D. Yahr (Eds.), *The Thalamus.* Columbia University Press, New York, pp. 255 – 282.

Araki, T. and Endo, K. (1976) Short latency EPSPs in pyramidal tract cells evoked by stimulation of the centrum medianum-parafascicular complex and the nucleus ventralis anterior of the thalamus. *Brain Res.,* 113: 405 – 410.

Asanuma, H. and Rosen, I. (1972) Topographic organization of cortical efferent zones projecting to distal forelimb muscles in the monkey. *Exp. Brain Res.,* 16: 507 – 520.

Asanuma, H. and Sakata, H. (1967) Functional organization of a cortical efferent system examined with focal depth stimulation in cats. *J. Neurophysiol.,* 30: 35 – 54.

Baev, K.V. (1971) Convergence of corticospinal and rubrospinal influences on cervical motoneurons. *Neirofiziologiya,* 3: 599 – 608.

Botteron and Cheney, P.D. (1989) Corticomotoneuronal postspike effects in averages of unrectified EMG activity. *J. Neurophysiol.,* 62: 1127 – 1139.

Brodal, (1981). *Neurological Anatomy in Relation to Clinical Medicine.* Oxford University Press, Oxford.

Burke, R.E., Jankowska, E. and Bruggencati, G. (1970) A comparison of peripheral and rubrospinal synaptic input to slow and fast twitch motor units of triceps surae. *J. Physiol. (Lond.),* 207: 709 – 732.

Buys, E.J., Lemon R.N., Mantel, G.W.H. and Muir, R.B. (1986) Selective facilitation of different hand muscles by single corticospinal neurones in the conscious monkey. *J. Physiol.,* 381: 529 – 549.

Chang, H.T., Ruch, T.C. and Ward, A.A. (1947) Topographical representation of muscles in motor cortex in monkeys. *J. Neurophysiol.,* 10: 39 – 56.

Cheney, P.D. (1980) Response of rubromotoneuronal cells identified by spike-triggered averaging of EMG activity in awake monkeys. *Neurosci. Lett.,* 17: 137 – 142.

Cheney, P.D. (1985) Role of cerebral cortex in voluntary movements. A review. *Phys. Ther.,* 65: 624 – 635.

Cheney, P.D. and Fetz E.E. (1980) Functional classes of

primate corticomotoneuronal cells and their relation to active force. *J. Neurophysiol.*, 44: 773 – 791.

Cheney, P.D., Kasser R.J. and Fetz, E.E. (1985) Motor and sensory properties of primate corticomotoneuronal cells. In: A.W. Goodwin and I. Darian-Smith (Eds.), *Hand Function and the Neocortex, Experimental Brain Research, Supplement 10,* Springer-Verlag, Berlin, Heidelberg, pp. 211 – 231.

Cheney, P.D., Mewes, K. and Fetz, E.E. (1988) Encoding of motor parameters by corticomotoneuronal (CM) and rubromotoneuronal (RM) cells producing postspike facilitation of forelimb muscles in the behaving monkey. *Behav. Brain Res.*, 28: 181 – 191.

Cheney, P.D. and Fetz, E.E. (1985) Comparable patterns of muscle facilitation evoked by individual corticomotoneuronal (CM) cells and by single intracortical microstimuli in primates: evidence for functional groups of CM cells. *J. Neurophysiol.*, 53: 786 – 804.

Cheney, P.D. and Mewes, K. (1985) Changes in corticomotoneuronal (CM) postspike facilitation of EMG activity associated with logarithmic and square transformation of the EMG signal. *Neurosci. Abstr.*, 11: 1275.

Cheney, P.D. and Mewes, K. (1986) Encoding of movement parameters by rubromotoneuronal cells. *Neurosci. Abstr.*, 12: 1303.

Cheney, P.D., Kasser, R. and Holsapple, J. (1982) Reciprocal effect of single corticomotoneuronal cells on wrist extensor and flexor muscle activity in the primate. *Brain Res.*, 247: 164 – 168.

Clough, J.F.M., Kernell, D. and Phillips, C.G. (1968) The distribution of monosynaptic excitation from the pyramidal tract and from primary spindle afferents to motoneurons of the baboon's hand and forearm. *J. Physiol.*, 198: 145 – 166.

Cope, T.C., Fetz, E.E. and Matsumura, M. (1987) Cross-correlation assessment of the synaptic strength of single Ia fibre connections with lumbar motoneurones in the cat. *J. Physiol.*, 390: 161 – 188.

Coulter, J.D., Ewing, L. and Carter, C. (1976) Origin of primary sensorimotor cortical projections to lumbar spinal cord of cat and monkey. *Brain Res.*, 103: 366 – 372.

Delong, M.R. and Strick, P.L. (1974) Relation of basal ganglia, cerebellum and motor cortex units to ramp and ballistic movements. *Brain Res.*, 71: 327 – 335.

Elger, C.E., Speckmann, E.-J., Caspers, H. and Janzen, R.W.C. (1977) Cortico-spinal connections in the rat I. Monosynaptic and polysynaptic responses of cervical motoneurons to epicortical stimulation. *Exp. Brain Res.*, 28: 385 – 404.

Enberg, I. (1963) Effects from the pyramidal tract on plantar reflexes in the cat. *Acta Physiol. Scand.*, 59: (Suppl. 213). 39.

Evarts, E.V. (1966) Methods for recording activity of individual neurons in moving animals. *Methods Med. Res.*, 11: 241 – 261.

Evarts, E.V. (1968) Relation of pyramidal tract activity to force exerted during voluntary movement. *J. Neurophysiol.*, 31: 14 – 27.

Fetz, E.E. and Cheney, P.D. (1980) Postspike facilitation of forelimb muscle activity by primate corticomotoneuronal cells. *J. Neurophysiol.*, 44: 751 – 772.

Fetz, E.E., Cheney, P.D. and German, D.G. (1976) Corticomotoneuronal connections of precentral cells detected by postspike averages of EMG activity in behaving monkeys. *Brain Res.*, 14: 505 – 510.

Fetz, E.E. and Gustafsson, B. (1983) Relation between shapes of post-synaptic potentials and changes in firing probability of cat motoneurons. *J. Physiol. (Lond.)*, 341: 387 – 410.

Fetz, E.E., Cheney, P.D., Mewes, K. and Palmer, S. (1989) Control of forelimb muscle activity by populations of corticomotoneuronal and rubromotoneuronal cells. *Prog. Brain Res.*, 80: 437 – 449.

Fortier, P.A., Flament, D. and Fetz, E.E. (1989) Relationships between primate corticomotoneuronal cells and their target forearm motor units during torque tracking. *Neurosci. Abstr.*, 15: 788.

Fritsch, G. and Hitzig, E. (1870) Uber die electrische Erregbarkeit des Grosshirns. *Archs. Anat. Physiol. Wiss. Med.*, 37: 300 – 332. (Translation by Bonin, G. *The Cerebral Cortex,* C.C. Thomas, Springfield, IL. pp. 73 – 96.)

Fritz, N., Illert, M., Kolb, F.P., Lemon, R.N., Muir, R.B., van der Burg, J., Wiedemann, E. and Yamaguchi, T. (1985) The cortico-motoneuronal input to hand and forearm motoneurones in the anesthetized monkey. *J. Physiol. (Lond.)*, 366: 20P.

Georgopoulos, A.P. (1988) Neural integration of movement: role of motor cortex in reaching. *FASEB J.*, 2: 2849 – 2857.

Georgopoulos, A.P., Caminiti, R,., Kalaska, J.F. and Massey, J.T. (1983) Spatial coding of movement: a hypothesis concerning the coding of movement direction by motor cortical populations. *Exp. Brain Res. (Suppl.)* 7: 327 – 336.

Georgopoulos, A.P., Kalaska, J.F., Crutcher, M.D., Caminiti, R. and Massey, J.T. (1984) The representation of movement direction in the motor cortex: single cell and population studies. In: G.M. Edelman, W.M. Cowan and W.E. Gall, (Eds.), *Dynamic Aspects of Neocortical Function,* John Wiley and Sons, New York, pp. 501 – 524.

Ghez C. and Kubota, K. (1977) Activity of red nucleus neurons associated with skilled forelimb movement in the cat. *Brain Res.*, 129: 383 – 388.

Ghez, C. and Vicaro, D. (1978) Discharge of red nucleus neurons during voluntary muscle contraction: Activity patterns and correlations with isometric force. *J. Physiol.*, (Paris), 74: 283 – 285.

Gibson, A.R., Houk, J.C. and Kohlerman, N.J. (1985a) Magnocellular red nucleus activity during different types of limb movement in the macaque monkey. *J. Physiol.*, 358: 527 – 549.

Gibson, A.R., Houk, J.C. and Kohlerman, N.J. (1985b) Relation between red nucleus discharge and movement parameters in trained macaque monkeys. *J. Physiol.*, 358:

551 – 570.

Grillner, S. Hongo, T. and Lund, S. (1971) Convergent effects on alpha motoneurons from the vestibulospinal tract and a pathway descending in the medial longitudinal fasciculus. *Exp. Brain Res.,* 12: 457 – 479.

Holstege, G. (1987) Some anatomical observations on the projections from the hypothalamus to brainstem and spinal cord: an HRP and autoradiographic tracing study in the cat. *J. Comp. Neurol.,* 260: 98 – 126.

Hongo, T., Jankowska, E. and Lundberg, A. (1969) The rubrospinal tract. I. Effects on alpha motoneurones innervating hindlimb muscles in cats. *Exp. Brain Res.,* 7: 344 – 364.

Houk, J.D., Gibson, A.R., Harvey, C.F., Kennedy, P.R. and Van Kan, P.L.E. (1988) Activity of primate magnocellular red nucleus related to hand and finger movements. *Behav. Brain Res.,* 28: 201 – 206.

Humphrey, D.R., Schmidt, E.M. and Thompson, W.D. (1970) Predicting measures of motor performance from multiple cortical spike trains. *Science,* 179: 758 – 762.

Humphrey, D.R. and Rietz, R.R. (1976) Cells of origin of corticorubral projections from the arm area of primate motor cortex and their synaptic actions in the red nucleus. *Brain Res.,* 110: 162 – 169.

Illert, M., Lundberg, A. and Tanaka, R. (1976a) Integration in descending motor pathways controlling the forelimb in the cat. 1. Pyramidal effects on motoneurons. *Exp. Brain Res.,* 26: 509 – 519.

Illert, M., Lundberg, A. and Tanaka, R. (1976b) Integration in descending motor pathways controlling the forelimb in the cat. 2. Convergence on neurons mediating disynaptic corticomotoneuronal execution. *Exp. Brain Res.,* 26: 521 – 540, 1976.

Illert, M. and Wiedemann, E. (1984) Pyramidal actions in identified radial motor nuclei of the cat. *Pflugers Archiv., Eur. J. Physiol.,* 401: 132 – 142.

Jankowska, E. and Roberts, W.J. (1972) Synaptic actions of single interneurones mediating reciprocal Ia inhibition of motoneurones. *J. Physiol. (Lond.),* 222: 623 – 642.

Jankowska, E. and Tanaka, R. (1974) Neuronal mechanisms of the disynaptic inhibition evoked in primate spinal motoneurones from the corticospinal tract. *Brain Res.,* 75: 163 – 166.

Jankowska, E., Padel, Y. and Tanaka, R. (1975) Projections of pyramidal tract cells to alpha motoneurons innervating hindlimb muscles in the monkey. *J. Physiol.,* 249: 637 – 667.

Jankowska, E., Padel, Y. and Tanaka, R. (1976) Disynaptic inhibition of spinal motoneurones from the motor cortex in the monkey. *J. Physiol. (London),* 258: 467 – 487.

Janzen, R.W.C., Speckmann, E.-J., Caspers, H. and Elger, C.E. (1977) Cortico-spinal connections in the rat. II. Oligosynaptic and polysynaptic responses of lumbar motoneurons to epicortical stimulation. *Exp. Brain Res.,* 28: 405 – 420.

Jasper, H., Ricci, G.F. and Doane, B. (1958) Patterns of cortical neurone discharge during conditioned response in monkeys. In: G. Wolstenholme and C. O'Connor (Eds.), *Neurological Basis of Behavior.* Little Brown; Boston.

Jones, E.G. and Wise, S.P. (1977) Size, laminar and columnar distribution of efferent cells in the sensory-motor cortex of primates. *J. Comp. Neurol.,* 175: 391 – 438.

Kalaska, J.F., Cohen, D.A., Hyde, M.L. and Prud'homme, M. (1989) A comparison of movement direction-related versus load direction related activity in primate motor cortex, using a two dimensional reaching task. *J. Neurosci.,* 9: 2080 – 2102.

Kasser, R.J. and Cheney, P.D. (1985) Characteristics of corticomotoneuronal postspike facilitation and reciprocal suppression of EMG activity in the monkey. *J. Neurophysiol.,* 53: 959 – 978.

Kasser, R.J. and Cheney, P.D. (1983) Double-barreled electrode for simultaneous iontophoresis and single unit recording during movement in awake monkeys. *J. Neurosci. Methods,* 7: 235 – 242.

Kohlerman, N.J., Gibson, A.R. and Houk, J.C. (1982) Velocity signals related to hand movements recorded from red nucleus neurons in monkeys. *Science,* 217: 857 – 860.

Kwan, H.C., MacKay, W.A., Murphy, J.T. and Wong, Y.C. (1978) Spatial organization of precentral cortex in awake primates. II. Motor outputs. *J. Neurophysiol.,* 41: 1120 – 1131.

Landgren, S., Phillips, C.G. and Porter, R., (1962a) Minimal synaptic actions of pyramidal impulses on alpha motoneurones of the baboon's hand and forearm. *J. Physiol. (Lond.),* 161: 91 – 111.

Landgren, S., Phillips, C.G. and Porter, R. (1962b) Cortical fields of origin of the monosynaptic pyramidal pathways to some alpha motoneurones of the baboon's hand and forearm. *J. Physiol. (Lond.),* 161: 112 – 125.

Lawrence, D.G. and Kuypers, H.G.J.M. (1968a) The functional organization of the motor system in the monkey. I. The effects of bilateral pyramidal tract lesions. *Brain,* 91: 1 – 14.

Lawrence, D.G. and Kuypers, H.G.J.M. (1968b) The functional organization of the motor system in the monkey. II. The effects of lesions of the descending brain-stem pathways. *Brain,* 91: 15 – 36.

Lemon, R.N., Mantel, G.W.H. and Muir, R.B. (1986) Corticospinal facilitation of hand muscles during voluntary movement in the conscious monkey. *J. Physiol.,* 381: 497 – 527.

Lemon, R.N. and Muir, R.B. (1983) Cortical addresses of distal muscles: a study in the conscious monkey using the spike-triggered averaging technique. *Exp. Brain Res.,* Suppl. 7: 230 – 238.

Lemon, R.N. and Porter, R. (1976) Afferent input to movement related precentral neurones in conscious monkey. *Proc. R. Soc. B.,* 194: 313 – 339.

Mantel, G.W.H. and Lemon, R.N. (1987) Cross-correlation reveals facilitation of single motor units in thenar muscles by single corticospinal neurones in the conscious monkey. *Neurosci. Lett.*, 77: 113 – 118.

McCurdy, M.L., Hansma, D.I., Houk, J.C. and Gibson, A.R. (1984) Cat red nucleus projects to digit extensor motoneurons. *Neurosci. Abstr.*, 10: 744.

Mewes, K. and Cheney, P.D. (1986) Characteristics of rubromotoneuronal postspike effects in EMG activity of wrist and hand muscles in the behaving monkey. *Neurosci. Abstr.*, 12: 1303.

Mewes, K., Widener, G.W. and Cheney, P.D. (1987) Comparison of postspike and poststimulus facilitation of forearm muscle EMG activity from red nucleus sites in the monkey. *Neurosci. Abstr.*, 13: 245.

Muir, R.B. and Lemon, R.N. (1983). Corticospinal neurones with a special role in precision grip. *Brain Res.*, 261: 312 – 316.

Murray, E.A. and Coulter, J.D. (1981) Organization of corticospinal neurons in the monkeys. *J. Comp. Neurol.*, 195: 339 – 365.

Palmer, S. and Fetz, E.E. (1985a) Discharge properties of primate forearm motor units during isometric muscle activity. *J. Neurophysiol.*, 54: 1178 – 1193.

Palmer, S. and Fetz, E.E. (1985b) Effects of single intracortical microstimuli in motor cortex on activity of identified forearm motor units in behaving monkeys. *J. Neurophysiol.*, 54: 1194 – 1212.

Peterson, B.W. (1979) Reticulospinal projections to spinal motor nuclei. *Ann. Rev. Physiol.*, 41: 127 – 140.

Peterson, B.W., Pitts, N.G. and Fukushima, K. (1979) Reticulospinal connections with limb and axial motoneurons. *Exp. Brain Res.*, 36: 1 – 20.

Peterson, B.W., Pitts, N.G., Fukushima, K. and Mackel, R. (1978) Reticulospinal excitation and inhibition of neck motoneurons. *Exp. Brain Res.*, 32: 471 – 489.

Phillips, C.C. and Porter, R. (1964) The pyramidal projection to motoneurons of some muscle groups of the baboon's forelimb. *Prog. Brain Res.*, 12: 222 – 242.

Phillips, C.G. and Porter, R. (1977) *Corticospinal neurones. Their role in movement.* Monographs of the Physiological Society. Academic Press, London.

Preston, J.B. and Whitlock, D.G. (1961) Intracellular potentials recorded from motoneurons following precentral gyrus stimulation in primate. *J. Neurophysiol.*, 24: 91 – 100.

Preston, J.B., Shende, M.C. and Uemura, K. (1967) The motor cortex pyramidal system: patterns of facilitation and inhibition on motoneurons innervating limb musculature of cat and baboon and their possible adaptive significance. In: M.D. Yahr and D.P. Purpura (Eds.), *Neurophysiological Basis of Normal and Abnormal Motor Activities.* Raven Press, New York.

Purpura, D.P., Shofer, R.J. and Musgrave, F.S. (1964) Cortical intracellular potentials during augmenting and recruiting responses. II. Patterns of synaptic activities in pyramidal and nonpyramidal tract neurons. *J. Neurophysiol.*, 27: 133 – 151.

Roland, P.E., Larsen, B. Lassen, N.A. (1980) Supplementary motor area and other cortical areas in organization of voluntary movements in man. *J. Neurophysiol.*, 43: 118 – 136.

Schmidt, E.M., Jost, R.G. and Davis, K.K. (1975) Reexamination of the force relationship of cortical cell discharge patterns with conditioned wrist movements. *Brain Res.*, 83: 213 – 223.

Shapovalov, A.I. (1973) Extrapyramidal control of primate motoneurons. In: J.E. Desmedt (Ed.), *New developments in electromyography and clinical neurophysiology*, 3: Karger: Basel, 145 – 158.

Shapovalov, A.I., Karamjan, O.A., Kurchavyi, G.G. and Repina, Z.A. (1971) Synaptic actions evoked from the red nucleus on the spinal alpha motoneurons in the Rhesus monkey. *Brain Res.*, 32: 325 – 348.

Shapovalov, A.I. (1972) Extrapyramidal monosynaptic and disynaptic control of mammalian alpha-motoneurons. *Brain Res.*, 40: 105 – 115.

Smith, A.M., Hepp-Reymond, M.-C. and Wyss, U.R. (1975) Relation of activity in precentral cortical neurons to force and rate of force change during isometric contractions of finger muscles. *Exp. Brain Res.*, 23: 315 – 332.

Smith, W.S. and Fetz, E.E. (1989) Effects of synchrony between primate corticomotoneuronal cells on post-spike facilitation of muscles and motor units. *Neurosci. Lett.*, 96: 76 – 81.

Thach, W.T. (1978) Correlation of neural discharge with pattern and force of muscular activity, joint position, and direction of intended next movement in motor cortex and cerebellum. *J. Neurophysiol.*, 41: 654 – 676.

Tower, S.S. (1940) Pyramidal lesion in the monkey. *Brain*, 63: 36 – 90.

Wilson, V.J. and Yoshida, M. (1969) Comparison of effects of stimulation of Deiters nucleus and the medial longitudinal fasciculus on neck, forelimb, and hindlimb motoneurons. *J. Neurophysiol.*, 32: 742 – 758.

Wilson, V.J., Yoshida, M. and Schor, R.A. (1970) Supraspinal monosynaptic excitation and inhibition of thoracic back motoneurons. *Exp. Brain Res.*, 11: 282 – 295.

Yu, H. DeFrance, J.F., Iwata, N., Kitai, S.T. and Tanaka, T. (1972) Rubral inputs to facial motoneurons in cat. *Brain Res.*, 42: 220 – 224.

G. Holstege (Ed.)
Progress in Brain Research, Vol. 87

CHAPTER 12

Forebrain nuclei involved in autonomic control

A.D. Loewy

Department of Anatomy and Neurobiology, Washington University School of Medicine, St. Louis, MO 63110, U.S.A.

Introduction

Certain cell groups of the forebrain play an important role in maintaining homeostasis by controlling neuroendocrine and autonomic functions. These regions include the hypothalamus, the basal forebrain and the cerebral cortex. The anatomical connections of many of these areas have been determined using anterograde and retrograde transport methods. The picture that has emerged is that there is a set of nuclei which are interconnected and have been termed the central autonomic network. Apart from its reciprocal interconnections, this network innervates both the vagal and sympathetic preganglionic neurons and thus, regulates autonomic functions (see Loewy, 1990 for review). The objective of this chapter is to provide a brief summary of this field with an emphasis on cardiovascular regulation. More detailed discussions of the anatomical connections and functions of these forebrain areas may be found in reviews by Price et al. (1987), Swanson (1987), and Cechetto and Saper (1990).

Background

Interest in the forebrain as a CNS site that regulates autonomic functions can be traced back to 1909 when Karplus and Kreidl began their pioneering physiological mapping studies. These investigators used the electrical stimulation method to determine the location of autonomic centers in the diencephalon. They found a highly reactive region localized in the subthalamic nucleus which they thought was a sympathetic center controlling pupillary dilation and blood pressure (Karplus and Kreidl, 1910). We now know that this interpretation is probably incorrect. These investigators used the electrical stimulation technique and as we now know this method is not an optimal tool for localizing functions within CNS cell groups, because when an electrical current is applied to a CNS region it can activate both cell bodies and fibers of passage. Karplus and Kreidl were well aware of this problem and attempted to deal with it by using animals that had been chronically decorticated. This was done to eliminate the possibility that descending cortical pathways travelling in the cerebral peduncle were activated. However, their experiments did not eliminate the possibility that additional nearby fiber systems were activated. For example, the other descending brain stem pathways arising from the amygdala and/or the hypothalamus travel in close proximity to their stimulation site and were not excluded in their study. Similarly, ascending pathways which traverse or project to this region may have been antidromically activated by their procedures. While these experiments are no longer viewed as providing definitive information, this work stands as an important initial contribution to the field of autonomic control because it raised the idea of that higher CNS levels regulated the sympathetic preganglionic neurons.

This field remained dormant for 25 years until Ranson and his co-workers made a detailed electrical stimulation mapping study of the forebrain of the cat in order to determine the sites involved in blood pressure control (Kabat, Magoun and Ranson, 1935). They found two pressor zones: one was the periventricular region of the hypothalamus and the other was the area containing the zona incerta and the lateral hypothalamic area. In addition, a depressor area was found at more rostral sites which included the medial preoptic area and the septal area. More contemporary electrical stimulation studies have provided similar results and have been summarized by Mancia and Zanchetti (1981). Like the early investigations of Karplus and Kreidl, these studies served to reenforce the idea of a hierarchical pattern of central autonomic control, but the actual information provided in them is now largely discounted because of the uncertainties in the interpretation associated with data generated with the electrical stimulation technique.

In the last decade, the technology for studying central autonomic pathways has improved markedly. Detailed anatomical maps have been constructed and in some cases, the putative neurotransmitters involved have been elucidated with the immunohistochemical method. The microinjection technique has become the method of choice for studying the function of central autonomic cell groups because nanoliter amounts of various chemicals which activate or inhibit only cell bodies can be injected into discrete CNS nuclei (Goodchild et al., 1982; Neil and Loewy, 1982; Blessing and Reis, 1983). Excitatory amino acids such as glutamic, homocysteic, or kainic acid or inhibitory agents like GABA, glycine, or related agonists and antagonists can be used respectively to excite or inhibit specific sets of CNS neurons. When this method is coupled with the autoradiographic method, it may be used in a even more precise manner to localize the injection site and correlate it with a specific anatomical region (Spencer et al., 1988, 1989). The remainder of this chapter will focus on the more contemporary advances in the field of central autonomic control.

Forebrain cell groups innervating sympathetic and vagal preganglionic neurons

The autonomic outflow of both the sympathetic and parasympathetic systems is regulated by a variety of cell groups in the brain stem and forebrain. The axoplasmic transport methods have provided considerable information regarding which CNS cell groups innervate the preganglionic neurons, but these studies have provided only a limited understanding of these neural circuits because the techniques do not provide any information on the functional nature of the connections. For example, if a particular forebrain CNS area is shown to project to the upper thoracic intermediolateral cell column (IML), it has not been possible to determine whether this pathway regulates sympathetic preganglionic neurons involved with pupillomotor, cardiovascular, or pilomotor functions. Only a few studies have attempted to circumvent this problem. For example, one approach has been to first retrogradely label the sympathetic preganglionic neurons that innervate a particular structure like the adrenal gland, and then to use the immunohistochemical method in conjunction with the first method to visualize various putative neurotransmitter containing fibers in relationship to somata of the sympathoadrenal preganglionic neurons (Appel et al., 1987). A similar approach was used by Hosoya (1983) to study the hypothalamic inputs to the superior salvatory nucleus neurons. However, these combined histological approaches are usually quite difficult to perform and for this reason most investigators have tended not to use them. As a result, relatively little information exists on the pattern of innervation of the specific functional classes of autonomic preganglionic neurons.

The CNS cell groups that innervate the sympathetic preganglionic neurons have been studied extensively with axoplasmic transport methods (see reviews by Loewy, 1982 and Coote, 1988). As mentioned above, these studies failed to provide an understanding of the functional significance of these connections. To circumvent this problem, the retrograde transneuronal viral cell body labeling method has been used to study the CNS cell groups that innervate specific sets of sympathetic preganglionic neurons (Strack et al., 1989a). By making localized injections of a suspension containing live pseudorabies virus (PRV), a herpes virus endemic to pigs, into various sympathetic ganglia or the adrenal gland in rats, and allowing sufficient time for the virus to be first to be retrogradely transported in the sympathetic preganglionic neurons and then to be transferred transneuronally to the second order neurons that synapse on the sympathetic preganglionic neurons, we have been able to elucidate with immunohistochemical techniques the CNS regions which innervate the specific sets of sympathetic preganglionic neurons. As a result of this work, a general idea has emerged: five areas of the brain innervate all levels of the sympathetic outflow. These areas include the paraventricular hypothalamic nucleus, A5 noradrenergic cell group, caudal raphe region, rostral ventrolateral medulla, and ventromedial medulla (Fig. 1). This observation seems to be true for all levels of the sympathetic outflow. However, other areas of the brain also innervate sympathetic preganglionic neurons. Some of these areas appear to provide unique innervation of specific types of sympathetic preganglionic neurons. For example, we found that when the superior cervical ganglion or the stellate ganglion were injected with PRV, retrograde transneuronal cell body labeling was also found in the mesencephalic central gray matter and the lateral hypothalamic area. With the stellate ganglion experiments, however, a much larger number of cells was found in the lateral hypothalamic area than was seen after the superior cervical ganglion experiments. Also, after stellate ganglion experiments, neurons in the ventral zona incerta and posterior periventricular hypothalamic region were transneuronally labeled as well. These projections appear unique to the sympathetic preganglionic neurons which innervate the stellate ganglion – the major source of sympathetic ganglion cells innervating the heart. These results provide suggestive evidence that some specific CNS areas regulate cardiac function. Physiological studies have also been performed that support the idea. For example, stimulation of the lateral hypothalamic area causes a reduction in cardiac output (Spencer et al., 1989), and stimulation of the zona incerta a decrease in heart rate (Spencer et al., 1988), and stimulation of the posterior periventricular hypothalamic area causes hypotension and bradycardia (Spencer et al., 1990).

The inputs to the vagal preganglionic nuclei have been studied with the retrograde cell body labeling technique (ter Horst et al., 1984). Figure 2 shows the pattern of retrograde cell body labeling in the forebrain after an horseradish peroxidase (HRP)

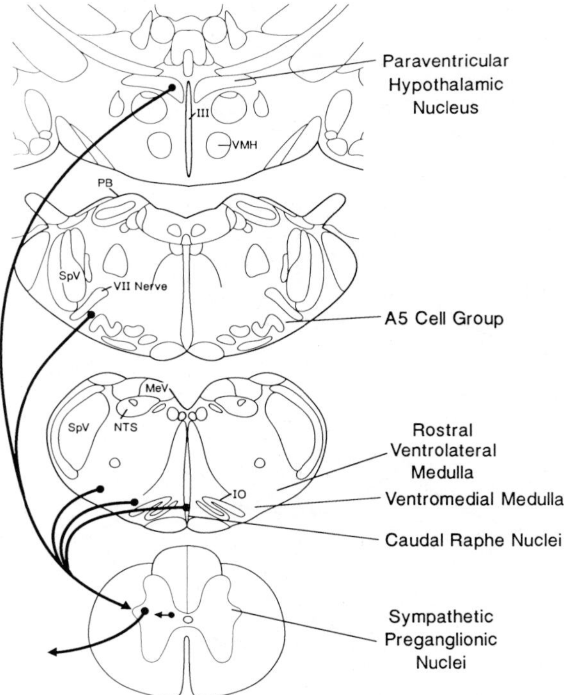

Fig. 1. The general pattern of innervation of the sympathetic outflow as demonstrated by transneuronal cell body labeling after PRV infections of the sympathetic ganglia or adrenal gland. This pattern was seen after PRV infections of the superior cervical, stellate, celiac, and L5 sympathetic ganglia, as well as the adrenal gland. Reproduced from Strack et al., *Brain Res.,* 491 (1989) 156 – 162.

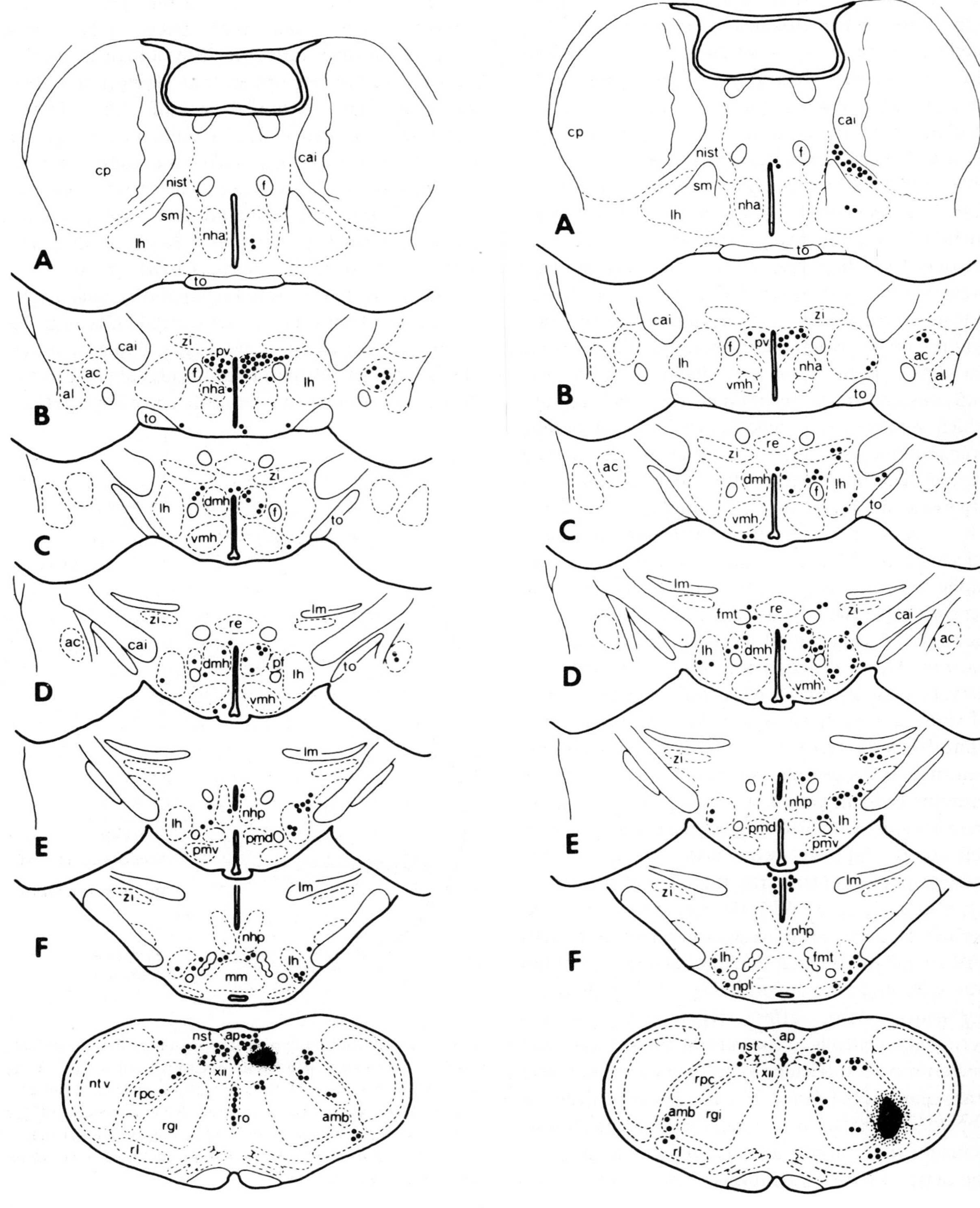
cp
nist
sm
lh
nha
f
cai
A
to
cai
zi
pv
ac
al
f
nha
lh
B
to
lh
dmh
zi
f
vmh
to
C
zi
lm
re
ac
cai
dmh
pf
lh
to
vmh
D
lm
nhp
lh
pmv
pmd
E
zi
lm
nhp
lh
mm
F
nst
ap
x
XII
ntv
rpc
rgi
ro
amb
rl
cp
cai
nist
f
sm
lh
nha
A
to
cai
zi
lh
f
pv
nha
ac
vmh
al
B
to
re
zi
ac
dmh
f
lh
to
vmh
C
lm
fmt
re
zi
cai
ac
lh
dmh
vmh
D
zi
nhp
pmd
lh
pmv
E
zi
lm
nhp
lh
fmt
npl
F
nst
ap
x
XII
rpc
amb
rgi
rl

injection in the dorsal vagal nucleus and after an HRP injection in the region of the nucleus ambiguus. The vagal outflow from the dorsal vagal nucleus is thought to be involved mainly in control of gastrointestinal functions while the cardioinhibitory neurons are found mainly in the area of the nucleus ambiguus (see Loewy and Spyer, 1990 for review). Both of these areas receive inputs from the paraventricular hypothalamic nucleus, dorsomedial hypothalamic nucleus, lateral hypothalamic area, and central nucleus of the amygdala. In addition, the area of the nucleus ambiguus also receives input from the zona incerta and bed nucleus of the stria terminalis (See however, Holstege, Chapter 14 this volume). The role these CNS sites provide in autonomic processing and in control of specific vagal functions remains unknown.

Hypothalamus

Paraventricular hypothalamic nucleus

The paraventricular hypothalamic nucleus (PVH) is involved in a variety of autonomic and endocrine functions. It is composed of three functional parts (Swanson, 1987). First, the magnocellular portion contains vasopressin and oxytocin neurons which send their axons to the posterior pituitary. Second, the medial parvocellular and periventricular portions are made up of corticotropin releasing hormone and thyrotropin releasing hormone containing neurons that project to the median eminence and release peptides which act as local hormones to affect specific cells in the anterior pituitary. Third, the dorsal and lateral parvocellular areas of the PVH contain neurons that provide descending connections to the autonomic nuclei of the brain stem and spinal cord. In keeping with the theme of this chapter, the present discussion will focus only on the autonomic part of the PVH.

The most detailed information on the descending connections of the PVH can be found in an anterograde transport study published by Luiten et al. (1985) and is shown in Fig. 3. In this study, small iontophoretic injections of the kidney bean lectin *Phaseolus vulgaris* leucoagglutinin (PHA-L) were made in the PVH. After several days survival, the immunohistochemical method was used to reveal minute details of PVH neurons and their axons including the terminals. The PVH projects to all the autonomic relay centers of the lower brain stem, including the autonomic premotor nuclei such as the A5 noradrenergic cell group and the rostral ventrolateral medulla. These nuclei provide direct projections to the vagal and sympathetic preganglionic neurons. On the basis of these findings, as well as other studies, this nucleus has all the connectional properties which would suggest that it may function as the "master controller" of the autonomic nervous system. However, this does not mean that each PVH autonomic neuron connects in a diffuse manner with all of these autonomic sites. In contrast, it is quite likely that neurons in specific parts of the autonomic PVH are organized in a highly specialized way. This has

Fig. 2. Retrogradely labeled cell bodies are found in the forebrain of the rat after HRP injections in the dorsal vagal nucleus (left) or the area of the nucleus ambiguus (right). *Abbreviations:* aa, anterior amygdaloid nucleus; ac, central amygdaloid nucleus; amb, nucleus ambiguus, ap, area postrema; dmh, dorsomedial hypothalamic nucleus; h_2, Forel's field 'h_2'; hl, lateral habenular nucleus; lc, locus coeruleus; lh, lateral hypothalamic area; ncu, cuneiform nucleus; nha, anterior hypothalamic nucleus; nhp, posterior hypothalamic nucleus; nist, interstitial nucleus of stria terminalis; npd, dorsal parabrachial nucleus; npl, lateral mammillary nucleus, pars posterior; npv, ventral parabrachial nucleus; nsc, suprachiasmic nucleus; nst, solitary tract nucleus; ntd, dorsal tegmental nucleus; ntdl, dorsal tegmental nucleus, pars lateralis; pf, perifornical nucleus; pmd, dorsal premammillary nucleus; pmv, ventral premammillary nucleus; pv, paraventricular nucleus; rd, dorsal raphe nucleus; rgi, nucleus reticularis gigantocellularis; rl, lateral reticular nucleus; ro, nucleus raphe obscurus; rpc, nucleus reticularis parvocellularis; sd, dorsal septal nucleus; sgc, substantia grisea centralis; sl, lateral septal nucleus; snr, substantia nigra, pars reticulata; vmh, ventromedial hypothalamic nucleus; zi, zona incerta; X, dorsal motor vagus nucleus. Reproduced from ter Horst et al., *J. Autonom. Nerv. System,* 11, 59–75, (1984), with permission of the authors and publisher.

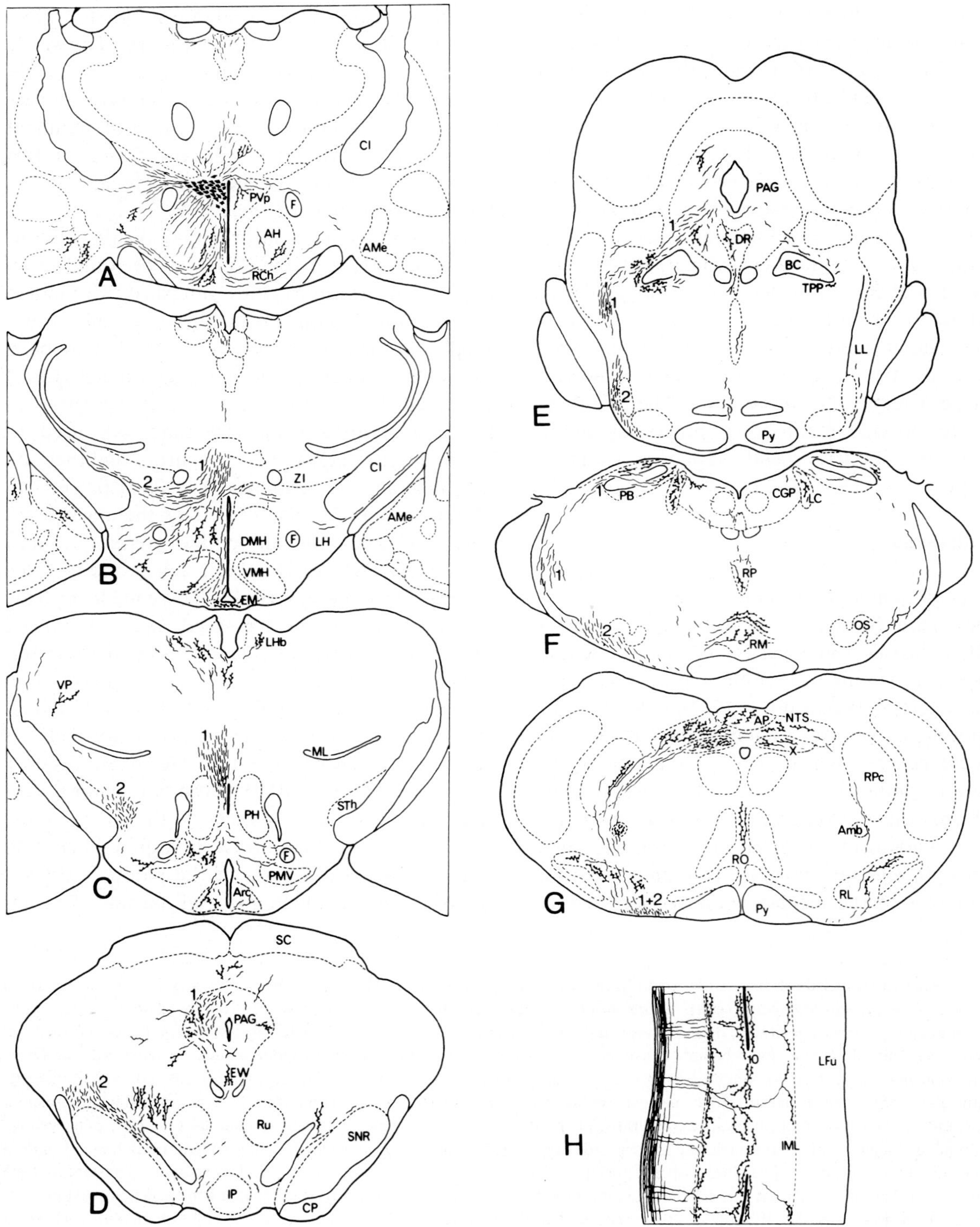

Fig. 3. Descending projections arising from the paraventricular hypothalamic nucleus. Reproduced from Luiten et al., *Brain Res.*, 329 (1989) 374 – 378.

been demonstrated for the PVH projections to the IML where a topographic projection pattern of innervation to specific sets of sympathetic preganglionic neurons has been demonstrated with the retrograde transneuronal viral transport method (Strack et al., 1989a). A "ganglion" specific pattern of transneuronal retrograde cell body labeling may be demonstrated in the PVH. As shown in Fig. 4, the neurons innervating the upper thoracic IML lie in the medial aspect of the PVH while those innervating the lower thoracic IML lie in its lateral part. While there are a number of unresolved issues related to the specificity of the transneuronal viral transport technique, these data clearly support the contention that the descending PVH projection in the spinal cord is organized in a specific fashion.

A variety of different transmitters are involved in the PVH→IML pathway affecting the adrenal gland (Strack et al., 1989b). This may be true for other descending PVH→IML systems as well. The function of these different transmitters is unknown, but when oxytocin or vasopressin are applied iontophoretically to rat sympathetic preganglionic neurons, they cause inhibition of ongoing sympathetic neural activity (Gilbey et al., 1982). When these same peptides are applied to cat sympathetic preganglionic neurons these produce excitatory effects (Backman and Henry, 1984). Whether this difference relates to species variations or is a reflection that different classes of sympathetic preganglionic neurons with different types of receptors were activated in these two experiments is uncertain. This issue needs to be reexamined, particularly since neurotransmitters involved in the PVH spinal system may be quite extensive as was shown for the innervation of the sympathoadrenal preganglionic neurons (Strack et al., 1989a).

The PVH is thought to be involved in cardiovascular regulation. L-glutamate stimulation of the PVH in rats causes a decrease in blood pressure which is mediated by sympathetic inhibition (Yamashita et al., 1987). PVH stimulation produces a non-uniform effect on the sympathetic outflows: renal nerve activity is decreased and adrenal sympathetic nerve activity increased (Katafuchi et al., 1988). The effect on heart rate is controversial. Yamashita et al. (1987) reported that L-glutamate stimulation of the PVH has no effect on heart rate, but Darlington et al. (1988)

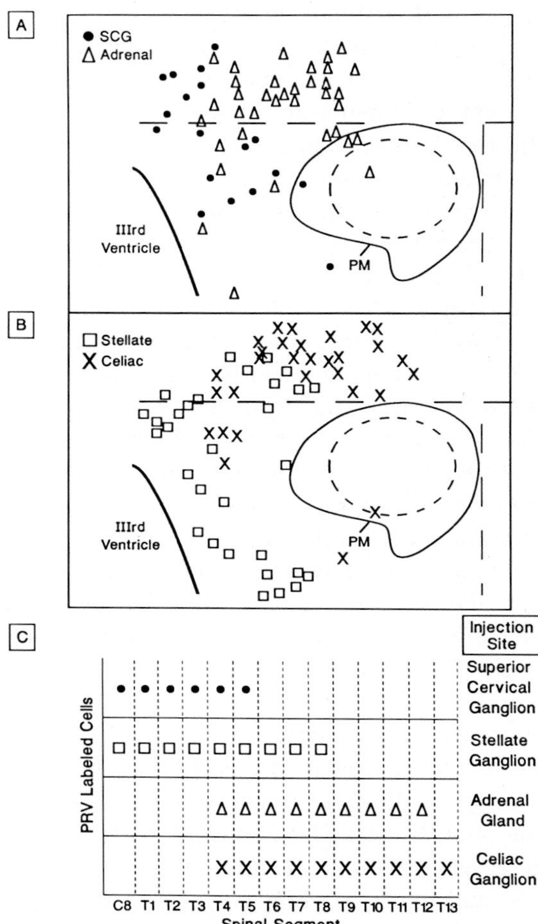

Fig. 4. Topographic organization of the paraventricular hypothalamic neurons that project to different sympathetic outflows as determined after viral infections of the various sympathetic ganglia and the adrenal gland. (A) Pattern of cell body infections seen after PRV infections of the superior cervical ganglion and adrenal gland. (B) Pattern of cell body labeling after injections in the stellate and celiac sympathetic ganglia. (C) Spinal segmental distribution of sympathetic preganglionic neurons labeled after viral infection of the various sympathetic ganglia for comparison with the cell body labeling in the PVH. Reproduced from Strack et al., *Brain Res.*, 491 (1989) 156–162.

observed that the same chemical agent causes bradycardia with no change in blood pressure. The reason for this discrepancy is unknown.

Other studies have been performed that support the idea that the PHV regulates the cardiovascular system. Three examples will be cited. First, when lidocaine is injected into the PVH, it causes an increased level of inhibition of the lumbar sympathetic nerve activity that is elicited during baroreceptor stimulation (Patel and Schmid, 1988). Heart rate changes are not affected. Second, bilateral kainic acid lesions of the PVH reverse hypertension that develops following aortic nerve denervation (Zhang and Ciriello, 1985). Third, bilateral electrolytic lesions of the PVH (which destroyed cell bodies as well as incoming and passing by fibers) affect development of hypertension in spontaneously hypertensive rats (SHR) (Ciriello et al., 1984). The PVH-lesioned rats have lower blood pressure and heart rates than control SHRs. One to 3 months after the lesions, Ciriello and coworkers report that the arterial pressure in the PVH-lesioned animals increases, but remains lower than the blood pressure of the control SHRs. These results suggest that the PVH may be important in the initial phase and in the full expression of the hypertension in the SHR.

Lateral hypothalamic area

The lateral hypothalamic area (LHA) is involved in a variety of different functions such as feeding (Anand and Brobeck, 1951), insulin release (Berthoud et al., 1980), and cardiovascular control (Hilton and Redfern, 1986; Gelsema et al., 1989; Spencer et al., 1989). To date, the majority of these studies have been focused on establishing the role of this area in cardiovascular regulation. Before discussing the evidence supporting this idea, it is worth briefly reviewing the anatomy of the descending projections which arise from the LHA.

Anatomical studies (Berk and Finkelstein, 1982; Hosoya and Matsushita, 1981; Holstege, 1987) using the autoradiographic technique have established that the LHA projects extensively to forebrain, brain stem, and spinal cord areas implicated in autonomic functions (Fig. 5). These areas of termination include the bed nucleus of the stria terminalis, PVH, central gray matter, parabrachial nucleus, nucleus of the solitary tract, the bulbar lateral tegmental field, the ventral medulla and the intermediate zone and IML. The LHA receives inputs from many of these same areas as well. This nucleus and the interconnected nuclei form part of a central autonomic network (see Loewy, 1990 for review).

In order to determine the role this nucleus may play in cardiovascular control, we made an extensive study of the effects of L-glutamate stimulation of the LHA on cardiovascular function in the rat (Spencer et al., 1989). Stimulation of this area causes a decrease in blood pressure, heart rate, and cardiac output and seems to affect only one peripheral vascular bed – the coronary circulation (Fig. 6). The bradycardia is mediated by both β-adrenergic and muscarinic mechanisms. The hypotension is due to a decrease in cardiac output, not a decrease in total peripheral resistance. In addition, stimulation of the LHA causes a reduction in coronary blood flow. It was demonstrated that if heart rate is held constant by electrical pacing of the heart, L-glutamate stimulation of the LHA still causes a fall in blood pressure that is due to a fall in cardiac output. The cardiac output reduction is mediated by both β-sympathetic or parasympathetic mechanisms as determined by dual pharmacological blockade experiments, but when either limb of the autonomic nervous system was blocked alone, the change in cardiac output could not be produced. Under these latter conditions, it seems that some type of compensatory mechanism is operative. The exact central neural circuits and their transmitters involved in this response are unknown, but may be an area of potential importance in the field of hypertension.

Posterior hypothalamus

The idea of what role the posterior hypothalamus plays in autonomic control has undergone a significant revision in the last 5 years. Prior to this

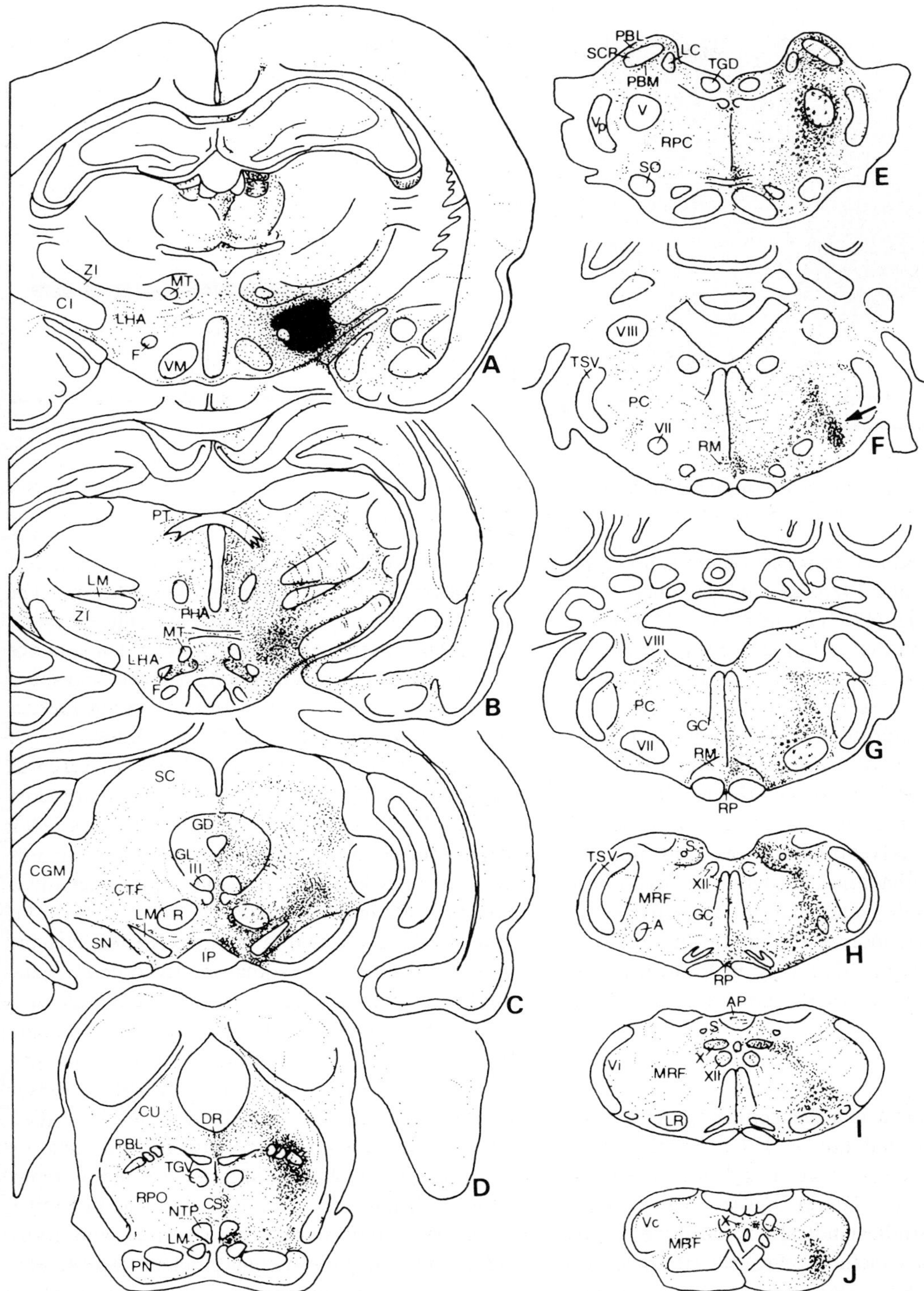

Fig. 5. The descending projections arising from the lateral hypothalamic area. Reproduced from Hosoya and Matsushita, *Neurosci. Lett.*, 24 (1981) 111 – 116.

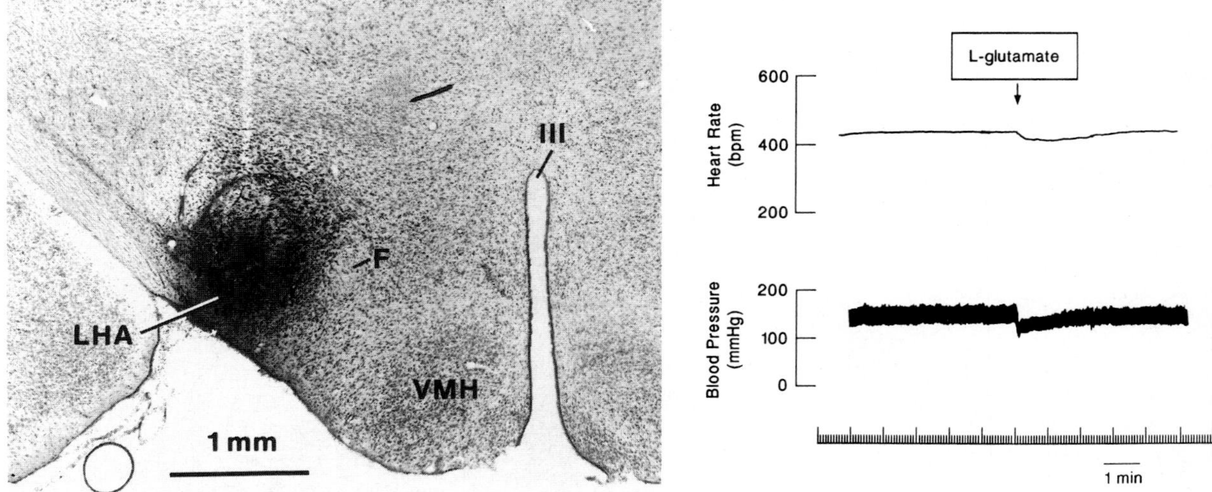

Fig. 6. L-Glutamate stimulation of the lateral hypothalamic area causes a decrease in blood pressure, heart rate, and cardiac output. Reproduced from Spencer et al., *Am. J. Physiol.,* 257 (1989) 540 – 552.

period, it was thought that this region is a pressor area (Kabat et al., 1985; as well as others), but studies by Bandler (1982) in the cat and Hilton and Redfern (1986) in the rat failed to confirm this finding. They found that after microinjections of excitatory amino acids in the posterior hypothalamus, either no response was elicited or a depressor response was found. Gelsema et al. (1989) and Spencer et al. (1990) confirmed this result. The latter showed that the most cardioreactive zone was the posterior periventricular area and not the posterior hypothalamic nucleus as had been previously thought. The anatomical pathways involved in this response are unknown and it is somewhat surprising that very little information exists on connections of the posterior hypothalamus.

Zona incerta

The zona incerta is a diencephalic nucleus that lies between the thalamus and the hypothalamus. Its medial and ventral edges merge with the fields of Forel and the lateral hypothalamic areas. Physiological studies indicate it subserves many diverse functions including arousal (Parmeggiani and Franzini, 1973; Startzl et al., 1951), feeding (Kendrick and Baldwin, 1986), drinking (Mok and Mogenson, 1986, 1987), locomotion (Mogenson et al., 1985) and gonadotropin release (James et al., 1987). The anatomical connections of this area are quite complex and it is distinctly possible that there are specialized subnuclei within the zona incerta that are involved in these different functions.

Afferents to this region arise from the cerebral cortex (especially prefrontal, motor, and somatosensory I and II areas), mesencephalic reticular formation, central gray matter, parabrachial nuclei, dorsal column nuclei, and spinal trigeminal nucleus (Shammah-Lagnado et al., 1985). The zona incerta projects to a number of CNS sites involved in regulation of somatomotor functions, including the globus pallidus, the mesencephalic premotor nuclei (viz., interstitial nucleus of Cajal, nucleus of Darkschewitsch), the inferior olivary nucleus, and cervical ventral horn (Ricardo, 1981). This region also provides a direct input to cardiac sympathetic preganglionic neurons, projects to both vagal motor nuclei, and receives inputs from the lower brain stem visceral relay nuclei including the nucleus tractus solitarius (Ricardo and Koh, 1981) and the parabrachial nucleus (Saper and Loewy, 1980; Shammah-Lagnado et al., 1985).

A number of studies have been directed at trying to understand the role of the zona incerta. Most of the studies suggest that some of the cells in this area are involved in control of water balance. For example, some zona incerta neurons alter their firing after intracarotid arterial injections of hypertonic saline (Tanaka and Seto, 1988) and these neurons project to the subfornical organ – a circumventricular organ involved in control of water intake (see Johnson and Loewy, 1990 for review). Other neurons in this area receive convergent inputs from angiotension II-receptive neurons in the

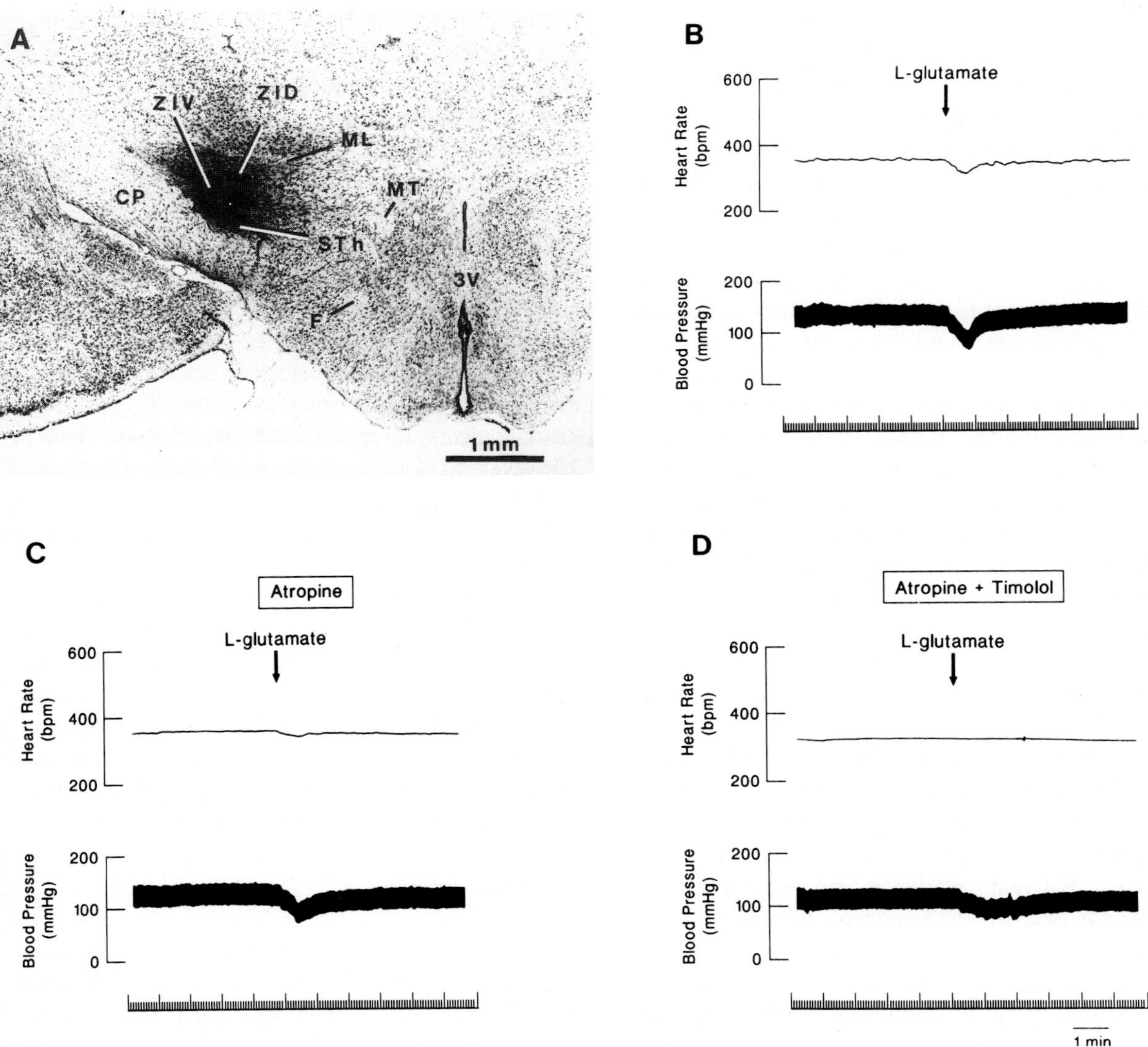

Fig. 7. (A) Photomicrograph showing a ventral zona incerta stimulation site as determined by the autoradiographic method. (B) Polygraph record showing a blood pressure and heart rate decrease after a 15 nl injection of 500 mM L-glutamate into the ventral zona incerta. (C) After i.v. atropine methyl nitrate, the heart rate response elicited by L-glutamate stimulation of the ventral zona incerta was attenuated, but the blood pressure response was only mildly reduced. (D) After combined muscarinic and β-adrenergic blockade of the heart, L-glutamate stimulation of the ventral zona incerta caused only a decrease in blood pressure. This response was ~50% of control value (cf. B and D). Reproduced from Spencer et al., *Brain Res.*, 458 (1988) 72–81.

subfornical organ and possibly osmoreceptors in the basal forebrain (Mok and Mogenson, 1987). Rats with zona incerta lesions show a marked reduction in water intake after intracellular dehydration produced by intraperitoneal injections of hypertonic saline, but appear normal in response to subcutaneous injections of polyethylene glycol which produces extracellular hypovolemia (Walsh and Grossman, 1976). As with many of the other forebrain autonomic nuclei, the details regarding the neural pathways subserving these functions are unknown.

L-glutamate stimulation of the zona incerta causes hypotension and bradycardia in rats (Spencer, Sawyer and Loewy, 1988). The bradycardia is mediated mainly via the vagal outflow because it is almost completely eliminated after atropine methyl nitrate treatment (Fig. 7). β-Blockade with timolol caused a further reduction in the response. In a series of L-glutamate microinjection experiments, it was found that the most sensitive cardioreactive region lies in the ventral zona incerta (Fig. 7). Control injections made ventral to this area which involved the subthalamic nucleus and dorsal to it, involving the dorsal zona incerta produced virtually no cardiovascular change.

Basal forebrain

Certain nuclei in the basal forebrain are thought to be involved in neural regulation of autonomic functions. The two most likely candidates are the amygdala and the bed nucleus of the stria terminalis. Current evidence suggests that the amygdala and the bed nucleus of the stria terminalis are essentially the same neuroanatomical structure. These two forebrain nuclei become subdivided during brain development by the stria terminalis and some nuclei of the basal forebrain such as the ventral palladium (De Olmos et al., 1985; Holstege et al., 1985). The central amygdaloid nucleus and the lateral part of the bed nucleus of the stria terminalis are similar in terms of their afferent and efferent connections and their chemoarchitecture (Holstege et al., 1985; Hopkins and Holstege, 1978; Gray and Magnuson, 1987). Both of these nuclei appear to be part of the central autonomic network with interconnections with the lower brain stem autonomic cell group like the parabrachial nucleus and nucleus tractus solitarius as well as other sites.

The function of these CNS regions is unclear and to date only relatively few studies have been performed on the central amygdaloid nucleus and none on the bed nucleus of the stria terminalis. Despite this paucity of data, the central amygdaloid nucleus is thought to be involved in fear or stress-related functions which affect the autonomic nervous system. This has been deduced from behavioral studies following electrolytic lesions of the amygdala (e.g. Hitchcock and Davis, 1987; LeDoux et al., 1984). In support of this idea is the observation that chronic electrical stimulation of the amygdala has been shown to produce gastric ulcers (Henke, 1982; Ray et al., 1987). However, as with any electrical lesion or stimulation study concern has to be raised regarding whether the response is actually due to the cell bodies of the area or axonal systems projecting to or through it. To avoid this problem, Iwata et al. (1987) used L-glutamate chemical stimulation to activate the central nucleus of the amygdala and demonstrated that stimulation of this area causes an increase in heart rate and blood pressure. Because of only limited additional data, it is impossible at this stage to describe much more about the role of this area in autonomic function.

Cerebral cortex

The issue of whether the cerebral cortex influences the autonomic nervous system has been debated for over a century and has been reviewed by Cechetto and Saper (1990). Electrical stimulation of the motor cortex produces limb movements and these movements are accompanied by hypotension and an increase in limb blood flow (vasodilation). This debate centered over whether the cardiovascular response was due to direct activation of the sympathetic nervous system or is an indirect effect. This issue was resolved when it was demonstrated that the increase in blood flow in skeletal muscle is due to a hyperemia that occurred as a secondary response to the muscular contraction and is independent of the sympathetic nervous system (Hilton et al., 1979). Thus, the motor cortex is no longer regarded as a site that regulates the autonomic nervous system. However, other cortical areas have been shown to be involved in autonomic control.

The insular cortex is one these areas. Three lines of experimental evidence support this idea. First, microinjections of L-glutamic or kainic acid into this region produces an increase in blood pressure and heart rate (Ruggiero et al., 1987). Second, electrophysiological recordings have been made in insular cortex and it has been demonstrated that this area receives inputs from gustatory (Yamamoto et al., 1980; Pritchard et al., 1986; Kosar and Norgren, 1987) and other visceral nerves carrying information from gastric mechanoreceptors, arterial chemoreceptors, and baroreceptors (Cechetto and Saper, 1987). These inputs appear to be viscerotopically organized in a similar manner as the somatic sensory cortex. Third, the insular cortex receives inputs from several visceral relay centers including the ventroposteromedial parvocellular nucleus of the thalamus (VPMpc), the lateral hypothalamic area, and parabrachial nucleus. Finally, the insular cortex projects to four autonomic regions implicated in autonomic control including the central nucleus of the amygdala, lateral hypothalamic area, parabrachial nucleus, and nucleus tractus solitarius (see Cechetto and Saper, 1990 for review).

The medial prefrontal cortex is another area involved in autonomic processing, although the evidence supporting this view is far less conclusive than the information that has been accumulated on the insular cortex. Briefly, this cortical area receives inputs from a number of limbic areas including the prelimbic, insular, and entorhinal cortices, the hippocampus and the amygdala, and other areas including the ventroposteromedial parvocellular thalamic nucleus (VPMpc), lateral hypothalamic area, parabrachial nucleus, and nucleus of the solitary tract. It projects to most of these areas as well (Terreberry and Neafsey, 1987). To date, the physiological studies of this region that have been published have relied on electrical stimulation or lesion methods, and thus it is difficult to interpret the significance of these findings (Cechetto and Saper, 1990). This area of the cerebral cortex should provide fertile ground for future physiological studies.

Summary

Several key regions of the forebrain are involved in regulation of autonomic functions (Fig. 8). These areas include the several areas within the hypothalamus (viz., paraventricular hypothalamic nucleus, lateral hypothalamic area, posterior periventricular area, and zona incerta), the basal forebrain (viz., central nucleus of the amygdala and bed nucleus of the stria terminalis), and the cerebral cortex (viz., insular and medial prefrontal

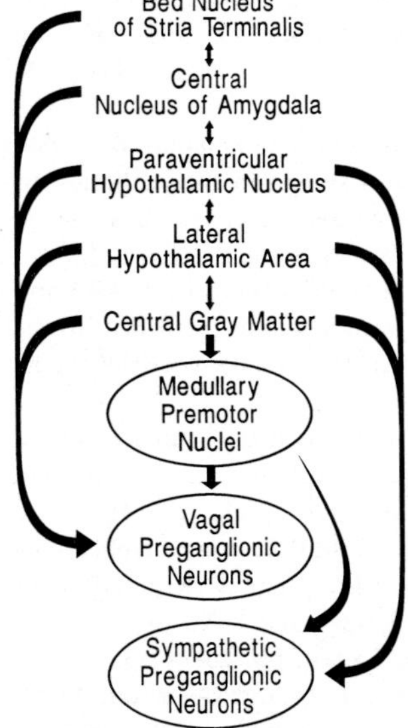

Fig. 8. Summary of the interconnections of forebrain autonomic cell groups and potential pathways that regulate the vagal and sympathetic preganglionic neurons.

cortex). All these areas have been implicated on anatomical grounds to be part of a central autonomic network involving multiple interconnecting circuits. Apart from these complex interconnections, most of these areas project to the lower brain stem where they are capable of influencing the cell groups which innervate the vagal and sympathetic preganglionic neurons or in some cases, like the paraventricular hypothalamic nucleus and the lateral hypothalamic area, provide direct projections to these neurons.

References

Anand, B.K. and Brobeck, J.R. (1951) Hypothalamic control of food intake. *Yale J. Biolog. Med.* 24, 123 – 140.

Appel, N.M., Wessendorf, M.W. and Elde, R.P. (1987) Thyrotropin-releasing hormone in spinal cord: coexistence with serotonin and with substance P in fibers and terminals apposing identified preganglionic sympathetic neurons. *Brain Res.,* 415, 137 – 143.

Backman, S.B. and Henry, J.L. (1984) Effects of oxytocin and vasopressin on thoracic sympathetic preganglionic neurones in the cat. *Brain Res. Bull.,* 13, 679 – 684.

Bandler, R. (1982) Induction of "rage" following microinjections of glutamate into midbrain but not hypothalamus of cats. *Neurosci. Lett.,* 30, 183 – 188.

Berk, M.L. and Finkelstein, J.A. (1982) Efferent connections of the lateral hypothalamic area of the rat: an autoradiographic investigation. *Brain Res. Bull.,* 8, 511 – 526.

Berthoud, H.-R., Bereiter, D.A. and Jeanranaud, B. (1980) Role of the autonomic nervous system in the mediation of LHA electrical stimulation-induced effects on insulinemia and glycemia. *J. Autonom. Nerv., System,* 2, 183 – 198.

Blessing, W.W. and Reis, D.J. (1983) Evidence that GABA and glycine-like inputs inhibit vasodepressor neurons in the caudal ventrolateral medulla of the rabbit. *Neurosci. Lett.,* 37, 57 – 62.

Cechetto, D.F. and Saper, C.B. (1987) Evidence for a viscerotopic sensory representation in the cortex and thalamus in the rat. *J. Comp. Neurol.,* 252, 27 – 45.

Cechetto, D.F. and Saper, C.B. (1990) Role of the cerebral cortex in autonomic function. In: Central Regulation of Autonomic Function, A.D. Loewy and K.M. Spyer (eds.), Oxford University Press, New York, pp. 208 – 223.

Ciriello, J., Kline, R.L., Zhang, T.X. and Caverson, M.M. (1984) Lesions of the paraventricular nucleus alter development of spontaneous hypertension in the rat. *Brain Research,* 310, 355 – 359.

Darlington, D.N., Shinsako, J. and Dallman, M.R. (1988) Paraventricular lesions: hormonal and cardiovascular responses to hemorrhage. *Brain Research,* 439, 289 – 301.

DeOlmos, J., Alheid, G.F. and Beltramino, C.A. (1985) Amygdala, vol. 1 In: G. Painos (Ed.), *The Rat Nervous System.* Academic Press, New York; pp. 223 – 307.

Gelsema, A.J., Roe, M.J. and Calaresu, F.R. (1989) Neurally mediated cardiovascular responses to stimulation of cell bodies in the hypothalamus of the rat. *Brain Res.,* 482, 67 – 77.

Gilbey, M.P., Coote, J.H., Fleetwood-Walker, S. and Peterson, D.F. (1982) The influence of the paraventriculo-spinal pathway, and oxytocin and vasopressin on sympathetic preganglionic neurons. *Brain Res.,* 251, 283 – 290.

Goodchild, A.K., Dampney, R.A.L. and Bandler, R. (1982) A method for evoking physiological responses by stimulation of cell bodies but not axons of passage, within a localized region of the central nervous system. *J. Neurosci. Methods,* 6, 351 – 363.

Gray, T.S. and Magnuson, D.J. (1987) Neuropeptide neuronal efferents from the bed nucleus of the stria terminalis and central nucleus of amygdala to the dorsal vagal complex in the rat. *J. Comp. Neurol.,* 262, 365 – 374.

Henke, P.G. (1982) The telencephalic limbic system and experimental gastric pathology: A review. *Neurosci. Biobehav. Rev.,* 6, 381 – 390.

Hilton, S.M. and Redfern, W.S. (1986) A search for brain stem cell groups integrating the defense reaction in the rat. *J. Physiol. (London),* 378, 213 – 228.

Hilton, S.M., Spyer, K.M. and Timms, R.J. (1979) The origin of the hindlimb vasodilation evoked by stimulation of the motor cortex in the cat. *J. Physiol.,* 287, 545 – 557.

Hitchcock, J.M. and Davis, M. (1987) Fear-potential startle using an auditory conditioned stimulus: Effect of lesions of the amygdala. *Physiolog., Behavior,* 39, 403 – 408.

Holstege, G. (1987) Some anatomical observations on the projections from the hypothalamus to brainstem and spinal cord. An HRP and autoradiographic tracing study. *J. Comp. Neurol.,* 260: 98 – 126.

Holstege, G., Meiners, L. and Tan, K. (1985) Projections of the bed nucleus of the stria terminalis to the mesencephalon, pons, and medulla oblongata in the cat. *Exp. Brain Res.,* 58, 379 – 391.

Hopkins, D.A. and Holstege, G. (1978) Amygdaloid projections to the mesencephalon, pons and medulla oblongata in the cat. *Exp. Brain Res.,* 32, 529 – 547.

Hosoya, Y. and Matsushita, M. (1981) Brainstem projections from the lateral hypothalamic area in the rat, as studied with autoradiography. *Neurosci. Lett.,* 24, 111 – 116.

Hosoya, Y., Matsushita, M. and Sugiura, Y. (1983) A direct hypothalamic projection to the superior salvatory nucleus neurons in the rat. A study using anterograde autoradiographic and retrograde HRP methods. *Brain Res.,* 266, 329 – 333.

Iwata, J., Chida, K. and LeDoux, J.E. (1987) Cardiovascular

responses elicited by stimulation of neurons in the central nucleus of amygdala in awake but not anesthetized rats resemble conditioned emotional responses. *Brain Res.,* 418, 183 – 188.

James, M.D., MacKensie, F.J., Touhy-Jones, P.A. and Wilson, C.A. (1987) Dopaminergic neurones in the zona incerta exert a stimulatory control on gonadotropin release via D_1 dopamine receptors. *Neuroendocrinol., (Basel),* 45, 348 – 355.

Johnson, A.K. and Loewy, A.D. (1990) Circumventricular organs and their role in visceral functions. In: A.D. Loewy and K.M. Spyer (Eds.), *Central Regulation of Autonomic Functions.* Oxford University Press, New York, pp. 247 – 267.

Kabat, H., Magoun, H.W. and Ranson, S.W. (1935) Electrical stimulation of points in the forebrain and midbrain: the resultant alterations in blood pressure. *Arch. Neurol., (Chicago),* 34, 931 – 955.

Karplus, J.P. and Kreidl, A. (1909) Gehirn und Sympathicus, I. Mitteilung. Zwischen hirnbasis und Halosympatheticus. *Pflügers Arch. Ges. Physiol.,* 129, 138 – 144.

Karplus, J.P. and Kreidl, A. (1910) Gehirn und Sympathicus. I. Ein sympathicuszentrum im Zwischenhirn. *Pflügers Arch. Ges. Physiol.,* 135, 401 – 416.

Katafuchi, T., Oomura, Y. and Kurosawa, M. (1988) Effects of chemical stimulation of paraventricular nucleus on adrenal and renal nerve activity in rats. *Neurosci. Lett.,* 86, 195 – 200.

Kendrick, K.M. and Baldwin, B.A. (1986) The activity of neurones in the lateral hypothalamus and zona incerta of the sheep responding to the sight or approach of food is modified by learning and satiety and reflects food preference. *Brain Res.,* 375, 320 – 328.

Kosar, E., Grill, H.J. and Norgren, R. (1986) Gustatory cortex in the rat. I. Physiological properties and cytoarchitecture. *Brain Res.,* 379, 329 – 341.

LeDoux, J.E., Sakaguchi, A. and Reis, D.J. (1984) Subcortical efferent projections of the medial geniculate nucleus mediate emotional responses conditioned to acoustic stimuli. *J. Neurosci.,* 4, 683 – 698.

Loewy, A.D. (1990) Central autonomic pathways. In: A.D. Loewy and K.M. Spyer (Eds.), *Central Regulation of Autonomic Functions.* Oxford University Press, New York, pp. 88 – 103.

Loewy, A.D. and Spyer, K.M. (1990) Vagal preganglionic neurons. In: A.D. Loewy and K.M. Spyer (Eds.), *Central Regulation of Autonomic Functions.* Oxford University Press, New York, pp. 68 – 87.

Luiten, P.G.M., ter Horst, G.J., Karst, H. and Steffens, A.B. (1985) The course of paraventricular hypothalamic efferents to autonomic structures in medulla and spinal cord. *Brain Res.,* 329, 374 – 378.

Mancia, G. and Zanchetti, A. (1981) Hypothalamic control of autonomic functions. In: P.J. Morgane and J. Panksepp (Eds.), *Handbook of the Hypothalamus,* Vol. 3B, Dekker, New York, pp. 147 – 202.

Mogenson, G.J., Swanson, L.W. and Mu, M. (1985) Evidence that projections from substantia innominata to zona incerta and mesencephalic locomotor region contribute to locomotor activity. *Brain Res.,* 334, 65 – 76.

Mok, D. and Mogenson, G.J. (1986) Contribution of zona incerta to osmotically induced drinking in rats. *Am. J. Physiol.,* 251, R823 – R832.

Mok, D. and Mogenson, G.J. (1987) Convergence of signals in the zona incerta for angiotensin mediate and osmotic thirst. *Brain Res.,* 407, 332 – 340.

Neil, J.J. and Loewy, A.D. (1982) Decreases in blood pressure in response to L-glutamate microinjections into the A5 catecholamine cell group. *Brain Res.,* 241, 271 – 278.

Nosaka, S., Yamamoto, T. and Tamai, S. (1982) Vagal cardiac preganglionic neurons: distribution, cell types, and reflex discharge. *Am. J. Physiol.,* 243, R92 – R98.

Nosaka, S., Yamamoto, T. and Yasunaga, K. (1979) Localization of vagal cardioinhibitory preganglionic neurons with rat brain stem. *J. Comp. Neurol.,* 186, 79 – 92.

Parmeggiani, P.L. and Franzini, C. (1973) On the functional significance of subcortical single unit activity during sleep. *Electroencephalog. Clin. Neurophysiol.,* 34, 495 – 508.

Patel, K.P. and Schmid, P.G. (1988) Role of paraventricular nucleus (PVH) in baroreflex-mediated changes in lumbar sympathetic nerve activity and heart rate. *J. Autonom. Nerv. System,* 22, 211 – 219.

Price, J.L., Russchen, F.T. and Amaral, D.G. (1987) The limbic region. II. The amygdaloid complex. In: A. Bjorklund, T. Hokfelt, and L.W. Swanson (Eds.), *Chemical Neuroanatomy, Vol. 5, Integrated Systems of the CNS, Part I.* Elsevier, Amsterdam, pp. 279 – 388.

Ray, A., Henke, P.G. and Sullivan, R. (1987) The central amygdala and immobilization stress-induced gastric pathology in rats: neurotensin and dopamine. *Brain Res.,* 409, 398 – 402.

Ricardo, J. (1981) Efferent connections of the subthalamic region in the rat. II. The zona incerta. *Brain Res.,* 214, 43 – 60.

Ruggiero, D.A., Mraovitch, S., Grenata, A.R., Anwar, M. and Reis, D.J. (1987) Role of insular cortex in cardiovascular functions. *J. Comp. Neurol.,* 257, 189 – 207.

Shammah-Lagnado, S.J., Negrao, N. and Ricardo, J.A. (1985) Afferent connections of the zona incerta: a horseradish peroxidase study in the rat. *Neuroscience,* 15, 109 – 134.

Spencer, S.E., Sawyer, W.B. and Loewy, A.D. (1988) L-Glutamate stimulation of the zona incerta in the rat decreases heart rate and blood pressure. *Brain Res.,* 458, 72 – 81.

Spencer, S.E., Sawyer, W.B. and Loewy, A.D. (1989) Cardiovascular effects produced by L-glutamate stimulation of the lateral hypothalamus area. *Am. J. Physiol.,* 257, H540 – H552.

Spencer, S.E., Sawyer, W.B. and Loewy, A.D. (1990) L-glutamate mapping of cardioreactive areas in the rat posterior hypothalamus. *Brain Res.,* 511, 149 – 157.

Startzl, T.E., Taylor, C.W. and Magoun, H.W. (1951) Ascending conduction in reticular activating system, with special reference to the diencephalon. *J. Neurophysiol.,* 14, 461 – 477.

Strack, A.M., Sawyer, W.B., Hughes, J.H., Platt, K.B. and Loewy, A.D. (1989a) A general pattern of CNS innervation of the sympathetic outflow demonstrated by transneuronal pseudorabies viral infections. *Brain Res.,* 491, 156 – 162.

Strack, A.M., Sawyer, W.B., Platt, K.B. and Loewy, A.D. (1989b) CNS cell groups regulating the sympathetic nervous outflow to adrenal gland as revealed by transneuronal cell body labeling with pseudorabies virus. *Brain Res.,* 491, 274 – 296.

Swanson, L.W. (1987) The hypothalamus. In: A. Bjorklund, T. Hokfelt and L.W. Swanson (Eds.), *Chemical Neuroanatomy, Vol. 5, Integrated Systems of the CNS,* Part I, Elsevier, Amsterdam, pp. 1 – 124.

Tanaka, J. and Seto, K. (1988) Neurons in the lateral hypothalamic area and zona incerta with ascending projections to the subfornical organ area in the rat. *Brain Res.,* 456, 397 – 400.

ter Horst, G.J., Luiten, P.G.M. and Kuypers, F. (1984) Descending pathways from hypothalamus to dorsal motor vagus or ambiguus nuclei in the rat. *J. Autonom. Nerv. System,* 11, 59 – 75.

Terreberry, R.R. and Neafsey, E.J. (1987) The rat media frontal cortex projects directly to autonomic regions of the brain stem. *Brain Res. Bull.,* 17, 639 – 649.

Walsh, L.L. and Grossman, S.P. (1976) Zona incerta lesions impair osmotic but not hypovolemic thirst. *Physiol. Behavior,* 16, 211 – 215.

Yamamoto, T., Matsuo, R. and Kawamura, Y. (1980) Localization of cortical gustatory area in rats and its role in taste discrimination. *J. Neurophysiol.,* 44, 440 – 455.

Yamashita, H., Kannan, H., Kasai, M. and Osaka, T. (1987) Decrease in blood pressure by stimulation of the rat hypothalamic paraventricular nucleus with L-glutamate or weak current. *J. Autonom. Nerv. System,* 19, 229 – 234.

Zhang, T.-X. and Ciriello, J. (1985) Kainic acid lesions of paraventricular nucleus neurons reverse the elevated arterial pressure after aortic baroreceptor denervation in the rat. *Brain Res.,* 358, 334 – 338.

G. Holstege (Ed.)
Progress in Brain Research, Vol. 87

CHAPTER 13

Integration of somatic and autonomic reactions within the midbrain periaqueductal grey: Viscerotopic, somatotopic and functional organization

Richard Bandler, Pascal Carrive and Shi Ping Zhang

Brain-Behavior Laboratory, Department of Anatomy, The University of Sydney, Sydney, NSW, Australia 2006

Introduction

Considerable evidence suggests that the cell dense region surrounding the midbrain aqueduct, the midbrain periaqueductal grey region (PAG), is a crucial neural substrate for the integration of an animal's reactions to threatening or stressful stimuli. It has been known since the work of Hunsperger (1956) and Skultety (1963), that electrical stimulation within the midbrain PAG or the adjacent tegmentum elicits, in the freely moving cat, behavior characteristic of a cat's natural defense reactions (i.e., threat display, attack and flight). As well, electrical stimulation within the PAG or adjacent tegmentum of the acute, anesthetized cat evokes cardiovascular changes, including increased arterial pressure, tachycardia, and regional blood flow changes characteristic of defense (Abrahams et al., 1960; Eliasson et al., 1954; Lindgren, 1955; Lindgren, et al., 1956). Similar results have been reported for the rat, monkey and a number of other species (see Bandler, 1988, for a recent review). That such stimulation affects an intrinsic midbrain circuitry, rather than simply exciting descending fibres of passage (e.g., from hypothalamus or amygdala) is suggested by the findings that the integrated patterns of somatic and autonomic changes characteristic of defensive reactions can be elicited by midbrain electrical stimulation or natural stimuli: (i) in the precollicular decerebrate cat (Bard and Macht, 1958; Keller, 1932); (ii) after either large hypothalamic or amygdaloid lesions (Fernandez DeMolina and Hunsperger, 1962; Kelly et al., 1946); or, (iii) after surgical isolation of the hypothalamus (Ellison and Flynn, 1968; Gellen et al., 1972). As well, lesions which extensively damage the PAG either eliminate or dramatically attenuate defense reactions evoked by nociceptive stimuli, by confrontation with another animal, or by electrical stimulation of the hypothalamus or the amygdala (Blanchard et al., 1981; Edwards and Adams, 1974; Fernandez DeMolina and Hunsperger, 1962; Hunsperger, 1956; Skultety, 1963). Until recently, however, little information has been available concerning, either the representation within the PAG of the individual components of defense reactions; or how, within the PAG, the individual somatic and autonomic components are integrated into defense reactions.

The discovery that electrical and chemical stimulation of the PAG evoked analgesia (Liebeskind et al., 1973; Mayer et al., 1971; Reynolds, 1969; Urca et al., 1980; Yaksh et al., 1976) focused additional interest on the PAG and led to many new studies of the cytoarchitecture, connectional and chemical organization of the PAG. These studies have indicated: (i) that neurons containing different neurotransmitters and neuropeptides are found within distinct parts of the PAG (e.g., Beitz et al., 1983; Moss and Basbaum, 1983; Moss et al., 1983; Reichling et al., 1988); (ii) that PAG projection neurons are localized to distinct parts of the PAG (Holstege, 1988; Rose, 1981; ter Horst et al., 1984); (iii) that specific afferents have restricted PAG termination zones (Blomqvist and Wiberg, 1985; Yezierski, 1988). Overall, however, there has been a lack of success in elucidating with tract tracing, immunohistochemical and autoradiographic receptor binding techniques, the neural organization underlying the complex physiological functions mediated by the PAG. One obvious difficulty is that in contrast to brain regions for which the neural representation of a specific sensory input or a specific motor output is an obvious focus of study, in a brain region implicated in as many different functions as the PAG, it is often not clear which are the most relevant functional units for analysis.

A premise of the work to be described here is that the great diversity of PAG output functions makes an understanding of its functional organization prerequisite to the study of its neural organization. In the work that follows we will consider first the results of studies from our laboratory which have employed the technique of intracerebral stimulation with excitatory amino acids (EAA) in order to map the diverse functional output zones that exist within the PAG. Next, the results of anatomical studies of the PAG efferents, which may mediate certain outputs will be considered. Finally, data pertaining to the afferent regulation of the functionally diverse PAG regions will be discussed.

Functional organization within the PAG

As electrical stimulation excites cell bodies and axons of passage, the exact location of the neuronal cell bodies which mediate the reactions evoked by midbrain electrical stimulation cannot be determined from such studies. The intracerebral microinjection of EAA (e.g., L-glutamic acid, L-aspartic acid, D,L-homocysteic acid, kainic acid) represents a well accepted method for selectively exciting neuronal cell bodies (and their dendritic processes) within the central nervous system (Goodchild et al., 1982; Lipski et al., 1988). Therefore, in order to investigate the PAG functional organization mediating defense reactions, microinjections of EAA were made at sites in the midbrain of the cat and behavioral and cardiovascular variables measured. Experiments were carried out in both the unanesthetized decerebrate cat and the intact, freely moving cat.

Experiments in the decerebrate cat

The use of an unanesthetized, unparalyzed decerebrate preparation made it possible to study simultaneously both the cardiovascular and certain of the somatomotor changes characteristic of defense. The decerebration procedure involved the removal of the entire forebrain, except for the ventral portion of the hypothalamus. It was carried out, in the halothane anesthetized cat, by the use of a suction-diathermy procedure (Carrive et al., 1987, 1989a; Korner et al., 1969). Prior to decerebration, while under anesthesia, cats were instrumented for the recording of arterial pressure (via a catheter in the right femoral artery), heart rate (derived from the pulsatile pressure signal), and blood flows, measured via electromagnetic flow probes, placed around two of the following arteries: left external iliac artery, left renal artery, left superior mesenteric artery, left common carotid artery. After completion of the decerebration, anesthesia was discontinued. Experimental observation did not begin until at least 30 min later. Behavioral responses were recorded on videotape for later analysis. In order to determine if the evoked cardiovascular changes were secondary to movement or respiratory changes, additional experiments were undertaken in decerebrate cats which were paralyzed with Flaxedil (15 mg/kg, i.m.) and artificially ventilated. For intracerebral chemical stimulation, a stainless steel injection cannula (o.d. 0.28 mm, i.d. 0.18 mm) was inserted vertically into the midbrain and microinjections of D,L-homocysteic acid (DLH) were made at sites within and surrounding the PAG. The standard injection was 40 nmol of DLH in a volume of 0.20 μl of phosphate buffer (0.02M, pH 7.4). Injections were usually made at 3 to 6 sites along a track and the sites were separated by approximately 0.50 mm (for further details see Carrive et al., 1987, 1989a).

The PAG can be roughly divided into a rostral two-thirds, which because it lies in front of the tentorium cerebri (which in the cat is made of bone) has been referred to as the pretentorial PAG, and a caudal one-third, which because it lies beneath the tentorium has been referred to as the subtentorial PAG. The pretentorial PAG extends from approximately A5.2 to A0.6, and the subtentorial PAG from A0.6 to P2.0 (Fig. 1). In order to insert the injection cannula vertically into the subtentorial PAG, it was necessary to first remove the tentorium cerebri.

Arterial pressure

Microinjections of DLH were made at sites, in and surrounding the PAG of the decerebrate cat. As seen in Fig. 2, DLH microinjections made at sites within a longitudinal column, lateral to the midbrain aqueduct, extending from approximately A3.3 to P1.5, evoked a 20 – 50% increase in arterial pressure. In contrast, DLH microinjections made at sites, within a longitudinal column, ventrolateral to the midbrain aqueduct, extending from approximately A2.0 to P1.5, evoked a 5 – 25% decrease in arterial pressure. Apart from these regions, microinjections of DLH within the rest of the PAG or the adjacent midbrain tegmen-

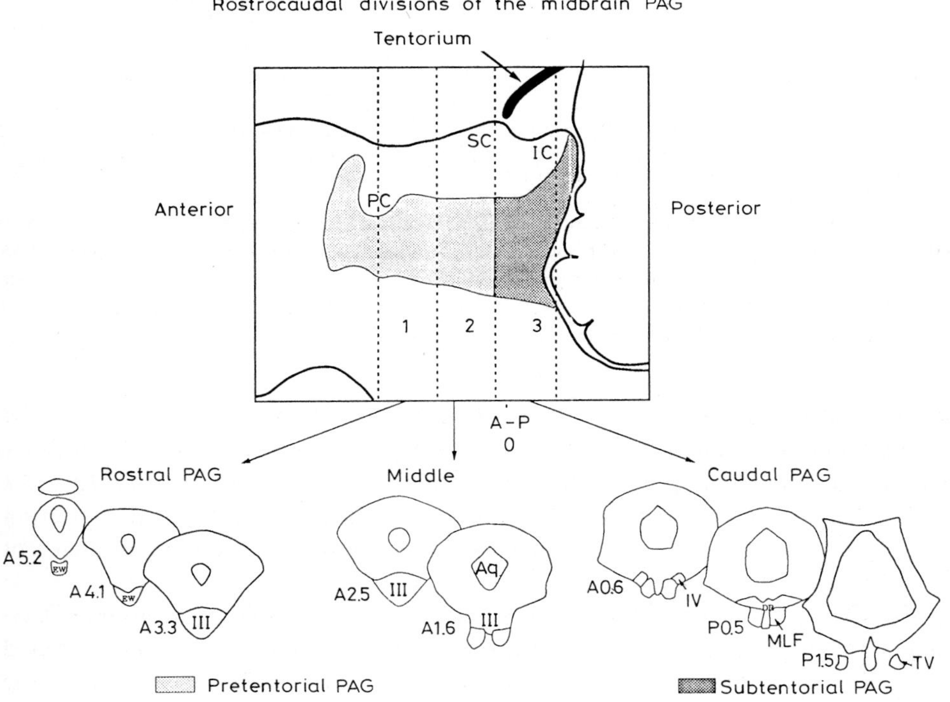

Fig. 1. Parasagittal representation of the midbrain of the cat showing the PAG (shaded), with respect to the bony tentorium cerebri. The rostral and middle one-third of the PAG constitute the pretentorial PAG (light shading). The caudal third of the PAG corresponds to the subtentorial PAG (darker shading). Coordinates are in mm (anterior or posterior) from the interaural plane (Berman, 1968).

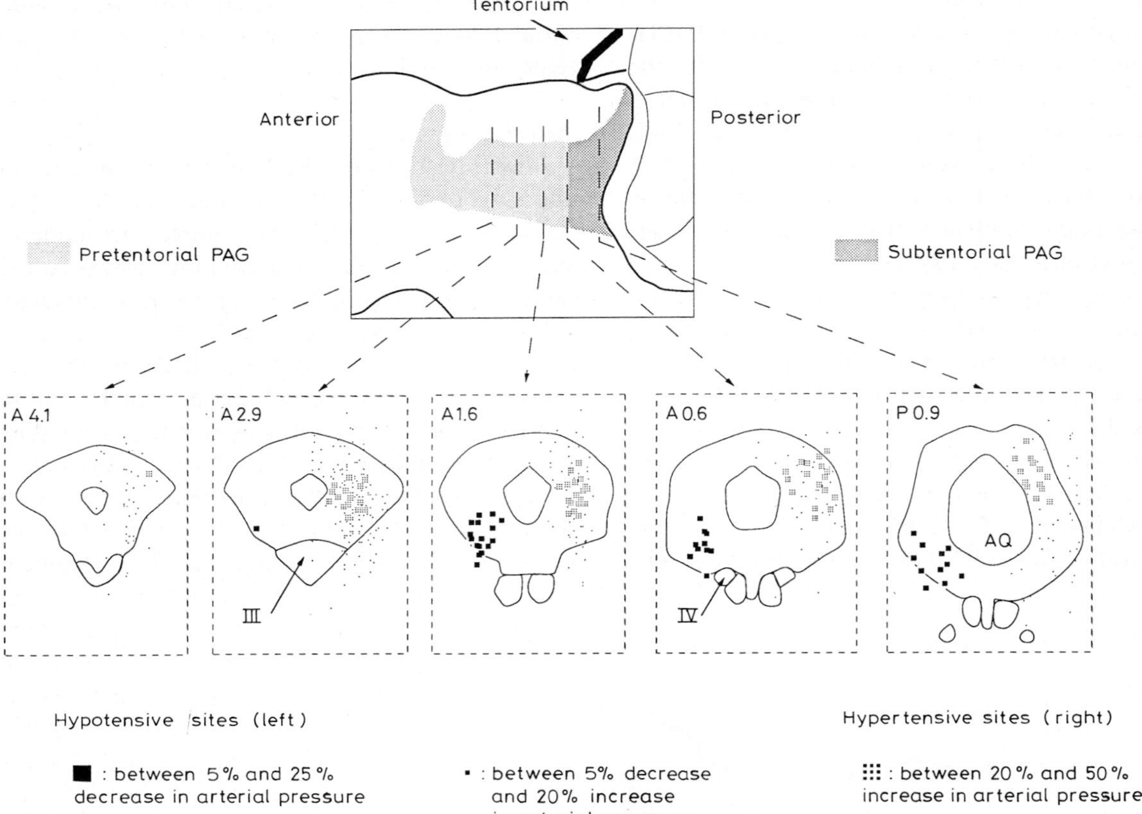

Fig. 2. (Top): schematic parasagittal view of the PAG showing the extent of the pretentorial and subtentorial portions of the PAG. (Bottom): a series of 5 representative coronal sections, drawn with reference to the atlas of Berman (1968), showing the location of the centers of the sites at which arterial blood pressure changes were evoked following microinjections of DLH, in the decerebrate cat. Sites at which hypotensive reactions were evoked are plotted on the left side. Sites at which no change in arterial presure or hypertensive reactions were evoked are plotted on the right side (reproduced from Fig. 2 of Carrive et al., 1991a).

tum had no significant effect on blood pressure. Paralysis and artifical ventilation did not alter the hypertensive or hypotensive reactions evoked by DLH microinjection within the lateral or ventrolateral PAG.

Since DLH, like other EAA, excites cell bodies and their dendritic processes (but not axons of passage), these results suggest that the evoked reactions are mediated by direct excitation of "pressor" or "depressor" neurons found near the tip of the injection cannula in the lateral and ventrolateral PAG. In support of this interpretation are the following observations: (i) the hypertensive and hypotensive effects were always the primary effect evoked by DLH microinjection; (ii) these effects were usually evoked within the first 10 – 15 s post-injection, and (iii) a lowering of the injection cannula 0.50 – 1.0 mm often resulted in different effects.

To summarize, these results indicate that PAG neurons modulating arterial pressure are restricted topographically to the caudal two-thirds of the PAG. PAG "pressor neurons" are found lateral to the midbrain aqueduct within a longitudinal column extending from approximately A3.3 to P1.5. PAG "depressor" neurons are found ventrolateral to the midbrain aqueduct, within a somewhat rostrocaudally compressed longitudinal column extending from approximately A2.0 to P1.5.

Changes in regional vascular beds

Distinct patterns of changes in regional blood flows accompanied the hypertensive and hypotensive reactions evoked respectively from the pretentorial and subtentorial PAG (Carrive and Bandler 1991a,b; Carrive et al., 1987, 1989a).

Pretentorial PAG hypertensive pattern As seen in Fig. 3, the hypertensive reaction evoked from the pretentorial PAG was accompanied by a large decrease in iliac conductance (30 – 50%). There was, as well, a small to moderate decrease in renal or superior mesenteric conductance (5 – 30%). Common carotid flow was studied only in the paralyzed preparation. It was found that DLH evoked a large increase in common carotid conductance (30 – 60%) at sites at which iliac constriction and hypertension were also evoked (Fig. 4, left). It should be noted, that in the decerebrate preparation common carotid blood flow almost exclusively supplies extracranial vascular beds, since the intracranial vasculature (i.e., forebrain) had been largely removed. Each of the blood flow changes occurred during the early stages of the reaction (first 10 – 20 s) and were not secondary to movement, since they could be evoked also in the paralyzed preparation. The region at which DLH evoked this hypertensive pattern was restricted to the part of the pretentorial PAG, lateral to the aqueduct, between approximately A3.3 to A1.0 (Fig. 5).

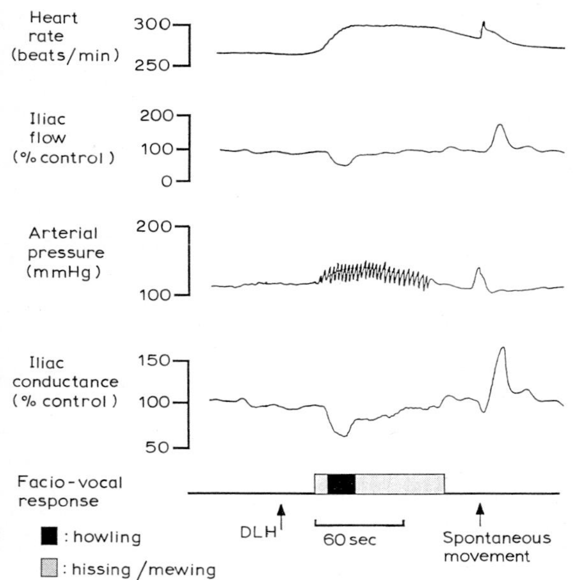

Fig. 3. Example of cardiovascular changes evoked from the lateral, pretentorial PAG of the unparalyzed, decerebrate cat. The first arrow indicates the point where a DLH microinjection (40 nmol) was made. The period of intense facio-vocal reaction (howling) is indicated by dark shading, and was preceeded and followed by a period of moderate facio-vocal reaction (hissing/mewing). Note that the period of howling was accompanied by a marked decrease in iliac conductance (reproduced from Fig. 2, of Carrive et al., 1987).

Subtentorial PAG hypertensive pattern As seen in Fig 6A, a quite different pattern of regional blood flow changes accompanied the hypertensive reaction evoked from the subtentorial PAG. Specifically, there were substantial decreases in renal or superior mesenteric conductances (30 – 50%) and a large increase in external iliac conductance (100 – 200%). This pattern was also obtained in the paralyzed preparation, indicating that the regional blood flow changes were not secondary to movement (Fig. 6B). Again, common carotid flow was only studied in the paralyzed preparation. It was found also that DLH injected in the subtentorial PAG evoked a substantial decrease in carotid conductance (20 – 40%) at sites at which hypertension and iliac dilation were also evoked (Fig. 4, right).

The external iliac vasodilation was mediated by both sympathetic, cholinergic vasodilator nerves and circulating catecholamines acting on β-adrenergic receptors on skeletal muscles arteries, since: (i) intravenous injection of the muscarinic receptor blocker, atropine sulphate (0.45 mg/kg), eliminated the sharp, early occurring vasodilation component, but spared the component of vasodilation which was slower in onset and more gradual in ocurrence (Fig. 7); (ii) intravenous injection of the β-adrenoreceptor antagonist, propranolol (0.3 mg/kg) eliminated the late component of the external iliac vasodilation (Fig. 7). Results from these experiments also suggest that the subtentorial PAG neurons regulating the cholinergic and adrenergic components of the iliac vasodilation are topographically separable. That is, the early occurring, atropine sensitive vasodilation was evoked from sites dorsal to those at which the late occurring, propranolol sensitive vasodilation was evoked (Fig. 7).

As seen in Fig. 5, the subtentorial PAG region at which DLH injection evoked this hypertensive pattern was restricted to the region, dorsolateral to the midbrain aqueduct, between approximately A0.6 and P1.5.

PAG hypotensive patterns As seen in Fig. 8 two distinct patterns of regional blood flow changes accompanied the fall in blood pressure (5 – 25 mm Hg) evoked from the ventrolateral PAG (Carrive and Bandler, 1991a). The same patterns were obtained in both the unparalyzed and paralyzed decerebrate preparation and for purposes of presentation these data have been pooled. In these experiments blood flows were recorded only for

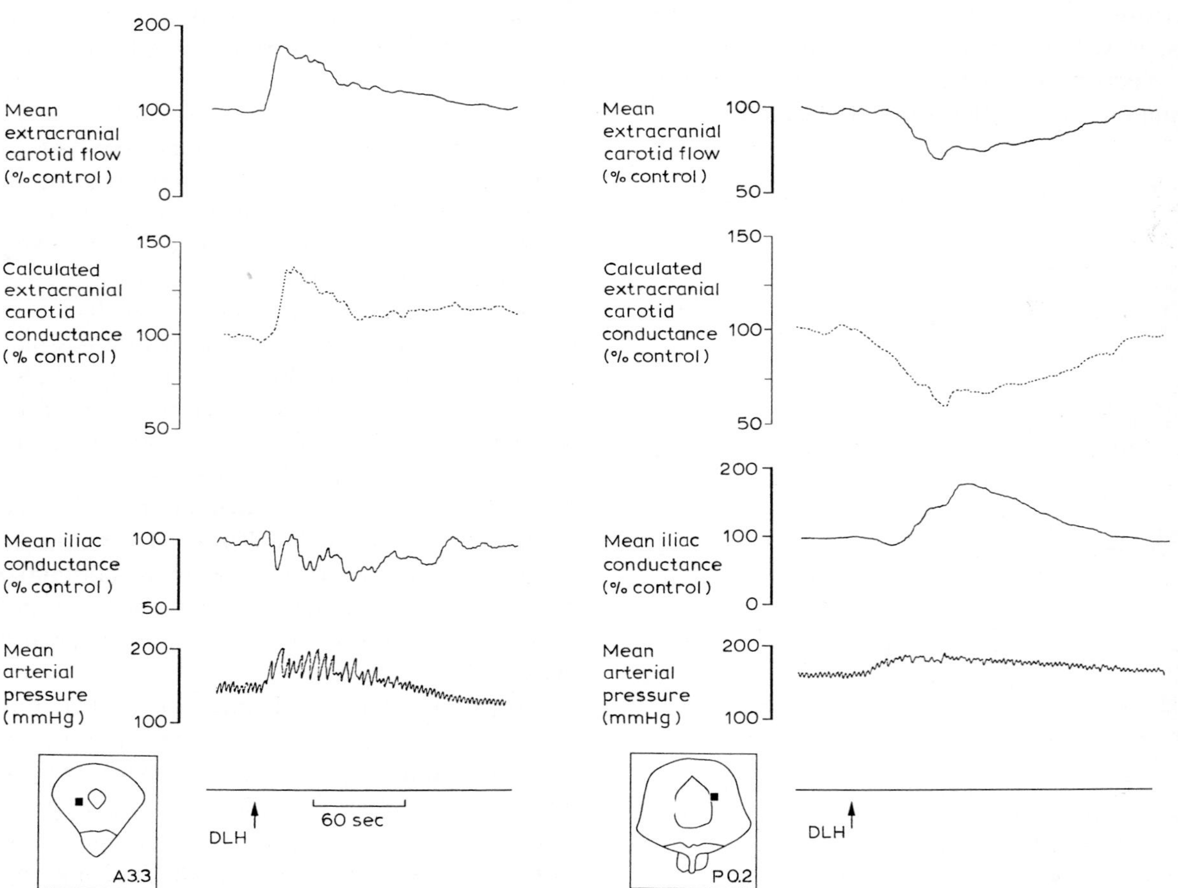

Fig. 4. Changes in mean carotid flow, calculated carotid conductance mean iliac conductance and mean arterial pressure evoked in the paralyzed, unanesthetized decerebrate cat following DLH microinjection in the pretentorial PAG, A3.3 (left panel) or the subtentorial PAG, P0.2 (right panel). Each arrow indicates the start of the DLH microinjection (40 nmol.) (reproduced from Fig. 1, of Carrive and Bandler, 1991b).

the external iliac and renal arteries. For one hypotensive pattern, the fall in arterial pressure was associated with a significant increase in iliac conductance, but no significant change in renal conductance (Fig. 8, left panel and Fig. 9); whereas, a second hypotensive pattern was characterized by a significant increase in renal conductance, but no significant change in iliac conductance, (Fig. 8, right panel and Fig. 9). Further, the two hypotensive patterns were evoked from sites located in different parts of the ventrolateral PAG. Thus, the sites at which the hypotensive reaction was characterized by an increase in iliac conductance were located mostly in the rostral (pretentorial) part of the PAG hypotensive area; whereas, the sites at which DLH injection evoked a hypotensive reaction characterized by an increase in renal conductance were located preferentially in the caudal (subtentorial) part of the PAG hypotensive area (Fig. 10).

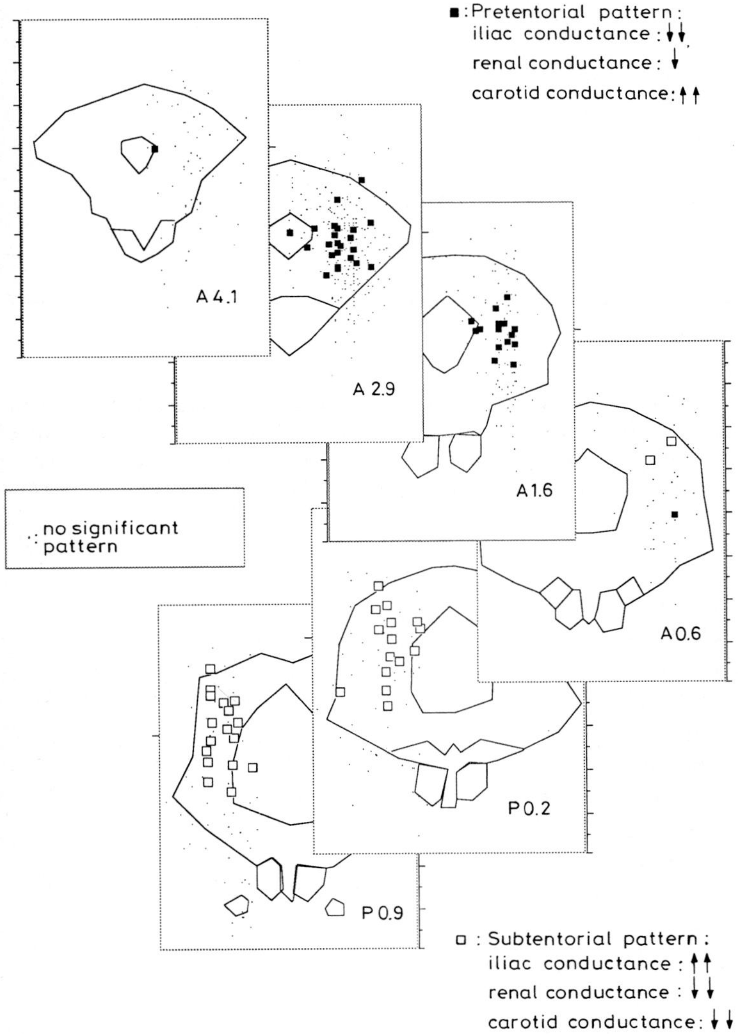

Fig. 5. Coronal sections through the PAG of the cat (Berman, 1968) showing the distribution of sites at which DLH microinjection evoked a pretentorial cardiovascular pattern, a subtentorial cardiovascular pattern, or no clear cardiovascular pattern.

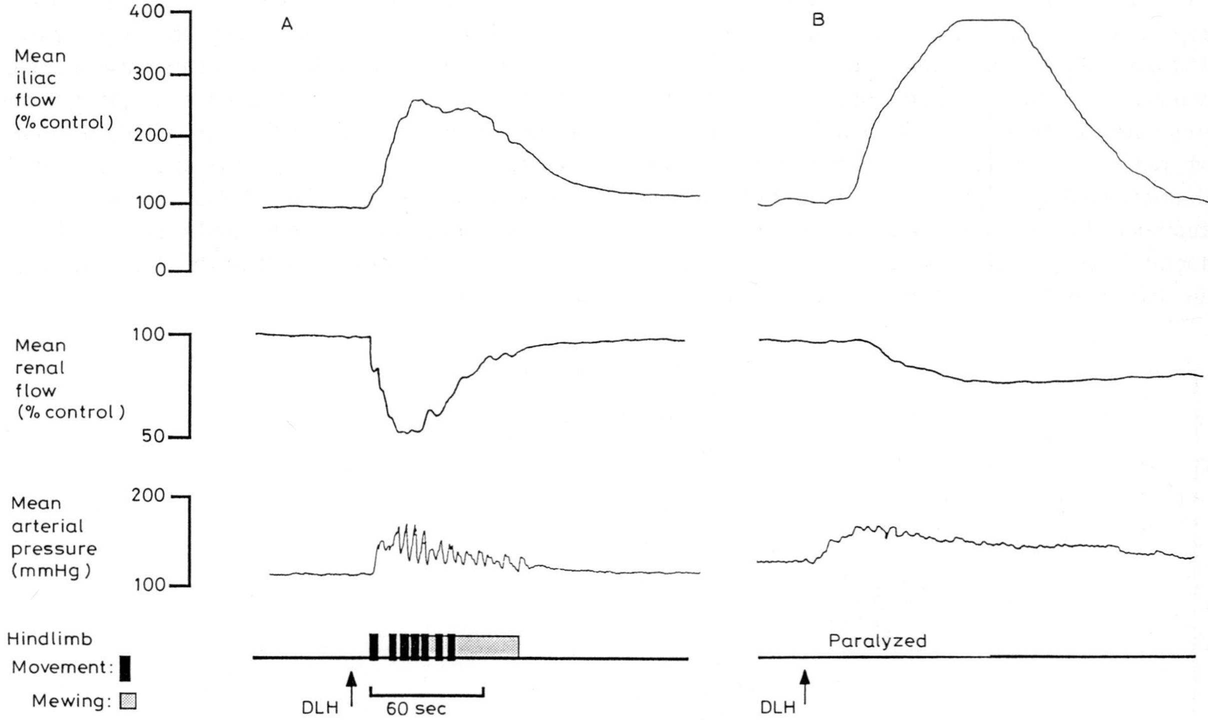

Fig. 6. Examples of the patterns of changes in mean iliac flow, mean renal flow and mean arterial pressure evoked by DLH microinjection in the lateral subtentorial PAG of the unparalyzed (A) or paralyzed (B) decerebrate cat. Each burst of hindlimb movement in the unparalyzed preparation is indicated by dark shading. A period of vocalization (i.e., mewing) is indicated by the lighter shading. Each arrow indicates the start of a DLH microinjection (40 nmol.) (reproduced from Fig. 1 of Carrive et al., 1989a).

In summary, the ventrolateral PAG hypotensive area can be divided roughtly into two halves. A rostral half, centered at approximately A1.6, which contains a majority of sites at which DLH injection evokes a hypotensive reaction characterized by an increase in iliac conductance, but no significant changes in renal conductance; and a caudal half, centered at approximately P0.5, which contains a majority of sites at which the DLH-evoked hypotensive reaction is characterized by an increase in renal conductance, but no significant change in iliac conductance.

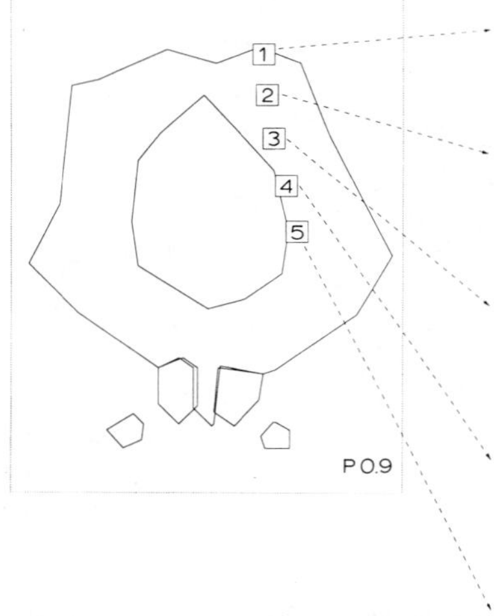

Viscerotopic organization

Although activation of neurons in the ven-

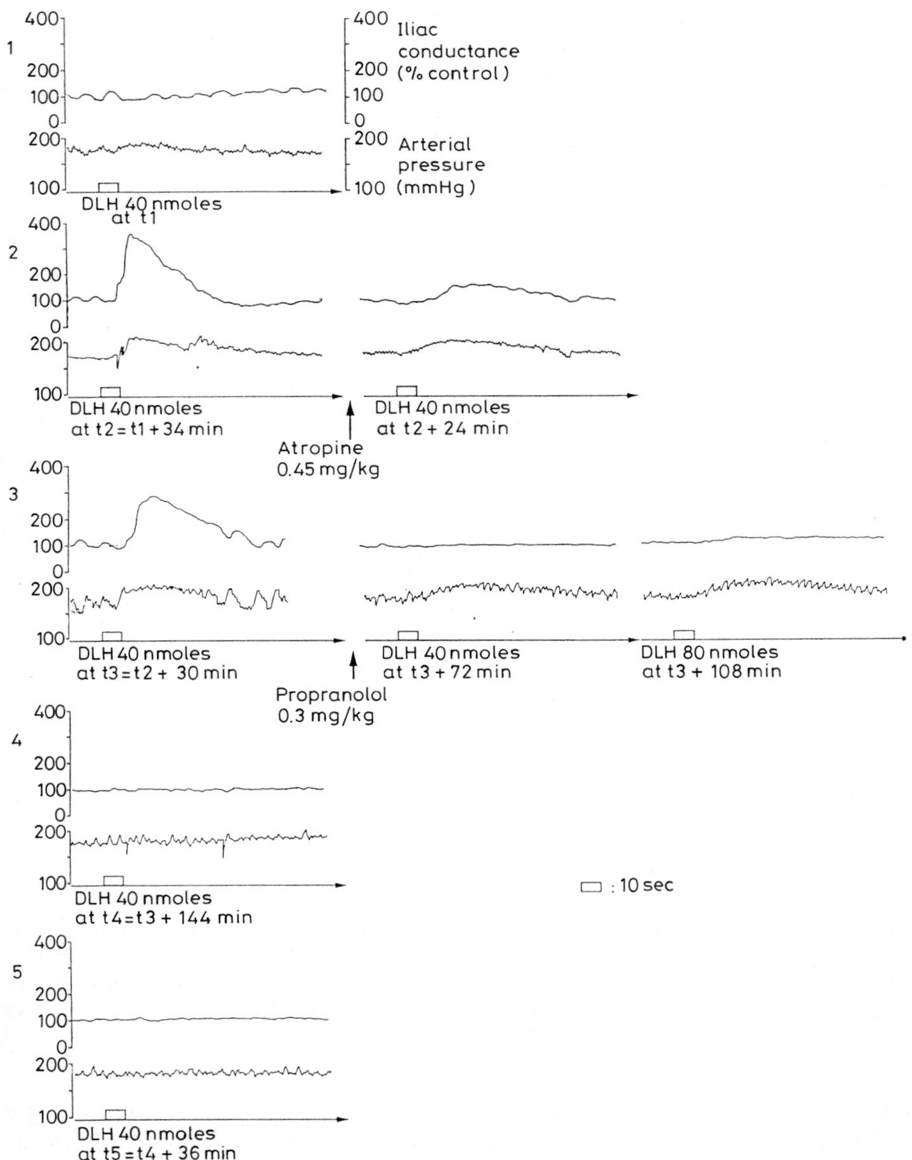

Fig. 7. Examples of the changes in iliac conductance and arterial pressure evoked in the paralyzed decerebrate cat by repeated DLH microinjections made at 5 sites along a track through the subtentorial PAG. A first (sharp) vasodilatory effect (site 2) was blocked by an intravenous injection of atropine sulphate. A second vasodilatory effect (site 3) was blocked by an intravenous injection of propranolol. The time at which each DLH microinjection was performed is indicated on the abscissa.

trolateral PAG evoked effects on sympathetic vasomotor tone (i.e., hypotension) which were the opposite of the effects of excitation of lateral PAG neurons (i.e., hypertension), the regional flow data indicate a similar viscerotopic organization for both the hypertensive (lateral) and hypotensive (ventrolateral) columns of the PAG. That is, changes in hindlimb vasomotor tone were evoked when DLH injections were made at sites in the rostral or pretentorial portion of both the

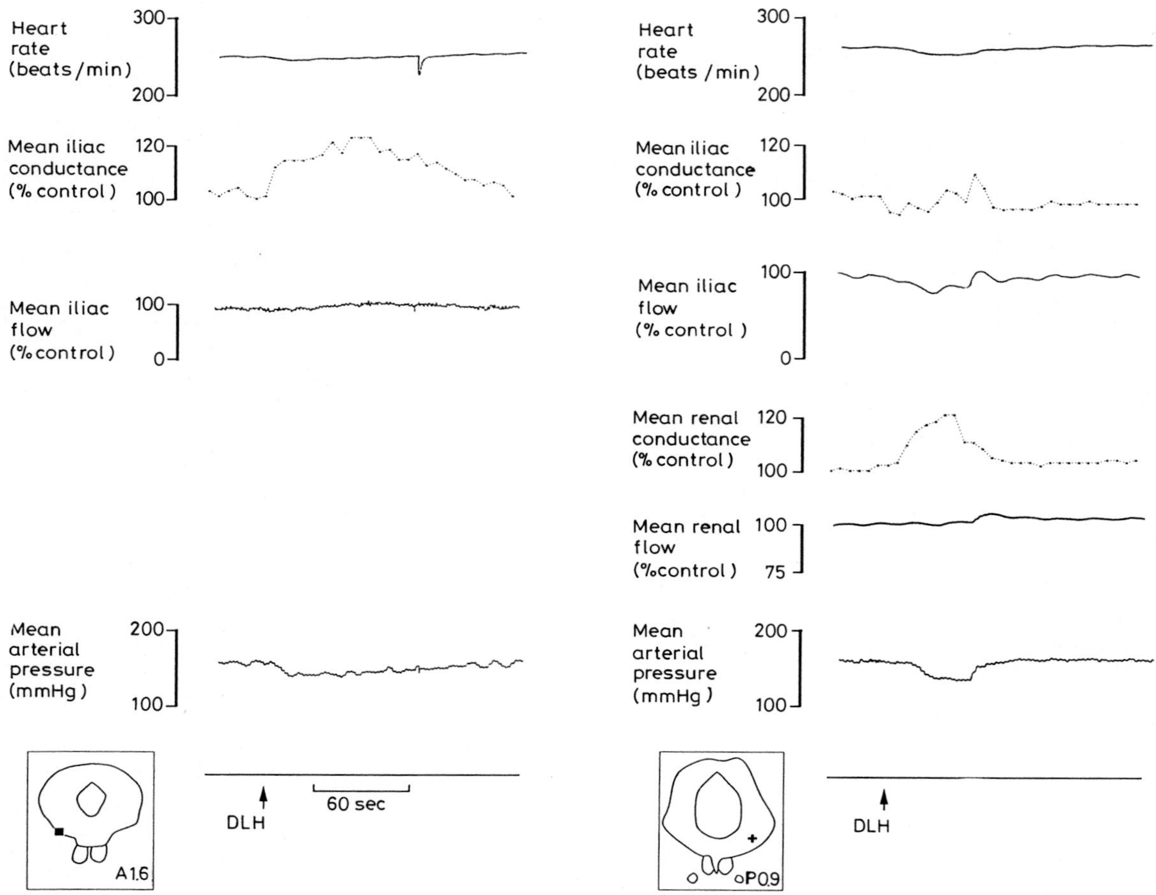

Fig. 8. Examples of the two patterns of hypotensive cardiovascular changes evoked by DLH microinjection in the ventrolateral PAG of the unparalyzed, decerebrate cat. The left panel indicates the hypotensive pattern characterized by an increase in iliac conductance. The right panel indicates the hypotensive pattern characterized by an increase in renal conductance. The location of the centers of each microinjection are indicated on coronal sections of the PAG. The arrows indicate the start of the DLH microinjections (40 nmol) (reproduced from Fig. 1 of Carrive and Bandler, 1991a).

hypertensive (lateral) and hypotensive (ventrolateral) columns of the PAG; whereas, renal vasomotor tone was selectively altered when DLH injections were made in the caudal or subtentorial portion of both the hypertensive and hypotensive columns of the PAG. These findings are illustrated schematically in Fig. 11.

As well, the results suggest a separate viscerotopic representation, within the lateral PAG, for the regionally specific vasodilation in skeletal muscle beds. Thus, a sharp vasodilation in the extracranial vascular bed (i.e., common carotid artery in the decerebrate preparation), but not the hindlimb vascular bed, was evoked by DLH injection in the lateral pretentorial PAG; whereas, a vasodilation in the hindlimb vascular bed, but not the extracranial vascular bed, was evoked by DLH injections made in the lateral subtentorial PAG. These findings are illustrated schematically in Fig. 12.

Somatic changes

Microinjections of DLH were made at 263 sites in the unparalyzed decerebrate cat. Significant somatic effects were evoked at 105 sites. The observed effects consisted of vocalization, facial movement and hindlimb movement.

Facio-vocal changes

Howling At 32 sites, DLH microinjection evoked howling alone, or howling mixed with hissing. Howling usually began within the first 5 – 20 sec post-injection and was the most intense sound evoked from the PAG. During each howl, the cat's mouth opened wide and the lips were retracted. When hissing occurred, the position of the mouth and lips remained the same, but the sides of the tongue curled upward. Howling was associated with an observable contraction of abdominal muscles. As the intensity of the reaction weakened, howling usually changed to mewing (see below). As seen in Fig. 13 the sites at which DLH injection evoked howling were found only within the pretentorial PAG, primarily between A3.3 – A1.0.

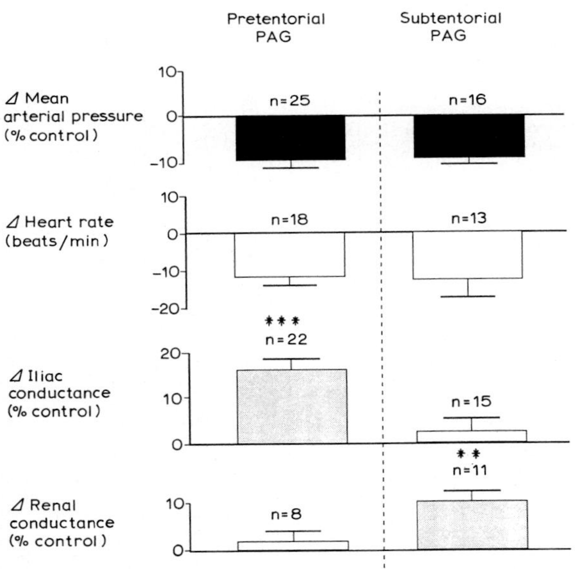

Fig. 9. Histograms showing the changes (mean +/− SEM) in mean arterial pressure, heart rate, iliac conductance and renal conductance evoked by microinjection of DLH into the pretentorial and subtentorial PAG hypotensive area. ** $P < 0.01$, *** $P < 0.001$ (*t*-test) (reproduced from Fig. 3 of Carrive and Bandler, 1991a).

Hissing Hissing, by itself, was evoked at 23 other sites. These sites were also found within the pretentorial PAG, but primarily dorsal and rostral to sites at which howling was evoked (Fig. 13).

Mewing At the remaining 50 sites mewing alone, or mewing mixed with an occasional hiss or growl was evoked by DLH injection. Mewing and growling were associated with only a partial opening of the mouth, and the sound produced was usually not as intense as howling. The sites from which mewing was evoked were found both in the pretentorial and subtentorial PAG (Fig. 13). The intensity of the mewing evoked from the subtentorial PAG sites was generally stronger than that evoked from the pretentorial PAG and occasionally the mewing evoked from the subtentorial PAG ap-

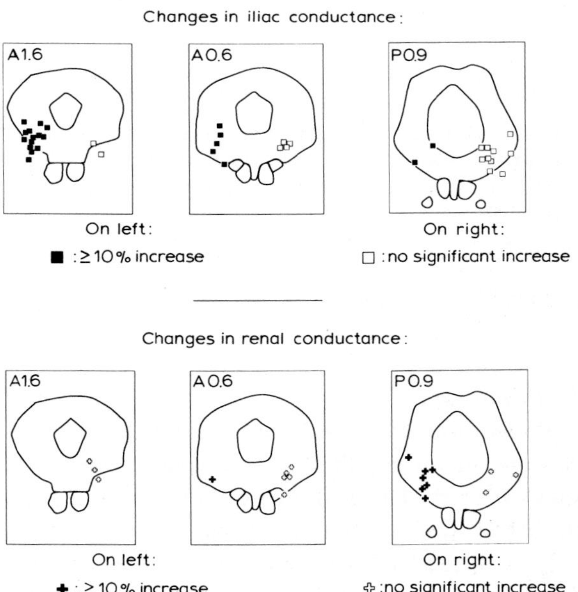

Fig. 10. Series of 3 representative coronal sections, through the caudal PAG, showing the location of the centers of the sites at which DLH microinjection evoked a hypotensive effect associated with an increase in iliac conductance (upper row) and an increase in renal conductance (lower row). Sites at which a significant increase in conductance was evoked are represented on the left. Sites at which no significant change in conductance was evoked are represented on the right (reproduced from Fig. 5 of Carrive and Bandler, 1991a).

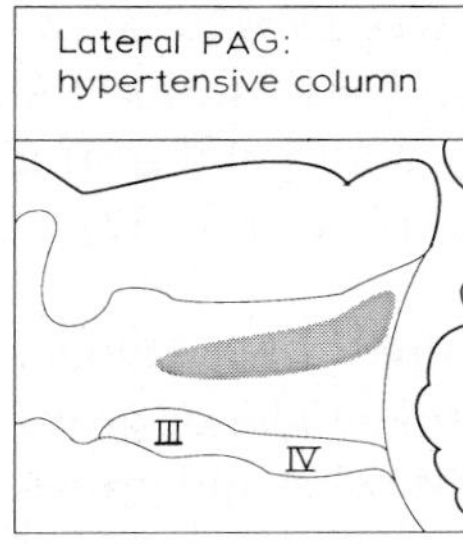

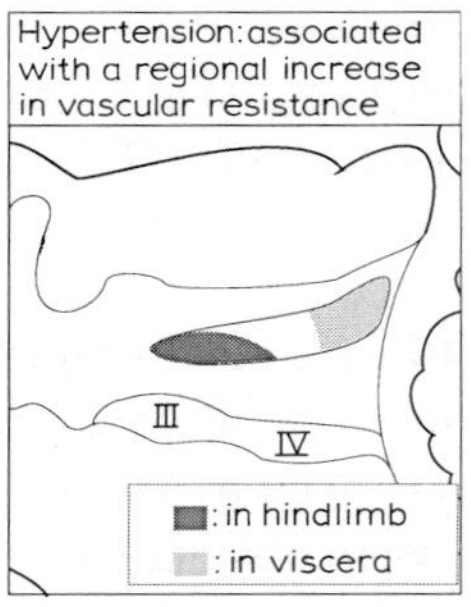

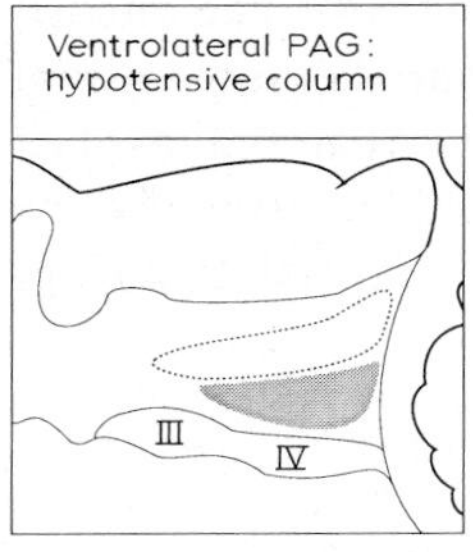

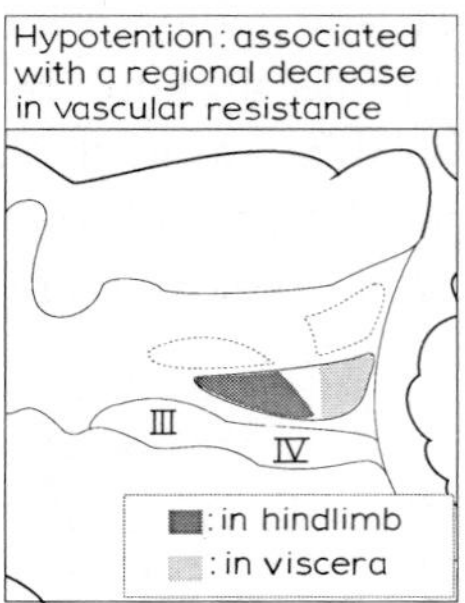

Fig. 11. Schematic parasagittal representation of the parallel viscerotopic organization within the hypertensive (lateral) and hypotensive (ventrolateral) parts of the pretentorial and subtentorial PAG.

proached the intensity of the howling evoked from the pretentorial PAG.

Limb movements

Pretentorial PAG An increase in extensor muscle tone in the hindlimb was regularly evoked at sites within the lateral pretentorial PAG. At 7 sites, the effect was so pronounced that the trunk of the animal lifted off the operating table. Intense vocalization (i.e., howling) was usually evoked at the same time. Such a tonic increase in hindlimb extensor tone was not observed if DLH injections were made in the subtentorial PAG.

Subtentorial PAG At 22 sites within the subtentorial PAG, DLH microinjection evoked $1-6$ bursts of hindlimb movement. These sites were restricted to the region lateral and dorsolateral to

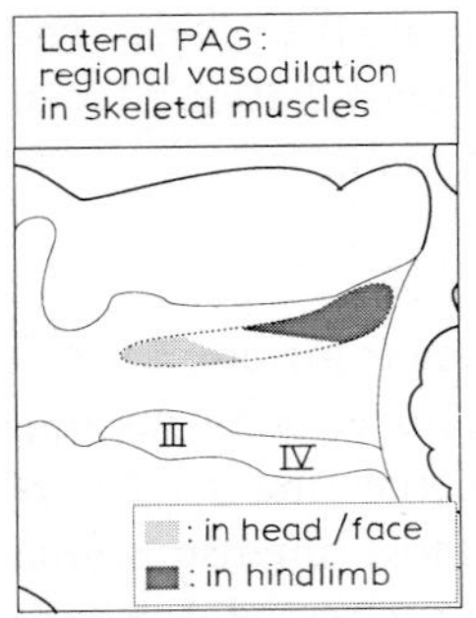

Fig. 12. Schematic parasagittal representation of the regional vasodilation in skeletal muscle associated with DLH microinjection within the pretentorial and subtentorial parts of the lateral PAG.

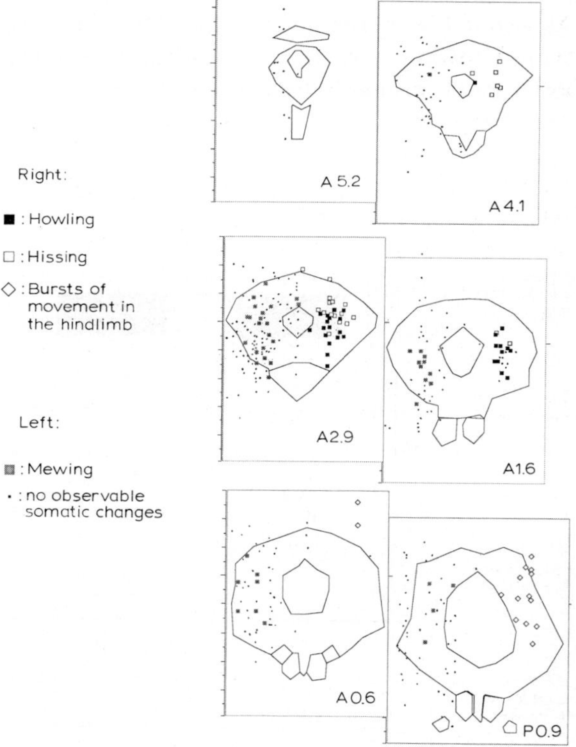

Fig. 13. Coronal sections through the PAG of the cat (Berman, 1968) showing the distribution of sites, in the decerebrate, at which DLH microinjection evoked somatic changes. Sites at which howling, hissing or hindhimb movement was evoked are represented on the right. Sites at which no observable somatic changes or mewing was evoked are represented on the left.

the aqueduct, between P0.2 – P1.5 (Fig. 13). Each burst of movement, which lasted only a few seconds, consisted of a series of 2 – 5 flexion-extensions of the hindlimb. The hindlimb movement was sometimes accompanied by vocalization (i.e., mewing).

Integration of somatic and autonomic reactions in the decerebrate cat

Lateral pretentorial PAG To summarize, within the lateral pretentorial PAG, DLH microinjection evoked a co-ordinated pattern of cardiovascular and facio-vocal changes. The pattern, in its strongest form, comprised howling (sometimes mixed with hissing) and an increase in arterial pressure and heart rate, associated with a strong hindlimb skeletal muscle vasoconstriction, and a moderate vasoconstriction in visceral beds (Fig. 14). This pattern was evoked by DLH injection within a restricted part of the lateral PAG, centered at approximately A2.5 (compare Figs. 5 and 13). It should be noted that the onset of the howling coincided well with the time of the most intense cardiovascular changes (see Fig. 3). More moderate facio-vocal responses (e.g., hissing alone or mewing) were associated with more moderate cardiovascular changes (Fig. 14), and were evoked from a more extensive part of the lateral pretentorial PAG (Figs. 5 and 13). DLH injections which failed to evoke facio-vocal changes did not evoke significant cardiovascular changes (Fig. 14). Although carotid flow was studied only in the paralyzed preparation, DLH injections made within the pretentorial PAG, which evoked a significant increase in carotid conductance, also evoked a substantial iliac vasoconstriction and a rise in arterial pressure (Fig. 15). This suggests that the increase in extracranial carotid conductance constitutes a component of the pretentorial PAG hypertensive reaction.

Lateral subtentorial PAG At sites within a restricted part of the lateral subtentorial PAG, DLH microinjection evoked a different co-ordinated pattern of somatomotor and cardiovascular changes. The pattern, in its strongest form, consisted of 2 – 6 short bursts of strong hindlimb movement, a rise in arterial pressure, tachycardia, a large visceral vasoconstriction, and a large hindlimb skeletal muscle vasodilation (Fig. 16). This pattern was evoked by DLH injection within the lateral/dorsolateral subtentorial PAG, between approximately A0.2 – P1.5 (compare Figs. 5 and 13). The onset of the iliac vasodilation was always tightly linked with the onset of hindlimb movements (Fig. 6A). However, the possibility that the vasodilation was secondary to movement was ruled out by the experiments which

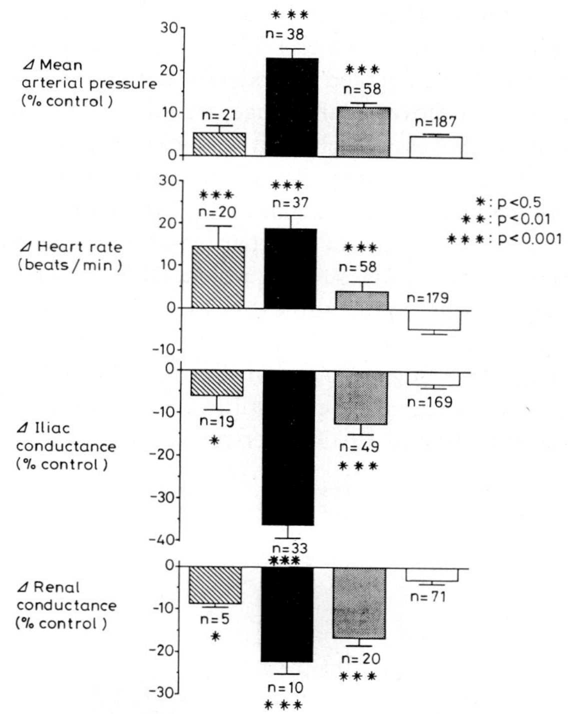

Fig. 14. Histograms showing the DLH-evoked changes (mean +/− SEM) in mean arterial pressure, heart rate, mean iliac conductance and mean renal conductance, which accompanied the different types of facio-vocal reactions evoked from the pretentorial PAG. Statistical significance was assessed by the Mann-Whitney U-test.

demonstrated that the same cardiovascular changes were evoked by DLH injection in the subtentorial PAG of the paralyzed decerebrate cat (Fig. 6B). Sites at which DLH evoked only 1 burst of movement evoked a moderate but similar pattern of cardiovascular change; whereas, no significant cardiovascular changes were observed following DLH injection at sites at which movement was not evoked (Fig. 16). Again, although carotid flow was studied only in the paralyzed preparation, subtentorial PAG sites at which DLH evoked a carotid constriction also evoked a large increase in iliac conductance and a rise in arterial pressure (Fig. 15), suggesting that constriction of extracranial vasculature constitutes a component of the subtentorial PAG hypertensive reaction.

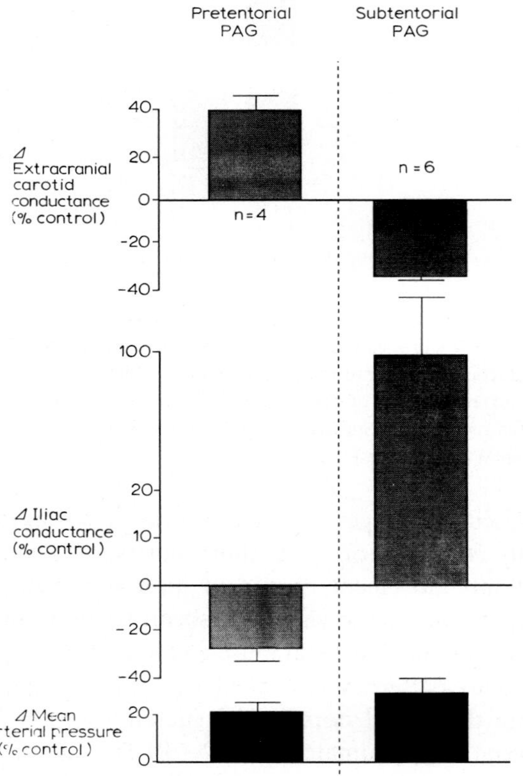

Fig. 15. Histograms showing the changes (mean +/− SEM) in mean arterial pressure and mean iliac conductance which accompanied the changes in mean extracranial carotid conductance evoked by DLH microinjection within the pretentorial and subtentorial parts of the lateral PAG.

Ventrolateral PAG In the unparalyzed decerebrate cat, hypotensive reactions were not accompanied by any movement. Further, in the few cases in which spontaneous movements were observed prior to the DLH injection, they ceased during the

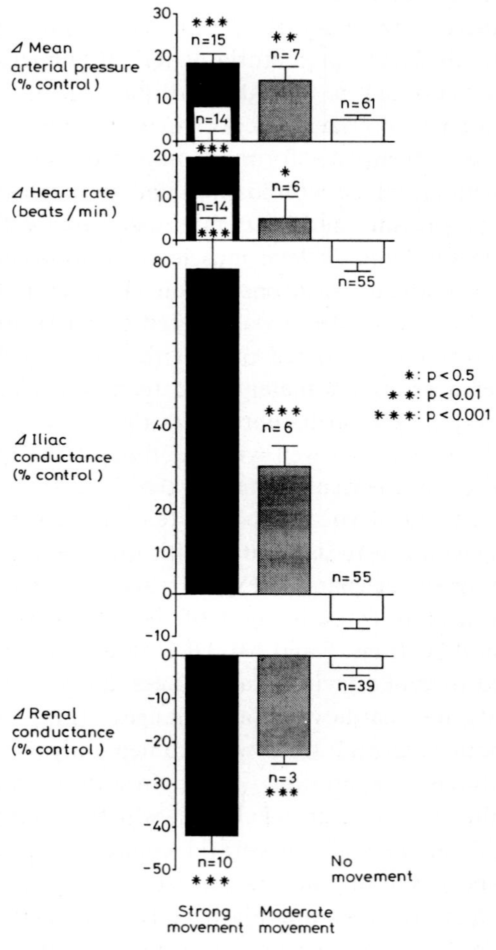

Fig. 16. Histograms showing the DLH-evoked changes (mean +/− SEM) in mean arterial pressure, heart rate, mean iliac conductance and mean renal conductance associated with hindlimb movement evoked from the subtentorial PAG. Strong and moderate movement refer respectively to the occurrence of multiple (2−6), or a single burst of hindlimb movement. Statistical significance was assessed by the Mann-Whitney U-test.

period of hypotension, but reappeared at the end of the hypotensive period.

Experiments in the freely moving cat

One week prior to study of the behavioral changes evoked by EAA injection, cats were anesthetized (sodium pentobarbital, 40 mg/kg), secured in a stereotaxic frame, and 2 – 4 guide tubes, through which guide cannulae could be later implanted into the midbrain PAG, were cemented over holes drilled stereotaxially in the skull. An approach in the coronal plane was used for the implantation of the pretentorial midbrain guide tubes. However, for the subtentorial midbrain, because the bony tentorium precluded a stereotaxic approach in the coronal plane, the guide tubes were positioned at an angle of 20° from the vertical. Guide cannulae implantation and EAA microinjections were made in accordance with the procedure described previously (for details see Bandler, 1982; Bandler and Carrive, 1988; Zhang et al., 1990). A standard injection, 20 – 80 nmol of DLH in 0.20 – 0.40 μl of phosphate buffer 0.02 M, pH 7.4) was used. Prior to making a chemical injection the protective cap covering the guide cannulae assembly was removed and a stylet withdrawn from a guide cannula. The cat was then allowed to move freely about the test cage (approx 1.8 m × 1.0 m × 1.0 m). The cat's behavior during this time was recorded on videotape. An analysis of this period was used to establish a mean control level of behavior following pre-injection handling. Each cat's behavior from the start of a DLH injection, until the end of the experimental period (2 – 6 min) was observed and videotape recorded. For some experiments the experimental period was extended for up to 30 min, and intermittent video recordings were made during this time. The occurrence of different behavioral items, during the first 2 – 4 min of the experimental period, were encoded from the video recordings, the encoder being blind to the location of the DLH injection site. Data were processed for each item with respect to frequency and/or duration. The following items were individually encoded: *General movement:* turning of the head; arching of the back; nonlocomotory limb movement; nibbling, licking, scratching any part of its own body; *Locomotion:* walking; backing; circling; running; *Escape movement:* rearing, sometimes accompanied by pawing movements at the side of the test cage; *Jumps:* jumps, directed usually to the top or sides of the test cage; *Vocalization:* hissing; howling; mewing or growling. The position of the ears, the size of the pupils and the degree of piloerection also were noted.

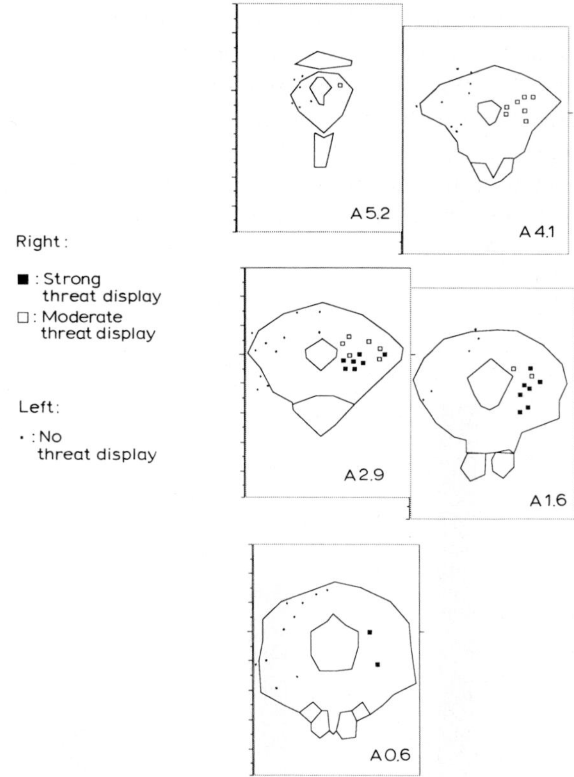

Fig. 17. Coronal sections through the PAG of the cat (Berman, 1968) showing the distribution of sites, at which DLH microinjection evoked a threat display. The centers of the sites at which either a strong threat display (associated with howling), or a moderate threat display (associated with hissing) was evoked, are represented on the right side. Sites at which no significant effect was evoked are represented on the left.

Lateral Pretentorial PAG

DLH injections made at sites within a longitudinal column, lateral to the midbrain aqueduct, extending from approximately A4.5 to A1.0, elicited a reaction which consisted of moderate pupillary dilation and piloerection, vocalization (howling usually mixed with hissing; hissing alone) and dependent on the specific site, retraction of the ears and/or arching of the back. The reactions characterized by howling were the most intense and the longest in duration (howl 97.7s vs. hiss alone 61.2 s, *t*-test, $P < 0.5$).

The sites at which DLH injection evoked a strong threat display, associated with howling, were localized to a restricted part of the pretentorial PAG, lateral to the aqueduct, between A3.3 to A1.0 (Fig. 17). The moderate threat display, associated with hissing alone, was evoked from a more dorsal and rostral extent of the lateral, pretentorial PAG (Fig. 17). At other sites, DLH microinjection evoked mewing and mild alerting or was without effect.

Lateral subtentorial PAG

In contrast, DLH injections made at 9 sites in the lateral subtentorial PAG evoked a strong "flight" reaction, characterized by: rapid running around the cage (primarily in a direction contralateral to the site of injection), multiple jumps and attempts to escape from the test cage, moderate pupil dilation and piloerection, and occasional mewing (Fig. 18). This reaction lasted approximately 120 s, the individual components of the reaction declining in parallel (Fig. 19). At 56 other sites DLH injection evoked a moderate flight reaction (Fig. 18).

The sites from which a strong flight reaction was evoked were localized to a restricted part of the subtentorial PAG, lateral to the aqueduct, between P0.0 – P1.2 (Fig. 20). Sites at which a moderate flight reaction was evoked included the subtentorial PAG region lateral and dorsolateral to the aqueduct, between A1.0 and P1.5, as well as a number of sites in the tegmentum laterally and dorsolaterally adjacent to the PAG (Fig. 20).

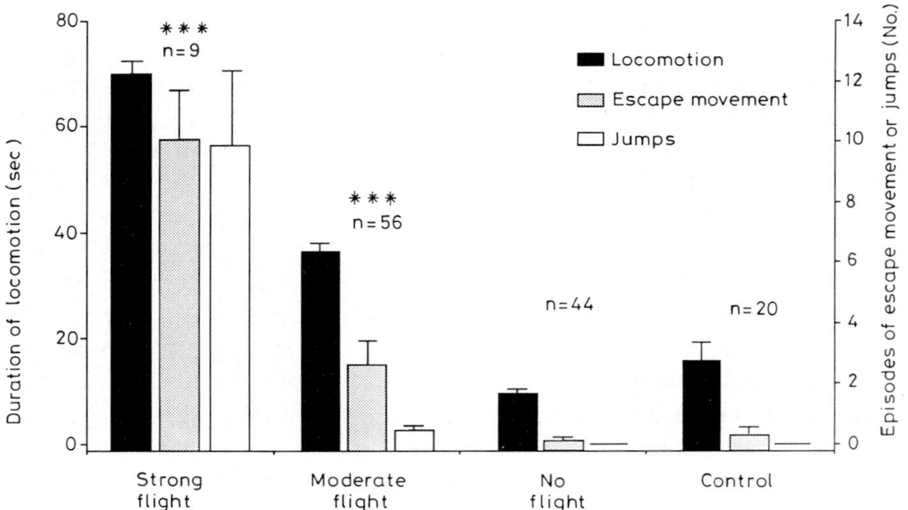

Fig. 18. Histogram showing the DLH evoked changes (mean +/− SEM) in duration of locomotion, number of episodes of escape movements and number of jumps. Sites were arbitrarily divided into three groups on the basis of the duration of locomotion (strong, ≥ 61 s of locomotion; moderate, 21 – 60 s of locomotion; no, 4 – 20 s of locomotion). Control levels of locomotion, escape movements and jumps were determined from analysis of videotape records of the behavior of cats ($N = 20$) during the pre-injection, post-handling period Significance between groups was assessed by the Mann-Whitney U-test. *** $P < 0.001$ (reproduced from Fig. 1 of Zhang et al., 1990).

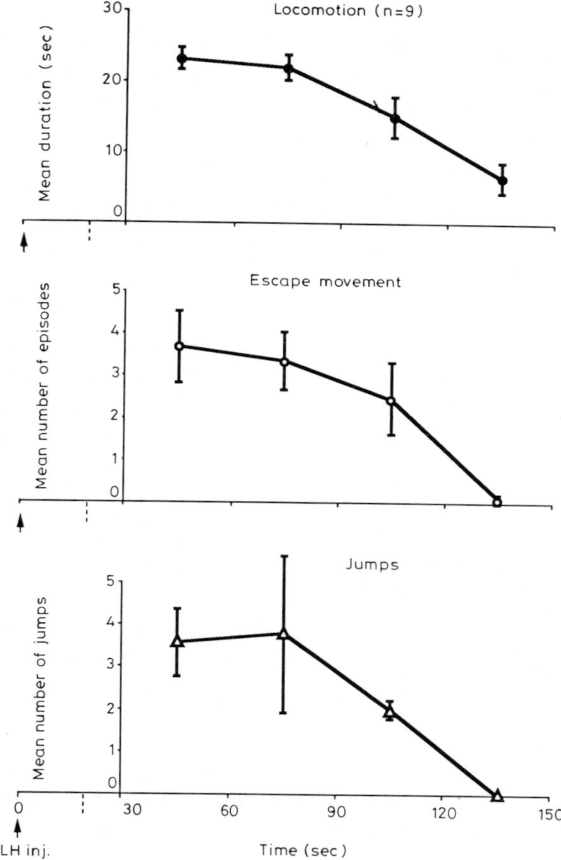

Fig. 19. Line graphs showing, at the strong flight sites ($N = 9$), for each 30 s period, the DLH-evoked (mean +/− SEM) duration of locomotion, number of episodes of escape movements and number of jumps. Each arrow indicates the start of the DLH injection (80 nmol) and each dashed line indicates when the cat was released by the experimenter (reproduced from Fig. 2 of Zhang et al., 1990).

Ventrolateral Subtentorial PAG

In contrast to the flight behavior evoked from the lateral subtentorial PAG, DLH injections made at 49 sites in the ventrolateral subtentorial PAG evoked significantly less locomotion (mean 1.1 s) than during the control period following pre-injection handling (mean 15.8 s) (Fig. 21). DLH injection at 17 of these sites evoked also a period of profound inactivity, during which time the cat did not turn its head, lick, scratch, groom or move its limbs. At another 22 sites a period of moderate inactivity was evoked. The combination of suppression of both locomotion and general movement has been called immobility (Fig. 21). As strong immobility sites the period of suppression of locomotion lasted for 2 to 2.5 min, post-DLH injection. The period of inactivity, however, lasted for 4 to 8 min post-injection.

As seen in Fig. 20, the sites at which a strong immobility reaction was evoked were confined to the PAG region, ventrolateral to the aqueduct, between A1.0 – P1.2. A number of strong immobility sites, were also located in the tegmentum adjacent to the ventrolateral PAG. The reaction of moderate immobility was evoked from sites in the same ventrolateral midbrain region (Fig. 20).

Functional localization within the midbrain PAG

Two defense regions in the lateral PAG

The results of these studies in the freely moving and decerebrate cat demonstrate, for the first time, that two different patterns of defense (threat display and flight) are mediated by pools of neurons in different parts of the PAG. Neurons whose excitation evoke the most intense form of threat display are found, lateral to the aqueduct, in a region centered at approximately the A2.5 level, in the pretentorial PAG. This region appears to be identical to the pretentorial PAG region at which DLH injections in the decerebrate cat evoke howling and a hypertensive reaction associated with a strong iliac vasoconstriction and an extracranial vasodilation (Fig. 22). In contrast, neurons whose excitation evokes a strong flight reaction are found, lateral to the aqueduct, in a region centered at approximately the P0.5 level, in the subtentorial PAG. This region appears to be identical to the subtentorial PAG region at which DLH injection in the decerebrate cat evokes repetitive bursts of hindlimb movement and a hypertensive reaction characterized by increased vascular resistance in visceral and extracranial vascular beds and a large hindlimb skeletal muscle vasodilation (Fig. 22).

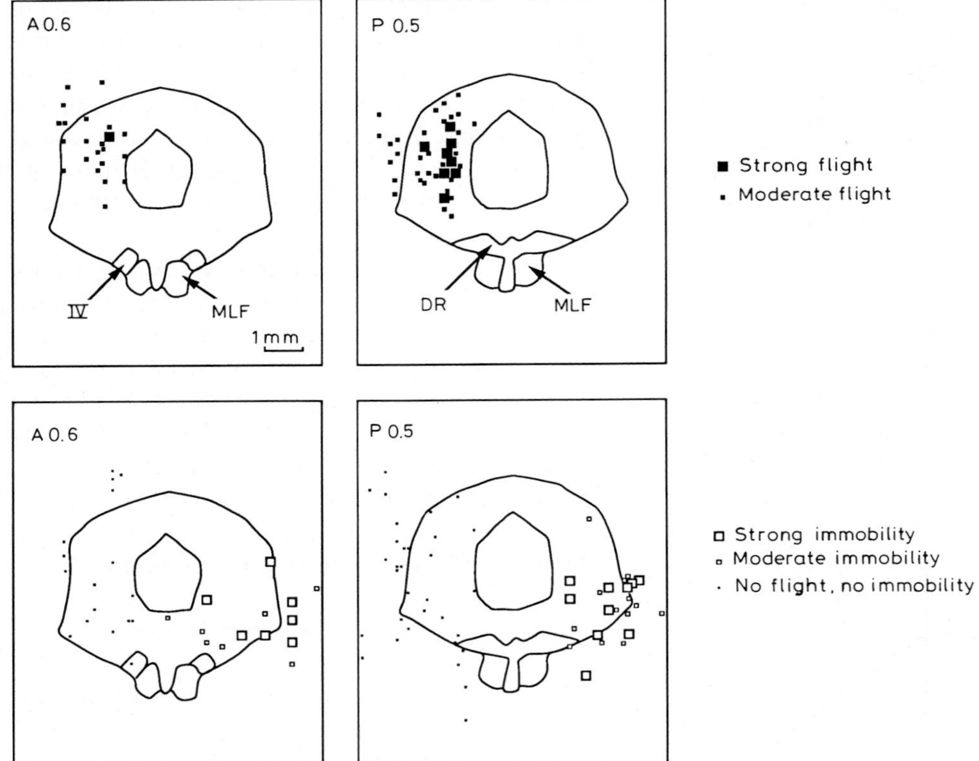

Fig. 20. Two representative coronal sections (Berman, 1968) showing the centers of the sites, within the subtentorial midbrain PAG, at which either flight (top row) or immobility (bottom row) was evoked by DLH microinjection in the freely moving cat.

In a series of now classic studies in the conscious, freely moving, instrumented cat, Zanchetti, Mancia and colleagues (Adams et al., 1969, 1971; Mancia and Zanchetti, 1981; Mancia et al., 1972, 1974; as well as other workers, Martin et al., 1976), observed that if confronted by a familiar threatening stimulus (e.g. another threatening cat), a cat's initial response during the early stage of confrontation consisted of a threat display (but neither attack nor flight) and a cardiovascular reaction characterized by iliac vasoconstriction, and small to moderate increases in renal and superior mesenteric resistance. If the threatening stimulus were allowed to come closer, however, the cat began to defend itself with vigorous limb movements and a different cardiovascular pattern was evoked. This new cardiovascular reaction was characterized by an increase in arterial pressure, an iliac vasodilation and renal and superior mesenteric vasoconstriction. It should be noted that the results of these studies, in the freely moving cat, are in conflict with the view of Hilton and colleagues (Abrahams et al., 1964; Hilton, 1979, 1982), derived largely from experiments with anesthetized cats, that a single cardiovascular pattern, defined by an increase in arterial pressure, iliac vasodilation and visceral vasoconstriction, is characteristic of the defense reactions of threat display, attack and flight from their early alerting stage, onwards.

There is an obvious similarity between the defense reactions evoked by DLH injections made in the pretentorial and subtentorial PAG, and the integrated somatic and autonomic reactions evok-

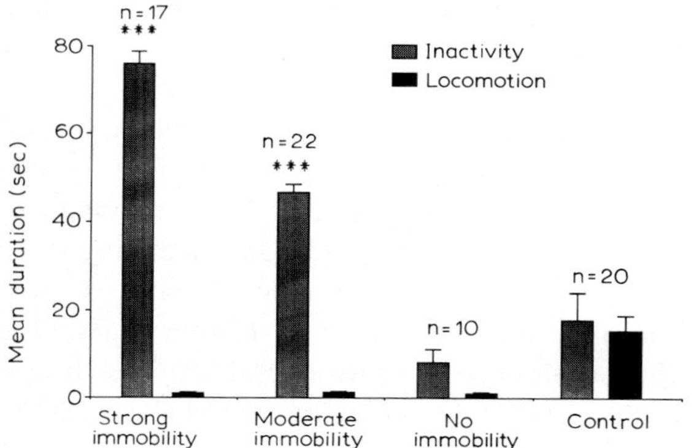

Fig. 21. Histogram showing the DLH-evoked changes (mean +/− SEM) in the duration of inactivity (absence of licking, grooming, scratching, head and limb movements) and locomotion. Sites were arbitrarily divided into three groups on the basis of the duration of inactivity (strong, ≥ 61 s of inactivity; moderate, 30 − 60 s of inactivity; no, ≤ 29 s of inactivity). Control levels of locomotion and inactivity were determined from analysis of videotape records of the behavior of cats (N = 20) during the pre-injection, post-handling period. Significance between groups was assessed by the Mann-Whitney U test, *** P < 0.001 (reproduced from Fig. 3 of Zhang et al., 1990).

ed in the conscious, freely moving cat confronted by a familiar, threatening stimulus. Our data, then, strongly support the view, first espoused by Zanchetti, Mancia and colleagues, that different defense reactions are characterized by distinct and different cardiovascular reactions. Of more significance, however, our data indicate for the first time, the location of neurons, in restricted parts of the midbrain PAG, that mediate the different patterns of integrated somatic and autonomic reactions characteristic of the defense reactions of threat display and flight.

It is likely that the patterns of regional blood flow changes associated with these different defense reactions help to redistribute blood to those beds with the highest metabolic demands. This appears to be achieved in a similar manner for each of the defense reactions studied. Thus, following EAA microinjection in the lateral pretentorial PAG, the onset of an intense threat display is associated with vasodilation in the extracranial vasculature (and intense facio-vocal activity), but vasocontriction in other less active skeletal muscle beds (e.g., hindlimb). Similarly, the flight response, evoked from the lateral subtentorial PAG, is associated with a large vasodilation in hindlimb skeletal muscle vascular beds (and intense hindlimb movement), but vasoconstriction in renal, superior mesenteric and extracranial vascular beds.

To summarize then, the organization of the

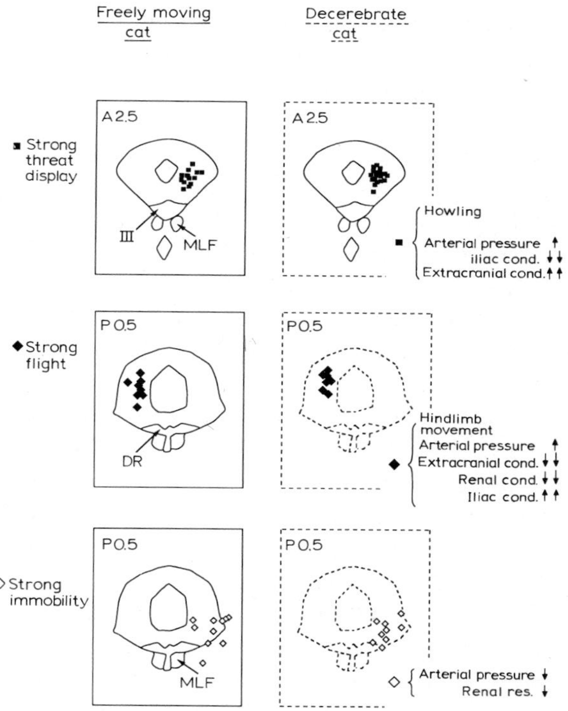

Fig. 22. (Left column): Representative coronal sections through the midbrain of the cat (Berman, 1968) showing the centers of the sites of DLH microinjections, within the midbrain PAG, which evoked in the freely moving cat: strong threat display (top row); strong flight (middle row); strong immobility (bottom row). (Right column): Representative coronal sections through the midbrain of the cat (Berman, 1968) showing the centers of the sites of the DLH microinjections, within the midbrain PAG, which in the decerebrate cat evoked: a pretentorial hypertensive reaction associated with howling (top row); a subtentorial hypertensive pattern associated with strong hindlimb movement (middle row); a subtentorial hypotensive reaction (bottom row).

defense reactions (threat display, flight) evoked by EAA microinjections, within the lateral part of the pretentorial and subtentorial PAG, includes: (i) the excitation of "viscerotopically organized" PAG neurons, mediating regionally specific vasoconstrictor and vasodilatory effects; (ii) the excitation of "somatotopically organized" PAG neurons, mediating regionally specific changes in facio-vocal and hindlimb activity. A major question which remains to be answered is whether the integrated somatic and autonomic output arises from: (i) excitation of PAG output neurons which have collateralized efferent projections; or (ii) excitation of separate but largely co-extensive populations of cells with individual projections.

A hypotensive region in the ventrolateral PAG

Our studies in the decerebrate and freely moving cat have delineated also a functionally distinct region, within the ventrolateral PAG (and the adjacent tegmentum), at which DLH injection evokes a strong immobility reaction. This appears to be the same region at which DLH microinjection in the decerebrate cat evokes a hypotensive reaction (Fig. 22). It is interesting to note that the ventrolateral part of the PAG is also the midbrain region within which analgesia has been most readily evoked by either electrical or chemical stimulation (e.g., Carstens et al., 1980; Fardin et al., 1984a; Lewis and Gebhart, 1977; Yaksh et al., 1976). It is not known if all of these changes (immobility, hypotension and analgesia) are components of a single pattern. One possibility is that together, these effects might contribute to a response which would assist the recovery of an animal which had been injured during a stressful encounter (see Duggan, 1983, for a further discussion of this idea). It remains to be determined, of course, if these effects are evoked simultaneously by EAA microinjection within the ventrolateral subtentorial PAG region.

A preliminary model of output organization in the PAG

The integrated somatic and autonomic reactions evoked by EAA microinjections in the PAG of the unanesthetized decerebrate and freely moving cat indicate that PAG output neurons mediating such effects are localized to restricted parts of the caudal two-thirds of the PAG. More specifically, both the lateral and ventrolateral PAG each appear to contain a complex "mosaic-like" representation of both body territories and functions. Our present understanding suggests at least two levels of organization:

(i) Viscerotopic and somatotopic organization; with each "tile of the mosaic" (i.e., group of projection neurons) modulating a specific physiological parameter(s) (e.g., vasomotor tone, skeletal muscle activity) in a specific body territory (somatic or visceral). Projection neurons modulating the same physiological parameter(s) appear to be arranged along a rostrocaudal axis, forming longitudinal, viscerotopically and somatotopically organized functional columns (see Figs. 11 and 12).

(ii) Excitatory and inhibitory organization: Although the projection neurons located in the lateral and ventrolateral PAG have a similar topographical organization, and modulate the same physiological parameters, they appear to do so in opposite ways (i.e., lateral PAG – excitation; ventrolateral PAG – inhibition).

Anatomical studies of PAG efferent projections

Both degeneration and axonal transport techniques have been used to trace the routes and destination of efferent fibres, originating from the PAG, in a number of different species including the cat (Bandler, 1988; Bandler and Tork, 1987; Holstege 1988, 1989), the rabbit (Meller, 1987) and the monkey (Jurgens and Pratt, 1979; Mantyh,

1983). The main descending pathways as revealed in these studies are very similar. The descending projection consists of predominantely ipsilateral fibers which course laterally and ventrolaterally through the midbrain and pontine tegmentum. Within the pons, fibers terminate in the cuneiform nucleus, the parabrachial nuclei and the lateral pontine tegmentum. Other fibers pass caudally, and gradually turn in a ventromedial direction. Large numbers of fibers terminate in the medial and lateral reticular formation of the rostral ventral medulla. In the caudal medulla, the remaining fibers sweep laterally and terminate in the ambiguual-retroambiguual complex and in the lateral medullary reticular formation. A few fibers can be followed to the level of the cervical and upper thoracic spinal cord.

PAG projections to the rostral ventrolateral medulla

In earlier experiments undertaken in our laboratory, WGA-HRP (50-150 nl, 1.5% solution) was used as an anterograde tracer, and injected at pretentorial PAG sites at which DLH microinjection had elicited a strong threat display (Bandler, 1988; Bandler et al., 1985a; Carrive et al., 1988). One region found to receive an input from the PAG was the so-called "pressor region" of the rostral ventrolateral medulla (see Figs. 24A and 25A). In the cat, this region contains a discrete longitudinal column of spinally projecting cells, which has been called the subretrofacial (SRF) nucleus (Dampney et al., 1987; McAllen et al., 1987). It is thought that the SRF nucleus plays a crucial role in the tonic and phasic control of arterial pressure (Ciriello et al., 1986; Dampney et al., 1985; Ross et al., 1984); and, it has been suggested that the cardiovascular changes evoked from the PAG may be mediated, at least in part, by this direct pathway to the SRF nucleus (Carrive et al., 1988).

Recently, it was suggested that the SRF nucleus was viscerotopically organized with respect to its control over specific vascular beds (Dampney and McAllen, 1988; Lovick, 1987). That is, the relative contribution of each vascular bed, to the increase in arterial pressure evoked by EAA injection in the SRF nucleus, varied according to the site of injection. For example, EAA injection made in the caudal part of the SRF nucleus evoked an increase in arterial pressure associated with a vasoconstriction in hindlimb muscle (Fig. 23); whereas, EAA injection made in the rostral part of the SRF nucleus evoked an increase in arterial pressure associated with a renal vasoconstriction (Fig. 23). EAA injection in the rostral part of the SRF nucleus evoked also a delayed vasodilation in hindlimb muscle (Fig. 23). It was further shown that this delayed iliac vasodilation, although atropine insensitive, was significantly attenuated by propanolol, suggesting that neurons in the rostral part of the SRF nucleus may modulate the release of catecholamines from the adrenal medulla (Lovick, 1987).

The finding that distinct patterns of vascular changes were topographically organized within the SRF nucleus raised the possibility that the different cardiovascular patterns evoked from the pretentorial and subtentorial PAG, might be mediated by projections to viscerotopically organized subgroups of cells within the SRF nucleus. To study this question retrogradely transported fluorescent-labeled microspheres were injected into physiologically identified sites in the rostral and caudal parts of the SRF nucleus, and the retrograde labeling in the PAG was examined (Carrive and Bandler, 1991a). Fluorescent microspheres were used because of their very limited spread at the site of injection (Katz et al., 1984). Two such injections sites are shown in Fig. 23 (bottom panel). A computer assisted three-dimensional reconstruction of the retrograde labelling in the PAG, after such tracer injections, is shown in Figs. 24C and 25C. The PAG neurons labeled, after injection of retrograde tracer into the SRF, formed three longitudinal columns; (1) a dorsomedial column; (2) a lateral column, which appears to correspond to the PAG hypertensive area; and (3) a ventrolateral column, which appears to

Parasagittal section of Rostral Ventrolateral medulla.

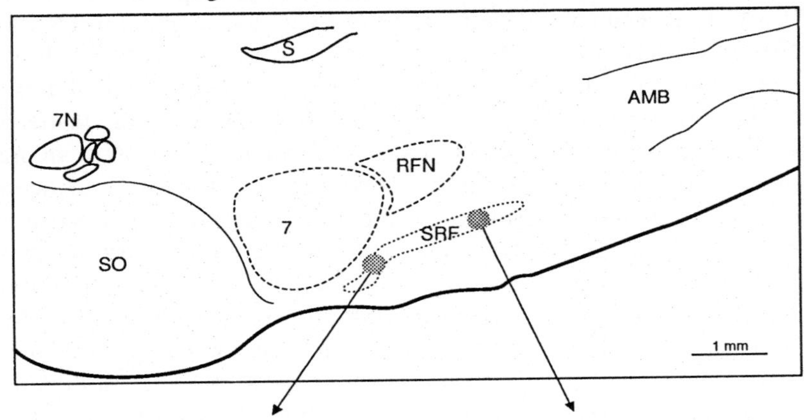

Cardiovascular effects evoked by Glutamate injection into:
the ROSTRAL SRF | the CAUDAL SRF

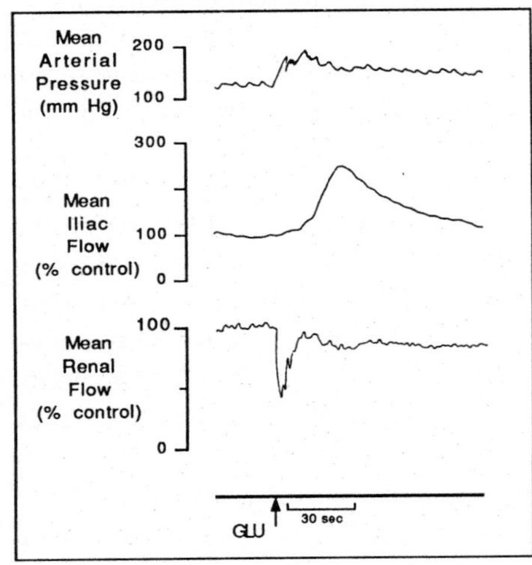

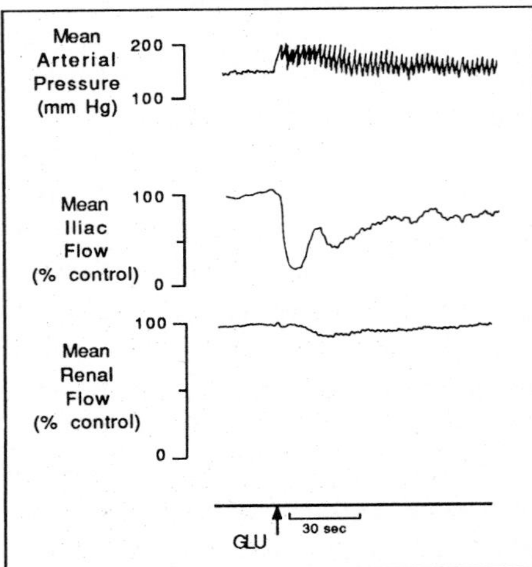

Retrograde fluorescent tracer injection sites in the rostral and caudal SRF.

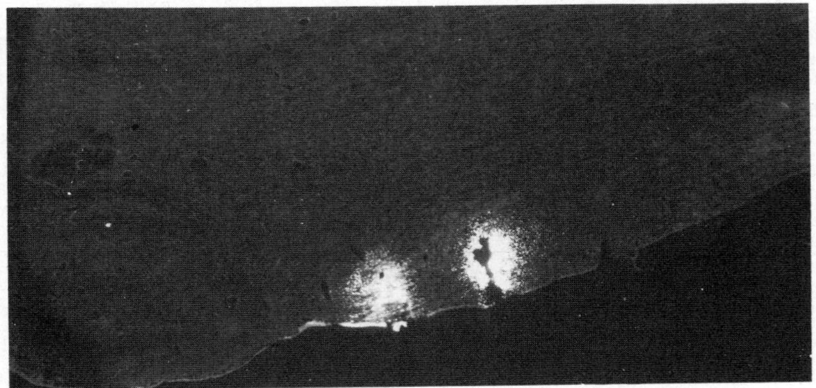

correspond to the PAG hypotensive area. Further, there was compelling anatomical evidence of viscerotopic organization within these columns of lateral and ventrolateral PAG cells. Thus, as seen in Fig. 25C, following tracer injection in the caudal part of the SRF nucleus (green patch), labeled PAG neurons (green dots) were found in the rostral portions of both the lateral and ventrolateral columns. In contrast, following tracer injection in the rostral part of the SRF nucleus (red patch), labeled PAG neurons (red dots) were found in the caudal portions of both the lateral and ventrolateral columns. No such viscerotopic organization was apparent for the dorsomedial PAG.

There is a remarkable correspondence between the viscerotopic organization of the PAG-SRF projections and the patterns of regional vascular changes evoked by DLH microinjection in the PAG. As summarized in Fig. 26, the rostral part of the lateral and ventrolateral PAG (A2.5, A0.6): (i) contains neurons projecting specifically to the caudal (iliac constrictor) part of the SRF nucleus (Fig. 26, middle row); and, (ii) is the region at which DLH microinjection selectively alters hindlimb vascular resistance (Fig. 26, bottom row). Conversely, it is the caudal part of the lateral and ventrolateral PAG regions (P0.9) that: (i) contains neurons projecting specifically to the rostral (renal) part of the SRF nucleus (Fig. 26, top row); and, (ii) is the region at which DLH microinjection selectively alters renal vascular resistance (Fig. 26, bottom row). Thus, both anatomical and physiological data suggest that lateral and ventrolateral midbrain PAG neurons, like sympathetic preganglionc neurons in the spinal cord (Janig, 1985) and presympathetic neurons in the SRF nucleus of the medulla (Dampney and McAllen, 1988; Lovick, 1987), consist of subgroups which are viscerotopically organized.

A simple model of the neuronal connections of the PAG with the SRF nucleus is drawn schematically in Fig. 27. According to this model, excitation of "pressor" or "depressor" neurons, in the rostral or caudal parts of the lateral and ventrolateral PAG, evokes respectively an increase or decrease in sympathetic vasomotor tone, via an overall excitatory or inhibitory effect on the same subgroups of SRF presympathetic neurons. Although this model provides perhaps the simplest explanation of these findings, it is possible, of course, that other more indirect pathways may mediate these effects. For example, there are extensive projections from the PAG to the parabrachial pons and the nucleus raphe magnus (Abols and Basbaum, 1981; Bandler, 1988; Holstege, 1988). The parabrachial pons (Kolliker-Fuse n.), in turn, projects to both the SRF nucleus (Dampney et al., 1987) and the intermediolateral (IML) column (Holstege, 1988) and has been implicated in cardiovascular function (Darlington and Ward, 1985; Mraovitch et al., 1982). The nucleus raphe magnus also projects quite heavily to the IML (Holstege, 1988) and has been implicated in cardiovascular functions (Haselton et al., 1988a,b; McCall, 1984). Little is known, however, about viscerotopic organization within these alternate pathways.

PAG projections to the nucleus retroambigualis

Following WGA-HRP injections in the pretentorial PAG, at sites at which DLH had evoked a strong threat display, another region found to receive a substantial projection, was the nucleus retroambiguualis (NRA) (Bandler, 1988) (see Figs. 24B and 25B). In a recent study, using tritiated leucine as an anterograde tracer, Holstege (1989)

Fig. 23. (Upper Panel): Drawing of a parasagittal section (Lat. 3.7) of the rostral ventrolateral medulla. Injections sites in the rostral and caudal parts of the subretrofacial (SRF) nucleus are indicated. Middle Panel: Patterns of cardiovascular changes evoked from the rostral and caudal SRF by microinjection of sodium glutamate (GLU), 22 nl, 500 mM. (Lower Panel): Photomicrograph of a parasagittal section showing injection sites of retrograde fluorescent tracers in the rostral (rhodamine microspheres) and the caudal (fluorescein microspheres) parts of the SRF. At each site a glutamate microinjection had previously elicited the cardiovascular pattern characteristic of the rostral or caudal SRF.

also observed that the PAG projected heavily to the NRA. Additionally, Holstege (1989; and this volume) reported that the NRA projects to spinal motor neuronal groups innervating intercostal and abdominal muscles, and brain stem motor neuronal groups innervating mouth-opening and perioral muscles, the pharynx, soft palate, tongue and larynx. Based on these anatomical data Holstege suggested further that the NRA be considered a premotor nucleus for the control of vocalization. Retrograde labeling in the midbrain following WGA-HRP injection into the NRA was also studied (Holstege, 1989). As seen in Fig. 28: (i) within the PAG labeled neurons were largely restricted to the caudal two-thirds of the lateral PAG; and, (ii) the distribution of retrogradely labeled PAG neurons matches well the distribution of PAG sites at which DLH microinjection evoked vocalization in both the freely moving and the decerebrate cat (compare Figs. 13 and 17 with Fig. 28).

To summarize, it has been suggested that the NRA may function as a premotor integrating center for vocalization, in much the same manner as the SRF is a premotor center for the control of sympathetic vasomotor tone. The anatomical data (Holstege, 1989) indicate also that the NRA is topographically organized with respect to its motor neuronal targets, much as the SRF has been found to be topographically organized with respect to its control over specific vascular beds. Finally, both the NRA and the SRF receive a significant input from the PAG.

General organization of descending projections from the PAG

As well as the projections to the SRF and the NRA, it has been reported that the lateral and ventrolateral parts of the caudal two-thirds of the PAG have substantial projections to the n. raphe magnus, n. raphe pallidus, n. raphe obscurus, and to the lateral region of the medullary reticular formation (Fardin et al., 1984b; Holstege, 1988;

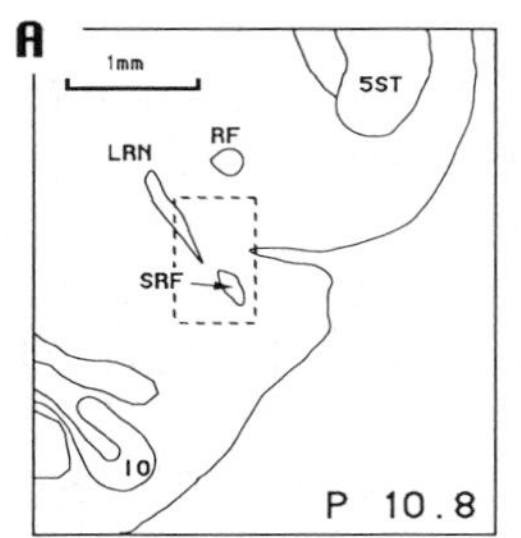

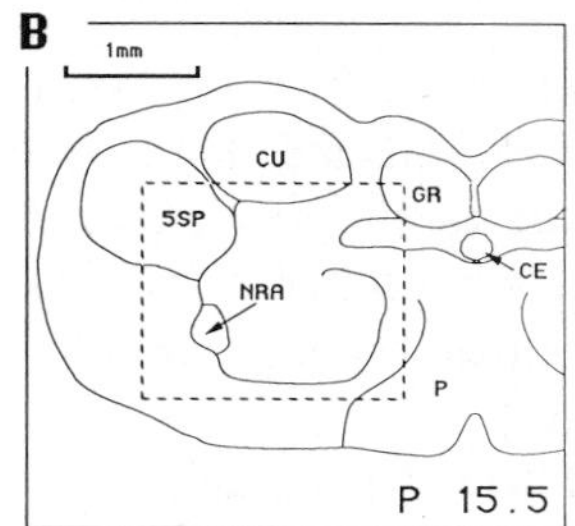

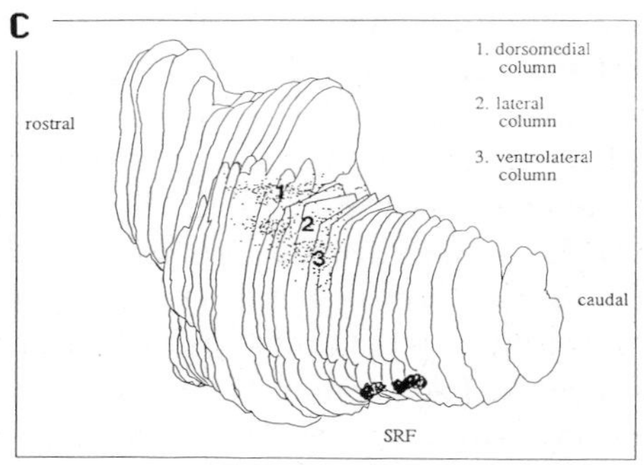

Fig. 24 (A). Coronal section through the region of the rostral ventrolateral medulla. (B). Coronal section through the region of the caudal medulla. (C). Computer assisted three-dimensional reconstruction of the distribution of labeled neurons in the PAG following injection of fluorescent microspheres into the rostral and caudal parts of the SRF nucleus. The labeled midbrain PAG neurons forms 3 longitudinal columns, from top to bottom: 1. a dorsomedial column; 2. a lateral column; 3. a ventrolateral column.

Fig. 25. (Top left): Darkfield photomicrograph of anterograde labeling in the caudal part of the ipsilateral SRF nucleus (refer to Fig. 24A) following a WGA-HRP injection made at a pretentorial PAG site from which a DLH microinjection evoked a strong threat display. (Top right): Darkfield photomicrograph of anterograde labeling in the NRA and adjacent reticular formation (refer to Fig. 24B) following a WGA-HRP injection made at a pretentorial PAG site at which a DLH microinjection evoked a strong threat display. (Bottom): Pattern of labeling inside the PAG columns following injection of retrogradely transported fluorescent microspheres in the rostral (red patch) and caudal (green patch) parts of the SRF pressor nucleus. (refer to Fig. 24C) (reproduced from Fig. 6 of Carrive et al., 1990).

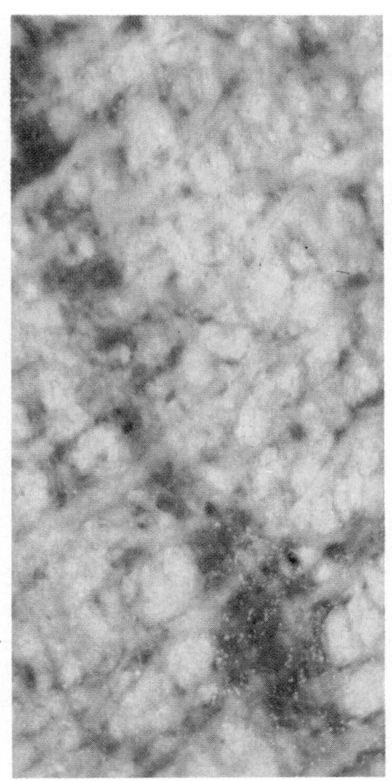

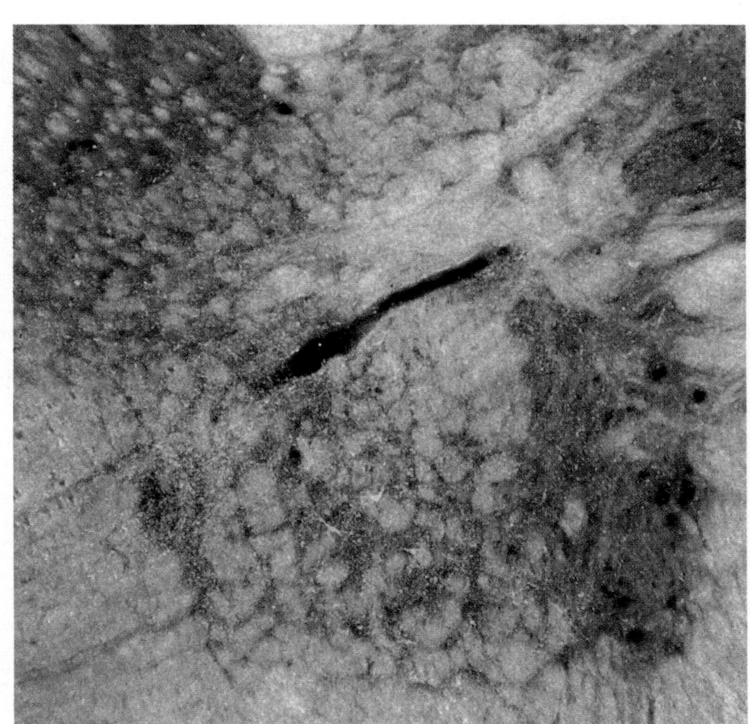

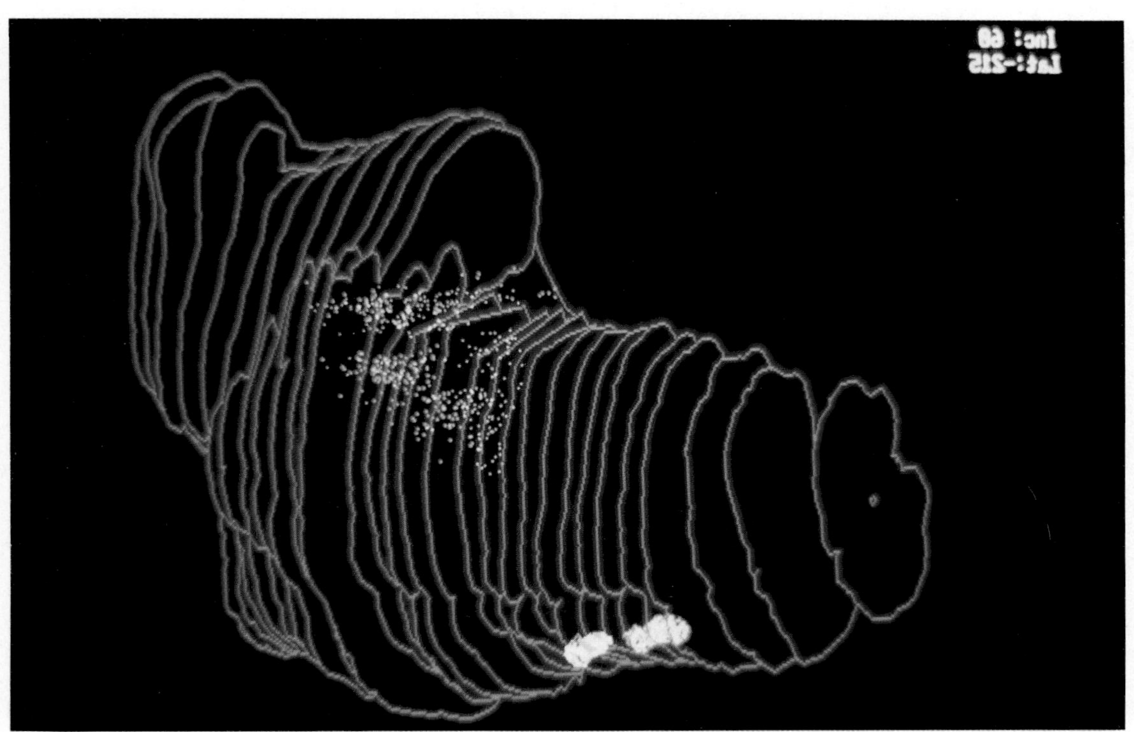
Inc: 60
Lat:-215

Pattern of PAG retrograde labelling after tracer injection into:

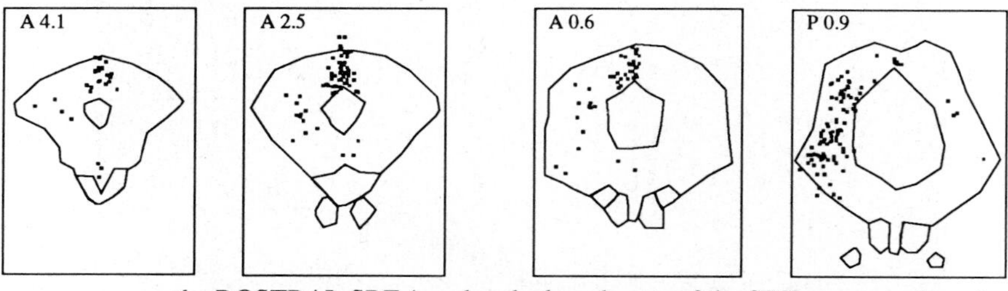

- the ROSTRAL SRF (renal and adrenal parts of the SRF pressor column)

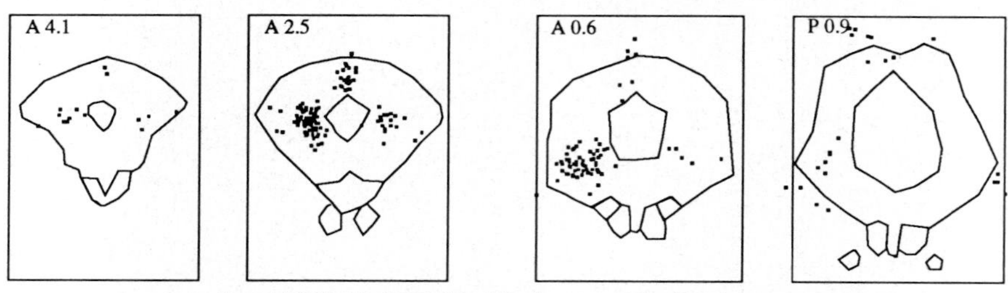

- the CAUDAL SRF (hindlimb part of the SRF pressor column)

Functional organization in the PAG:

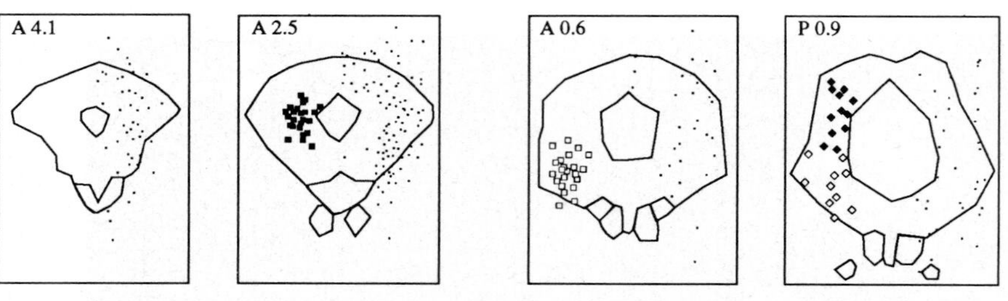

HYPERTENSIVE reaction associated with :

■ : a ↑ in **iliac** resistance
◆ : a ↑ in **renal** resistance
+ release of circulating
cathecholamines

HYPOTENSIVE reaction associated with :

□ : a ↓ in **iliac** resistance ◇ : a ↓ in **renal** resistance

Fig. 26. (Top and middle row): Representative coronal sections of the PAG (Berman, 1968) showing the distribution of labeled neurons following injection of fluorescent microspheres into the rostral (top row) or caudal (middle row) parts of the SRF nucleus. Ipsilateral is to the left, contralateral is to the right. Each PAG section is a reconstruction from 15 consecutive 30 μm sections. (Bottom row): Location of the centers of the sites at which changes in vasomotor tone in iliac and renal beds were evoked by DLH microinjection. The sites at which DLH injection evoked significant changes are represented on the left side of each section. Filled symbols indicate an increase in vasomotor tone (> 40% increase in resistance), and open symbols represent a decrease in vasomotor tone (between 4 and 20% decrease in resistance). Those sites at which DLH microinjection failed to evoke a significant change in vasomotor tone are indicated on the right of each section.

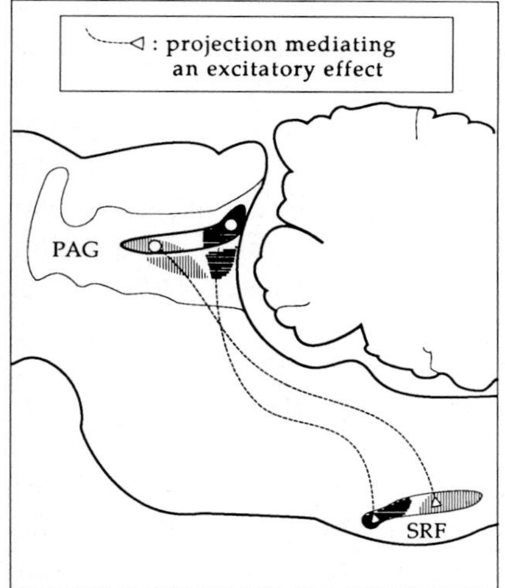

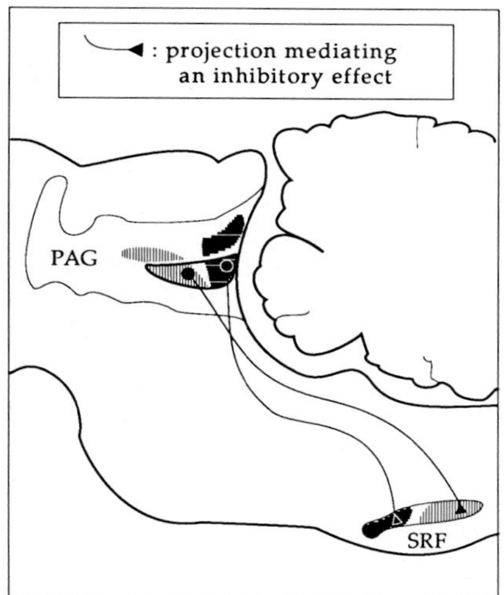

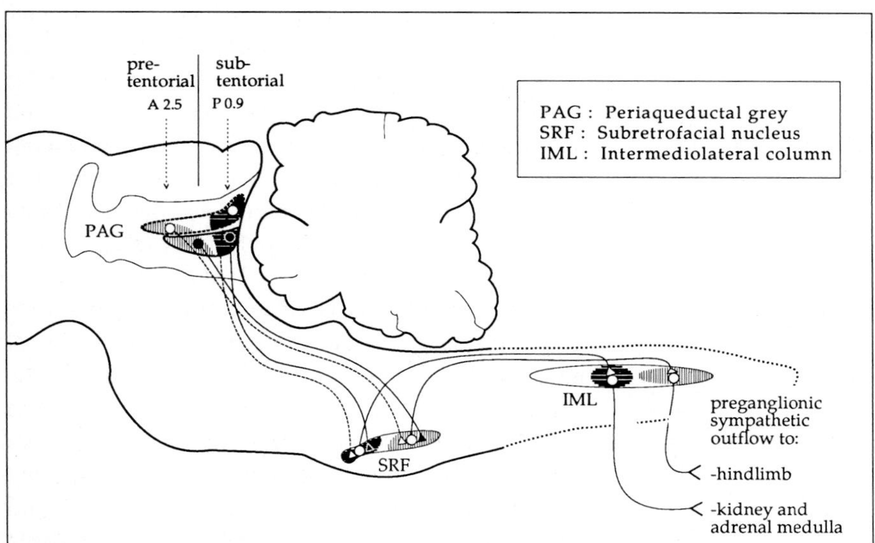

Fig. 27. Schematic diagram of pathways which may mediate the decrease and increase of vasomotor tone in the renal and hindlimb vascular beds following excitation of neurons in the lateral or ventrolateral PAG (reproduced from Fig. 8 of Carrive and Bandler, 1991a).

Holstege and Tan, 1988; Mantyh, 1983). The n. raphe magnus and the lateral medullary reticular formation are known to project to both the dorsal horn and intermediolateral cell column of the spinal cord; and the n. raphe pallidus and n. raphe obscurus (as well as adjacent parts of medullary reticular formation) project to the intermediate gray and the ventral horn of the spinal cord (Bowker et al., 1988; Holstege, 1987, 1988; Kuypers and Maisky, 1975; Willis, 1988). As no significant direct projections have been found from the PAG to brain stem or spinal cord motor nuclei (Holstege, 1988, 1989; Mantyh, 1983; although see Thoms and Jürgens, 1987), it seems clear that pontine and medullary cell groups (such as the SRF, NRA, n. raphe magnus) provide the

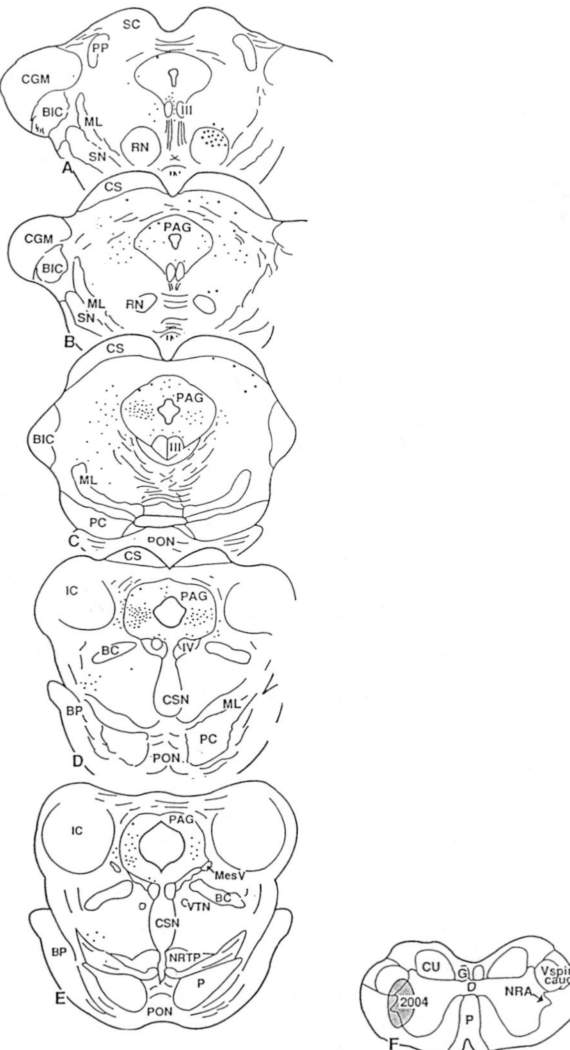

Fig. 28. Pattern of retrograde labeling in the midbrain PAG and adjacent tegmentum (sections (A – E) following a WGA-HRP injection into the NRA (section F) (reproduced with permission from Fig. 1 of Holstege, 1989).

major anatomical substrate through which the PAG modulates, second order afferent, and somatic and autonomic motor neuronal activity.

Afferent regulation of PAG output

The data considered thus far clearly indicate that projections neurons to the lower brain stem are restricted to topographically distinct parts of the PAG (i.e., lateral and ventrolateral to the aqueduct) and that the lateral and ventrolateral PAG consist of distinct functional regions. As the PAG receives a diverse set of forebrain, brain stem and spinal cord afferents, this raises the question of whether the functionally distinct PAG regions receive selective afferent inputs

Spinal cord and spinal trigeminal nucleus

It is most appropriate in the context of this volume, to note that it was William Mehler who drew attention, first, to the existence of a major spinomesencephalic pathway, including a substantial projection to the PAG (Mehler, 1962; Mehler et al., 1960). More recent studies (Blomqvist and Wiberg, 1985; Wiberg and Blomqvist, 1984; Wiberg et al., 1986; Yezierski, 1988) have revealed that not only is the PAG a major spinal and spinal trigeminal afferent recipient zone, but further that these afferents: (i) terminate in distinct PAG regions, and (ii) are somatotopically organized.

The distribution within the PAG of anterogradely transported WGA-HRP injected unilaterally into lumbar and cervical enlargements of the spinal cord, or pars caudalis (laminar portion) of the spinal trigeminal nucleus of the cat is illustrated in Fig. 29. It can be seen that in the subtentorial PAG, lumbar spinal afferents terminate (largely) contralaterally within restricted dorsolateral and ventrolateral zones, which delineate remarkably well those PAG regions from which flight-hypertension (dorsolateral) and immobility-hypotension (ventrolateral) have been evoked by EAA microinjection (compare Figs. 22 and 29). More rostrally in the PAG, afferents from cervical spinal cord and laminar spinal trigeminal nucleus terminate in a restricted region, lateral to the aqueduct, within the pretentorial PAG. This terminal zone corresponds precisely to the PAG region at which a threat display and hypertension is evoked by EAA microinjection (compare Figs. 22 and 29). Although the trigeminal input ter-

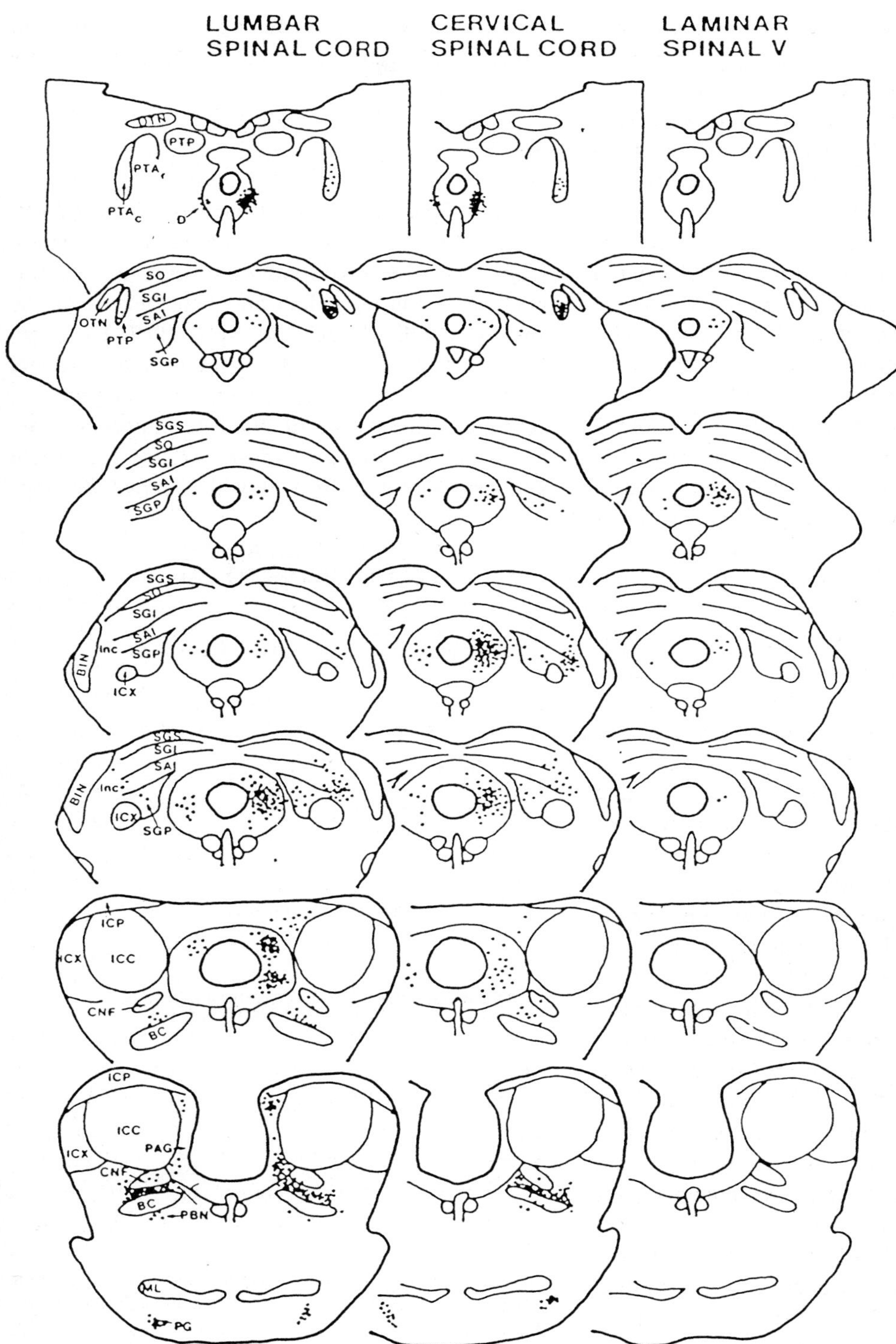

Fig. 29. Coronal sections through the midbrain of the cat showing the distribution of anterograde labeling following a unilateral WGA-HRP injection into either the lumbar spinal cord, cervical spinal cord, or the laminar spinal trigeminal nucleus. Contralateral is to the right; ipsilateral is to the left. Note the somatotopic organization of the projections to the PAG (reproduced with permission from Fig. 1 of Blomqvist and Wiberg, 1985).

minates most rostrally, it should be noted that trigeminal afferents do not extend into the rostral one-third of the PAG (Fig. 29). In other words, spinal and spinal trigeminal afferents are restricted to those regions within the caudal two-thirds of the PAG at which somatic and autonomic changes are evoked by EAA microinjection.

It is known that spinomesencephalic projections arise largely from laminae I and IV/V of the spinal cord, with smaller contributions from laminae VII and X (Lima and Coimbra, 1989; Liu, 1983; Menetrey et al., 1982; Swett et al., 1985). The projection from the laminar part of the spinal trigeminal also arises primarily from lamina I (Mantyh, 1982; Wiberg et al., 1986). Mesencephalic projecting lamina I neurons have been reported to be mostly nociceptive-specific, whereas mesencephalic-projecting lamina IV/V neurons generally possess a wide dynamic range, responding to both noxious and non-noxious stimuli (Hylden et al., 1986; Yezierski et al., 1987). The predominantly nociceptive nature of the somatic afferent input to the PAG, and in particular, the restricted termination zones within the lateral and ventrolateral PAG, obviously suggest that this pathway may play an important role in mediating an organism's reactions to noxious stimuli (i.e., the integrated somatic and autonomic response; the activation of descending pain modulatory mechanisms). The significance of the somatotopic specificity of the spinal and spinal trigeminal projections to the PAG remains for now obscure. It should be noted, however, that the subtentorial PAG regions, which receive input from lumbar (and cervical) spinal cord, are also the regions at which DLH microinjection evokes either flight or immobility; reactions which are associated with either strong limb movement or an absence of limb movement. In contrast, the pretentorial PAG region, which receives input from the laminar spinal trigeminal nucleus (and cervical spinal cord), is also the region at which DLH microinjection evokes a threat display, associated with strong facio-vocal activity. Thus, there appears to be a correlation, within the PAG, of the somatotopy of the afferent input and the region of the body in which skeletal muscle activity is most affected by DLH microinjection.

Forebrain

Hypothalamus and central nucleus of amygdala:

The PAG receives also a significant projection from both the hypothalamus, and the central nucleus of the amygdala and bed nucleus of the stria terminalis (Enoch and Kerr, 1967; Holstege, 1987; Holstege et al., 1985; Hopkins and Holstege, 1978; Krieger et al., 1979). As summarized schematically in Fig. 30, these termination zones are largely restricted to those parts of the lateral and ventrolateral PAG at which threat display/

"LIMBIC FOREBRAIN" PROJECTIONS TO PAG

FROM PREFRONTAL AND CINGULATE CORTEX

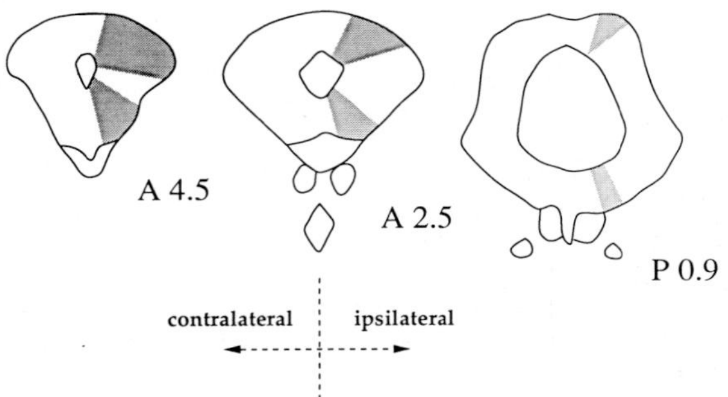

FROM AMYGDALA, BED NUCLEUS OF STRIA TERMINALIS, HYPOTHALAMUS

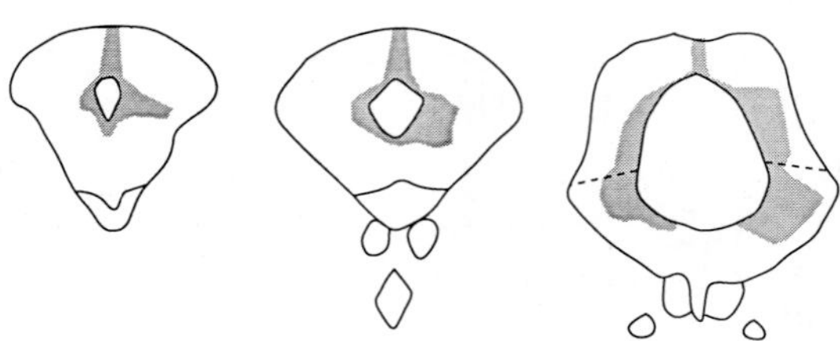

Fig. 30. Summary schematic diagram showing the regional distribution of afferents from the "limbic forebrain" to the PAG. The stippled areas represent the regions of anterograde labeling in the PAG. In all cases the site of anterograde tracer injection was on the right side. See text for references.

flight-hypertension (lateral) and immobility-hypotension (ventrolateral) are evoked by DLH microinjection.

Prefrontal cortex and cingulate gyrus:

In contrast, the prefrontal and cingulate cortices do not appear to project extensively to the lateral and ventrolateral parts of the PAG. Instead afferents from these limbic cortical regions terminate in the dorsolateral and ventromedial parts of the PAG, and especially in the rostral one-third of the PAG (Fig. 30) (Bragin et al., 1984; Hardy and Leichnetz, 1981; Segal et al., 1983; Wyss and Sripanidkulchai, 1984). Both our own studies (Carrive et al., 1988, 1989b), and those of others (Holstege, 1988, 1989), indicate further that neither the dorsolateral nor the ventromedial regions of the PAG project to cell groups in the pons, medulla or spinal cord. The dorsolateral PAG region has been recently found, however, to project to the cuneiform nucleus in the caudal midbrain of the rat (Redgrave et al., 1988).

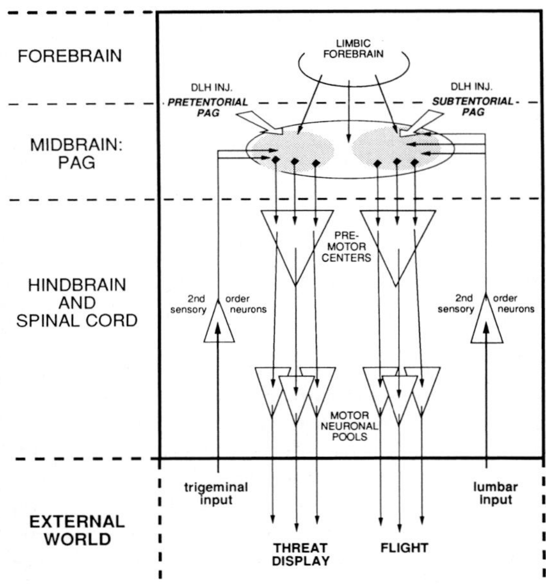

Fig. 31. Summary diagram depicting certain of the afferent and efferent pathways connecting the PAG with the periphery. See text for explanation.

General organization of limbic afferents to the PAG

Although not extensive, the data that are available suggest that there may exist a clear segregation in the distribution of "limbic" afferents to the PAG (Fig. 30). That is, limbic cortical regions (prefrontal cortex, cingulate gyrus) appear to project predominantly to those parts of the PAG, at which DLH microinjections do not evoke significant autonomic or somatic effects, and which, in turn, do not project to the lower brainstem. In contrast, subcortical limbic structures (i.e., hypothalamus, central nucleus of amygdala and bed nucleus of the stria terminalis) project to those parts of the PAG at which DLH microinjections evoke integrated somatic and autonomic reactions, and which project extensively to the lower brainstem.

Co-ordination of somatic and autonomic reactions: the role(s) of the PAG?

The data presented indicate that the caudal two-thirds of the PAG is an important region for the co-ordination of somatic and autonomic reactions. This part of the PAG consists of a number of functionally distinct regions (lateral and ventrolateral), each of which may be not more than two synapses removed from the periphery, on both the input and output sides. The proximity of these PAG neurons to the periphery suggests that each of these PAG regions may be considered an integrating center located at the top of a series of "reflex loops". The afferent limb of each reflex loop could be the spinomesencephalic or spinal trigeminomesencephalic pathways. The efferent limbs would be the multiple pathways which connect distinct PAG regions with specific premotor neuronal pools in the pons and medulla (Fig. 31).

Considerable progress has been made in the analysis of the functional organization of the efferent pathways originating within the PAG (e.g., PAG projections to the SRF, NRA and n. raphe magnus). The functional organization of the afferent pathways to the PAG and the specific role(s) played by these pathways, however, remains elusive. As discussed above, the nociceptive nature of the somatic afferent input to the PAG has led to considerable speculation (e.g., Basbaum and Fields, 1984; Hylden et al., 1986; Lima and Coimbra, 1989) that these pathways play important roles in mediating certain of the responses characteristic of an organism's reaction to noxious stimuli (e.g., visceral reflexes, integrated defense reactions, pain modulation). Other data, to be considered in the following section, suggest, in addition, that the effect(s) of afferent input transmitted along these pathways is critically dependent on the ongoing state of neural activity in the PAG.

The PAG as a "state-dependent" reflex center

After unilateral microinjection of pmol doses of kainic acid (KA) (Bandler and Carrive, 1988; Depaulis et al., 1989), or GABA antagonists (Bandler et al., 1985a; Depaulis and Vergnes, 1986; DiScala et al., 1984), into the lateral PAG of the cat and/or the rat, a clear asymmetry in the evoked defense reactions is usually observed. For example, following KA injection into the lateral, pretentorial PAG of the cat (Bandler and Carrive, 1988), it was found that light touch on the contralateral side of the body increased the intensity of the threat display and often evoked directed striking or biting. In contrast, tactile stimulation of the ipsilateral side of the body rarely evoked such effects. Light touch anywhere on the body in the absence of PAG stimulation, either was without effect, or evoked only a mild orienting reaction.

Similarly, in the rat, following KA injection into the lateral, pretentorial PAG (Depaulis et al., 1989), tactile stimuli applied to the contralateral side of the body evoked defensive reactions, whereas tactile stimuli applied to the ipsilateral side of the body did not. Interestingly, even on the contralateral half of the body, the effects of tactile stimulation, applied to different body regions, were different. As seen in Fig. 32, tactile stimulation of the contralateral head of the rat elicited the most intense and long-lasting reaction, whereas a less intense reaction was elicited by tactile stimulation of the contralateral forelimb. No reaction was observed, however, after tactile stimulation of the contralateral flank or the contralateral hindlimb. These results may recall the observations that, in the cat, the lateral, pretentorial PAG receives a predominantely contralateral spinal trigeminal and contralateral spinomesencephalic input from the lower cervical (i.e., forelimb) region of the spinal cord. We would suggest therefore that, in these experiments, the appearance of a lateralized and somatotopically specific defensive reactivity is due to the combination of: (i) increased pretentorial PAG neural activity following the unilateral injection of KA; and further, (ii) a specific augmentation of pretentorial PAG neural activity brought about by tactile stimulation of the contralateral

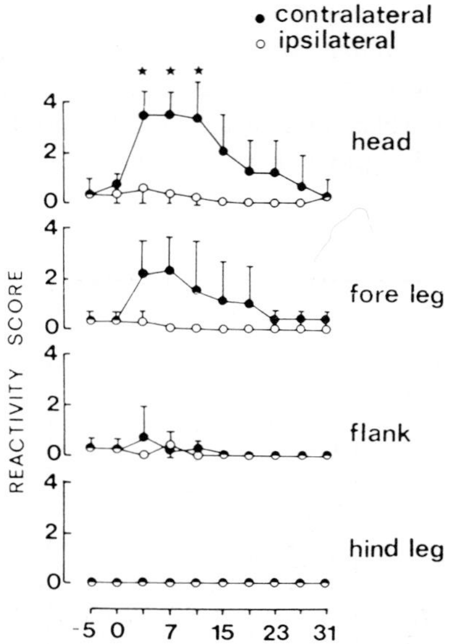

Fig. 32. Defensive reactivity score (mean +/− SEM) to tactile stimulation following microinjection of 40 pmol of kainic acid in the lateral pretentorial PAG of the rat (N = 7). Tactile stimulation (with a 1 cm dia. nylon brush) was applied at 4 different body sites each, on the contralateral and ipsilateral sides of the body. As indicated on the abscissa, rats were tested 5 min before and immediately prior to the KA injection; 3 min after the KA injection, and then at 4 min intervals until the end of the experiment (31 min post-KA injection). * $P < 0.05$, ipsi vs. contra, Wilcoxon text. For details see Depaulis et al., 1989 (reproduced with permission from Fig. 6 of Depaulis et al., 1989).

head/forelimb. In other words: (i) tactile stimulation of the ipsilateral head/forelimb is largely without effect because the predominantly crossed spinal trigeminal and cervical spinal afferents project to the "non-KA" injected side of the pretentorial PAG; and (ii) tactile stimulation of the hindlimb (either ipsilateral or contralateral) is without effect because lumbar spinal afferents, for the most part, project to the subtentorial PAG. To summarize then, a normally non-provocative stimulus (e.g., light touch of the contralateral head/forelimb) evoked a defensive reaction only if the PAG region receiving this afferent input has already been "activated".

Obviously, in these experiments the lateralized and somatotopically-specific defensiveness was the product of an artificial and localized excitation of the pretentorial PAG. Nonetheless, such an experimental distortion is useful precisely because it provides dramatic evidence of the interaction between a somatotopically specific afferent input and a highly localized PAG excitation. In terms of predictability, regularity and presumed underlying anatomical connections (see Fig. 31), it may be useful to consider such effects as "PAG state-dependent" reflexes.

To summarize, then, we have found that excitation of restricted pools of neurons, located within distinct parts of the pretentorial or subtentorial PAG, evokes distinct and different patterns of integrated somatic and autonomic changes. We are suggesting further that, in the natural situation, excitation of the same PAG neuronal pools (perhaps by descending limbic forebrain input) "enables" PAG reflex-circuitry which prepares the organism to respond in quite specific ways to certain stimuli (e.g., flight if the hind end is touched vs. threat display if the animal is approached or touched around the head). It is quite clear, therefore, that the defence reactions evoked by PAG stimulation are composed not solely of responses or reflexes that are inextricably bound together in rigid sequences. Rather, that during excitation of the PAG the animal is "prepared" so that from among a number of possible defensive responses, the actual response chosen is determined by its immediate environment. It should be noted that such a formulation is quite consistent with the ethological viewpoint that behavior depends on a dynamic interplay between the animal, its mood (i.e., the "state" of its central nervous system) and its environment (with respect to defensive behavior see for example Leyhausen, 1979). Whether certain of the "inhibitory" functions of the ventrolateral PAG (e.g., immobility, hypotension) are expressed in a similar manner remains to be studied.

Acknowledgements

The research from our laboratory reported in this chapter was supported by grants from the Australian National Health and Medical Research Council, The Harry Frank Guggenheim Foundation (USA) and The Clive and Vera Ramaciotti Foundation (Australia). The authors wish to acknowledge the valued collaboration of Dr. R.A.L. Dampney and Dr. A. Depaulis and the technical assistance of J. Polson.

Abbreviations

AQ, midbrain aqueduct; AMB nucleus ambiguus; CE, central canal; CU,cuneate nucleus; DLH, D,L-homocysteic acid; DR, dorsal raphe nucleus; EW, Edinger Westphal nucleus; GR, gracile nucleus; IC, inferior colliculus; III, oculomotor nucleus; IO, inferior olivary nucleus; IV, trochlear nucleus; LRN, lateral reticular nucleus; MLF, medial longitudinal fasciculus; P, pyramids; PAG, midbrain periaqueductal grey matter; PC, posterior commissure; RF, retrofacial nucleus; S, solitary tract; SC, superior colliculus; SO, superior olivary nucleus; SRF, subretrofacial nucleus; TV, ventral tegmental nucleus (Gudden); 5SP, laminar spinal trigeminal nucleus; 5ST, spinal tract of the trigeminal nerve; 7, facial nucleus; 7N, facial nerve.

References

Abrahams, V.C., Hilton, S.M. and Zbrozyna, A.W. (1960) Active muscle vasodilatation produced by stimulation of the brain stem: its significance in the defence reaction. *J. Physiol. (Lond.),* 154: 491 – 513.

Abrahams, V.C., Hilton, S.M. and Zbrozyna, A.W. (1964) The role of active muscle vasodilatation in the alerting stage of the defence reaction. *J. Physiol. (Lond.),* 171: 491 – 513.

Abols, I.A. and Basbaum, A.I. (1981) Afferent input to the rostral medulla of the cat: A neural substrate for midbrain-medullary interactions in the modulation of pain. *J. Comp. Neurol.,* 201: 285 – 297.

Adams, D.B., Baccelli, G., Mancia, G. and Zanchetti, A. (1969) Cardiovascular changes during naturally elicited fighting behavior in the cat. *Am. J. Physiol.,* 216: 1226 – 1235.

Adams, D.B., Baccelli, G., Mancia, G. and Zanchetti, A. (1971) Relation of cardiovascular changes in fighting to emotion and exercise. *J. Physiol. (Lond.),* 212: 321 – 326.

Bandler, R. (1982) Induction of rage following microinjections of glutamate into midbrain but not hypothalamus of cats. *Neurosci. Lett.,* 30: 183 – 188.

Bandler, R. (1988) Brain mechanisms of aggression as revealed by electrical and chemical stimulation: Suggestion of a central role for the midbrain periaqueductal grey region. In: A. Epstein and A. Morrison (Eds.), *Progress in Psychobiology and Physiological Psychology, Vol. 13.* Academic Press, New York, pp. 67 – 154.

Bandler, R. and Carrive, P. (1988) Integrated defence reaction elicited by excitatory amino acid injection in the midbrain periaqueductal grey region of the unrestrained cat. *Brain Res.,* 439: 95 – 106.

Bandler, R., Depaulis, A. and Vergnes, M. (1985a) Identification of midbrain neurons mediating defensive behaviour in the rat by microinjections of excitatory amino acids. *Behav. Brain Res.,* 15: 107 – 119.

Bandler, R., McCulloch, T. and Dreher, B. (1985b) Afferents to a midbrain periaqueductal grey region involved in the "defence reaction" in the cat as revealed by horseradish peroxidase: I. The telencephalon. *Brain Res.,* 330: 109 – 119.

Bandler, R. and Tork, I. (1987) Midbrain periaqueductal grey region in the cat has afferent and efferent connections with solitary tract nuclei. *Neurosci. Lett.,* 74: 1 – 6.

Bard, P. and Macht, M.B. (1958) The behaviour of chronically decerebrate cats. In: G.E.W. Wolstenholme and C.M. O'Connor (Eds.), *CIBA Foundation Symposium on Neurological Basis of Behaviour.* Churchill, London, pp. 55 – 75.

Basbaum, A.I. and Fields, H.L. (1984) Endogenous pain control systems: brainstem spinal pathways and endorphin circuitry. *Ann. Rev. Neurosci.,* 7: 309 – 338.

Beitz, A.J., Shepard, R.D. and Wells, W.E. (1983) The periaqueductal gray-raphe magnus projection contains somatostatin, neurotensin and serotonin but not cholecystokinin. *Brain Res.,* 261: 132 – 137.

Berman, A.L. (1968) *The brainstem of the cat.* A cytoarchitectonic atlas with stereotaxic coordinates. Madison: The University of Wisconsin Press.

Blanchard, D.C., Williams, G., Lee, E.M.C. and Blanchard, R.J. (1981) Taming of wild Rattus norvegicus by lesions of the mesencephalic central gray. *Physiol. Psychol.,* 9: 157 – 163.

Blomqvist, A. and Wiberg, M. (1985) Some aspects of the anatomy of somatosensory projections to the cat midbrain. In: M.J. Rowe and W.D. Willis, (Eds.), *Development, organization, and processing in somatosensory pathways.* Alan R. Liss, New York, pp. 215 – 222.

Bowker, R.M., Abbott, L.C. and Dilts, R.P. (1988) Peptidergic neurons in the nucleus raphe magnus and the nucleus gigantocellularis: their distributions, interrelationships, and projections to the spinal cord. *Prog. Brain Res.,* 77: 95 – 127.

Bragin, E.O., Yeliseeva, Z.V., Vasilenko, G.F., Meizerov, E.E., Chuvin, B.T. and Durinyan, R.A. (1984) Cortical projections to the periaqueductal grey in the cat: A retrograde horseradish peroxidase study. *Neurosci. Lett.,* 51: 271 – 275.

Carlton, S.M., Chung, J.M., Leonard, R.B. and Willis, W.D. (1985) Funicular trajectories of brain stem neurons projecting to the lumbar spinal cord in the monkey (Maccaca fascicularis): a retrograde labeling study. *J. Comp. Neurol.,* 241: 382 – 404.

Carrive, P. and Bandler, R. (1991a) Viscerotopic organization of neurons subserving hypotensive reactions within the midbrain periaqueductal grey: a correlative functional and anatomical study. *Brain Res.* (in press).

Carrive, P. and Bandler, R. (1991b) Control of hindlimb blood flow by the midbrain periaqueductal grey of the cat. *Exp. Brain Res.* (in press).

Carrive, P., Dampney, R.A.L. and Bandler, R. (1987) Excitation of neurones in a restricted region of the midbrain periaqueductal grey elicits both behavioural and cardiovascular components of the defence reaction in the unanaesthetized decerebrate cat. *Neurosci. Lett.,* 81: 273 – 278.

Carrive, P., Bandler, R. and Dampney, R.A.L. (1988) Anatomical evidence that hypertension associated with the defence reaction in the cat is mediated by a direct projection from a restricted portion of the midbrain periaqueductal grey to the subretrofacial nucleus of the medulla. *Brain Res.,* 460: 339 – 345.

Carrive, P., Bandler, R. and Dampney, R.A.L. (1989a) Somatic and autonomic integration in the midbrain: A distinctive pattern evoked by excitation of neurones in the subtentorial portion of the midbrain periaqueductal grey region. *Brain Res.,* 483: 251 – 258.

Carrive, P., Bandler, R. and Dampney, R.A.L. (1989b) Viscerotopic control of regional vascular beds by discrete groups of neurons within the midbrain periaqueductal gray. *Brain Res.,* 493: 385 – 390.

Carstens, E., Klump D. and Zimmermann, M. (1980) Time course and effective sites for inhibition from midbrain periaqueductal gray of spinal dorsal horn neuronal responses to cutaneous stimuli in the rat. *Exp. Brain Res.*, 38: 425 – 430.

Ciriello, J., Caverson, M.M. and Polosa, C. (1986) Function of the ventrolateral medulla in the control of the circulation. *Brain Res. Rev.*, 11: 359 – 391.

Dampney, R.A.L. and McAllen, R.M. (1988) Differential control of sympathetic fibres supplying hindlimb skin and muscle by subretrofacial neurones in the cat. *J. Physiol. (Lond.)*, 395: 41 – 56.

Dampney, R.A.L., Czachurski, J., Dembowsky, K., Goodchild, A.K. and Seller, H. (1987) Afferent connections and spinal projections of the pressor region in the rostral ventrolateral medulla of the cat. *J. Auton. Nerv. Syst.*, 20: 73 – 86.

Dampney, R.A.L., Goodchild, A.K. and McAllen, R.M. (1987) Vasomotor control by subretrofacial neurones in the rostral ventrolateral medulla. *Can. J. Physiol., Pharmacol.* 65: 1572 – 1579.

Dampney, R.A.L., Goodchild, A.K. and Tan, E. (1985) Vasopressor neurones in the rostral ventrolateral medulla of the rabbit. *J. Auton. Nerv. Syst.*, 14: 239 – 254.

Darlington, D.N. and Ward, D.G. (1985) Rostral pontine and caudal mesencephalic control of arterial pressure and iliac, celiac and renal vascular resistance. II. Separate control and topographic organization. *Brain Res.*, 361: 301 – 308.

Depaulis, A. and Vergnes, M. (1986) Elicitation of intraspecific defensive behaviors in the rat by microinjection of picrotoxin, a GABA antagonist, into the midbrain periaqueductal gray matter. *Brain Res.*, 367: 87 – 95.

Depaulis, A., Bandler, R. and Vergnes, M. (1989) Characterization of pretentorial periaqueductal gray neurons mediating intraspecific defensive behaviors in the rat by microinjections of kainic acid. *Brain Res.*, 486: 121 – 132.

Di Scala, G., Schmitt, P. and Karli, P. (1984) Flight induced by infusion of bicuculline methiodide into periventricular structures. *Brain Res.*, 309: 199 – 208.

Duggan, A.W. (1983) Injury, pain and analgesia. *Proc. Aust. Physiol. Pharmacol. Soc.* 14: 218 – 240.

Edwards, M.A. and Adams, D.B. (1974) Role of the midbrain central gray in pain-induced defensive boxing of rats. *Physiol. Behav.*, 13: 113 – 121.

Eliasson, S., Lindgren, P. and Uvnas, B. (1954) The hypothalamus, a relay station of the sympathetic vasodilator tract. *Act. Physiol. Scand.*, 31: 290 – 300.

Ellison, G.D. and Flynn, J.P. (1968) Organized aggressive behavior in cats after surgical isolation of the hypothalamus. *Arch. Ital. Biol.*, 106: 1 – 20.

Enoch, D.M. and Kerr, F.W.L. (1967) Hypothalamic vasopressor and vesicopressor pathways. II. Anatomic study of their course and connections. *Arch. Neurol.*, 16: 307 – 320.

Fardin, V., Oliveras, J.-L. and Besson, J.-M. (1984a) A reinvestigation of the analgesic effects induced by stimulation of the periaqueductal gray matter in the rat. I. The pruduction of behavioral side effects together with analgesia. *Brain Res.*, 306: 105 – 123.

Fardin, V., Oliveras, J.-L. and Besson, J.-M. (1984b) Projections from the periaqueductal gray matter to the B_3 cellular area (nucleus raphe magnus and nucleus reticularis paragigantocellularis) as revealed by the retrograde transport of horseradish peroxidase in the rat. *J. Comp. Neurol.*, 223: 483 – 500.

Fernandez De Molina, A. and Hunsperger, R.W. (1962) Organization of the subcortical system governing defence and flight reactions in the cat. *J. Physiol. (Lond.)*, 160: 200 – 213.

Gellen, B., Gyorgy, L. and Doda, M. (1972) Influence of the surgical isolation of the hypothalamus on oxotremorine-induced rage reaction and sympathetic response in the cat. *Act. Physiol. Acad. Sci. Hung.*, 42, 195 – 202.

Goodchild, A.K., Dampney, R.A.L. and Bandler, R. (1982) A method for evoking physiological responses by stimulation of cell bodies, but not axons of passage, within localized regions of the central nervous system. *J. Neurosci. Methods*, 6: 351 – 363.

Hardy, S.G.P. and Leichnetz, G.R. (1981) Cortical projections to the periaqueductal gray in the monkey: anterograde and orthograde horseradish peroxidase study. *Neurosci. Lett.*, 22: 97 – 101.

Haselton, J.R., Winters, R.W., Liskowsky, D.R., Haselton, C.L., McCabe, P.M. and Schneiderman, N. (1988a) Cardiovascular responses elicited by electrical and chemical stimulation of the rostral medullary raphe of the rabbit. *Brain Res.*, 453: 167 – 175.

Haselton, J.R., Winters, R.W., Liskowsky, D.R., Haselton, C.L., McCabe, P.M. and Schneiderman, N. (1988b) Anatomical and functional connections of neurons of the rostral medullary raphe of the rabbit. *Brain Res.*, 453: 176 – 182.

Hilton, S.M. (1979) The defence reaction as a paradigm for cardiovascular control. In: C. Brooks, K. Koisumi and A. Sato (Eds.), *Integrative Functions of the Autonomic Nervous System.* University of Tokyo Press, Tokyo, pp. 443 – 449.

Hilton, S.M. (1982) The defence-arousal system and its relevance for circulatory and respiratory control. *J. Exp. Biol.*, 100: 159 – 174.

Holstege, G. (1987) Some anatomical observations on the projections from the hypothalamus to brainstem and spinal cord: an HRP and autoradiographic tracing study in the cat. *J. Comp. Neurol.*, 260: 98 – 126.

Holstege, G. (1988) Direct and indirect pathways to lamina I in the medulla oblongata and spinal cord of the cat. *Prog. Brain Res.*, 77: 47 – 94.

Holstege, G. (1989) An anatomical study on the final common pathway for vocalization in the cat. *J. Comp. Neurol.*, 284: 242 – 252.

Holstege, G. and Tan, J. (1988) Projections from the red nucleus and surrounding areas to the brainstem and spinal cord in the cat. An HRP and autoradiographic tracing study. *Behav. Brain Res.,* 28: 33 – 57.

Holstege, G., Meiners, L. and Tan, K. (1985) Projections of the bed nucleus of the stria terminalis to the mesencephalon, pons, and medulla oblongata in the cat. *Exp. Brain Res.,* 58: 379 – 391.

Hopkins, D.A. and Holstege, G. (1978) Amygdaloid projections to the mesencephalon, pons, and medulla oblongata in the cat. *Exp. Brain Res.,* 32: 529 – 547.

Hunsperger, R.W. (1956) Affektreaktionen auf elektrische Reizung in Hirnstamm der Katze. *Acta. Helv. Physiol. Pharmacol.* 14: 70 – 92.

Hylden, J.L.K., Hayashi, H., Dubner, R. and Bennett, G.J. (1986) Physiology and morphology of the lamina I spinomesencephalic projection. *J. Comp. Neurol.,* 247: 505 – 515.

Janig, W. (1985) Organization of the lumbar sympathetic outflow to skeletal muscle and skin of the cat hindlimb and tail. *Rev. Physiol. Biochem. Pharmacol.,* 102: 119 – 213.

Jurgens, U. and Pratt, R. (1979) Role of the periaqueductal grey in vocal expression of emotion. *Brain Res.,* 167: 367 – 378.

Katz, L.C., Burkhalter, A. and Dreyer, W.J. (1984) Fluorescent latex microspheres as a retrograde neuronal marker for in vivo and in vitro studies of visual cortex. *Nature,* 310: 498 – 500.

Keller, A.D. (1932) Autonomic discharges elicited by phsyiological stimuli in midbrain preparations. *Am. J. Physiol.,* 100: 576 – 586.

Kelly, A.H., Beaton, L.E. and Magoun, H.W. (1946) A midbrain mechanism for facio-vocal activity. *J. Neurophysiol.,* 9: 181 – 189.

Korner, P.I., Uther, J.B. and White, S.W. (1969) Central nervous integration of the circulatory and respiratory responses to arterial hypoxemia in the rabbit. *Circ. Res.,* 24: 757 – 776.

Krieger, M.S., Conrad, L.C.A. and Pfaff, D.W. (1979) An autoradiography study of the efferent connections of the ventromedial nucleus of the hypothalamus. *J. Comp. Neurol.,* 183: 785 – 816.

Kuypers, H.G.J.M. and Maisky, V.A. (1975) Retrograde transport of horseradish peroxidase from spinal cord to brain stem cell groups in the cat. *Neurosci. Lett.,* 1: 9 – 14.

LeDoux, J.E. (1987) Emotion. In: V.F. Plum (Ed.), *Handbook of Physiology: Nervous System.* American Physiological Society, Washington D.C., pp. 419 – 459.

Lewis, V.A. and G.F. Gebhart (1977) Evaluation of the periaqueductal central gray (PAG) as morphine-specific locus of action and examination of morphine-induced and stimulation-produced analgesia at coincident PAG loci. *Brain Res.,* 124: 283 – 303.

Leyhausen, P. (1979) *Cat behavior. The predatory and social behavior of domestic and wild cats.* Garland Press, New York.

Liebeskind, J.C., Guilbaud, G., Besson, J.-M. and Oliveras, J.-L. (1973) Analgesia from electrical stimulation of the periaqueductal gray matter in the cat: behavioural observations and inhibitory effects on spinal cord interneurons. *Brain Res.,* 50: 441 – 446.

Lima, D. and Coimbra, A. (1989) Morphological types of spinomesencephalic neurons in the marginal zone (lamina I) of the rat spinal cord, as shown after retrograde labelling with cholera toxin subunit B. *J. Comp. Neurol.,* 279: 327 – 339.

Lindgren, P. (1955) The mesencephalon and the vasomotor system. *Act. Physiol. Scand.,* 35 (Suppl 121): 1 – 183.

Lindgren, P., Rosen, A., Strandberg, P. and Uvnas, B. (1956) The sympathetic vasodilator outflow – a cortico-spinal autonomic pathway. *J. Comp. Neurol.,* 105: 95 – 109.

Lipski, J., Bellingham, M.C., West, M.J. and Pilowsky, P. (1988) Limitations of the technique of pressure microinjection of excitatory amino acids for evoking responses from localized regions of the CNS. *J. Neuronsci. Methods,* 26: 169 – 179.

Liu, R.P.C. (1983) Laminar origins of spinal projection neurons to the periaqueductal gray of the rat. *Brain Res.,* 264: 118 – 122.

Lovick, T.A. (1987) Differential control of cardiac and vasomotor activity by neurones in nucleus paragigantocellularis lateralis in the cat. *J. Physiol. (Lond.),* 389: 23 – 35.

Mancia, G. and Zanchetti, A. (1981) Hypothalamic control of autonomic functions. In: P.J. Morgane and J. Panksepp (Eds.), *Handbook of the Hypothalamus.* Marcel Dekker, New York, pp. 147 – 201.

Mancia, G., Baccelli, G. and Zanchetti, A. (1972) Hemodynamic responses to different emotional stimuli in the cat: Patterns and mechanisms. *Am. J. Physiol.,* 223: 925 – 933.

Mancia, G., Baccelli, G. and Zanchetti, A. (1974) Regulation of renal circulation during behavioral changes in the cat. *Am. J. Physiol.,* 227: 536 – 542.

Manyth, P.W. (1982 Forebrain projections to the periaqueductal gray in the monkey, with observations in the cat and rat. *J. Comp. Neurol.,* 204: 349 – 363.

Mantyh, P.W. (1983) Connections of the midbrain periaqueductal gray in the monkey. II. Descending efferent connections. *J. Neurophysiol.,* 49: 582 – 594.

Martin, J., Sutherland, C.J. and Zbrozyna, A.W. (1976) Habituation and conditioning of the defence reactions and their cardiovascular components in cats and dogs. *Pflugers Arch.,* 365: 37 – 47.

Mayer, D.J., Wolfe, T.L., Akil, H., Carder, B. and Liebeskind, J.C. (1971) Analgesia from electrical stimulation in the brainstem of the rat. *Science,* 174: 1351 – 1354.

McAllen, R.M., Dampney, R.A.L. and Goodchild A.K. (1987) The sub-retrofacial nucleus and cardiovascular control. In:

F.R. Calaresu, J. Ciriello, C. Polosa and L.P. Renaud, (Eds.), *Organization of the autonomic nervous system: central and peripheral mechanisms.* A. Liss, New York, pp. 215 – 225.

McCall, R.B. (1984) Evidence for a serotonergically mediated sympathoexcitatory response to stimulation of medullary raphe. *Brain Res.,* 311: 131 – 139.

Mehler, W.R. (1962) The anatomy of the co-called "pain tract" in man: An analysis of the course and distribution of the ascending fibers of the fasciculus anterolateralis. In: J.D. Fench and R.W. Porter, (Eds.), *Basic research in paraplegia.* C.C Thomas, Springfield, IL, pp. 26 – 55.

Mehler, W.R., Feferman, M.E. and Nauta, W.J.H. (1960) Ascending axon degeneration following antero-lateral cordotomy. An experimental study in the monkey. *Brain,* 83: 718 – 749.

Meller, S.Y. (1987) *The anatomy of the periaqueductal gray in the rabbit.* Ph.D. Thesis, Univ. of Adelaide.

Menetrey, D., Chaouch, A., Binder, D. and Besson, J.-M. (1982) The origin of the spinomesencephalic tract is the rat. An anatomical study using the retrograde transport of horseradish peroxidase. *J. Comp. Neurol.,* 206: 193 – 207.

Moss, M.S. and Basbaum, A.I. (1983) The peptidergic organization of the cat periaqueductal gray. II. The distribution of immunoreactive substance P and vasoactive intestinal polypeptide. *J. Neurosci.,* 3: 1437 – 1449.

Moss, M.S., Glazer, E.L. and Basbaum, A.I. (1983) The peptidergic organization of the cat periaqueductal gray. I. The distribution of immunoreactive enkephalin-containing neurons and terminals. *J. Neurosci.,* 3: 603 – 616.

Mraovitch, S., Kumada, M. and Reis, D.J. (1982) Role of the nucleus parabrachialis in cardiovascular regulation in cat. *Brain Res.,* 232: 57 – 75.

Redgrave, P., Dean, P., Mitchell, I.J., Odekunle, A. and Clark, A. (1988) The projection from superior colliculus to cuneiform area in the rat. I. Anatomical studies. Exp. *Brain. Res.,* 72: 611 – 625.

Reichling, D.B., Kwiat, G.C. and Basbaum, A.I. (1988) Anatomy, physiology and pharmacology of the periaqueductal gray contribution to antinociceptive controls. Prog. *Brain Res.,* 77: 31 – 46.

Reynolds, D.V. (1969) Surgery in the rat during electrical analgesia induced by focal brain stimulation. *Science,* 164: 444 – 445.

Rose, J.D. (1981) Projections to the caudolateral medulla from the pons, midbrain and diencephalon in the cat. *Exp. Neurol.,* 72: 413 – 428.

Ross, C.A., Ruggiero, D.A., Park, D.H., Joh, T.H., Sved, A.F., Fernandez-Pardal, J., Saavedra, J.M. and Reis, D.J. (1984) Tonic vasomotor control by the rostral ventrolateral medulla: effect of electrical or chemical stimulation of the area containing C1 adrenaline neurons on arterial pressure, heart rate and plasma catecholamines and vasopressin. *J. Neurosci.,* 4: 474 – 494.

Segal, R.L., Beckstead, R.M., Kersey, K. and Edwards, S.B. (1983) The prefrontal corticotectal projection in the cat. *Exp. Brain Res.,* 51: 423 – 432.

Skultety, F.M. (1963) Stimulation of periaqueductal gray and hypothalamus. *Arch. Neurol.,* 8: 609 – 620.

Stokman, C.L. and Glusman, M. (1981) Directional interaction of midbrain and hypothalamus in the control of carbachol-induced aggression. *Aggress. Beh.,* 7: 131 – 144.

Swett, J.E. and Woolf, C.J. (1985) The somatotopic organization of primary afferent terminals in the superficial laminae of the dorsal horn of the rat spinal cord. *J. Comp. Neurol.,* 231: 66 – 77.

ter Horst, G.J., Luiten, P.G.M. and Kuipers, F. (1984) Descending pathways from the hypothalamus to dorsal motor vagus and ambiguus nuclei in the rat. *J. Auton. Nerv. Syst.,* 11: 59 – 75.

Thoms, G., and Jürgens, U. (1987) Common input to the cranial motor nuclei involved in phonation in squirrel monkey. *Exp. Neurol.,* 95: 85 – 99.

Urca, G., Nahin, R.L. and Liebeskind, J.C. (1980) Glutamate-induced analgesia: Blockade and potentiation by naloxone. *Brain Res.,* 192: 523 – 530.

Wiberg, M. and Blomqvist, A. (1984) The spinomesencephalic tract in the cat: its cells of origin and termination in patterns as demonstrated by the intraaxonal transport method. *Brain Res.,* 291: 1 – 18.

Wiberg, M., Westman, J. and Blomqvist A. (1986) The projection to the mesencephalon from the sensory trigeminal nuclei. An anatomical study in the cat. *Brain Res.,* 399: 51 – 68.

Willis, W.D. (1988) Anatomy and physiology of descending control of nociceptive responses of dorsal horn neurons: comprehensive review. *Prog. Brain. Res.,* 77: 1 – 29.

Wyss, J.M. and Sripanidkulchai, K. (1984) The topography of the mesencephalic and pontine projections from the cingulate cortex of the rat. *Brain Res.,* 293: 1 – 15.

Yaksh, T.L., Yeung, J.C. and Rudy, T.A. (1976) Systematic examination in the rat of brain sites sensitive to the direct application of morphine: observation of differential effects within the periaqueductal gray. *Brain Res.,* 114: 83 – 103.

Yezierski, R.P. (1988) Spinomesencephalic tract: projections from the lumbosacral spinal cord of the rat, cat, and monkey. *J. Comp. Neurol.,* 267: 131 – 146.

Yezierski, R.P., Sorkin, L.S. and Willis, W.D. (1987) Response properties of spinal neurons projecting to midbrain or midbrain-thalamus in the monkey. *Brain Res.,* 437: 165 – 170.

Zhang, S.P., Bandler, R. and Carrive, P. (1990) Flight and immobility evoked by excitatory amino acid microinjection within distinct parts of the subtentorial midbrain periaqueductal grey of the cat. *Brain Res.,* 520, 73 – 82.

G. Holstege (Ed.)
Progress in Brain Research, Vol. 87

CHAPTER 14

Descending motor pathways and the spinal motor system: Limbic and non-limbic components

Gert Holstege*

Department of Anatomy, University of California, San Francisco and NASA/Ames Research Center, Moffett Field, CA 94035 U.S.A.

Introduction

For a thorough understanding of the descending pathways of the motor system originating in the forebrain, knowledge about the anatomy and function of the structures in the more caudally located parts of the central nervous system is indispensable. In this paper an overview will be presented of these caudal structures in brainstem and spinal cord as far as they concern the motor system. After that the descending pathways belonging to the so-called somatic motor system are reviewed. Finally, a summary of the many newly discovered pathways related to the limbic system will be given. In the Conclusions section a concept will be presented, which subdivides the multitude of motor pathways into three motor systems. In this concept the motoneurons will be considered to belong to the peripheral motor system, (motor unit, which is the motoneuronal cell body-motor axon-muscle). The first motor system consists of the interneurons involved in motor reflex pathways. The second motor system contains the pathways of the so-called somatic motor system, while the third motor system comprises the motor pathways related to the limbic system. The second and third motor systems act upon the neurons of the first motor system and to a limited extent directly on motoneurons, but not on each other. The importance and strength of the third motor system, which, until recently, was virtually unknown, will be emphasized.

Somatic and autonomic motoneurons in spinal cord and brainstem

Somatic motoneurons in the spinal cord

The somatic motoneurons innervate striated muscles of body and limbs. They are located in the ventral part of the ventral horn of the spinal cord, called lamina IX by Rexed (1952; 1954). The motoneurons innervating one particular muscle form a group, occupying a circumscribed portion of lamina IX. Rostrocaudally such a cell group can extend from one segment, (for example the medial gastrocnemius and soleus motor nuclei in the cat, which are located within the confines of the L7 spinal segment (Burke et al., 1977), up to 19 segments (the longissimus dorsi muscle motoneuronal cell group, which, according to Holstege et al., (1987), extends from C8 to L5). The motoneuronal cell groups can be subdivided into a medial and a lateral motor column. The medial motor column is present throughout the length of the spinal cord and its motoneurons innervate the axial muscles, which include the neck muscles. In the cat the lateral motor column is only present at the levels C5 to the upper half of T1 (cervical enlargement) and from L4 to S1 (lumbosacral enlargement). Motoneurons in the cervical and

* *Present address:* Department of Anatomy and Embryology, Medical School, Rijksuniversiteit Groningen, Oostersingel 69, 9713 EZ, Groningen, The Netherlands.

lumbosacral lateral column innervate the muscles of the fore- and hind-limbs respectively.

The axial musculature, innervated by motoneurons in the medial motor column, consists of epaxial and hypaxial muscles. The epaxial muscles are innervated by branches of the dorsal rami of a spinal nerve and the hypaxial muscles by branches of the ventral rami. In the ventral horn, motoneurons innervating epaxial muscles are always located ventral to the motoneurons innervating hypaxial muscles (Sprague, 1948; Smith and Hollyday, 1983). The epaxial muscles function as extensors and lateral flexors of the head and vertebral column. They also fix the vertebral column and some of them (the rotators) rotate the vertebral column about its longitudinal axis.

Upper cervical cord. Motoneurons in the upper cervical cord innervate the neck muscles. Epaxial neck muscles are the biventer cervicis, complexus, the suboccipitally located rectus dorsalis capitis major, medius and minor, the obliquus capitis cranialis and caudalis, the splenius and longissimus capitis. They are mainly involved in extension or elevation of the head, although unilateral contraction of the biventer cervicis, complexus and splenius muscles draws the head dorsally and laterally. Examples of hypaxial neck muscles are the prevertebral muscles (longus capitis, rectus capitis ventralis and rectus capitis lateralis), the sterno- and cleidomastoid muscles and the trapezius. All hypaxial muscles are involved in ventral and lateral flexion of head and neck. The upper portion of the trapezius muscle, the clavotrapezius, overlies all dorsal neck muscles and acts as an extensor and rotator of the head. All three superficial muscles are innervated by the spinal accessory nerve. Several reports exist on the location of the neck muscle motoneuronal cell groups in the cat, which are summarized by Holstege and Cowie (1989). Figure 1 gives an overview of the location of these motoneurons in the upper cervical ventral horn, indicating that the epaxial muscle motor cell groups are situated ventral to the hypaxial muscle motoneurons. Holstege and Cowie (1989) have emphasized the fact that the action, structure and fiber composition of the clavotrapezius, splenius and cleidomastoid muscles (Richmond and Abrahams, 1975) appear best suited to produce rapid or phasic torsional movements of the head such as might occur during orienting movements (Callister et al., 1987). On the other hand, the biventer cervicis, occipitoscapularis, semispinalis cervicis and rectus capitis dorsalis and probably

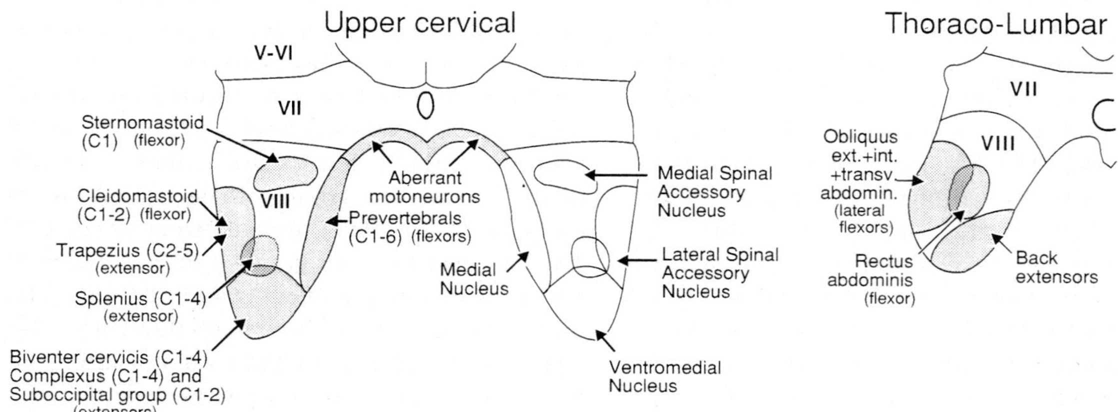

Fig. 1. Schematic representation of the combined C1 – 4 and T10 – L2 spinal segments. The motoneuronal cell groups innervating specific neck and axial muscles are shown. The general action of these muscles and the precise cervical cord location of the neck muscle motoneurons are also indicated. It must be emphasized that the cell groups not only contain motoneurons but also interneurons, (from Holstege and Cowie, 1989).

capitis dorsalis and probably also the prevertebral muscles, are all involved in more tonic aspects of head position (Richmond and Abrahams, 1975; Richmond et al., 1985; Roucoux et al., 1985). Note that the subdivision of the neck muscles into muscles involved in phasic (orienting) and tonic (head position) function does not follow the subdivision into epaxial and hypaxial muscles, but motoneurons innervating phasic muscles are always located lateral to the motoneurons innervating tonic muscles (Fig. 1). Such a functional subdivision is important, because the descending pathways project differently to the upper cervical ventral horn (see later).

Phrenic nucleus. The phrenic nucleus occupies a special position among the somatic motoneuronal cell groups, because its motoneurons innervate the diaphragm. Although the diaphragm is an axial muscle, it plays an essential role in respiration, which function is virtually independent of that of the other axial muscles. In the cat the phrenic nucleus is located in the ventromedial part of the ventral horn at the level of the most caudal portion of C4 and throughout the rostro-caudal extent of C5 and C6 (Duron et al., 1979). Phrenic motoneurons at the C5 level preferentially innervate the costal region of the diaphragm, while those in the C6 portion of the nucleus innervate the crural region (Duron et al., 1979). There are almost no muscle spindles in the diaphragm (Duron et al., 1978) or γ-motoneurons in the phrenic nucleus. Propriospinal projections to the phrenic nucleus have not convincingly been demonstrated anatomically (see p. 000), but the nucleus receives a great number of afferent fibers from specific brainstem areas (see p. 000). Sterling and Kuypers (1967) found a remarkably high number of rostro-caudally oriented dendrites within the phrenic nucleus, and the cell somata were elongated in a rostro-caudal direction (Cameron et al., 1983). On the other hand, Cameron et al. (1983), using intracellular HRP staining techniques, confirmed that the majority of the dendrites extended rostro-caudally within the phrenic motor column, and showed some dendrites of phrenic motoneurons extending in dorsolateral and dorsomedial directions. Many of the dorsomedial dendrites cross the midline in the anterior commissure or through the central gray. The dorsolaterally directed dendrites form bundles upon entering the lateral funiculus with the dendrites from other phrenic motoneurons (Cameron et al., 1983).

Cervical enlargement. At the level of the C5 to T1 spinal segments in the cat the medial motor column is located in the ventral portion of the ventral horn. Only very few retrograde tracing studies exist about the exact location of the medial column motoneurons at this level. The epaxial muscle motoneurons, for example those innervating the longissimus dorsi, are located in the medial part of this area, while hypaxial muscle motoneurons such as those innervating the most rostral rectus abdominis, are located just lateral to the longissimus neurons (Holstege et al., 1987). Muscles with their origin at the vertebral column (latissimus dorsi) or chest (pectoralis and deltoid muscles), but with insertion on the humerus, produce forelimb movements (Crouch, 1969). Therefore they are not considered axial, but limb muscles. Sterling and Kuypers (1967) call them girdle muscles. Their motoneurons take part in the lateral motor column and are located in the ventral part of the ventral horn, lateral to the axial muscle motoneurons, and ventral to the intrinsic limb muscle motoneurons (Sterling and Kuypers, 1967; Holstege et al., 1987) (Fig. 2). A very special place is occupied by a cell group in the most ventrolateral part of the ventral horn, named nucleus X by Giovanelli Barilari and Kuypers (1969) or ventral motor nucleus by Matsushita and Ueyama (1973). Only recently (Baulac and Meininger, 1981; Haase and Hrycyshyn, 1985 and Theriault and Diamond, 1988b in the rat; Krogh and Towns, 1984 in the dog; Holstege et al., 1987 in the cat) this cell group has been demonstrated to contain motoneurons innervating the cutaneous trunci or cutaneus maximus muscle, which extends over the thoracic and abdominal

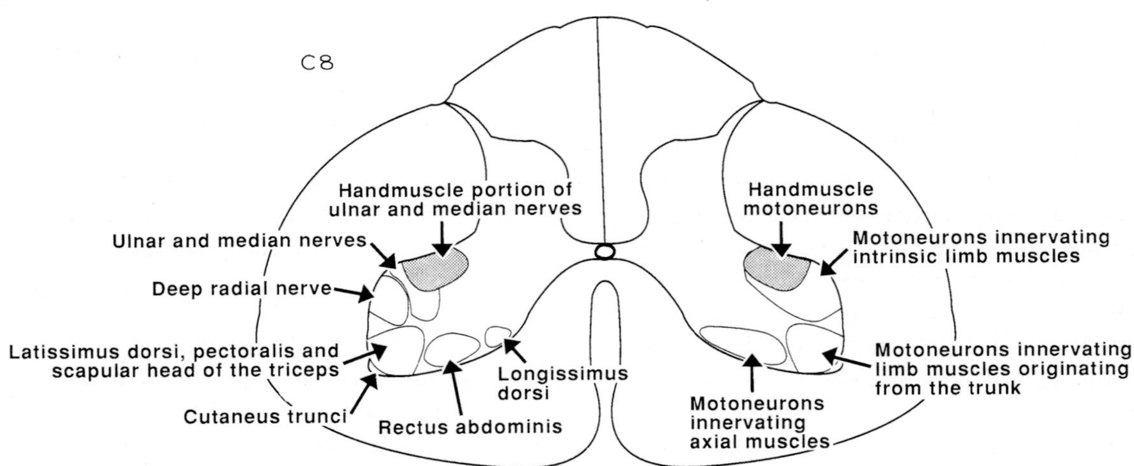

Fig. 2. Schematic overview of the location of the motorneuronal cell groups at the C8 level in the cat. The left side of the scheme shows the cell groups, the location of which has been studied using retrograde degeneration or tracing techniques (Sterling and Kuypers, 1967; Fritz et al., 1986a,b; Holstege et al., 1987 and Mc Curdy et al., 1988). On the right side of the scheme a more general subdivision into four motoneuronal cell groups has been made.

regions of the body, covering the underlying muscles like a veil (see Fig. 14). Motoneurons innervating muscles intrinsic to the forelimb are located more dorsally in the ventral horn, and the motoneurons innervating the most distal (hand-) muscles are located most dorsally (Fritz et al., 1986a,b; McCurdy et al., 1988) (Fig. 2). The difference in location between proximal and distal muscle motoneurons is nicely shown by Sterling and Kuypers (1967), who noted that the motoneurons of the scapular head of the triceps muscle were located more ventral in the ventral horn than those innervating the medial and lateral heads of this muscle, which are intrinsic to the forelimb.

Thoracic and upper lumbar spinal cord. At thoracic and upper lumbar levels, in rat and cat all the motoneurons belong to the medial motor column. Many of them innervate the epaxial extensor muscles of the trunk, and are located in greatly overlapping cell columns in the ventromedial portion of the ventral horn, largely segregated from the overlapping cell groups of the motoneurons innervating the hypaxial muscles which lie dorsolateral in the ventral horn (Brink et al., 1979; Smith and Hollyday, 1983; Miller, 1987; Holstege et al., 1987; Fetcho, 1987; Lipski and Martin-Body, 1987; Fig. 1). The hypaxial muscles include the abdominal (external and internal abdominal oblique, the transversus abdominis and the rectus abdominis) and the internal and external intercostal muscles. The abdominal muscles are involved in postural functions such as flexion and bending of the trunk, but they also play an important role in increasing the intra-abdominal pressure during defecation, vomiting and forced expiration (see Holstege et al., 1987 for review). Except for those innervating the rectus abdominis muscle, abdominal muscle motoneurons are scarce at upper thoracic levels, but are very numerous at low thoracic and upper lumbar segments (Holstege et al., 1987; Miller, 1987; Fig. 3). In the cat, at low thoracic and upper lumbar levels, the motoneuronal cell group innervating the rectus abdominis muscle (a medial hypaxial flexor) is located medial to the cell column of motoneurons innervating the other abdominal muscles, but dorsal to the epaxial muscle motoneurons (Miller, 1987; Holstege et al., 1987; Fig. 3). The intercostal muscles (internal and external) are inserted between adjacent ribs and their contraction decreases the distance between these ribs. The intercostal muscles are important for posture control, but they play a role in respiration also. Until recently it was generally been held that the external intercostal muscles are inspiratory in nature, while the internal intercostal muscles are expiratory. A recent study of Lipski and Martin-Body (1987) confirmed that all external intercostal motoneurons were inspiratory, but they also found that at upper thoracic levels three times as many internal intercostal motoneurons were inspiratory than expiratory. Apparently at upper thoracic levels expiratory motoneurons are scarce, since only a limited number of abdominal muscle motoneurons, which are all expiratory, was present at these levels (Holstege et al., 1987; Fig. 3). Conversely, at low thoracic levels all internal intercostal motoneurons were expiratory (47% of the total intercostal motoneuronal population). At these levels only very few external intercostal motoneurons were inspiratory (5% of the total intercostal motoneuronal population), while 48% of the intercostal motoneurons were non-respiratory (Lipski and Martin-Body, 1987). Furthermore the location of the expiratory intercostal motoneurons at low thoracic levels overlaps greatly with the location of the expiratory abdominal muscle motoneurons, which are quite numerous at these levels (Lipski and Martin-Body, 1987; Holstege et al., 1987; Miller, 1987). In conclusion, inspiratory motoneurons are mainly located at upper thoracic levels, and expiratory motoneurons at low thoracic and upper lumbar levels.

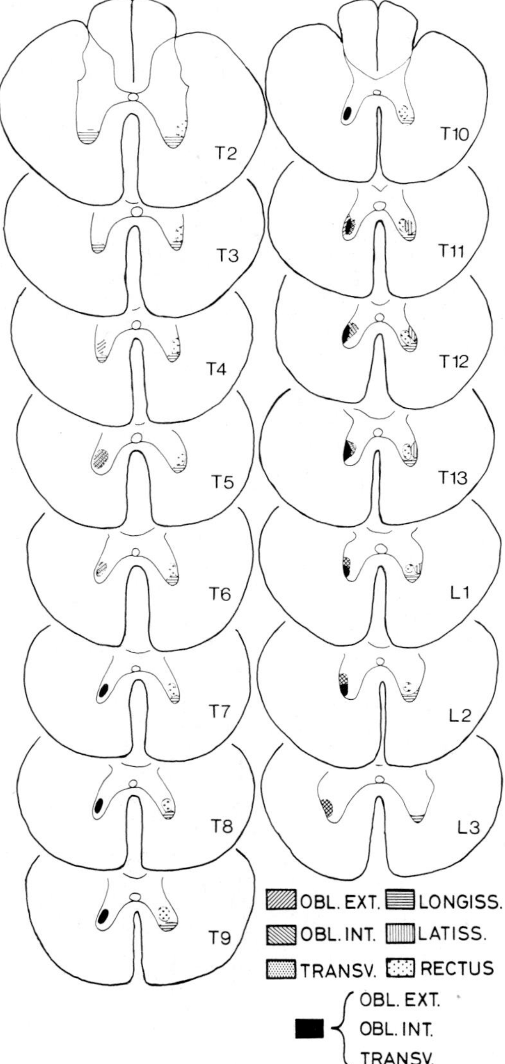

Fig. 3. Location of the motoneuronal cell groups innervating the hypaxial abdominal and latissimus dorsi muscles and the expaxial longissimus dorsi muscle (from Holstege et al., 1987).

Lumbosacral enlargement. The location of the motoneuronal cell groups at the lumbosacral enlargement (L4 to S1 in the cat) is very similar to the one of the cervical enlargement. The study of Romanes (1951) is still the most extensive on this subject, although there exist more recent retrograde HRP tracing studies of Burke et al. (1977) on the location of the medial gastrocnemius and soleus motor nuclei and Horcholle-Bossavit (1988) on the location of the peroneal motoneuronal cell groups. The position of the motoneuronal cell groups in the lumbosacral enlargement is very similar to that of the motoneurons in the cervical enlargement. For example, in both enlargements the motoneurons innervating the distal muscles of the limbs are located in the dorsal portions of the ventral horn, while those innervating proximal limb muscles occupy a more ventral position. Furthermore, the motoneurons of the most distal muscles are always located in the caudal part of the enlargement, for example at the level C8 – T1 for the small hand-muscle motoneuronal cell groups and at the level L7 – S1 for the small foot-muscle motoneurons. Trunk muscle motoneurons are always located within the medial column (Brink et al., 1979).

Nucleus of Onuf. Onufrowicz (1899), who called himself Onuf, described a group X in the ventral horn of the human sacral spinal cord, extending from the caudal S1 to the rostral S3 segments. According to Onuf, motoneurons in his nucleus X would be involved in erection and ejaculation, but they would also innervate the striated muscles of the urethral and anal sphincters. Romanes (1951) in the cat described a homologous cell group in the caudal half of the first and the rostral half of the second sacral segment and called it group Y. The cell group is now known as nucleus of Onuf (Fig. 4). Later retrograde HRP tracing studies in the cat (Sato et al., 1978; Mackel, 1979; Kuzuhara et al., 1980; Ueyama et al., 1984; Holstege and Tan,

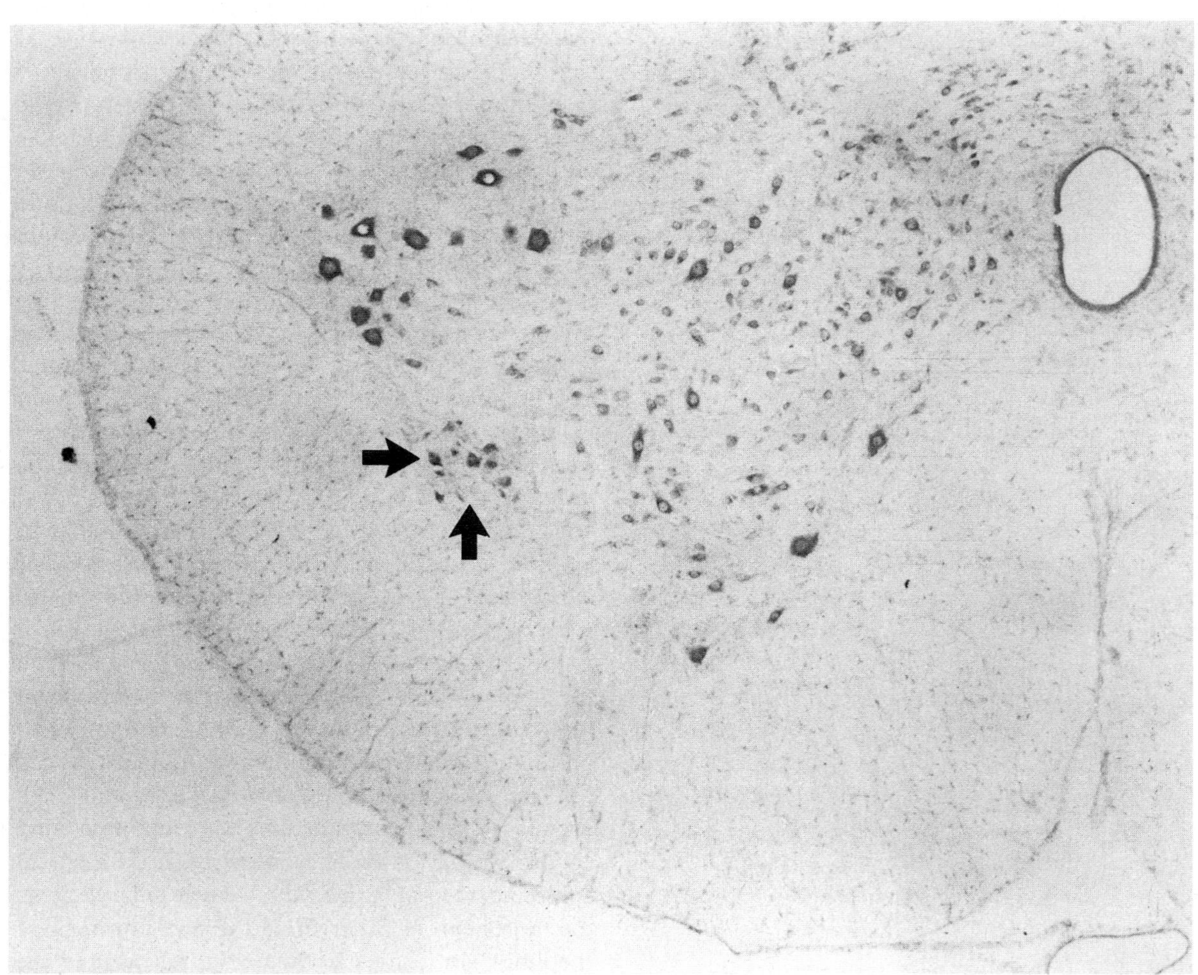

Fig. 4. Brightfield photomicrograph of the ventral horn of a section through the left ventral horn of the S1 spinal segment in the cat. The arrows indicate the nucleus of Onuf, (from Holstege and Tan, 1987).

1987) demonstrated that Onuf motoneurons, via the pudendal nerve, innervate the striated muscles of the pelvic floor, including the urethral and anal sphincters. Within Onuf's nucleus the dorsomedial motoneurons innervate the anal sphincter, while the ventrolateral motor cells innervate the urethral sphincter (Sato et al., 1978; Kuzuhara et al., 1980; Holstege and Tan, 1987; Pullen, 1988). The motoneurons in the nucleus of Onuf are characterized by their dense packing, their relatively small size (however, see Pullen, 1988), and their numerous longitudinal dendrites (Dekker et al., 1973). Although in cat (Sato et al., 1978; Mackel, 1979; Kuzuhara et al., 1980; Ueyama et al., 1984; Holstege and Tan, 1987), monkey (Roppolo et al., 1985) and man (Schrøder, 1981) Onuf's nucleus consists of a single motoneuronal pool, in rat it consists of two spatially separate motoneuronal groups, with those innervating the anal sphincter being located at the medial gray border just ventral to lamina X (Schrøder, 1980; McKenna and Nadelhaft, 1986).

There is evidence that Onuf motoneurons belong to a separate class of motoneurons. On the one hand they are somatic motoneurons, because they innervate striated muscles and are under voluntary control, but on the other hand they are autonomic motoneurons because; 1: cytoarchitectonically they resemble autonomic motoneurons (Rexed, 1954; Fig. 4); 2: they have an intimate relationship with sacral parasympathetic motoneurons (Holstege and Tan, 1987; Nadelhaft et al., 1980; Rexed, 1954); 3: they receive direct hypothalamic afferents (Holstege, 1987; Holstege and Tan, 1987) and 4: unlike the somatic motoneurons, but similar to the autonomic motoneurons, they are well preserved in the spinal cords of patients who have died from amyotrophic lateral sclerosis (ALS), (Mannen et al., 1977). Because the sacral autonomic (parasympathetic) motoneurons innervating the bladder are also spared in ALS patients, bladder and sphincter functions remain intact until the latest stages of the disease.

Autonomic motoneurons in the spinal cord

Sympathetic preganglionic motoneurons. The sympathetic motoneurons project to the chromaffin cells of the adrenal gland, and to the postganglionic neurons in the sympathetic trunk, the sympathetic chain of ganglion cells, in which the peripheral sympathetic system originates. In the rat the superior, middle and inferior (stellate) cervical ganglia receive their input from preganglionic motoneurons in the T1 – T5 spinal segments, with a minor contribution of C8 and T6 – T7 segments (Strack et al., 1988). The adrenal gland receives its sympathetic input from preganglionic cells in the T5 to T11 segments, with the emphasis on T8. The celiac, aortico-renal and superior mesenteric ganglia receive their main input from the T8 to T12 segments and the inferior mesenteric ganglion from the T13 – L2 segments (Strack et al., 1988). About 25% of the preganglionic cells in the T1 – T5 segments projecting to the cervical ganglia are located in the lateral funiculus, around 70% in the intermediolateral cell column (IML) and a total of 5% in the central autonomic cell group (CA) around the central canal (Rexed's (1954) lamina X) and in the area in between the IML and CA, called the intercalate nucleus (Strack et al., 1988; Fig. 5). The number of preganglionic motoneurons in the lateral funiculus, projecting to the other ganglia is much less numerous (≈ 5%), while, with the exception of the inferior mesenteric ganglion,

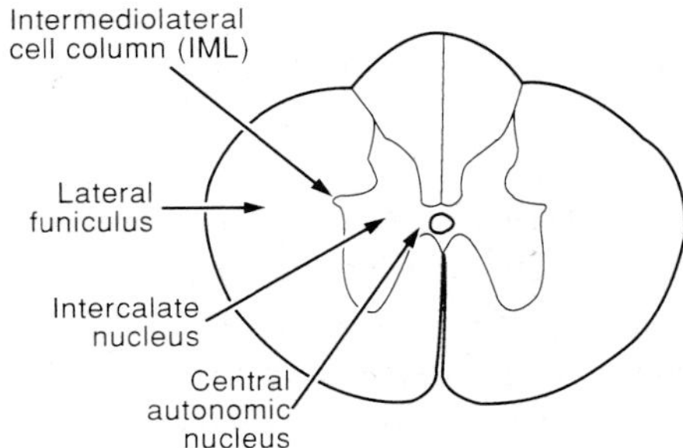

Fig. 5. Schematic drawing of a transverse section of the third thoracic segment of the spinal cord of the cat. The 4 different locations of sympathetic motoneurons are indicated.

≈ 90% of the preganglionic motoneurons are located in the IML. Around 70% of the preganglionic motoneurons projecting to the inferior mesenteric ganglion are located in the central autonomic nucleus and ≈ 25% in the IML. In the cat it is known that the sympathetic preganglionic motoneurons are segmentally organized (Rubin and Purves, 1980; Kuo et al., 1980). In the caudal C8 and rostral T1 segments of the cat preganglionic motoneurons are exclusively located in the dorsolateral funiculus (Henry and Calaresu, 1972; Chung et al., 1979). The highest concentration of neurons in the IML is at the T1 – T2 and at the L3 – L4 levels (Henry and Calaresu, 1972). In the lumbar cord the IML continues until the L4 level (Henry and Calaresu, 1972), but sympathetic motoneurons may also be present in the lateral part of the L5 intermediate zone (Jänig and McLachlan, 1986; Morgan et al., 1986), although not all cats have sympathetic motoneurons as caudal as L5 (Morgan et al., 1986). Many of them traverse the inferior mesenteric ganglia to make synaptic connections with terminal ganglia in the pelvic plexus as well as in the walls of their targets (bladder and genital organs). They run via the pelvic and hypogastric nerves, and innervate the bladder and genitals directly or indirectly via connections with the paravesical ganglia of the parasympathetic system (Hamburger and Norberg, 1965; Elbadawi, 1982). Sympathetic fibers have inhibitory effects on the detrusor muscle of the bladder and excitatory effects on the smooth musculature of the urethra and base of the bladder.

Parasympathetic preganglionic motoneurons. The parasympathetic preganglionic motoneurons in the sacral cord of the cat (S2 and S3 segments) innervate the detrusor muscle of the bladder and the colon. The motoneurons are organized into two groups, a lateral band of neurons, dorsoventrally oriented in the lateral part of lamina VII and a more medial group of neurons, the dorsal band, mediolaterally oriented in the lateral part of lamina V (Nadelhaft et al., 1980). The urinary bladder is innervated mainly by the lateral band of cells and the colon mainly by the dorsal band cells (Morgan et al., 1979; Holstege and Tan, 1987).

Somatic motoneurons in the brainstem

The motoneurons innervating the muscles of the head, such as the facial, chewing, tongue, pharynx and extra-ocular muscles are all located in the brainstem. They do not form a continuous rostrocaudal band of motoneurons such as in the spinal cord, but are subdivided into several distinct motoneuronal cell groups.

Extra-ocular muscle and retractor bulbi motoneuronal cell groups. The extra-ocular muscles are innervated by motoneurons in the oculomotor, trochlear and abducens nuclei, all of which are located dorsomedially in the tegmentum. The oculomotor nucleus is located in the rostral mesencephalon, the trochlear nucleus in the caudal mesencephalon and the abducens nucleus in the ponto-medullary transition zone. The oculomotor nucleus contains motoneurons innervating the ipsilateral medial rectus, inferior rectus and inferior oblique muscles and the contralateral superior rectus and levator palpebrae. Trochlear motoneurons innervate the contralateral superior oblique, and abducens motoneurons innervate the ipsilateral lateral rectus muscle (see Evinger, 1988 for review).

The accessory abducens or retractor bulbi nucleus in the cat is a loosely arranged motoneuronal cell group, just dorsal to the superior olivary complex (Fig. 6). The nucleus contains a total of about 100 (Grant et al., 1979; Spencer et al., 1980) motoneurons. They innervate the retractor bulbi muscle, an extraocular muscle divided into four slips, which attach themselves on the eyeball behind and beside the inferior and superior recti muscles. The four slips are thinner and shorter than the other extra-ocular muscles. Retractor bulbi muscles are present in most vertebrates, but not in apes and humans (Bolk et al., 1938). The functional role of the retractor

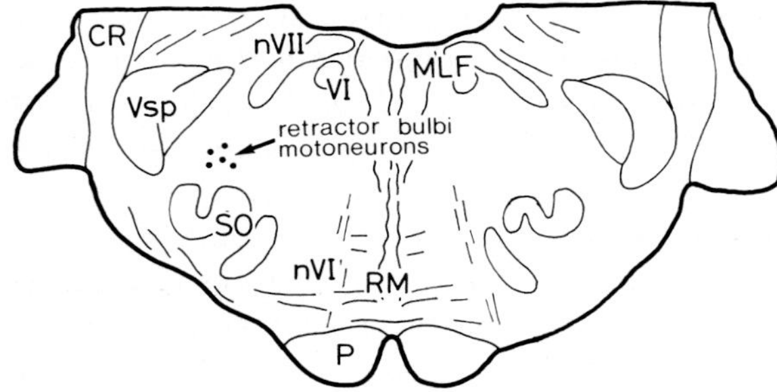

Fig. 6. Schematic drawing of a transverse section through the caudal brainstem at the level of the abducens (VI) and superior olivary nucleus (SO). The black dots indicate the position of the small accessory abducens or retractor bulbi nucleus, which consists of ≈ 100 motoneurons, (from Holstege et al., 1986).

bulbi muscles is purely eye-protection: it retracts the eyeball, forcing the intraorbital fat against the base of the nictitating membrane and causing the latter to sweep across the eyeball (Bach-y-Rita, 1971). This event is also called the nictitating membrane response. The retractor bulbi muscles do not contract independently of the orbicularis oculi (McCormick et al., 1982).

Jaw-closing and opening muscle motoneurons. In the cat the jaw-closing muscles masseter, temporalis and medial pterygoid muscles as well as the lateral pterygoid muscle, which is not a jaw closing muscle, are innervated by motoneurons in the dorsolateral two thirds of the motor trigeminal nucleus. The jaw-opening muscle motoneurons (anterior digastric and mylohyoid) are located in the ventromedial one third of this nucleus (Mizuno, et al., 1975; Batini et al., 1976). This region also contains the motoneurons innervating the tensor veli palatini (Keller et al., 1983). In the cat the posterior digastric muscle motoneurons, which send their axons via the facial nerve, are located in two separate small cell groups, one dorsal to the superior olivary complex and just medial to the VII nerve and one dorsal to the facial nucleus (Grant et al., 1981). The latter region also contains stylohyoid muscle motoneurons (Shohara and Sakai, 1983).

Facial muscle motoneurons. Motoneurons in the facial nucleus innervate the various facial muscles. In the cat the lateral and ventrolateral facial subnuclei contain the motoneurons innervating the muscles of the upper and lower mouth respectively. Motoneurons in the dorsomedial facial subnucleus innervate the ear or pinna muscles, and the dorsal portion of the facial nucleus (intermediate facial subnucleus) contains motoneurons innervating the muscles around the eye (Papez, 1927; Courville, 1966; Kume et al., 1978; Fig. 7). In other mammals slight variations in this subdivision are present (Komiyama et al., 1984 in the mouse; Hinrichsen and Watson, 1984; Klein and Rhoades, 1985 and Friauf and Herbert, 1985 in the rat; Dom et al., 1973 in the opossum; Provis, 1977 in the brush-tailed possum; Holstege and Collewijn, 1982 in the rabbit; Satoda et al., 1987 in the Japanese monkey). The facial nucleus contains mainly motoneurons, only a few non-motoneuronal cells have been detected. They project to the cerebellar flocculus (Røste, 1989).

Middle ear muscle motoneurons. In the cat, motoneurons innervating the tensor tympani, which send their axons via the motor trigeminal nerve, are located just ventral to the motor

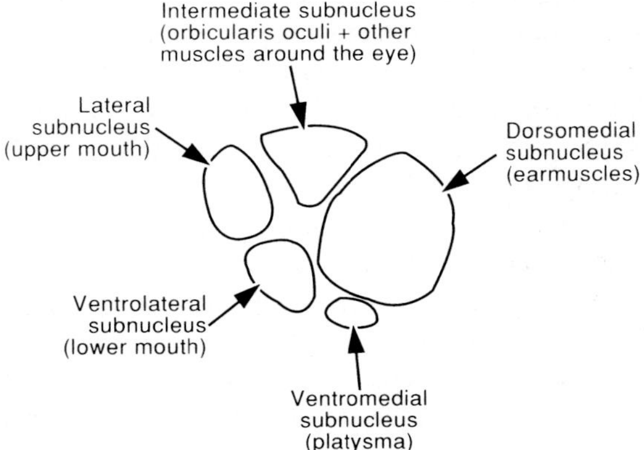

Fig. 7. Schematic drawing of a transverse section through the left facial nucleus. The different facial subnuclei and the muscles innervated by the motoneurons in these subnuclei are indicated.

trigeminal nucleus (Lyon, 1975; Mizuno et al., 1982; Keller et al., 1983; Friauf and Baker, 1985). Stapedius motoneurons, which send their axons via the facial nerve, are located in cell clusters around the traditional borders of the facial nucleus as well as dorsal to the lateral superior olivary nucleus (Lyon, 1978; Shaw and Baker, 1983; Joseph et al., 1985). In the squirrel monkey stapedius motoneurons are located ventromedial to the facial nucleus (Thompson et al., 1985). Recently it has been shown (McCue and Guinan, 1988; Guinan et al., 1989) in the cat that there is a spatial segregation of function within the stapedius motoneurons.

Somatic motoneurons belonging to the nucleus ambiguus. In the cat the somatic motoneurons in the nucleus ambiguus innervate the laryngeal, pharyngeal and soft palate muscles. The nucleus extends for a distance of 5 to 6 mm caudally from the facial nucleus. Laryngeal motoneurons are located in the caudal two thirds of the nucleus and lie dispersed in the ventrolateral part of the reticular formation. Motoneurons innervating pharynx and soft palate form a compact cell group, the dorsal group of the nucleus ambiguus. It is located 1.5 to 2.5 mm caudal to the facial nucleus. Pharyngeal motoneurons are also located in the more loosely arranged retrofacial part of the nucleus, situated just caudal to the facial nucleus. Furthermore, the retrofacial part of the nucleus ambiguus contains motoneurons innervating the cricothyroid muscles and the upper portion of the oesophagus (Lawn, 1966; Yoshida et al., 1981; Holstege et al., 1983; Davis and Nail, 1984). In the rat the oesophagus motoneurons are located in a compact cell group (Bieger and Hopkins, 1987), but in this animal certain palatal and upper pharyngeal muscles are absent (Cleaton-Jones, 1972; Bieger and Hopkins, 1987), which might simplify the motoneuronal arrangement in this species.

Tongue muscle motoneurons. Motoneurons innervating the intrinsic and extrinsic tongue muscles are located in the hypoglossal nucleus, which also contains motoneurons innervating the geniohyoid muscles (Uemura, 1979; Miyazaki et al., 1981). In the cat the geniohyoid muscle motoneurons are located in the most ventral portion of the rostral two thirds of the hypoglossal nucleus. The other extrinsic tongue muscle motoneurons (genioglossus, hyoglossus, and styloglossus) are located laterally in the hypoglossal nucleus. The intrinsic muscle motoneurons, which send their axons via the medial branch of the hypoglossal nerve, are located medially and ventrally in the nucleus, while the intrinsic muscle motoneurons, which send their axons via the lateral branch, are located in the dorsal portions of the nucleus (Uemura et al., 1979). This relatively complicated subdivision of the hypoglossal nucleus makes it impossible to subdivide the hypoglossal nucleus into tongue protrusion and a tongue retraction regions and further anatomic and physiological study is necessary to unravel a more precise subdivision within this motoneuronal pool.

Autonomic (parasympathetic) preganglionic motoneurons in the brainstem

Preganglionic motoneurons innervating iris and lens via the ciliary ganglion. Parasympathetic preganglionic motoneurons in the vicinity of the oculomotor nucleus innervate the ipsilateral ciliary ganglion, whose neurons control the iris and lens (ciliary body). Some may bypass the ciliary ganglion to innervate the iris or ciliary body directly (see Evinger, 1988 for review). All these preganglionic motoneurons are involved in the pupillary light reflex. In the cat the preganglionic motoneurons lie in the ipsilateral central gray dorsal to the oculomotor nucleus and in the tegmental area ventral to the oculomotor nucleus (Loewy et al., 1978; Toyoshima et al., 1980; Strassman et al., 1987). In the monkey (Burde and Loewy, 1980) the preganglionic motoneurons are located in the Edinger-Westphal nucleus and in the nucleus of Perlia, located between the somatic motoneuronal oculomotor nuclei (Olszewski and Baxter, 1954).

Preganglionic motoneurons innervating salivatory and lacrimal glands. The parasympathetic motoneurons innervating the parotid gland, via the minor petrosal nerve and the otic ganglion, as well as those innervating the submandibular and sublingual salivatory glands, via the chorda tympani, are all intermingled in the lateral tegmental field dorsal to the facial nucleus (Contreras et al., 1980 in the rat; Nomura and Mizuno, 1981, 1982; Hosoya et al., 1983 and Tramonte and Bauer, 1986 in the cat). The motoneurons innervating the lacrimal gland, via the greater petrosal nerve, are located slightly more rostrally and ventrally in the lateral tegmentum (Contreras et al., 1980).

Preganglionic motoneurons innervating the visceral organs. The parasympathetic motoneurons innervating the visceral organs (lung, heart, stomach and intestine) via the vagus nerve are located mainly in the dorsal vagal nucleus and in the ventral part of the medullary lateral tegmental field, i.e. the area of the nucleus ambiguus and retroambiguus (Nosaka et al., 1979; Weaver, 1980; Kalia and Mesulam 1980a,b; Kalia, 1981; Hopkins and Armour, 1982). A few neurons are present in the lateral tegmentum between both cell groups and in the upper cervical ventral horn (Kalia and Mesulam, 1980a,b). There is extensive overlap between the location of the neurons innervating the different viscera, although Hopkins and Armour (1982) and Plecha et al. (1988) indicate that almost 90% of the preganglionic neurons innervating the heart are located in the area of the nucleus ambiguus. It has always been difficult to give a precise description of the nuclei ambiguus and retroambiguus, because both nuclei consist of many different populations of motor (autonomic and somatic) and premotor cells. In the cat the only portion of the nucleus ambiguus that can easily be recognized as such in non-experimental Nissl sec-

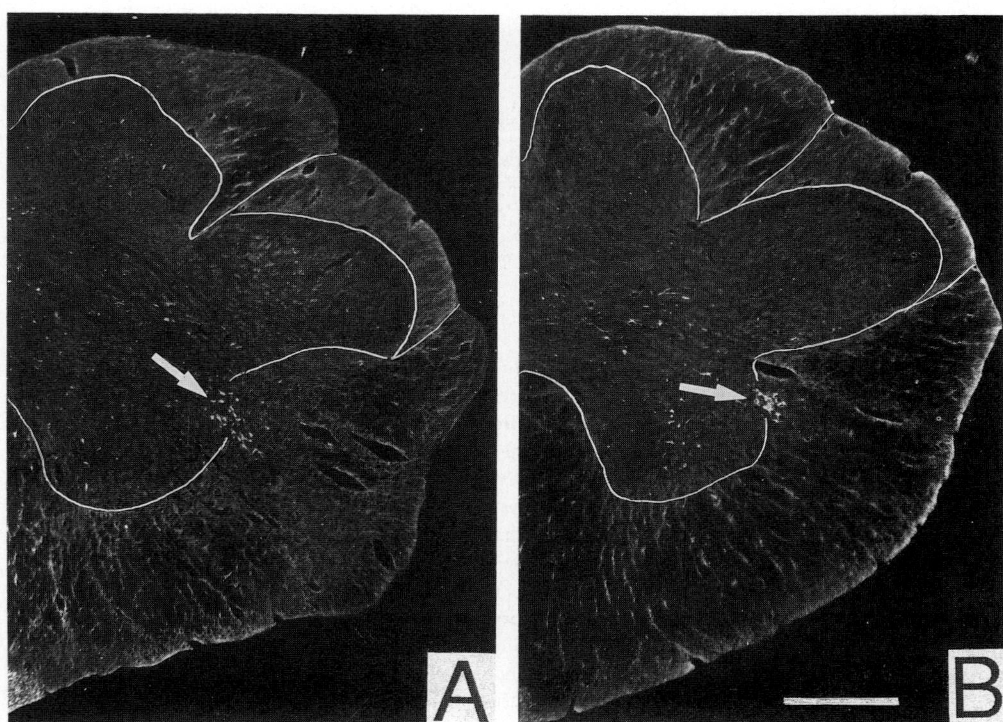

Fig. 8. Darkfield photomicrographs showing the HRP labeled neurons in the contralateral NRA (arrows) at the level of the caudal medulla (A) and medullospinal transition (B) after injection of HRP in the ipsilateral T1 spinal cord. Bar represents 1 mm.

tions is its dorsal group, containing motoneurons innervating pharynx and soft palate (Lawn, 1966; Yoshida et al., 1981; Holstege et al., 1983; Davis and Nail, 1984). Furthermore the caudal half of the nucleus retroambiguus (NRA), located at the border between gray and white matter at medullary levels caudal to the hypoglossal nucleus, forms a reasonably well circumscribed nucleus (Fig. 8). Kalia and Mesulam (1980a,b) reported that this nucleus contains vagal nerve parasympathetic preganglionic motoneurons. However, from their drawings the impression is gained that the parasympathetic neurons are not located within the confines of the nucleus retroambiguus, but just medial to it. The nucleus itself contains interneurons involved in expiration related systems (see Fig. 26). The fact that all other portions of the nuclei ambiguus and retroambiguus consist of neurons more or less scattered within the lateral tegmental field, makes a description of afferents to these nuclei practically useless without a precise identification of the motoneurons involved.

Local projections to motoneurons

Recurrent motoneuronal axon collateral projections to motoneurons

Recurrent collaterals of motoneurons innervating limb muscles terminate directly on local motoneurons innervating the same or synergistic muscles (Cullheim and Kellerth, 1978). Furthermore, motoneuronal axon collaterals project directly on local interneurons (Renshaw cells). Renshaw cells are located in the ventral horn medial to the motor nuclei (Jankowska and Lindström, 1971; Van Keulen, 1979; Fig. 9). They have an inhibitory effect on the same or synergistic α and γ motoneuronal cell groups from which they receive their afferents. This phenomenon is known as recurrent inhibition (see Baldissera et al., 1981 for review). Renshaw cells project via propriospinal pathways in the ventral funiculus (Fig. 9). Recurrent inhibition is especially strong in motoneuronal cell groups innervating proximal limb muscles, less strong in muscles of more distal parts of the limb (wrist or ankle) and absent in motoneuronal cell groups innervating the most distal limb musculature such as those innervating the phalanges of the forelimb (Hahne et al., 1988) or the small foot-muscles of the hindlimb (Cullheim and Kellerth, 1978). Apparently recurrent inhibition is primarily concerned with control of the

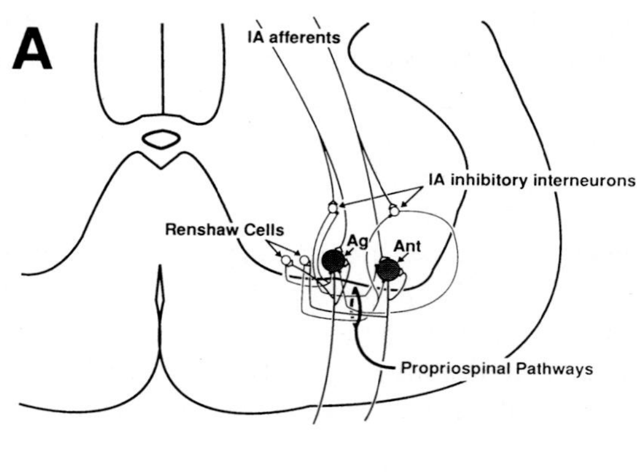

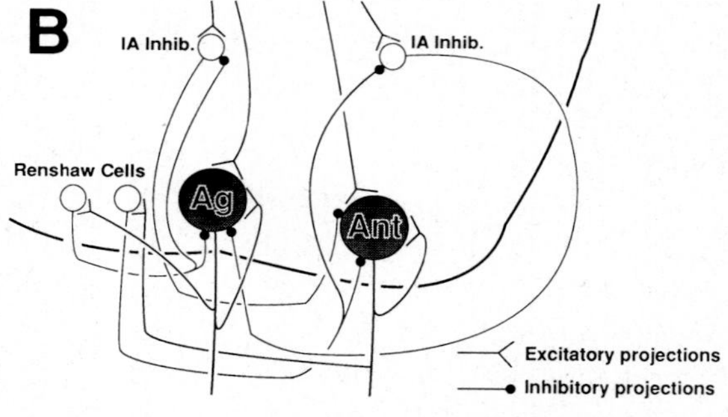

Fig. 9. In (A) a schematic drawing of the L7 ventral horn showing the recurrent axon collaterals, Renshaw cells, IA inhibitory interneurons and Ia afferent of two motoneurons innervating an agonist (Ag) and an antagonist (Ant) muscle respectively. Note that many of the neurons project via propriospinal pathways. In (B) a magnified view of the different projections is shown. Note that the motoneurons receive inhibitory input from their own axon collaterals and Renshaw cells as well as from the Ia inhibitory interneurons from the antagonist muscle. Excitatory input is derived from Ia afferents. It is known (Cullheim and Kellerth, 1978) that recurrent axon collaterals of a proximal muscle motoneuron project directly onto the somata or dendrites of other motoneurons innervating the same or synergistic muscles. Although indicated as such in the schematic drawing, it is not sure whether a motoneuron projects to its own dendrites or soma.

proximal muscles (limb position), rather than of the distal ones (movements of the digits).

Muscle spindle afferent projections to motoneurons

Muscle spindle afferent projections to motoneurons in the spinal cord. In the spinal cord group Ia muscle spindle afferents have an excitatory effect on motoneurons, innervating the same or synergistic muscle groups (Mendell and Henneman, 1971). Muscle spindles project directly (Brown and Fyffe, 1978; Ishizuka et al., 1979) or via interneurons (Jankowska et al., 1981) onto motoneurons. The Ia afferent projection system exists in proximal as well as in distal limb muscle control (Ishizuka et al., 1979; Fritz et al., 1978; 1984). Ia muscle spindle afferents not only have an excitatory effect on motoneurons, but also on the so-called Ia inhibitory interneurons which in turn have an inhibitory effect on motoneurons innervating muscles, antagonistic to the muscle from which the Ia muscle spindle afferents are derived. The Ia inhibitory interneurons are located in lamina VII of the spinal intermediate zone and project to the antagonist muscle motoneurons, mainly via propriospinal pathways (Jankowska and Lindström, 1972; Fig. 9). Thus, the IA afferents of a specific muscle excite the motoneurons of the same (homonymous) and synergistic muscles, and, via Ia inhibitory interneurons, inhibit the motoneurons of the antagonistic muscles (see Henneman and Mendell, 1981 and Baldissera et al., 1981 for reviews). Ia afferents also have an inhibitory influence on homonymous and synergistic muscle motoneurons (Fetz et al., 1979), but this inhibition is mediated by interneurons and not by direct projections to motoneurons.

Muscle spindle afferent projections to motoneurons in the brainstem. The neuronal cell bodies of the muscle spindle afferents are located in spinal ganglia outside the central nervous system. However, the ganglion cells of the muscle spindle afferents of the mouth closing muscles are located within the central nervous system. They are called mesencephalic trigeminal neurons and are mainly large-diameter globular cells with one process, although some of them are of smaller diameter. The mesencephalic trigeminal neurons, which combined form the mesencephalic trigeminal nucleus, are located at pontine and mesencephalic levels in the border area between periaqueductal gray (PAG) and the dorsally and laterally adjoining tegmentum. The peripheral processes of these cells first descend through the so-called mesencephalic trigeminal tract (Fig. 10A), and then via the motor root of the trigeminal nerve to the sensory receptors in the mouth closing muscles. The sensory signals are derived from the muscle spindles in the mouth closing muscles as well as from pressure receptors at the base of the teeth, the temporomandibular joint, gums and tongue. The muscle spindle afferents are located throughout the rostrocaudal extent of the mesencephalic trigeminal nucleus, while the pressure receptor ganglion cells are present in the caudal half of the nucleus. After a ^{3}H-leucine injection involving the rostral mesencephalic trigeminal nucleus, Holstege and Cowie (in preparation) found that the proximal processes pass caudally, first via the mesencephalic trigeminal tract (Fig. 10A), but at levels caudal to the motor trigeminal nucleus in the so-called Probst (1899) tract, which can be followed until the upper segments of the cervical cord (Figs. 10C – F). From this tract some fibers are distributed to the dorsolateral two thirds of the motor trigeminal nucleus (Fig. 10B), which contains mouth closing muscle motoneurons (See p. 315). Although the termination of muscle spindle afferents in the motor trigeminal nucleus was not very strong, it was more pronounced than the very weak projection reported by Luschei (1987). The detection of only a limited muscle spindle projection to the mouth closing motoneurons is in agreement with the finding of Appenteng et al. (1978), who triggered mouth closing muscle spindle afferents in the mesencephalic trigeminal nucleus. They found that the muscle spindles produced monosynaptic excitatory post synaptic potentials in only a small proportion of the mouth closing motoneurons. Much denser projections than to the motor trigeminal nucleus were found to the supratrigeminal and intertrigeminal regions (Fig. 10B), located just dorsal and lateral to the motor trigeminal nucleus (see also Luschei, 1987 and Shigenaga et al., 1988). Further caudally, Holstege and Cowie (in preparation) found that muscle spindle afferents in the Probst tract terminate only

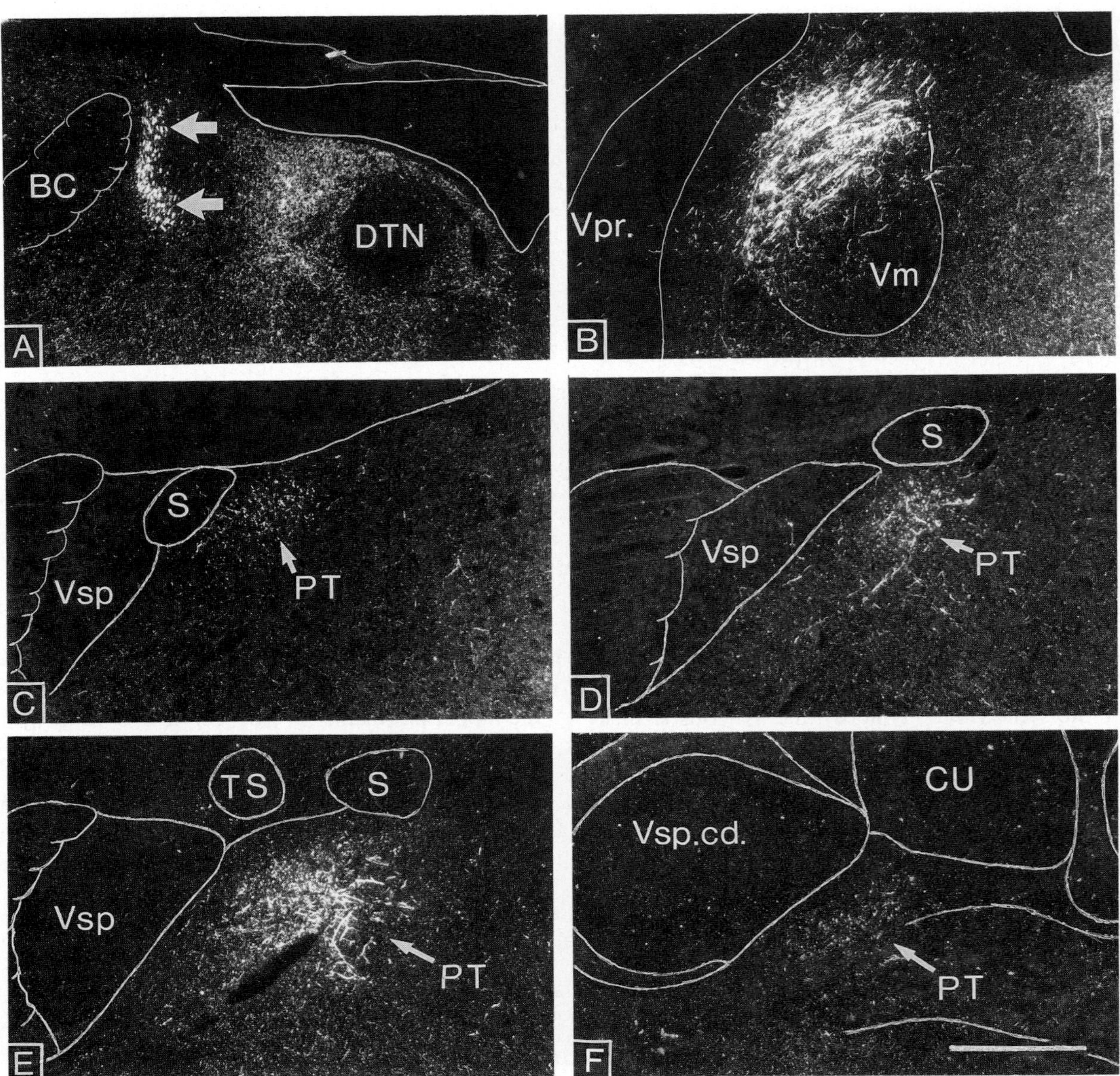

Fig. 10. Darkfield photomicrographs of the labeled fibers in the mesencephalic trigeminal tract (A) or Probst tract (Figs. C – F) after an injection of ^{3}H-leucine in the dorsolateral part of the pretentorial PAG and adjoining tegmentum, including the mes. V neurons at that level. Note the light projections to the dorsolateral two thirds of the motor trigeminal nucleus, the virtual absence of projections around the level of the facial nucleus, and the strong projections to the lateral tegmental field at the level of the hypoglossal nucleus (E).

to a very limited extent at levels around the facial nucleus (Fig. 10C), but strongly in the dorsal portion of the lateral tegmentum at the level of the hypoglossal nucleus (Fig. 10E). No labeled fibers were found in the trigeminal, solitary or hypoglossal nuclei. Projections to these nuclei may be derived from neurons in more caudal portions of the mesencephalic trigeminal nucleus receiving peri-oral pressure receptor afferents (Sirkin and Feng, 1987). Neurons in the dorsal portion of the lateral tegmentum at the level of the hypoglossal nucleus project to the hypoglossal nucleus and to the ventromedial one third of the motor trigeminal nucleus (Holstege and Kuypers, 1977; Holstege et al., 1977; Holstege and Blok, 1986), which area contains mouth opening muscle motoneurons (see p. 000, Fig. 11). Interneurons, which receive mouth closing muscle spindle afferents and project to mouth opening motoneurons, might serve as Ia inhibitory interneurons. However, after stimulating mouth closing muscle afferent fibers, Kidokoro et al. (1986) could not demonstrate such inhibitory effects in the antagonist digastric muscle motoneurons.

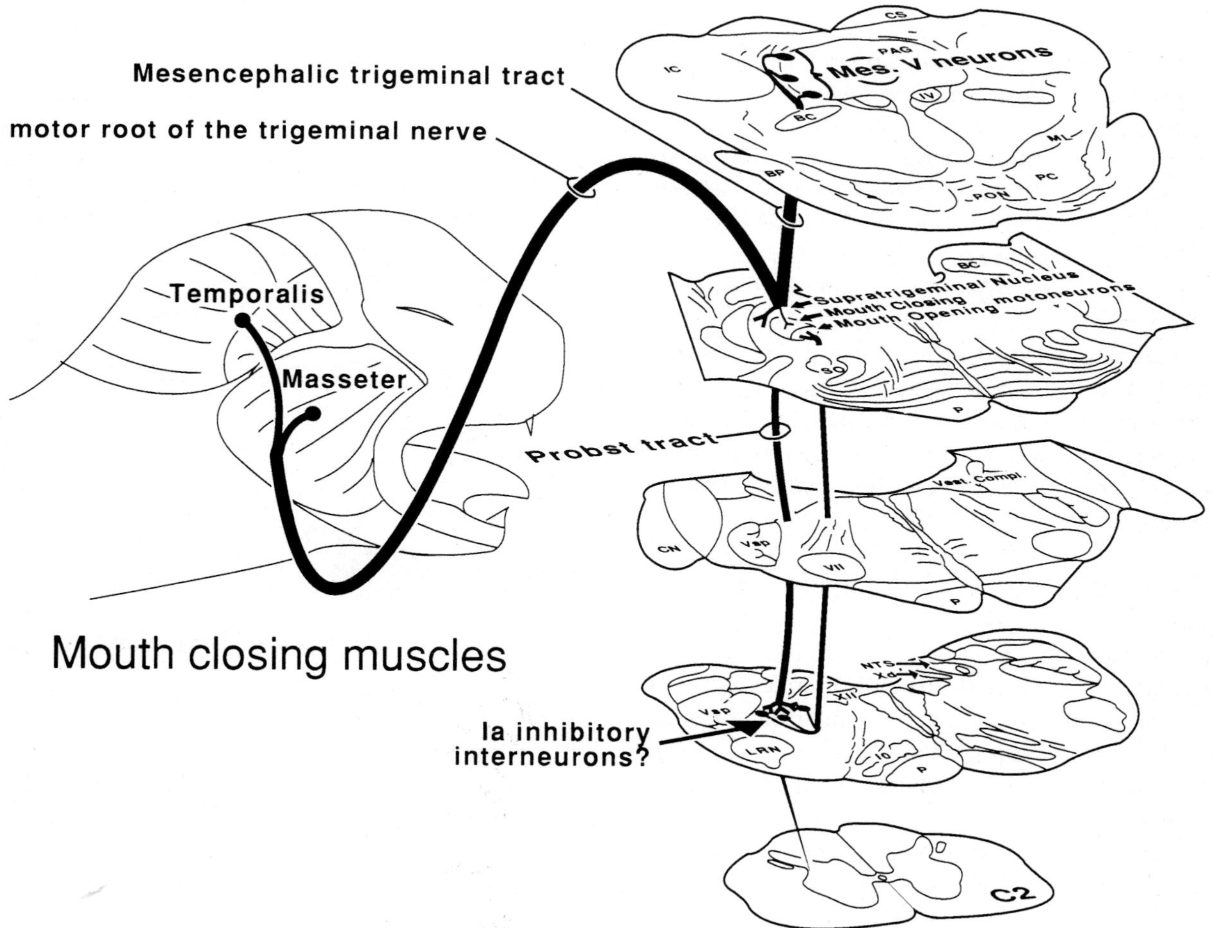

Fig. 11. Schematic drawing of the organization of the mesencephalic trigeminal nucleus and tract. The strongest projections from the Probst tract is at the level of the hypoglossal nucleus. Other tracing studies have indicated that neurons in this area project strongly to the mouth opening motoneurons in the motor trigeminal nucleus, but whether these neurons at the level of the hypoglossal nucleus play the role of Ia inhibitory neurons remains to be elucidated.

Propriospinal pathways

Projections from interneurons. With the exception of the Ia afferents, no direct primary afferent projections exist to the motoneurons. For example, stimulation of Ib tendon organ afferents of a specific muscle produces inhibition of the motoneurons of the same and synergistic muscles and excitation of motoneurons of antagonist muscles. These effects are mediated via excitation of interneurons in the intermediate zone, mainly laminae V and VI, which in turn project, via propriospinal pathways, to motoneurons (Czarkowska et al., 1976). Jankowska and McCrea (1983) demonstrated that both the excitatory and inhibitory interneuronal pathways to motoneurons are shared by Ia and Ib afferents.

Other primary afferents are derived from the skin and joints, and the group II and III muscle afferents. Their reflex pathways to motoneurons always include interneurons. In hindlimb segments of the cat the minimum linkage in reflex pathways from cutaneous afferents to motoneurons is trisynaptic (Lundberg, 1975), although in case of the forelimb disynaptic pathways seem to exist. The last order interneurons, projecting to the motoneurons, enter the funiculus at the same rostro-caudal level as their cell body is located. Within the funiculus they run rostrally and/or caudally to reenter the spinal gray at the level of their target motoneurons (Jankowska and Roberts, 1972). For such local pathways especially those parts of the dorsolateral, ventrolateral and ventral funiculi are involved, which border the gray matter. These parts are called fasciculi proprii or propriospinal pathways. Anatomic studies (Sterling and Kuypers, 1968; Rustioni et al., 1971; Molenaar et al., 1974; Molenaar, 1978) have indicated that the interneurons, located in different areas of the intermediate zone, project to different motoneuronal cell groups. Interneurons in the lateral part of laminae V and VI project via the dorsolateral funiculus to the dorsolateral motoneuronal cell group in the cervical or lumbosacral enlargement, which innervate distal limb muscles. Interneurons in the central part of the intermediate zone project via the ventrolateral funiculus to the ventrolateral motoneuronal cell group, innervating proximal limb muscles. Interneurons in the medial part of the intermediate zone, (lamina VIII and the medial part of lamina VII) project via the ventral funiculus, to the medial motoneuronal cell groups, innervating the axial and proximal muscles (Fig. 12). Within the cervical or lumbosacral enlargements such projections go from rostral to caudal and from caudal to rostral (Molenaar, 1978).

Projections from propriospinal neurons. According to Baldissera et al. (1981) there is a functional

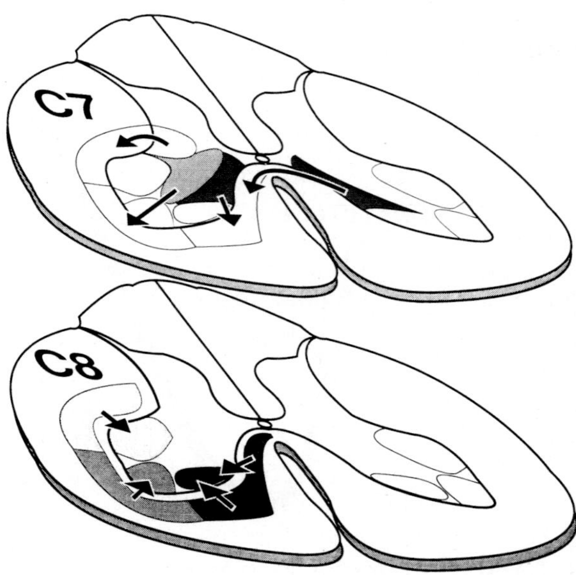

Fig. 12. Schematic illustration of the projections from interneurons in the C7 intermediate zone (laminae V-VII) via the propriospinal pathways to the motoneurons at the C8 level. Note that the neurons in the dorsolateral part of the intermediate zone project to the dorsolaterally located motoneuronal cell group innervating distal limb muscles. The interneurons in the central part of the intermediate zone project to motoneurons in the ventrolateral ventral horn, which innervate proximal limb muscles. Interneurons in the medial part of the intermediate zone on both sides of the spinal cord project to the motoneurons in the medial part of the ventral horn. These motoneurons innervate axial muscles. Note also that the C7 propriospinal fibers at the level of C8 shifted to a slightly more peripheral position in the funiculus.

difference between interneurons and propriospinal neurons. Interneurons are intercalated in reflex pathways of limb segments, while propriospinal neurons are located outside the limb segments, but project into them. The C3 – C4 neurons which relay supraspinal motor information to α-motoneurons in the C5 – T1 spinal cord (Illert et al., 1978) are examples of propriospinal neurons. Illert et al. (1978) demonstrated that, after a complete transection of the corticospinal tract at the level of C5, disynaptic excitatory postsynaptic potentials (EPSPs) in forelimb muscle motoneurons can still be evoked by stimulation of the contralateral pyramid or red nucleus, while they were abolished after a corticospinal tract transection at the level of C2. Alstermark et al. (1987), using intra-axonal injections of horseradish peroxidase, demonstrated C3 – C4 propriospinal projections to α-motoneurons and interneurons in the C6 – T1 spinal cord. Molenaar (1978) using the retrograde HRP technique found that only a limited number of labeled neurons in the C2 – C4 intermediate zone projected to α-motoneurons in the C5 – T1 spinal cord, but Holstege (1988b) and Holstege and Blok (1989), using the anterograde autoradiographic tracing technique, demonstrated that neurons in the intermediate zone of C2 project heavily to the C6 – T1 motoneuronal cell groups (Fig. 13), with the exception of the cutaneus trunci muscle motoneurons (see later). Thus, not only C3 – C4, but also C2 propriospinal neurons project to the C5 – T1 α-motoneurons. With regard to the functional importance of the upper cervical propriospinal projections to motoneurons, Alstermark et al. (1981; 1987) demonstrated that the propriospinal neurons, driven by cortico- and/or rubrospinal fibers, can produce target reaching movements in cats. During this movement the paw is brought in contact with the food. However, direct activation of the C5 – T1 inter- and motoneurons from the cortico- and/or rubrospinal tracts can also produce target reaching movements (Alstermark, 1987). Such direct activation is essential for food taking movements in cats, consisting of toe grasping and paw supination. Thus the upper cervical propriospinal neurons, when properly stimulated, can produce target reaching movements, but not the more precise food taking movements.

Propriospinal neurons as rhythm generators. During the scratch reflex (one limb) or locomotion (all four limbs) the limbs perform rhythmic movements, which are independent of the afferent signals from that limb. The main characteristics of the rhythmic movements of a limb are determined by its so-called spinal generator. During the scratch reflex only one generator is active, during locomotion, all four of them. The spinal generators consist of interneurons, which lie mainly in the lateral part of laminae V, VI and VII over the whole length of the cervical or lumbosacral enlargement. Renshaw cells and Ia inhibitory interneurons are not responsible for the basic pattern of rhythmic changes, (see Gelfand et al., 1988 for review). Grillner (1981) hypothesized that the spinal generator of a limb consists of several rhythm generators, each controlling one joint. The regulation of the rhythm generators is performed by means of tonic commands coming from higher brain centers. In all likelihood the diffuse descending systems, originating in the ventromedial medulla oblongata and projecting to all parts of the intermediate zone and motoneuronal cell groups, play an important role in this regulation (see pp. 371 and 374).

Long propriospinal projections. As pointed out earlier, the column of motoneurons innervating axial muscles extends from the caudal medulla oblongata (neck muscles) to the sacral cord (lower back muscles). Since they are often simultaneously active during certain proximal body movements, long propriospinal projections are necessary to coordinate such axial movements. Giovanelli Barilari and Kuypers (1969) and Molenaar and Kuypers (1978) have shown that there exist direct reciprocal connections between the cervical and lumbosacral spinal cord. The great majority of the neurons giving rise to such long propriospinal pro-

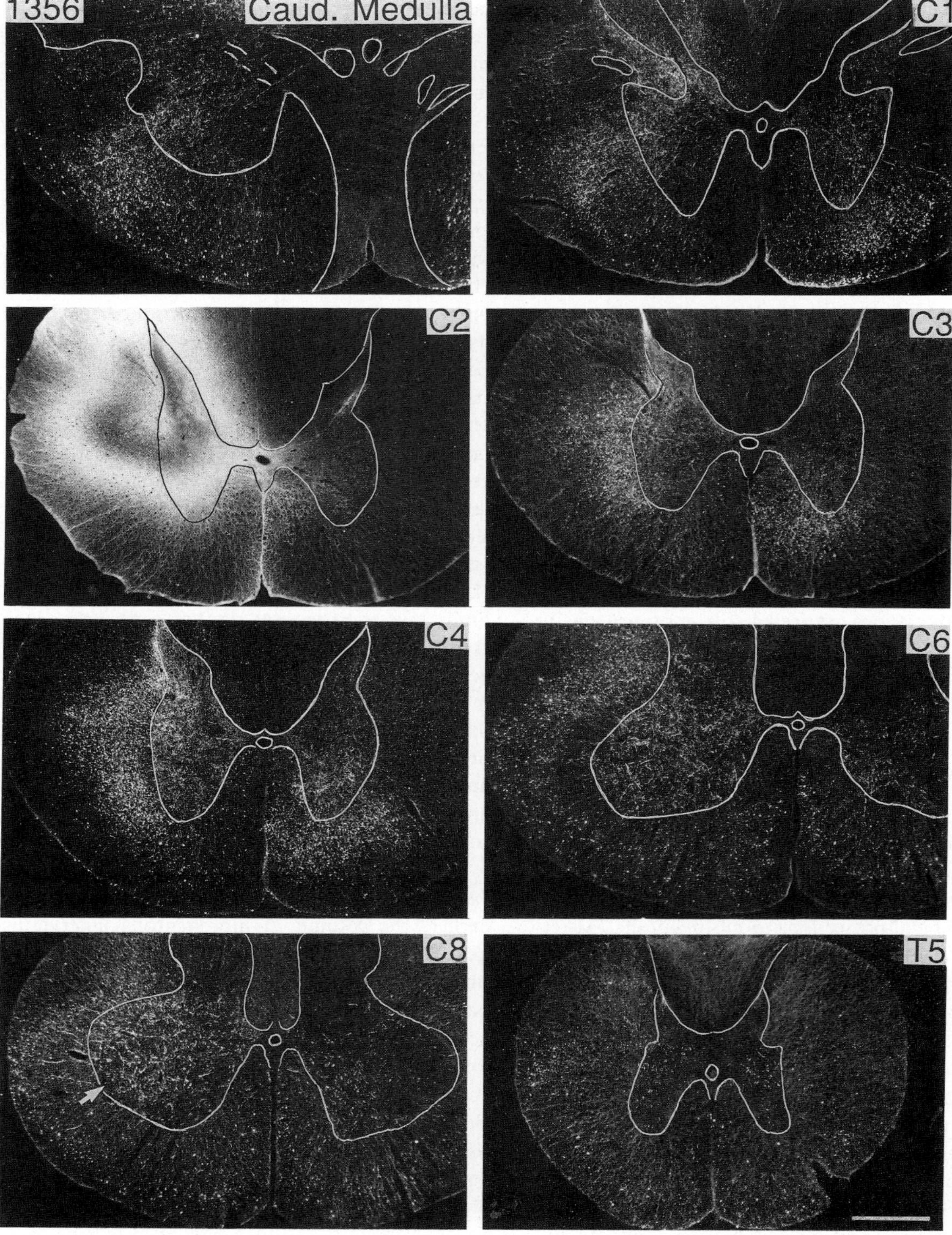
1356
Caud. Medulla
C1
C2
C3
C4
C6
C8
T5

jections are located in the medial part of the intermediate zone (lamina VIII and adjoining VII). They project bilaterally, but mainly ipsilaterally via the ventral funiculus, and probably play a role in establishing a functional unity of the axial and proximal musculature. A smaller number of neurons in the dorsolateral part of the cervical intermediate zone and a few in lamina I (Molenaar and Kuypers, 1978) send axons via the dorsolateral funiculus to the lumbar cord. The function of these projections is less clear, although it is known that stimulation of forelimb afferents evokes a sequence of excitation and inhibition in hindlimb motoneurons (for example to α-motoneurons of the flexor digitorum longus muscle (Schomburg et al., 1975)). In summary, long propriospinal pathways are probably involved in the coordination of axial muscle activity as well as in the coordination between fore- and hindlimbs.

Comparing the density of the short and long propriospinal projections, it is important to note that an injection of ^{3}H-leucine in the intermediate zone of a portion of the C2 or C6 intermediate zone produces many fibers terminating in the C8 – T1 motoneuronal cell groups (Holstege, 1988b; Fig. 13; Holstege and Blok, 1989), but only very few in the lumbar cord (Holstege, 1988b). After an injection of ^{3}H-leucine in the L7 spinal cord, which produces heavy labeling in for example the inferior olive, only very few labeled fibers were found in the medial part of the C8 intermediate zone (Holstege, unpublished observations). Thus, the long propriospinal projections are much weaker than the short propriospinal and interneuronal projections to motoneurons. It remains to be determined whether the coordination between fore- and hindlimbs relies entirely on the relatively weak long propriospinal projections, or on other projection systems as well.

Specific propriospinal projections. Giovanelli Barilari and Kuypers (1969) and Ueyama and Matsushita (1973) have demonstrated an ipsilateral projection from the thoracolumbar spinal cord to a specific motoneuronal cell group in the most ventrolateral portion of the C8 – T1 ventral horn. The cell group was called "group X" by Giovanelli Barilari and Kuypers (1969) and "ventral motor nucleus" by Ueyama and Matsushita (1973), indicating that it was not known which muscle was innervated by these motoneurons. It was later demonstrated (see p. 309) that the motoneurons in this cell group innervate the cutaneus trunci muscle (CTM). The CTM is a thin broad sheet of skeletal muscle just beneath the skin. It does not contain muscle spindles and receives its afferents from the overlying skin. Bilateral contraction of the muscle can easily be triggered by pinching the skin or in the cat by gentle displacement of the fur (CTM-reflex). The afferent information for this reflex is conveyed via the cutaneous nerves, which are segmentally organized. Physiological studies have shown that long ascending propriospinal pathways, originating in the thoracolumbar cord, exist between the cutaneous afferents and the CTM motor nucleus (Krogh and Denslow, 1979; Theriault and Diamond, 1988). Holstege and Blok (1989) in their study on the specific descending pathways to the CTM motor nucleus, combined the anatomic findings of Giovanelli Barilari and Kuypers (1969) and Ueyama and Matsushita, 1973 with the more recent physiological findings and produced a schematic diagram of the anatomy of the CTM reflex (Fig. 14).

Absence of propriospinal projections to certain motor nuclei

CTM motor nucleus. Short propriospinal

Fig. 13. Darkfield photomicrographs of the caudal medulla oblongata and 7 different levels of the cervical and upper thoracic cord after injection of ^{3}H-leucine in the lateral two thirds of the intermediate zone of the C2 spinal gray matter. Note the strong projections to the motoneuronal cell groups in the C6 and C8 ventral horn. Note also that from the injection site the descending propriospinal fibers gradually move to more peripheral parts of the funiculi. The arrow in C8 points to the CTM motor nucleus, which does not receive descending propriospinal pathways. Bar represents 1 mm.

pathways exist for almost all motoneuronal cell groups. However, the CTM motor nucleus, in contrast to the surrounding motoneuronal cell groups in the cervical enlargement, does not seem to receive projections from cervical interneurons (Holstege and Blok, 1989), although the nucleus receives many from more caudal regions (see p. 325 and Fig. 14). The lack of descending propriospinal pathways to the CTM motor nucleus is not surprising. CTM motoneurons are involved in totally different movements than the other motoneurons in the ventrolateral portion of the C8-upper T1 ventral horn, which innervate the muscles of the forelimb. The propriospinal afferent pathways from the cervical cord are mainly concerned with coordination of movements of the forelimb, in which the CTM does not play a role.

Phrenic nucleus. A second cell group that seems to receive only a small number of propriospinal fibers (if any) is the phrenic nucleus. Holstege (1988b) observed, in cases with relatively large injections of ^{3}H-leucine in the C1 and C2 spinal cord, strong projections to the C5 – T1 motoneuronal cell groups, but only very weak (if any) projections to the phrenic nucleus (Fig. 15). This observation is not unimportant, because Aoki et al. (1980) have reported that neurons in the C1 – C2 intermediate zone generate a spontaneous respiratory rhythm in cats two hours after a C1 spinal transection, but not after a C3 transection. On the other hand, Lipski and Duffin (1986) studied the C1 – C2 propriospinal inspiratory neurons, but could not find any evidence for synaptic connections between these cells and the phrenic motoneurons. They suggested a disynaptic pathway involving segmental interneurons, but Holstege (unpublished observations), in a case

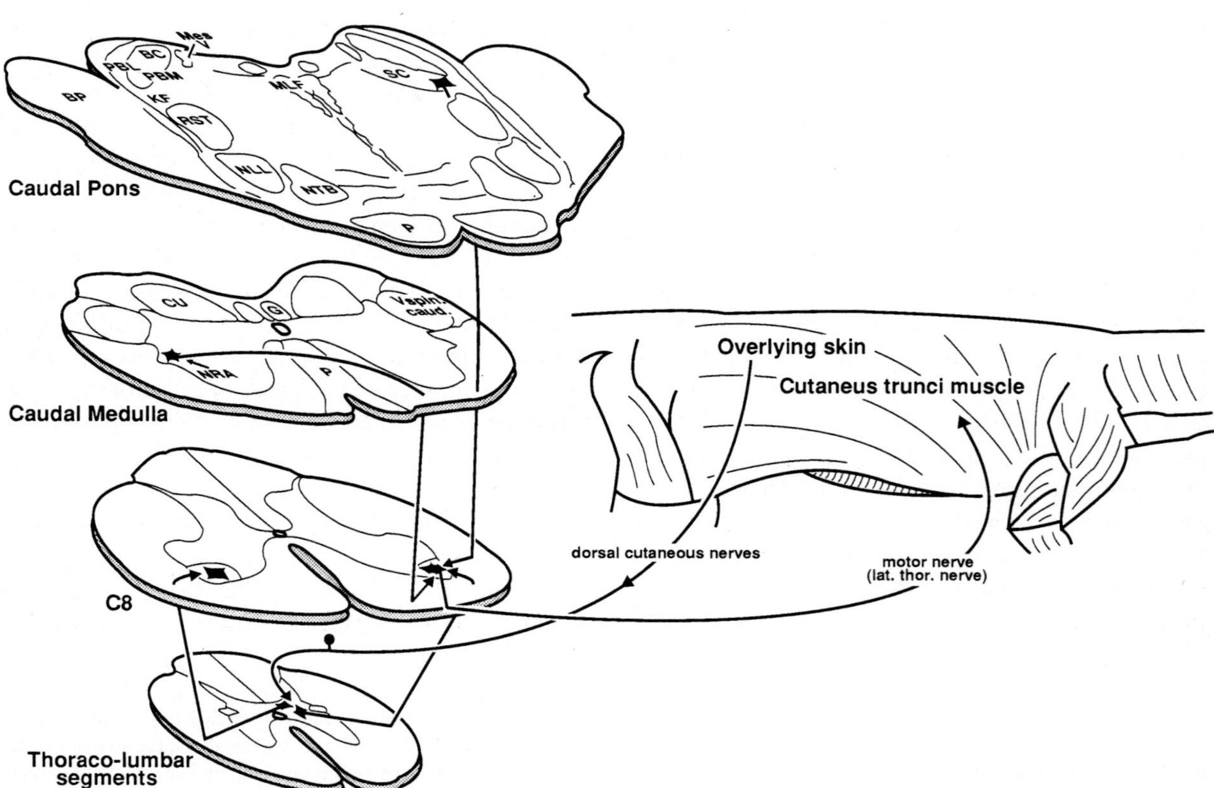

Fig. 14. Schematic representation of the pathways involved in the CTM reflex and the specific supraspinal projections to the CTM motor nucleus.

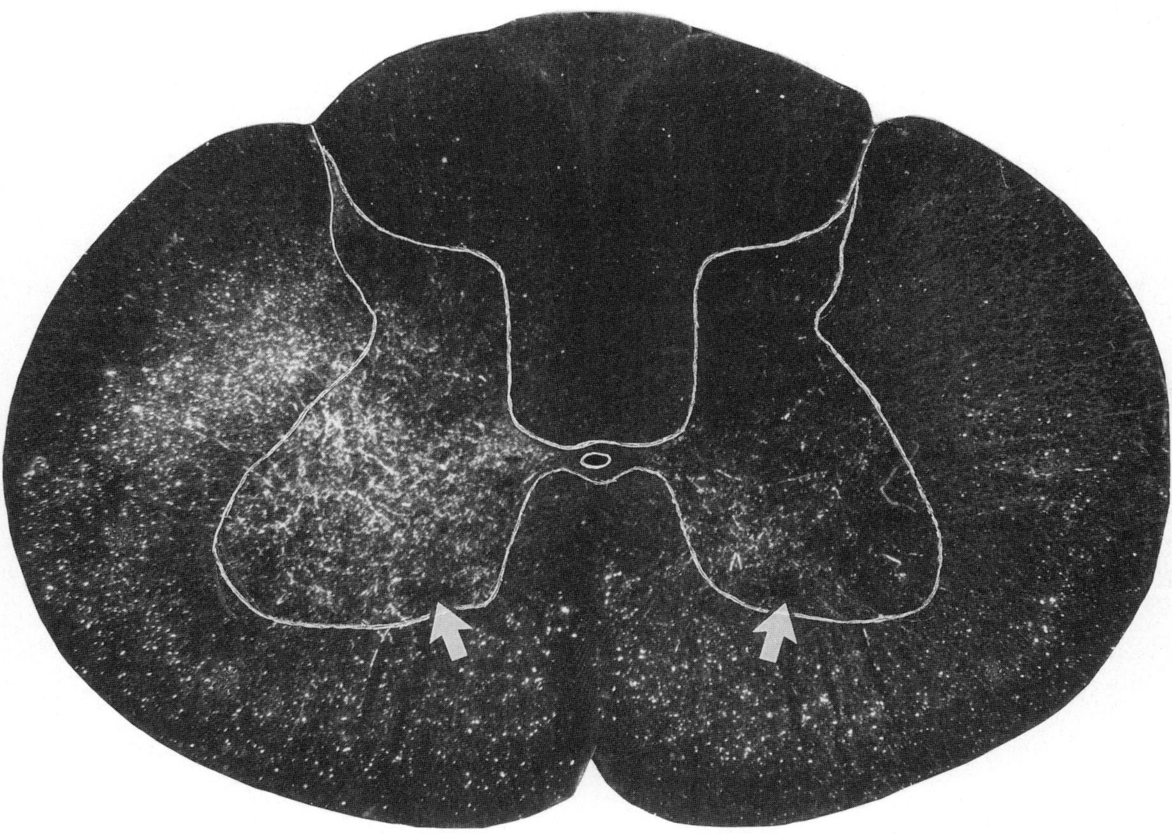

Fig. 15. Darkfield photomicrograph of a tranverse section of the C6 spinal cord after an injection of ^{3}H-leucine at the level of C2 (Fig. 13 C2). The arrows indicate the area of the phrenic nuclei, receiving virtually no labeled fibers from the C2 intermediate zone.

with a large ^{3}H-leucine injection in the segmental interneuronal zone at the upper C6 level, could not find well defined projections to the ipsi- or contralateral phrenic nucleus. Thus, it remains to be resolved how the C1 – C2 inspiratory interneurons of Aoki et al. (1980) control phrenic motoneurons. Possibly, propriospinal neurons in the thoracic cord project to the phrenic nucleus, because stimulation in spinal cats of the afferent fibers of the internal and external intercostal muscles elicits a polysynaptic reflex excitation of phrenic motoneurons, followed by a depression of spontaneous phrenic motor activity (Decima et al., 1969).

Onuf's nucleus. The third motoneuronal cell group which does not seem to receive propriospinal projections from more rostral levels is the nucleus of Onuf (Rustioni et al., 1971; Holstege and Tan, 1987) (Fig. 16). Similar to the descending propriospinal pathways to the CTM motor nucleus, the lack of descending interneuronal or propriospinal projections to Onuf's nucleus is not unexpected, because Onuf motoneurons are involved in completely different movements than the hindlimb innervating motoneurons surrounding Onuf's nucleus. The propriospinal afferent pathways from the lumbar cord are mainly concerned with coordination of movements of the hindlimb, in which Onuf's nucleus does not play a role.

However, Onuf motoneurons, innervating the pelvic floor muscles, have a very strong relationship with skin afferents. Stimulation of the

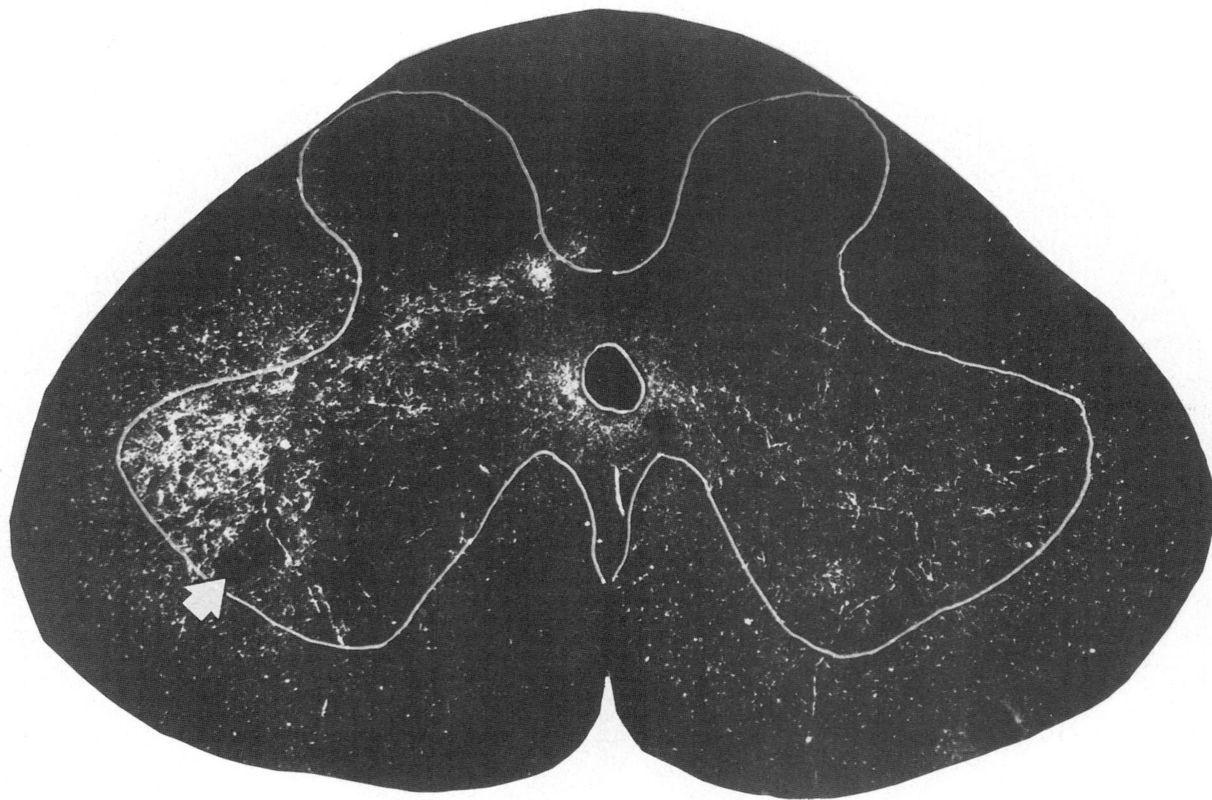

Fig. 16. Darkfield photomicrograph of a transverse section through the S1 spinal cord of the cat after an injection of ^{3}H-leucine at the level of L7. The arrow points to the nucleus of Onuf, receiving no labeled fibers from the L7 intermediate zone (from Holstege and Tan, 1987).

perianal skin gives rise to simultaneous reflex reactions of the anal, urethral and bulbocavernosus muscles (Pedersen, 1985). The afferent fibers enter the spinal cord via the pudendal nerve, in the cat in the segments S1, S2 and upper S3 (Ueyama et al., 1984), in the monkey in the segments L7 to S2 (Roppolo et al., 1985) and in humans in the segments S1 to S4 (Pedersen, 1985). In general the strongest afferent input enters the cord one segment caudal to the level of the nucleus of Onuf. Predictably, but not yet demonstrated, there exist projections from interneurons in the caudal sacral cord to the Onuf motoneurons, similar to the ascending projections from the thoracolumbar cord to the CTM motor nucleus.

The CTM, phrenic and Onuf's nuclei not only have in common that they receive only very few, if any, descending propriospinal fibers, but also that for all three of them the muscles they innervate contain only very few, if any muscle spindles, (see Theriault and Diamond, 1988a for the CTM motor nucleus, Duron et al., 1978 for the phrenic nucleus and Todd, 1964 and Gosling et al., 1981 for Onuf's nucleus). Furthermore all three motor nuclei have an exceptionally large number of longitudinally running dendrites within their nuclei (Dekker et al., 1973), and all three receive specific afferent projections from supraspinal structures (see later).

Propriobulbar pathways

The organization of the interneuronal projections to the trigeminal (V), facial (VII), ambiguus (X) and hypoglossal (XII) motor nuclei in the brainstem is not fundamentally different from the interneuronal and propriospinal projections in the spinal cord. This is not the case for the projections to the extra-ocular motor nuclei of the oculomotor, trochlear and abducens nerves and the ear muscle motoneurons in the facial nucleus, which form part of specific, mainly medially located premotor systems controlling eye-, head- and ear movements (see p. 351 – 358).

Going rostrally from the level of C1, the spinal intermediate zone (laminae V to VIII) is called reticular formation (subnuclei reticulares dorsalis and ventralis of Meessen and Olszewski, 1949). It contains interneurons projecting to the motoneurons in the upper cervical cord (Holstege, 1988b) and to the V, VII, X and XII motor nuclei (Holstege and Kuypers, 1977 and Holstege et al., 1977). Rostral to the level of the obex the reticular formation can be subdivided into a medial and a lateral tegmental field (Fig. 17). The lateral tegmental field extends rostrally into the parabrachial nuclei and the nucleus Kölliker-Fuse, and can be considered as the rostral extension of the spinal intermediate zone (Holstege et al., 1977). For example, the projections from the red nucleus and motor cortex in cat and monkey to the bulbar lateral tegmental field are continuous with the projections to the intermediate zone of the spinal cord (see p. 358 – 368). At medullary levels the bulbar lateral tegmental field involves the so-called parvocellular reticular formation, the lateral paragigantocellular reticular nucleus of Olszewski and Baxter (1954), (see also Martin et al., 1990) and the intermediate reticular nucleus, as defined by Paxinos and Watson (1985) in the rat. The lateral tegmental field adjoins the hypoglossal nucleus ventrolaterally, the facial nucleus dorsomedially and surrounds the nucleus ambiguus. At pontine levels the lateral tegmental field comprises area h of Meessen and Olszewski (1949), which surrounds the motor trigeminal nucleus, and the ventral part of the parabrachial nuclei and the nucleus Kölliker-Fuse. In general, interneurons located medially in the lateral tegmental field project bilaterally to the V, VII and XII motor nuclei, while neurons located laterally project ipsilaterally (Holstege et al., 1977). The medial tegmental field at the levels of pons and medulla is involved in eye-head coordination and gives rise to long descending pathways to the spinal cord, involved in regulating axial and proximal body movements (see p. 355 – 357) or level setting systems (see p. 371 – 374).

Interneuronal projections to the motor trigeminal nucleus. In the cat almost all afferent projections to the motor trigeminal nucleus are derived from the bulbar lateral tegmental field. There are only 3 exceptions; 1) the few afferents from the mesencephalic trigeminal ganglion cells to the mouth closing motoneurons (see p. 319 – 321; 2) fibers from the upper medullary ventromedial tegmentum, which project diffusely to all motoneuronal cell groups including the motor trigeminal nucleus (see p. 372) and 3) the motor cortex in monkey and humans, but not in cat, (Kuypers, 1958a,b,c,).

Interneurons projecting to the motor trigeminal

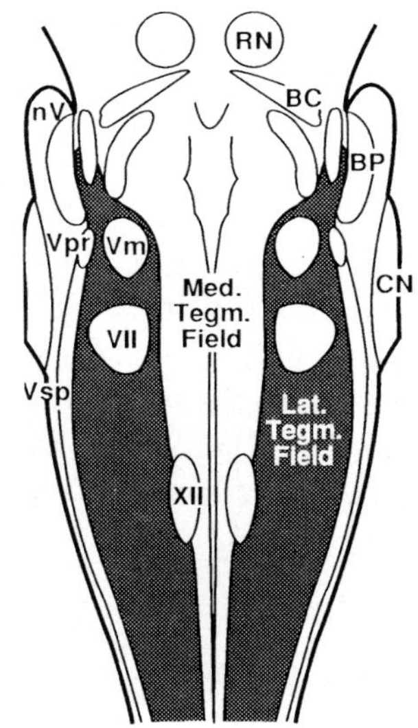

Fig. 17. Schematic drawing of the subdivision of the bulbar reticular formation into a medial and lateral tegmental field. The lateral tegmental field can be considered as the rostral extension of the spinal intermediate zone, containing interneurons for the motoneurons in brainstem and spinal cord. The medial tegmental field gives rise to descending pathways involved in postural and orienting movements and in level setting of all neurons in the spinal cord.

nucleus are not uniformly distributed throughout the lateral tegmental field. The mouth opening motoneurons receive their strongest projections from neurons in the lateral tegmentum at levels caudal to the obex (Holstege and Blok, 1986; Holstege, 1989). The mouth closing motoneurons receive their afferent projections mainly from neurons in more rostral parts of the lateral tegmental field, i.e. from the level of the hypoglossal nucleus rostrally until the supratrigeminal nuclei and the area of the ventral parabrachial nuclei and nucleus Kölliker-Fuse (Holstege and Kuypers, 1977; Holstege et al., 1977; Mizuno et al., 1983; Holstege and Blok, 1986; Travers and Norgren, 1983).

Furthermore, Holstege et al. (1983) demonstrated a very specific projection pattern, originating from neurons located just dorsal and dorsomedial to the superior olivary complex. These neurons project contralaterally to mouth opening motoneurons in the trigeminal nucleus, the geniohyoid motoneurons in the hypoglossal nucleus and soft palate and pharynx motoneurons in the dorsal group of the nucleus ambiguus (Fig. 18). The authors suggest that this projection pattern might play a role in the coordination of the first (buccopharyngeal) phase of swallowing. Physiological studies (Doty and Bosma, 1956; Miller, 1972) had demonstrated that the mylohyoid, geniohyoid and palatopharyngeal muscles were inhibited immediately prior to the swallowing act, which led Holstege et al. (1983) to speculate that this inhibition might be due to action of the pontine cell group.

Interneuronal projections to the hypoglossal nucleus. The afferents to the hypoglossal nucleus are organized in largely the same way as those to the motor trigeminal motoneurons, which suggests that a strong relationship exists between the motor control of tongue and jaw movements. With the exception of some diffuse projections originating in the medullary ventromedial tegmentum and some primary afferent fibers from the C1 – C3 dorsal roots (Holstege and Kuypers, 1977) all afferent projections to the hypoglossal nucleus are derived from the bulbar lateral tegmental field (Holstege et al., 1977; Travers and Norgren, 1983). Different levels of the lateral tegmental field project to different portions of the hypoglossal nucleus (Holstege, unpublished results). For instance, interneurons in the respiration related caudal part of the lateral tegmentum project to other parts of the hypoglossal nucleus (see also Sica et al., 1984) than interneurons in the rostral part of the lateral tegmental field, which are involved in coordinating mouth closing movements. However, the functional importance of these differences is difficult to assess, because, although some anatomic subdivisions have been described (see p. 316) within the hypoglossal nucleus of the cat, thorough knowledge about a functional subdivision (for example a different location in the hypoglossal nucleus for tongue protrusion and tongue retraction motoneurons) is still lacking. Only combined anatomic and physiological studies can reveal the meaning of the observed anatomic

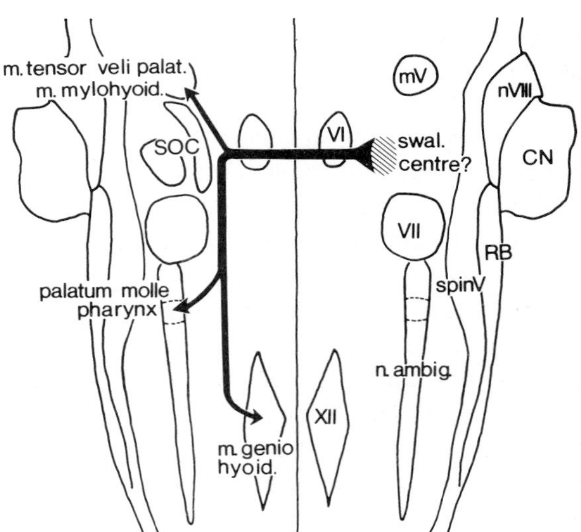

Fig. 18. Schematic drawing of the projections originating from neurons located just dorsomedial to the superior olivary complex. On the left side are indicated the muscles involved, on the right side the nuclei in which the motoneurons are located that innervate these muscles. It is suggested that this projection pattern might be involved in the first phase of swallowing.

differences in projections to the hypoglossal nucleus, (see for example the projection from the NRA to the hypoglossal nucleus in Fig. 22).

Interneuronal projections to the facial nucleus. The lateral tegmental field projects heavily to the facial nucleus. However, these projections differ strongly for each of the subnuclei, and will, therefore, be described for each subnucleus separately.

Interneuronal projections to the ear- and platysma muscle motoneuronal cell groups. The only portion of the lateral tegmental field projecting to the dorso- and ventromedial subnuclei, which contain ear and platysma muscle motoneurons respectively (Fig. 7), is its most caudal part, i.e. the area of the nucleus retroambiguus (NRA) (Holstege et al., 1977; Travers and Norgren, 1983; Holstege and Blok, 1989). These neurons probably form the rostral extent of a group of interneurons in the cervical cord projecting to the pinna- and platysma muscle motoneurons in the facial nucleus, because similar projections to the pinna muscle motoneuronal cell group are derived from the dorsal horn and intermediate zone at the level C1 – C4 (Mehler, 1969; Holstege and Kuypers, 1977; Nakano et al., 1986). These fibers ascend bilaterally (Holstege et al., 1977), (and not only contralaterally as suggested by Nakano et al., 1986), to terminate mainly ipsilaterally in the dorsomedial and ventromedial facial subnuclei (ear- and platysma muscle motoneuronal cell groups). The platysma muscle motoneurons receive their afferents from the C1 – C6 spinal cord (Mehler, 1969; Holstege and Kuypers, 1977). The ascending projections probably represent a similar pathway as the ascending propriospinal projections to the CTM motor nucleus (see p. 325). Neither the CTM nor the external ear and platysma muscles contain muscle spindles and these muscles use the overlying skin for there proprioceptive information. Afferent fibers from the skin overlying the external ear and platysma muscles reach the central nervous system via the auriculotemporal branch of the trigeminal nerve, and the C2 – C4 dorsal root fibers (pinna muscles) or the C2 – C6 dorsal root fibers (platysma muscle). The fibers of the auriculotemporal nerve terminate in the dorsal portion of the C1 – C3 dorsal horn (Panneton and Burton, 1981; Shigenaga et al., 1986), and the C2 – C6 dorsal roots fibers terminate mainly on interneurons in the C2 – C6 dorsal horn (Pfaller and Arvidsson, 1988). Such first order interneurons may project directly to the pinna and platysma muscle motoneurons in the facial nucleus (Holstege and Kuypers, 1977), but second order interneurons may also be involved. There exist other projections to the dorsomedial facial subnucleus, but they are derived from areas related to eye-head coordination (see p. 357).

Interneuronal projections to the orbicularis oculi and retractor bulbi muscle motoneuronal cell groups and the neuronal organization of the blink reflex. As for the ear and platysma muscles, the orbicularis oculi muscle does not contain muscle spindles and uses the overlying skin for its proprioception. The skin overlying the orbicularis oculi muscle and the cornea is innervated by the ophthalmic branch of the trigeminal nerve, the proximal fibers of which terminate in the ventral part of the spinal trigeminal nucleus (Panneton and Burton, 1981). Neurons in the ventral part of the spinal trigeminal nucleus project to the blink motoneurons, which are the orbicularis oculi and retractor bulbi motoneuronal cell groups (Takeuchi et al., 1979; Panneton and Martin, 1983; Holstege et al., 1986a,b; see p. 314 – 315). These disynaptic connections between trigeminal nerve afferents on the one hand and orbicularis oculi and retractor bulbi motoneurons on the other probably represent the R1 component of the blink reflex.

The blink reflex consists of two different reflexes; the orbicularis oculi reflex and the nictitating membrane response. The orbicularis oculi reflex in the cat consists of two EMG components (R1 and R2) (Lindquist and Martensson, 1970) and has latencies of 9 – 12 ms (R1) and 15 – 25 ms

(R2). R1 is ipsilateral in all vertebrates; R2 is bilateral in humans (Kugelberg, 1952), but ipsilateral in cats (Hiraoka and Shimamura, 1977). The nictitating membrane response, which is the retraction of the eyeball by the retractor bulbi muscles, also consists of two components similar to the orbicularis oculi reflex (Guégan and Horcholle-Bossavit, 1981). The nictitating membrane response is used in studying conditioned reflexes, because it provides the experimenter with a high degree of control over the sensory consequences of the unconditioned stimulus (Gormezano et al., 1962). Although the R1 reflex is disynaptic in mammals, in the lizard primary trigeminal afferents seem to project directly on retractor bulbi motoneurons (Barbas-Henry and Wouterlood, 1988), suggesting that in the lizard the R1 reflex is monosynaptic.

Holstege et al., (1986a,b) demonstrated a strong and specific ipsilateral projection to the blink motoneuronal cell groups from the ventrolateral pontine tegmental field, which they called the pontine blink premotor area (Fig. 19). It must be emphasized that this region, which forms part of the lateral tegmental field, lies outside the spinal trigeminal nucleus. It means that this projection cannot play a role in the disynaptic R1 component of the blink reflex.

Holstege et al. (1986a,b) also demonstrated specific projections from an area in the medial tegmentum at levels of the hypoglossal nucleus to the blink motoneuronal cell groups, which they called the medullary blink premotor area (Fig. 20). This region is not part of the lateral tegmental field, but belongs to the dorsal part of the medullary medial tegmentum, which plays an important role in eye- and neck muscle motor control (see p. 355 – 357). A similar projection to the retractor bulbi motoneuronal cell group has been described in the rabbit (Harvey et al., 1984). Holstege et al. (1986b) also observed projections from the medullary blink premotor area to the pontine blink premotor area (Fig. 20A, B). The projections from the medullary blink premotor area were mainly bilateral, but some ipsilateral projections were also observed (Holstege et al. 1988). Like the pontine blink premotor area, the medullary blink premotor area is not located in the spinal trigeminal nucleus and thus cannot be involved in the disynaptic organization of the R1 blink reflex component.

Both the pontine and medullary blink premotor areas are probably involved in the R2 blink reflex component because 1) The R2 reflex component is not disynaptic, but multisynaptic (Kugelberg, 1952; Lindquist and Martensson, 1970; Hiraoka and Shimamura, 1977; Ongerboer de Visser and Kuypers, 1978), and the response consists of

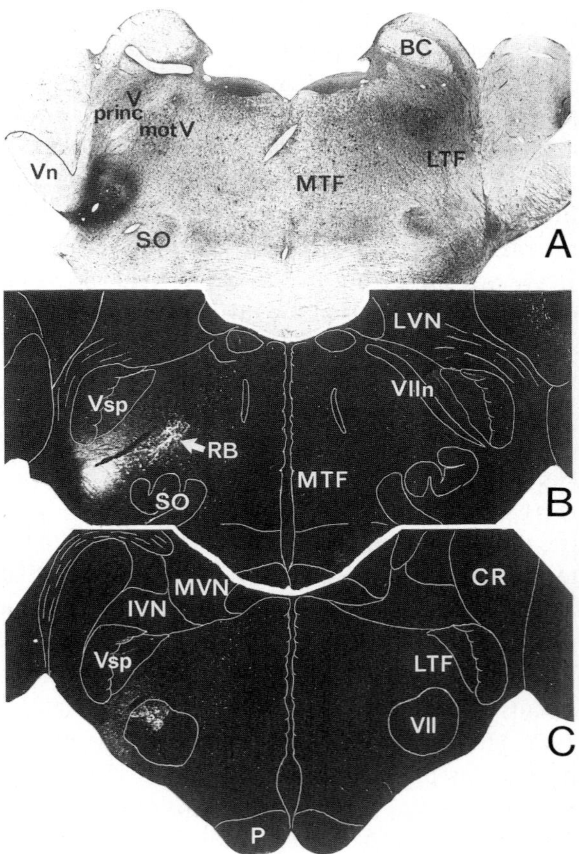

Fig. 19. Brightfield (A) and darkfield (B and C) photomicrographs of a case with an injection of ^{3}H-leucine in the caudal pontine ventrolateral tegmental field, not involving the trigeminal nucleus. Note the dense ipsilateral distribution of labeled fibers to the RB motoneuronal area (B) and the intermediate facial subnucleus (C), (from Holstege et al., 1986).

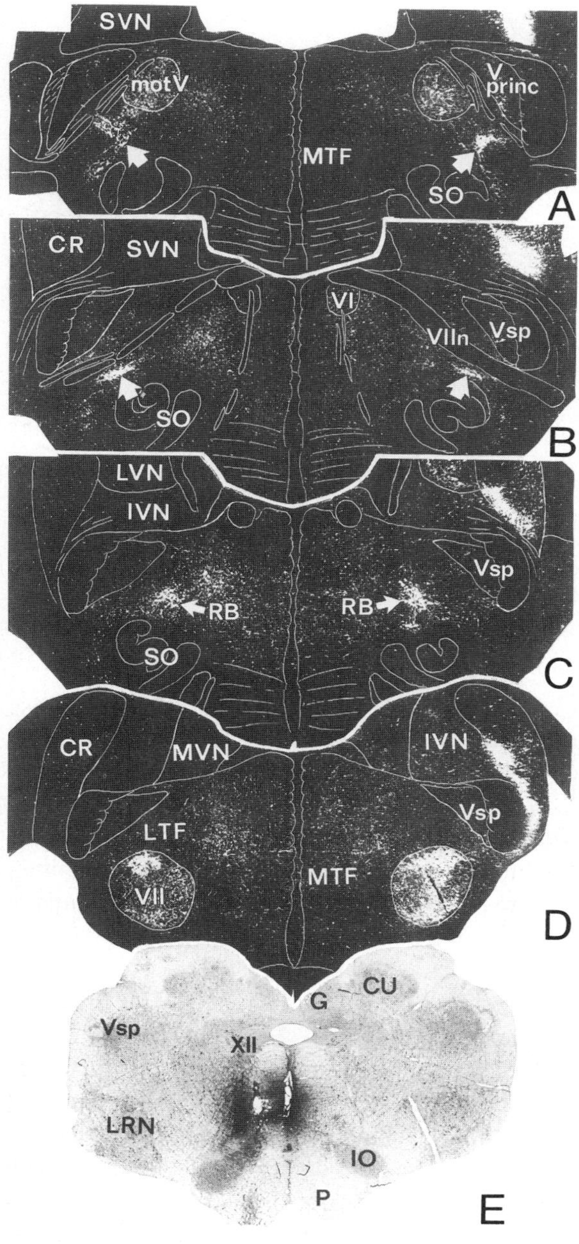

Fig. 20. Darkfield and brightfield photomicrographs of a case with an injection of ^{3}H-leucine in the medullary medial tegmentum at the level of the hypoglossal nucleus. Note the dense bilateral projection to the intermediate facial subnuclei (D), the RB motoneuronal cell group (C), and the pontine premotor blink area (arrows in A and B), (from Holstege et al., 1986).

several spikes (Berthier and Moore, 1983; Kugelberg, 1952); 2) The R2 blink reflex component, according to Shahani and Young (1972), is responsible for actual closure of the eyelids. For such a motor performance, strong projections to the blink motoneurons are necessary. Holstege et al. (1986a,b) found such connections only from the pontine and medullary blink premotor areas; 3) The medullary blink premotor area projects specifically to the pontine blink premotor area, indicating that both areas are involved in the same neuronal organization. For a description of the afferent projections to the pontine blink premotor area (from red nucleus, pretectum and medullary blink premotor area) and the medullary blink premotor area (from the superior colliculus and pontine medial tegmentum), which may play an important role in the R2 reflex, see Holstege et al. (1986b; 1988 and Fig. 21). There are also projections to the orbicularis oculi motoneurons that do not project to the retractor bulbi motoneurons. Such projections are derived from all levels of the bulbar lateral tegmental field from caudal medulla to the ventral parabrachial nuclei and nucleus Kölliker-Fuse (Holstege et al., 1986a). They probably play an important role in the relay of the cortical and lateral limbic control of the muscles around the eye.

Interneuronal projections to the motoneurons of the peri-oral muscles. Peri-oral muscles, like the other facial muscles, do not contain muscle spindles and depend on the overlying skin for their proprioception. According to Shigenaga et al. (1986) the afferent information of the peri-oral skin terminates in the rostral portion of the caudal spinal trigeminal nucleus, just caudal to the obex. However, peri-oral muscle motoneurons, located in the lateral and ventrolateral facial subnuclei, receive only a limited number of afferents from interneurons in the caudal spinal trigeminal nucleus itself, but very many from interneurons in the lateral tegmentum medially adjoining the caudal spinal trigeminal nucleus (Holstege et al., 1977; Erzurumlu and Killackey, 1979; Takeuchi et al.,

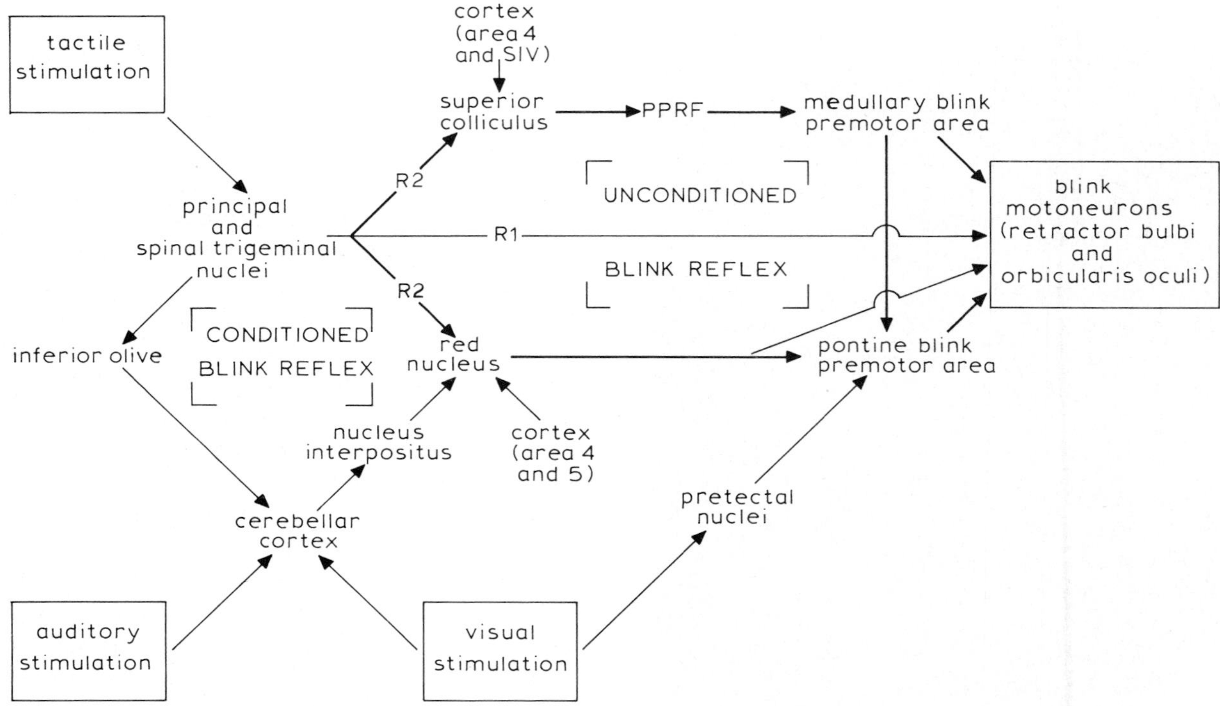

Fig. 21. Schematic representation of the pathways possibly involved in the anatomic framework of the R1 and R2 blink reflex components, (from Holstege et al., 1986).

1979; Panneton and Martin, 1983; Travers and Norgren, 1983). Although afferent projections to the peri-oral muscle motoneurons are derived from all levels of the lateral tegmental field, very strong projections originate in the most rostral portion of this area, the ventral parabrachial nuclei and the nucleus Kölliker-Fuse (Holstege et al., 1977; Takeuchi et al., 1979; Panneton and Martin, 1983; Travers and Norgren, 1983). Thus, similar to the organization of the afferents to the other facial muscle motoneurons, mainly second order neurons in the lateral tegmental field (intermediate zone) give rise to direct projections to motoneurons. Naturally, such second order interneurons receive also afferents from other sources, such as motor cortex, red nucleus and limbic system. Finally, neurons in the area of the NRA project mainly contralaterally to the ventrolateral facial subnucleus, innervating the muscles of the lower part of the mouth. Possibly, these projections take part in the expiration related system, which also projects mainly contralaterally to the mouth opening, pharynx, soft palate, and abdominal muscle motoneurons (Holstege, 1989).

Interneuronal projections to the dorsal group of the nucleus ambiguus. Most subgroups of the nucleus ambiguus of the cat consist of motoneurons scattered in the ventrolateral part of the medullary lateral tegmental field. In the cat only one subgroup, the dorsal group, is so compact that it can be easily recognized in Nissl stained sections (see p. 316). The dorsal group contains motoneurons innervating pharynx and soft palate. Direct projections to the dorsal group of the nucleus ambiguus have only been demonstrated to originate from a small number of areas. A light, but distinct projection is derived from a cell group dorsomedial to the superior olivary complex (see p. 330 – 331). From studying a large number of cases the

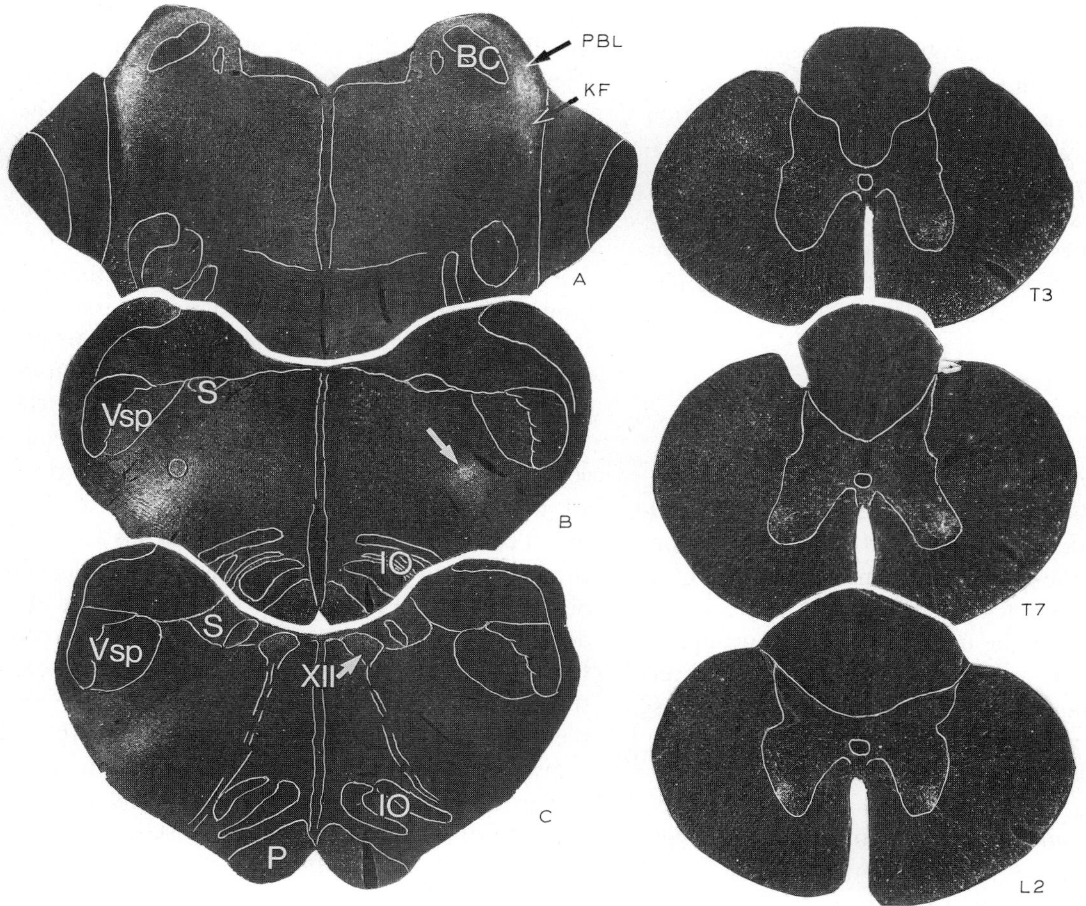

Fig. 22. Darkfield photographs of the caudal brainstem (A to C) and 3 segments (T3, T7 and L2) of the spinal cord after a relatively small injection ^{3}H-leucine in the caudal NRA. Note the strong bilateral projections to the lateral parabrachial nuclei and nucleus Kölliker-Fuse in A and the very strong projection to the contralateral dorsal group of the nucleus ambiguus in B (arrow). The projection to the ipsilateral dorsal group (in circle) is weaker. Note further the bilateral projection to the dorsal part of the hypoglossal nucleus in C and the strong projections to the intercostal and abdominal motoneuronal cell groups in the spinal cord, (from Holstege, G., 1989).

impression was gained that all other projections to the dorsal group of the nucleus ambiguus are derived from neurons in caudal parts of the medullary lateral tegmental field. From these projections, those from the caudal NRA are most numerous, especially contralaterally (Holstege, 1989; Fig. 22). Various studies have claimed that the nucleus ambiguus receives projections from the PAG and hypothalamus (Jürgens and Pratt, 1979; Mantyh, 1983; Saper et al., 1976; Ter Horst et al., 1984), but in none of these studies the precise subgroup of the nucleus ambiguus has been indicated. With respect to the dorsal group, it has been demonstrated that it receives no afferents from the PAG (Holstege, 1989), the hypothalamus (Holstege, 1987), or amygdala and bed nucleus of the stria terminalis (Holstege et al., 1985). Furthermore, the impression was gained that neither the ventral parabrachial nuclei/nucleus Kölliker-Fuse complex nor the lateral solitary nucleus project to the dorsal group (Holstege and Van Krimpen, 1986). These negative findings emphasize the importance of the caudal medullary lateral tegmental field, and especially the NRA as interneuronal link to the pharynx and soft palate motoneurons. The caudal NRA is strongly involved in expiration related activities (see p. 336 – 343) and that is probably also true for its projection to the pharynx motoneurons in the dorsal group of the nucleus ambiguus, because it has been shown that the pharynx muscles are involved in expiratory activities (Sherrey and Megirian, 1975).

Bulbospinal interneurons projecting to motoneurons

In the section Propriobulbar pathways (p. 328 – 336) it has been stated that the bulbar lateral tegmental field can be considered as the rostral continuation of the spinal intermediate zone. However, the bulbar lateral tegmental field not only contains interneurons for the motoneuronal cell groups V, VII, X and XII in the brainstem, but also for certain cell groups in the spinal cord, especially those involved in respiration, abdominal pressure, micturition and blood pressure.

Pathways controlling respiration and abdominal pressure

Chemoreceptors in the carotid body and the pulmonary stretch receptors form the most important peripheral afferents for the respiratory system. From the carotid body, which şenses arterial blood gases and pH, fibers terminate in the dorsomedial subnuclei of the solitary tract (Berger, 1980). These fibers have there cell bodies in the petrosal ganglion and pass via the glossopharyngeal and carotid sinus nerve. The pulmonary stretch receptors are located in the smooth muscle of the trachea, main bronchi and intrapulmonary airways. Peripheral afferent fibers innervating all these receptors, arise from cell bodies in the nodose ganglion and project to the nuclei of the solitary tract (Donoghue et al., 1982). The organization of the CTM (Fig. 14) and ear reflex pathways (see p. 331) indicate that the premotor interneurons are located close to the incoming afferent fibers. The same is true for the premotor interneurons of the respiratory motor output system. They are located in the caudal medulla, where the vagal nerve enters the brainstem, and not in the spinal cord. Therefore, the medullary projections to the respiratory motoneurons should not be considered as a specific supraspinal control system, but as a propriobulbospinal system.

Physiological studies have demonstrated that the brainstem neurons can be subdivided into inspiratory and expiratory neurons, although in the dorsolateral pons some inspiratory-expiratory phase-spanning neurons exist (see Feldman, 1986 for review). From the inspiratory neurons 50 – 90% project to the spinal cord, while almost all expiratory neurons project to the cord. The spinal cord projecting inspiratory neurons send excitatory fibers to the phrenic nucleus, while the expiratory neurons send excitatory fibers to the abdominal muscle motor nuclei. The expiratory fibers in the Bötzinger complex send inhibitory fibers to the phrenic nucleus. The importance of these pathways is exemplified by the finding that a transection at the spino-medullary junction completely abolishes respiratory movements of diaphragm, rib cage and abdominal muscles (St. John et al., 1981).

Projections to the phrenic nucleus. The phrenic nucleus, containing motoneurons innervating the diaphragm, is by far the most important motor nucleus for inspiratory activity. Although the phrenic nucleus receives only a limited number of descending propriospinal afferent connections (see p. 326 – 327), it receives very strong descending monosynaptic connections from four sources in the caudal brainstem: 1. The ventrolateral nucleus of the solitary tract; 2. The para-ambiguus nucleus/rostral NRA; 3. The Bötzinger-complex and 4. The ventrolateral parabrachial nuclei and nucleus Kölliker-Fuse.

Projections from the ventrolateral nucleus of the solitary tract. Physiological studies have pointed out the existence of direct monosynaptic excitatory inputs from the ventrolateral solitary nucleus (called dorsal respiratory group by investigators of the respiratory system) to the phrenic nucleus (Cohen et al., 1974; Hilaire and Monteaux, 1976; Davies et al., 1985a,b). Pulmonary vagal afferents terminate in the medial and dorsolateral subnuclei of the solitary tract nucleus and to a limited extent in the ventrolateral solitary nucleus (Donoghue et al., 1982; Berger and Averill, 1983). The neurons in the ventrolateral solitary nucleus, projecting to the phrenic nucleus, can be subdivided into R_α and R_β neurons. Pulmonary stretch receptors inhibit the R_α neurons and excite the R_β neurons (Von Baumgarten et al., 1957). The excitation of the R_β neurons is at least in part monosynaptic, but monosynaptic connectivity between pulmonary stretch receptors and the R_α neurons could not be demonstrated (Averill et al., 1984; Backman et al., 1984; Berger et al., 1985). Both R_α and R_β neurons have been shown to drive the spinal inspiratory neurons (phrenic and external intercostal) monosynaptically (Fedorko et al., 1983; Lipski et al., 1983; Lipski and Duffin, 1985).

Using anterograde tracing techniques, Loewy and Burton, (1978) and Holstege, G. and Kuypers, (1982) demonstrated such direct connections anatomically. Their finding was confirmed by Rikard-Bell et al., (1984) and Onai and Miura, (1986) using retrograde tracing techniques. According to Holstege (unpublished results), a contingent of labeled fibers crossed the midline just rostral to the obex and descended contralaterally via the dorsolateral, but mainly ventral funiculi until low thoracic levels. From these fibers, many terminate on both the somata and dendrites of the phrenic motoneurons at caudal C4 to C6 levels. Phrenic motoneuronal dendrites extend far into the lateral and ventrolateral funiculi and the medial and dorsal parts of the ventral funiculus (Cameron et al., 1983). The terminations on the phrenic motoneurons are so strong that terminations on the more distal portions of the dendrites are easily recognizable (Fig. 23). The projection to the contralateral phrenic motoneurons is slightly stronger than to the ipsilateral one. Part of the fibers terminating on ipsilateral phrenic motoneurons travel through the ipsilateral ventral funiculus. However, the impression is gained (Holstege, unpublished results) that the majority of the fibers terminating in the ipsilateral phrenic nucleus, descend via the contralateral ventral funiculus (Fig. 23), and recross in the ventral commissure of the C5 – C6 spinal level. This idea is further supported by the finding that a C2 hemi-infiltration with HRP resulted in only a few labeled neurons in the ipsilateral and many in the contralateral ventrolateral solitary nucleus (Holstege, unpublished results).

The R_α and R_β neurons not only receive afferent information from the pulmonary stretch receptors, but also from neurons in other parts of the solitary nucleus and from neurons in other parts of the brainstem (e.g. the Bötzinger neurons, see p. 338 – 339) and limbic system (see Fig. 58).

Projections from the para-ambiguus nucleus/ rostral NRA. Physiological studies have demonstrated that at levels around the obex, in the area of the nucleus ambiguus, a group of premotor

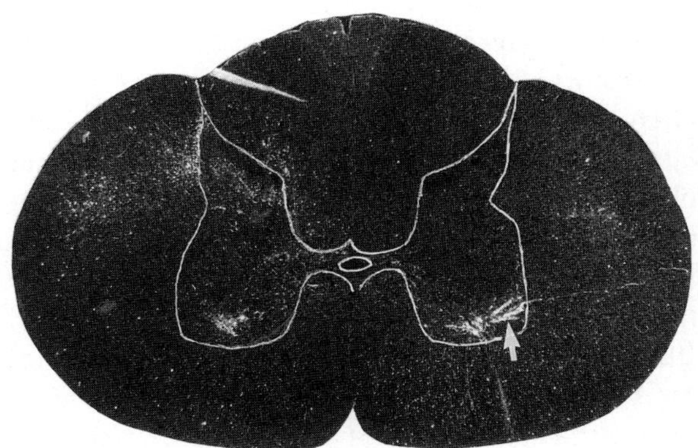

Fig. 23. Darkfield photomicrograph of a section through the C5 segment of the spinal cord in the cat, after a ^{3}H-leucine injection in the area of the lateral solitary nucleus on the left side. Note the strong bilateral projections to the phrenic motor nuclei and the heavy projection to the distal dendrites of the phrenic motoneurons on the contralateral side (arrow). Note also that almost all descending fibers in the ventral and ventrolateral funiculi are contralateral.

respiratory interneurons is located. This group is called the rostral retroambiguus or para-ambiguus or by scientists working in the respiratory system the ventral respiratory group. The rostral part of this group, (rostral to the obex), contains mainly inspiratory neurons, while the caudal portions, (caudal to the obex) contain mainly expiratory neurons. Especially at levels around the level of the obex the inspiratory and expiratory neurons are intermingled. Some of the inspiratory neurons maintain mono-, di-, or oligosynaptic excitatory projections to phrenic motoneurons (Merril, 1970; Cohen, 1974; Davies et al., 1985a,b) and, similar to the neurons in the ventrolateral solitary nucleus, they form a source of drive to inspiratory motoneurons (phrenic and external intercostal). Holstege, G. and Kuypers, (1982) and Holstege et al. (1984) were the first to demonstrate that neurons in this area indeed projected to the somata and dendrites of the phrenic motoneurons at caudal C4 to C6 levels, in an almost identical manner as the neurons in the ventrolateral solitary nucleus. Later anterograde (Feldman et al., 1985; Yamada et al., 1988) and retrograde (Rikard-Bell et al., 1984; Onai and Miura, 1986) tracing studies confirmed their findings. Holstege (unpublished observations), observed a rostrocaudal difference in the pathways to the phrenic and the intercostal motoneurons. The rostral portion of the rostral NRA project mainly via the dorsolateral and lateral funiculus, the caudal portions of the rostral NRA (at levels around the obex) project mainly via the ventral funiculus. Similar to the projections from the ventrolateral solitary nucleus, a substantial portion of the fibers terminating in the ipsilateral phrenic nucleus seems to be derived from the contralateral ventral funiculus, recrossing in the ventral commissure of the C5 and C6 segments (Holstege, unpublished results). The most caudal part of the NRA does not project to the phrenic nucleus (Holstege, 1989). There exist many different opinions about how many inspiratory neurons in the ventrolateral tegmentum project monosynaptically to the phrenic nucleus. Estimations range from 2 – 7% (Fedorko et al., 1983) via 25% (Merrill, 1974) and 28% (Sears et al., 1985) to 61% (Hilaire and Monteau, 1976). All other projections would be di- or oligosynaptic. In contrast to the physiological studies, anatomic tracing studies give the impression that most of the rostral retroambiguus/para-ambiguus projections to the phrenic nucleus are monosynaptic. They show specific pathways to the phrenic nucleus and very few projections to other portions of the cervical gray.

The finding of Holstege, G. and Kuypers, (1982); Feldman et al. (1985) and Holstege, G. (1989) that neurons in the caudal NRA also project to the phrenic nucleus, (according to Holstege, G. (1989) only the most caudal portion of the NRA does not project to the phrenic nucleus), seem to contradict the physiological findings of Merrill (1971). Merrill found no electrophysiologically identified expiratory neuron in the caudal NRA, which project to the phrenic nucleus. However, caudal NRA neurons, projecting to phrenic motoneurons may not be involved in expiration, but in vomiting, coughing and other abdominal straining activities. During vomiting and coughing the phrenic motoneurons are simultaneously active with the abdominal muscle motoneurons. Miller et al. (1987) found that neurons in the caudal NRA control vomiting, during which strong contractions of the abdominal muscle motoneurons take place. However, they also found that only one third of the expiratory neurons in the caudal NRA are active during vomiting. By making lesions in the upper cervical spinal cord, Newsom Davis and Plum (1972) were able to achieve a considerable reduction of the diaphragmatic component of the cough response, without any reduction of the diaphragmatic activity during rhythmic breathing. Furthermore, Newsom Davis (1970) showed that the descending pathways involved in producing hiccups in man was largely distinct from those concerned with rhythmic breathing.

Projections from the Bötzinger complex. The ventrolateral part of the lateral tegmental field of the medulla just caudal to the facial nucleus contains a group of neurons, called the Bötzinger complex. The name Bötzinger was chosen by participants at a symposium on the nucleus tractus solitarius in Heidelberg in honor of a German vineyard (Feldman, 1986). According to anterograde tracing studies of Holstege et al., (1984b); Ellenberger and Feldman, (1988) and Otake et al., (1988), Bötzinger neurons give rise to a specific bilateral projection to somata and dendrites of the phrenic nucleus by way of the contralateral dorsolateral funiculus. It was difficult to assess whether there were also descending fibers in the ipsilateral dorsolateral funiculus terminating in the ipsilateral phrenic nucleus, but the impression was gained that the ipsilateral phrenic nucleus receives fibers via the contralateral dorsolateral funiculus, recrossing at the C5/C6 level. Furthermore, Bötzinger neurons project bilaterally, but mainly contralaterally to the lateral solitary nucleus, and ipsilaterally to the NRA. Physiological studies have demonstrated that Bötzinger neurons are expiratory neurons, which, during the expiratory phase, monosynaptically inhibit the phrenic motoneurons (Merril and Fedorko, 1984) as well as the inspiratory neurons in the ventrolateral solitary nucleus (Merril et al., 1983) and rostral NRA (Fedorko and Merrill, 1984). It has been suggested that the Bötzinger projections to the caudal NRA

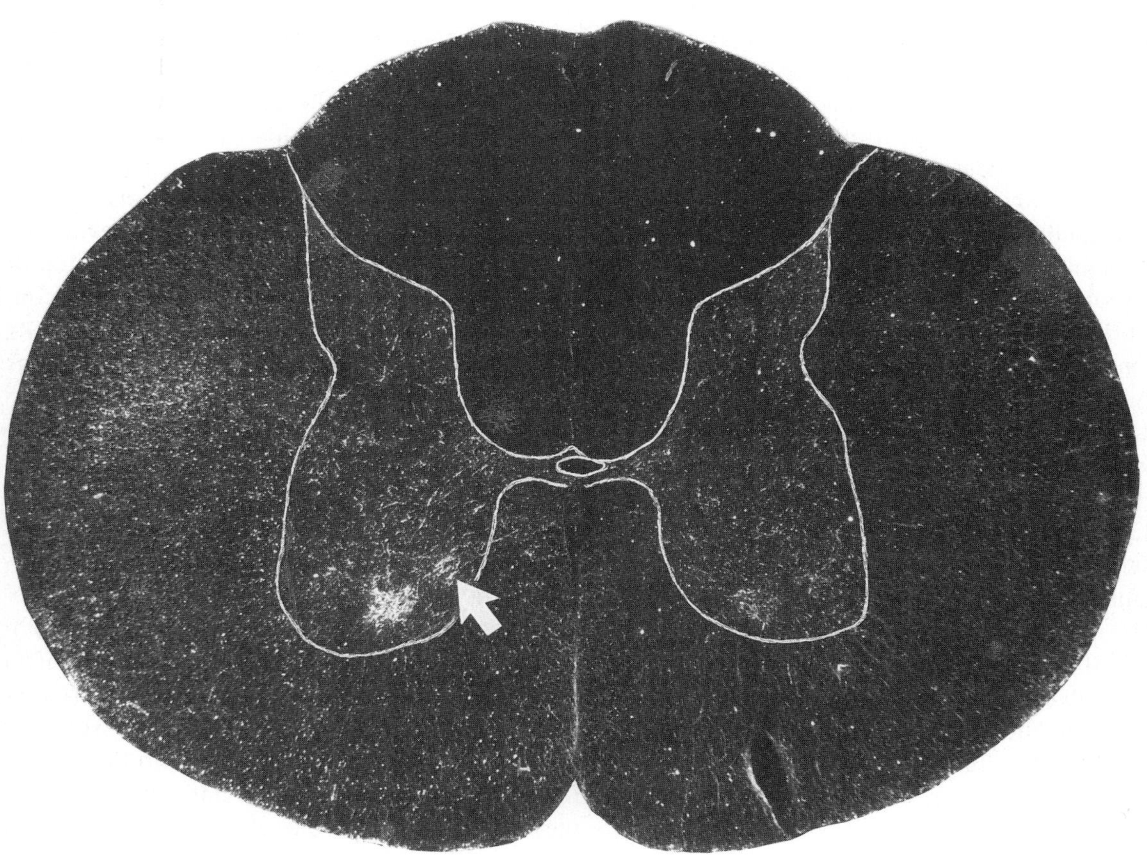

Fig. 24. Darkfield photomicrograph of a section through the C5 segment of the spinal cord in the cat, after a ^{3}H-leucine injection in the area of the ventral parabrachial nuclei and nucleus Kölliker-Fuse. Note on the left the strong ipsilateral projections to the phrenic nucleus and to the distral dendrites of the phrenic motoneurons (arrow). Note on the right the limited projection to the contralateral phrenic nucleus.

are excitatory (see Long and Duffin, 1986 for review).

Projections from the ventrolateral parabrachial nuclei and nucleus Kölliker-Fuse. A fourth source of phrenic nucleus afferents is the ventrolateral part of the parabrachial nuclei, including the area of the nucleus Kölliker-Fuse. This area was called pontine pneumotaxic center (Lumsden, 1923; Bertrand and Hugelin, 1971; Bertrand et al., 1974), but presently called pontine respiratory group by respiratory system investigators. According to anterograde tracing results of Holstege, G. and Kuypers, (1982), neurons in this area give rise to specific bilateral, but mainly ipsilateral projections to the somata and dendrites of the phrenic motoneurons (Fig. 24). Similar results were obtained by Rikard-Bell et al. (1984), using retrograde tracing techniques, but questioned by Onai and Miura (1986), who, after injecting HRP in the phrenic nucleus observed only sparse labeling in the dorsolateral pontine tegmentum. The last authors explained their failure to identify neurons in the dorsolateral pons by suggesting that the projections of this area to the phrenic nucleus were disynaptic, having a synaps in the NRA. However, transneuronal transport is difficult to obtain with the anterograde ^{3}H-leucine tracing technique (Grafstein and Laureno, 1973). It can only be observed in the case of extremely dense projections to certain areas, in which the silver grains are not only located around, but also over the cell bodies. An example is the retinal projection to the superior colliculus (Collewijn and Holstege, 1984), but even then the transneuronal fiber labeling is very weak. In none of the cases with dorsolateral pontine injections, silver grains were found over the cell bodies of the NRA (Holstege, unpublished observations), which excludes the possibility of labeling disynaptic projections from the dorsolateral pons to the phrenic nucleus.

Electrical stimulation in the area of the ventrolateral parabrachial nuclei and nucleus Kölliker-Fuse elicits different respiratory effects, depending on the phase, intensity and precise site of the stimulus. Stimulation in the dorsolateral pons (Cohen, 1971) revealed that dorsally in this area strong inspiratory facilitatory effects were obtained, while ventrally in this area, i.e. medial to the rubrospinal tract strong expiratory facilitatory effects were observed. The neurons projecting to the phrenic nucleus are located in the area between the inspiratory and expiratory facilitatory regions and at present it is unclear whether they have an excitatory or inhibitory effect on the phrenic motoneurons. Lesions in the dorsolateral pontine tegmentum produce so-called inspiratory apneusis, i.e. the inspiratory phase continues for abnormal length (Lumsden, 1923), which can sometimes lead to death by asphyxia. Later studies (Von Euler et al., 1976) demonstrated that a rise of body temperature causes a progressive shortening of apneustic duration after apneusis-promoting lesions in the area of the parabrachial nuclei and nucleus Kölliker-Fuse. Although the dorsolateral pons does not seem to contain the pneumotaxic centre, it exerts strong excitatory influence on the inspiratory switch-off mechanisms. Furthermore it may play an important role in the coordination of the respiratory functions with cardiovascular control functions (Mraovitch et al., 1982; Connelly and Wurster, 1985), also because neurons in the same dorsolateral pontine area project very strongly to the T1 – T3 intermediolateral cell column (Holstege and Kuypers, 1982).

Projections to the intercostal motoneurons. As indicated on p. 310 – 311, the intercostal motoneurons in the upper thoracic cord are mainly inspiratory and at caudal thoracic levels expiratory. Physiological studies of Davies et al. (1985a,b) and Duffin and Lipski, (1987) have demonstrated that the inspiratory brainstem neurons in the ventrolateral solitary nucleus and in the area of the rostral retroambiguus/paraambiguus not only project to the phrenic nucleus, but also to the intercostal motoneurons. Moreover, Davies et al. (1985a,b) found inspiratory neurons, that project to both the phrenic and intercostal motoneurons. The ventrolateral solitary nucleus projects contralaterally

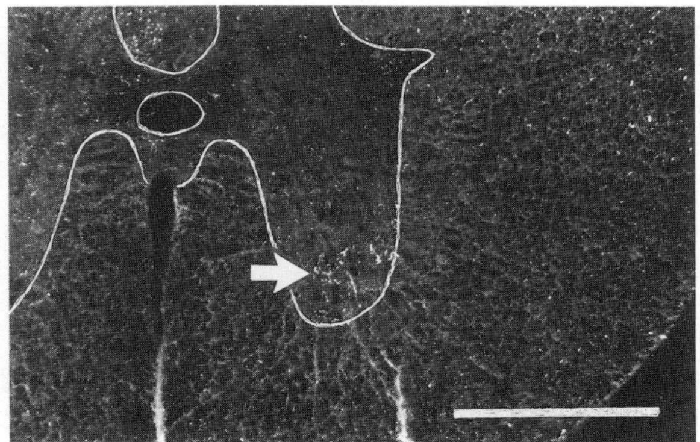

Fig. 25. Darkfield photomicrograph of a section through the T3 segment of the spinal cord in the cat, after a ^{3}H-leucine injection in the area of the lateral solitary nucleus on the left side. Note the projection in the contralateral ventral horn to motoneurons, probably innervating inspiratory intercostal muscles. Bar represents 1 mm.

to the upper thoracic ventral horn (Fig. 25) but fibers are scarce at mid-thoracic levels and absent beyond the level of T11 (Holstege, G. and Kuypers, 1982; Holstege, unpublished results). Merrill and Lipski, (1987) studied the retroambiguus projections to the external and internal intercostal motoneurons physiologically. They concluded that monosynaptic connections are rare (≈ 4%) and that most of them go via segmental interneurons, which would produce synchronized discharge of intercostal motoneurons. Anatomic tracing results of Holstege, G. and Kuypers, (1982) demonstrate that neurons in the area of the NRA just rostral to the obex project mainly contralaterally to large portions of the upper thoracic ventral horn, containing inter- and motoneurons. At caudal thoracic levels, however, the projections are very strong in the abdominal muscle motoneuronal cell groups. These projections are probably derived from expiratory neurons in the NRA. Projections from the Bötzinger complex to intercostal or abdominal muscle motoneurons were not observed, although Bongianni et al. (1988) have found inhibitory effects on the inspiratory external intercostal motoneurons, when they stimulated in the Bötzinger cell group. The dorsolateral pontine neurons, giving rise to specific projections to the phrenic nucleus, were not found to project to the inspiratory intercostal motoneurons (Holstege, unpublished results). The projections to the expiratory intercostal motoneurons are much more difficult to assess, because these motoneurons are intermingled with expiratory abdominal muscle motoneurons in the caudal thoracic cord. In all likelihood the expiratory intercostal motoneurons receive the same projections from the expiratory medullary neurons as the abdominal muscle motoneurons (see next section).

Projections to the cutaneus trunci, abdominal muscle and pelvic floor motor nuclei

Abdominal muscles not only play a role in the expiration phase of respiration, but also in straining of the abdomen in relation to coughing, vomiting, hiccups, parturition and defecation. Abdominal muscle motoneurons, located in the T5 to L3 spinal cord (see p. 310 – 311) receive strong monosynaptic afferent projections from the expiration related interneurons in the rostral as well as caudal parts of the NRA. Anatomic studies of Holstege, G. and Kuypers, (1982); Feldman et al. (1985) and Holstege G. (1989) show that the NRA gives rise to fibers, which cross the midline at the caudal medullary levels and travel via the contralateral ventral funiculus, to terminate on the somata and dendrites of the abdominal muscle motoneurons bilaterally, with a slight contralateral preponderance (Fig. 22). Holstege, G. (1989) and Holstege (unpublished observations) also observed that the caudal part of the rectus abdominis muscle motoneuronal cell column, which is located medial to the motoneurons innervating the other abdominal muscles (Holstege et al., 1987; Miller, 1987; Fig. 3), does not receive NRA projections. Apparently, the rectus abdominis muscle is not involved in abdominal straining related activities, which is in agreement with the finding of Ninane et al. (1988), that in the dog the rectus abdominis, unlike the other abdominal muscles, does not show phasic expiratory electromyographic (EMG) activity during respiration.

Thus, retrograde and anterograde tracing studies indicate that specific brainstem projections to the abdominal muscle motoneurons originate only in the NRA (from levels around the obex until C1). However, within the confines of the NRA neurons have different functions. Some are

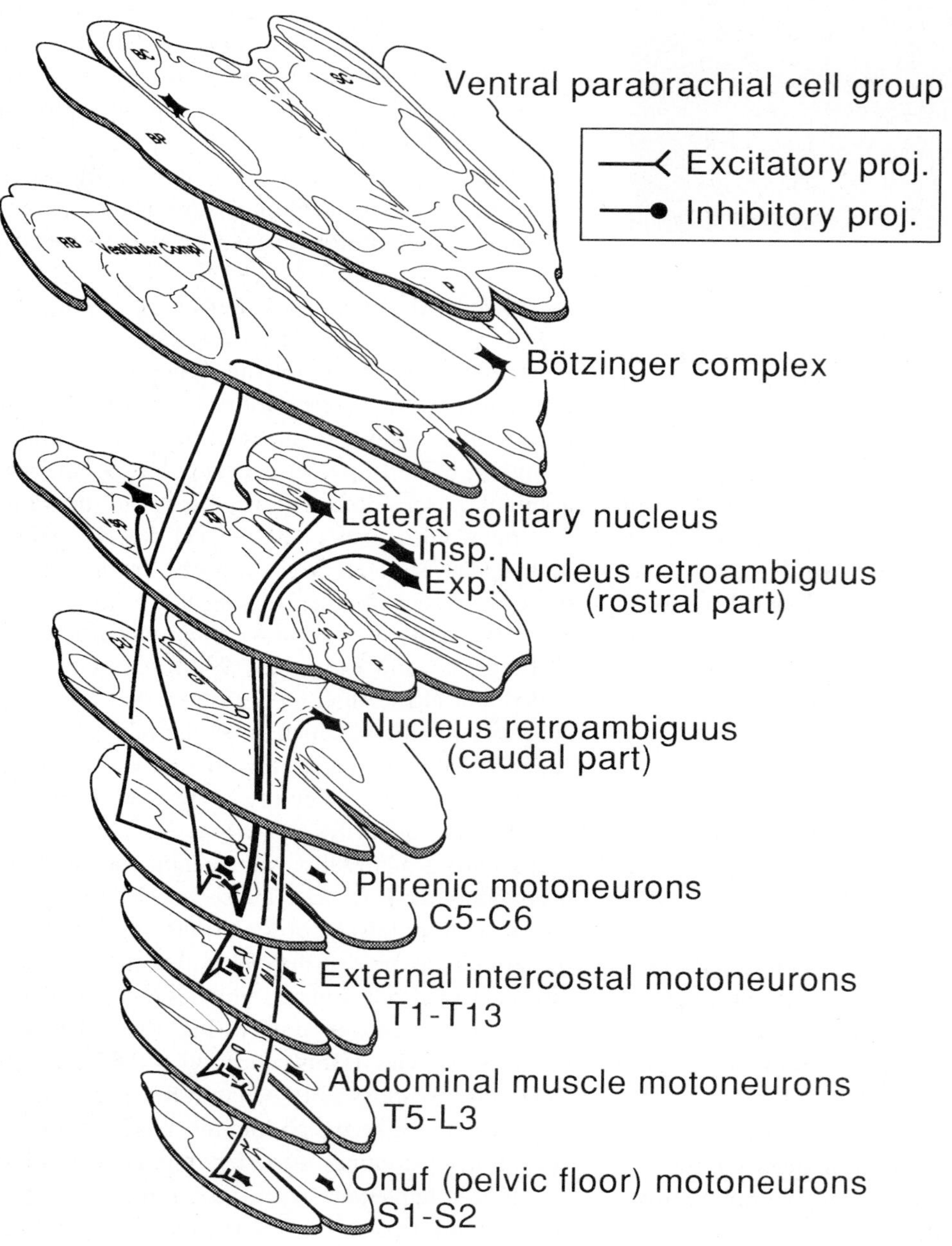

Fig. 26. Schematic overview of the pathways controlling respiration and abdominal pressure. Note that from the descending pathways originating in the medulla, only the contralateral ones are indicated, although there exist to a limited extent some ipsilateral pathways.

specifically involved in expiration and some others in vomiting and/or coughing or other abdominal straining activities. Only one third of the neurons seems to be active in more than one of these functions. The abdominal muscles also play a role in posture control. However, the supraspinal posture control areas are located in other parts of the brainstem (see p. 348 – 358) and do not involve the NRA.

The CTM motor nucleus also receives afferent fibers from the NRA, suggesting that the CTM is also involved in abdominal straining activities (Holstege and Blok, 1989; Fig. 14). Moreover, neurons in the ventral parabrachial nuclei and nucleus Kölliker-Fuse, which also send fibers to the ipsilateral phrenic nucleus and T1 – T3 intermediolateral cell column, project to the ipsilateral CTM motor nucleus (Holstege and Blok, 1989; Fig. 14). It remains to be determined whether the pontine projection to the CTM motor nucleus is respiration related.

A relatively small number of neurons in the most caudal portion of the caudal NRA project to the nucleus of Onuf, bilaterally but with a contralateral preponderance (Holstege and Tan, 1987). The involvement of the Onuf nucleus in this projection suggests that the pelvic floor also plays a role in abdominal straining and that neurons in the caudal NRA coordinates abdominal straining via direct projections to all abdominal wall muscle motoneurons, i.e. diaphragm, abdominal muscles and pelvic floor. Fig. 26 gives a schematic overview of the pathways controlling respiration and abdominal pressure.

Pathways involved in micturition control

The brainstem, via its long descending pathways to the sacral cord, is vital for coordinating muscle activity of bladder and bladder-sphincter, during normal micturition. The importance of the brainstem in micturition control is best shown by patients with spinal cord transection above the sacral level. They have great difficulty in emptying the bladder because of uncoordinated actions of the bladder and sphincter (detrusor-sphincter dyssynergia). Such disorders never occur in patients with neurologic lesions rostral to the pons, which indicates that the coordinatory neurons are located in the pontine tegmentum (Blaivas, 1982). Barrington showed as early as 1925 that these neurons are probably located in the dorsolateral part of the pontine tegmentum, because bilateral lesions in this area in the cat produced inability to empty the bladder. Later studies of Nathan and Smith (1958) supported this finding, which led to the concept that micturition can be considered as a spino-bulbo spinal reflex.

Recent anatomic studies in the rat (Loewy et al., 1979), opossum (Martin et al., 1979b); cat (Holstege et al., 1979; 1986c) and monkey (Westlund and Coulter, 1980) have shown that neurons in the dorsolateral pontine tegmentum, medial to the locus coeruleus, project directly and specifically to the sacral intermediolateral cell group (parasympathetic motoneurons) as well as to the sacral intermediomedial cell group, but not to the nucleus of Onuf (Fig. 27). The nucleus of Onuf receives specific projections from neurons in more lateral parts of the dorsolateral pontine tegmental field (Holstege et al., 1979; 1986c). The dorsolateral pontine tegmentum does not project to the sacral parasympathetic motoneurons (Fig. 27). In order to differentiate between the two different areas in the dorsolateral pons, Holstege et al. (1986c) called them the M- (medial) and L- (lateral) regions. The M-region probably corresponds with Barrington's (1925) area. Neither the M- nor the L-region projects to the lumbar intermediolateral (sympathetic) cell groups.

Electric stimulation in the M-region produces an immediate and sharp decrease in the urethral pressure and pelvic floor EMG, followed after about two seconds by a steep rise in the intravesical pressure (Holstege et al., 1986c), mimicking complete micturition (Fig. 28). The decrease in the urethral pressure cannot be caused by a direct M-region projection to the nucleus of Onuf, because such a projection does not exist (Holstege et al., 1979, 1986c). A study of Griffiths et al. (1989) suggests that the M- and L-regions may have

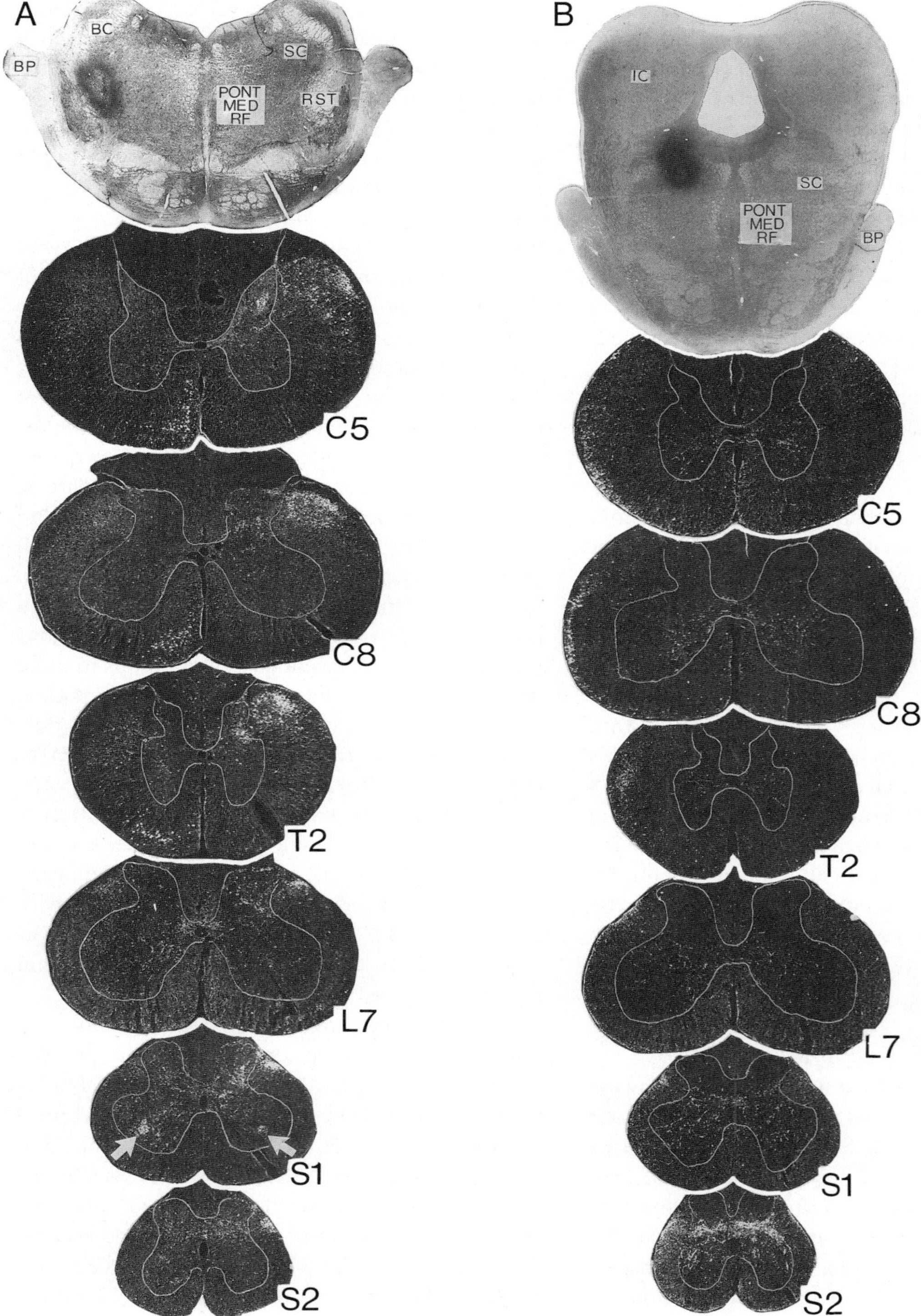
A
BC
SC
BP
PONT
MED
RF
RST
C5
C8
T2
L7
S1
S2
B
IC
SC
PONT
MED
RF
BP
C5
C8
T2
L7
S1
S2

reciprocal inhibitory connections. Stimulation in the L-region results in strong excitation of the pelvic floor musculature and an increase in the urethral pressure (Holstege et al., 1986c; Fig. 29). Bilateral lesions in the M-region result in a long period of urinary retention, during which detrusor activity is depressed and the bladder capacity increases. Bilateral lesions in the L-region give rise to inability to store urine. The urethral pressure decreases and due to absence of the inhibitory influence of the L-region on the M-region detrusor activity increases. The result is that the urine is expelled prematurely because of a combination of increased detrusor activity and decreased urethral pressure. Outside the episodes of detrusor activity the urethral pressure is not depressed below normal values (Griffiths et al. 1989). These observations suggest that during the filling phase the L-region has a continuous excitatory effect on the nucleus of Onuf, which inhibits urethral relaxation coupled with detrusor contraction. When micturition takes place, the M-region excites, via a direct pathway, the sacral parasympathetic motoneurons, but at the same time the M-region inhibits the L-region, which disinhibits sphincter relaxation so that micturition can take place.

Although patients with neurological lesions in the brain rostral to the pons never experience detrusor-sphincter dyssynergia, they suffer from lack of control of the initiation of micturition.

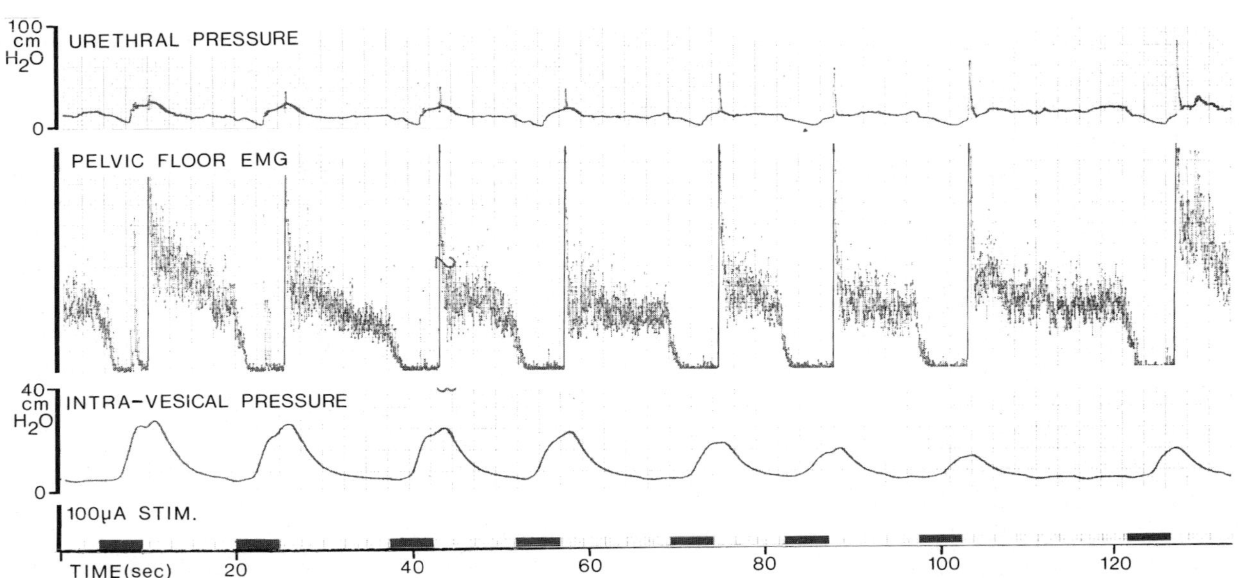

Fig. 28. Recordings of the urethral pressure, pelvic floor EMG, intravesical pressure, and stimulus timing during M-region stimulation in the cat. Note the immediate fall in urethral pressure and pelvic floor EMG after the beginning of the stimulus and the steep rise in the intravesical pressure about two seconds after the beginning of the stimulus. This pattern mimics complete micturition (from Holstege et al., 1986).

Fig. 27. Brightfield photomicrographs of autoradiographs showing the tritiated leucine injection areas and darkfield photomicrographs showing the spinal distributions of labeled fibers after an injection in the L-region (on the left) and after an injection in the M-region (on the right) in the cat. Note the pronounced projection to the nucleus of Onuf (arrows in the S1 segment) in the case with an injection in the L-region (left). Note also the dense distribution of labeled fibers to the sacral intermediolateral (parasympathetic motoneurons) and intermediomedial cell groups after an injection in the M-region (S2 segment on the right). Note further the contralateral pathway in the dorsolateral funiculus, terminating in lamina I, the outer part of II, and laminae V and VI throughout the length of the spinal cord (from Holstege et al., 1986).

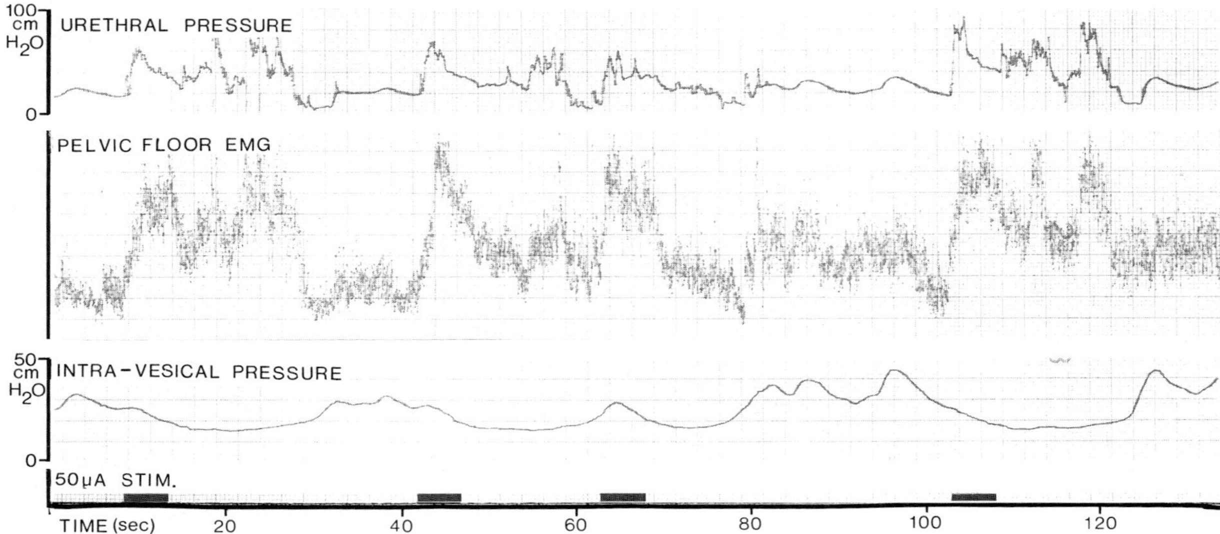

Fig. 29. Recordings of urethral pressure, pelvic floor EMG, intravesical pressure, and stimulus timing during L-region stimulation in the cat. At the beginning of each period of stimulation there is an immediate increase in the urethral pressure and the pelvic floor EMG. Note that the spontaneous detrusor contractions tend to be inhibited by the stimulation (from Holstege et al., 1986).

This raises the question of what determines the beginning of the micturition act. Obviously, precise information about the degree of bladder filling is conveyed to supraspinal levels, but specific sacral projections to the pontine micturition center have not been demonstrated. This suggests that other structures, rostral to the pontine micturition center, determine the initiation of micturition. Such structures would be expected to project specifically to the M-region of the pontine micturition center. Many clinical studies indicate that cortical (the medial frontal gyrus and anterior cingulate lobe) as well as subcortical structures (septum, preoptic region of the hypothalamus, and amygdala) are involved in control of the beginning of micturition. Experimentally, the only structure that has been demonstrated to project specifically to the M-region is the preoptic area in the cat (Holstege, 1987b; see p. 391). Stimulation in this area produces micturition-like contractions (Grossman and Wang, 1956), but it is not known whether it determines the beginning of micturition. It is possible that regions other than the preoptic area also project to the M-region. Furthermore, the fact that the pelvic floor, including the intrinsic external urethral sphincter, is under voluntary control, suggests that direct cortical projections to the nucleus of Onuf may exist. However, such projections have not been demonstrated convincingly. Figure 30 gives a schematic overview of the spinal and supraspinal structures involved in micturition control and their role in the neuronal framework of micturition.

Pathways specifically involved in cardiovascular control

The spinal cord motoneurons involved in cardiovascular control are the sympathetic motoneurons in the intermediolateral cell column (IML) (see p. 313 – 314). Afferent projections to these neurons originate in several parts of the medulla and pons. Strong afferent projections originate in the nucleus raphe magnus and pallidus, but these structures project diffusely to all parts of the spinal gray matter and not specifically to the IML. They are probably involved in level setting mechanisms of all spinal cord neurons (see p. 371 – 374). Physiological studies have indicated that the neurons specifically controlling cardiovascular functions are located in the ventrolateral part of the lateral tegmental field between inferior olive and facial nucleus. In several studies this area is referred to as the VLM (ventrolateral medulla), a large area extending from the level of the superior olivary nucleus to the most caudal extent of the lateral reticular nucleus. Although the whole area contains neurons which project to the IML (Loewy et al., 1981; Ross et al., 1984; Ciriello et al., 1986), the strongest projections are derived from an area in the rostral VLM, at the level of the caudal pole of the facial nucleus and just caudal to this nucleus. This area, some parts of which are located close to the ventrolateral surface of the medulla, is also called the subretrofacial nucleus. Subretrofacial neurons must not be mistaken by cells belonging to the Bötzinger complex, which are located in the retrofacial nucleus, dorsal and medial to the subretrofacial nucleus, and project to the phrenic nucleus (see p. 338 – 340). An injection of ^{3}H-leucine in this area shows thin labeled fibers descending in the lateral funiculus to terminate in the IML throughout its total length (T1 – L4) bilaterally, but at upper thoracic levels mainly ipsilaterally (Holstege, unpublished results; Fig. 31). The neurons in the subretrofacial nucleus take part in the rostral sympatho-excitatory VLM area, which is essential for the maintenance of the vasomotor tone and reflex regulation of the systemic arterial blood pressure (see Ciriello et al., 1986 for review). At least part of the cells in this area projecting to the IML contain substance P and phenylethanolamine *N*-methyltransferase, which catalyzes the synthesis of adrenalin (Lorenz et al., 1985). Lovick (1987) and Dampney and McAllen (1988) have shown that neurons in the rostral part of the subretrofacial nucleus project specifically to the IML neurons, innervating the kidney and adrenal medulla, while neurons in the caudal part of the subretrofacial nucleus innervate more caudal parts of the IML, with neurons innervating the hindlimb. Neurons in more caudal portions of the VLM, i.e. around the obex, have sympatho-inhibitory effects, probably by inhibiting neurons in the rostral VLM by means of release of noradrenalin (Ciriello et al., 1986).

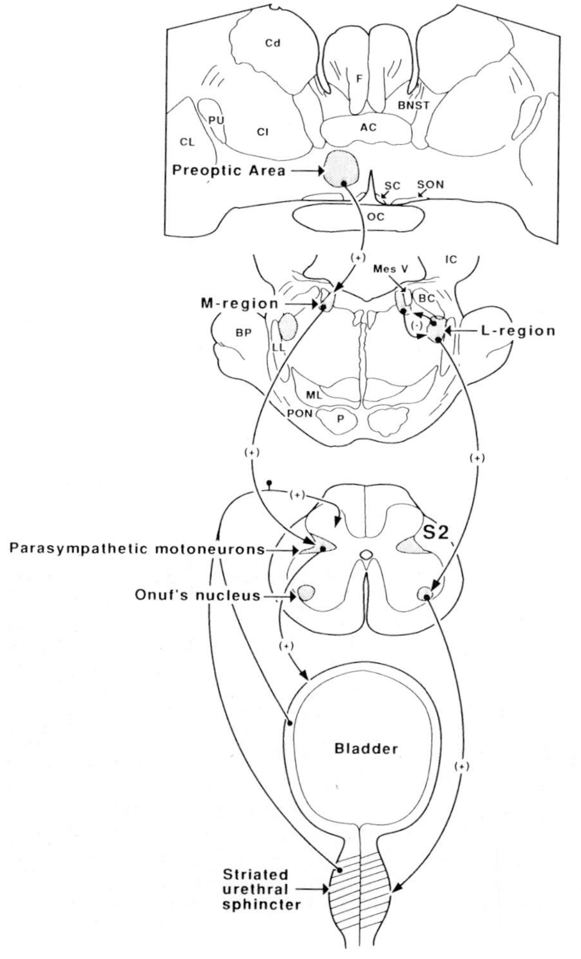

Fig. 30. Schematic representation of the spinal and supraspinal structures involved in micturition control. Excitatory pathways are indicated by "(+)", inhibitory projections by "(–)". (From Holstege and Griffiths, 1990).

Other bulbar areas projecting directly to the IML are the solitary nucleus (Loewy and Burton, 1978) and the lateral parabrachial nuclei and nucleus Kölliker-Fuse (Holstege, G. and Kuypers, 1982). The latter area projects specifically to the rostral (T1 – T3) portion of the IML, but the significance of these projections, and whether or not they play a role in cardiovascular control remains to be determined.

Descending pathways of somatic motor control systems

As pointed out earlier (p. 309 – 312) the somatic motoneurons in the cervical and lumbosacral enlargements of the spinal cord can be subdivided into lateral and medial columns. At upper cervical, thoracic and upper lumbar levels all motoneurons belong to the medial column. Motoneurons in the lateral motor column innervate the distal extremity muscles, i.e. the fore- and hindpaws in the cat (hands and feet in primates) and the distal portions of the fore- and hindlegs. Motoneurons in the medial column innervate proximal and axial musculature, such as muscles of neck, shoulder, trunk, hip and back. A similar mediolateral organization appears to exist in the propriospinal pathways (see p. 322) and in the descending pathways belonging to the somatic motor system. The medial motor column receives afferents mainly from cell groups in the brainstem which project via the ventral funiculus of the spinal cord (Petras, 1967; Holstege, G. and Kuypers, 1982a; Holstege, 1988b). They form the medial descending system. The lateral motor column receives its supraspinal fiber afferents mainly from red nucleus and cerebral motor cortex via the dorsolateral funiculus (lateral descending system) (Nyberg-Hansen and Brodal, 1964; Petras, 1967; Kuypers and Brinkman, 1970; Armand et al., 1985; Holstege, 1987; Holstege and Tan, 1988). They represent the lateral descending system.

The medial descending system

The function of the medial system is maintenance of erect posture (antigravity movements), integration of body and limbs, synergy of the whole limb and orientation of body and head (Kuypers, 1981). Within the medial system most of the proximal and axial muscles are simultaneously active, which explains why they are mutually connected via long propriospinal systems (see p. 323 – 325) and why supraspinal structures, projecting to inter- and motoneurons of the proximal and axial muscles are not clearly somatotopically organized. In order to control orientation of body and head, the medial system also determines the position of the eyes in space, which includes the position of the head on the trunk and the position of the eyes in the orbit. The following brainstem cell groups belong to the medial system: Field H of Forel, the interstitial nucleus of Cajal and surrounding reticular formation (INC-RF), the intermediate and deep layers of the superior colliculus, a cell group in the lateral PAG and adjacent tegmentum, the pontine and upper medullary

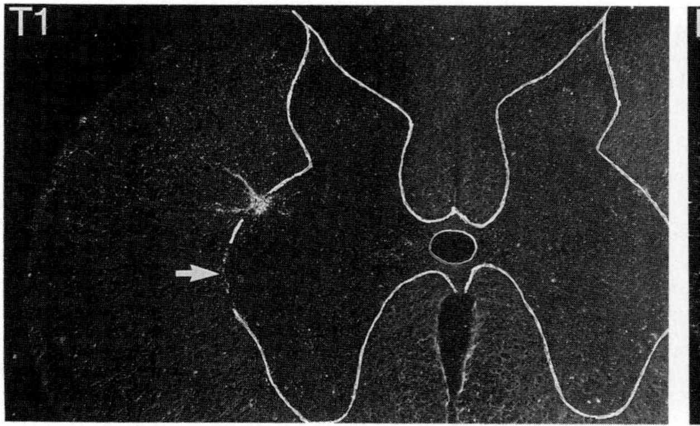

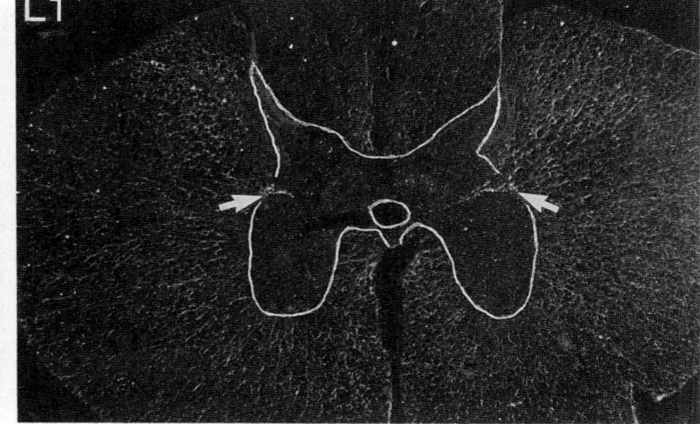

Fig. 31. Darkfield photomicrographs of a section through the T1 (left) and L1 (right) spinal segments after an injection of ^{3}H-leucine in the ventrolateral medulla (VLM) just caudal to the facial nucleus. The injection included the subretrofacial nucleus. Note the specific projections to the IML mainly ipsilaterally at T1, bilaterally at L1 (arrows). The arrow in T1 points to labeled fibers terminating on distal dendrites of the preganglionic motoneurons. Note also the specificity of the projection and the absence of other descending pathways.

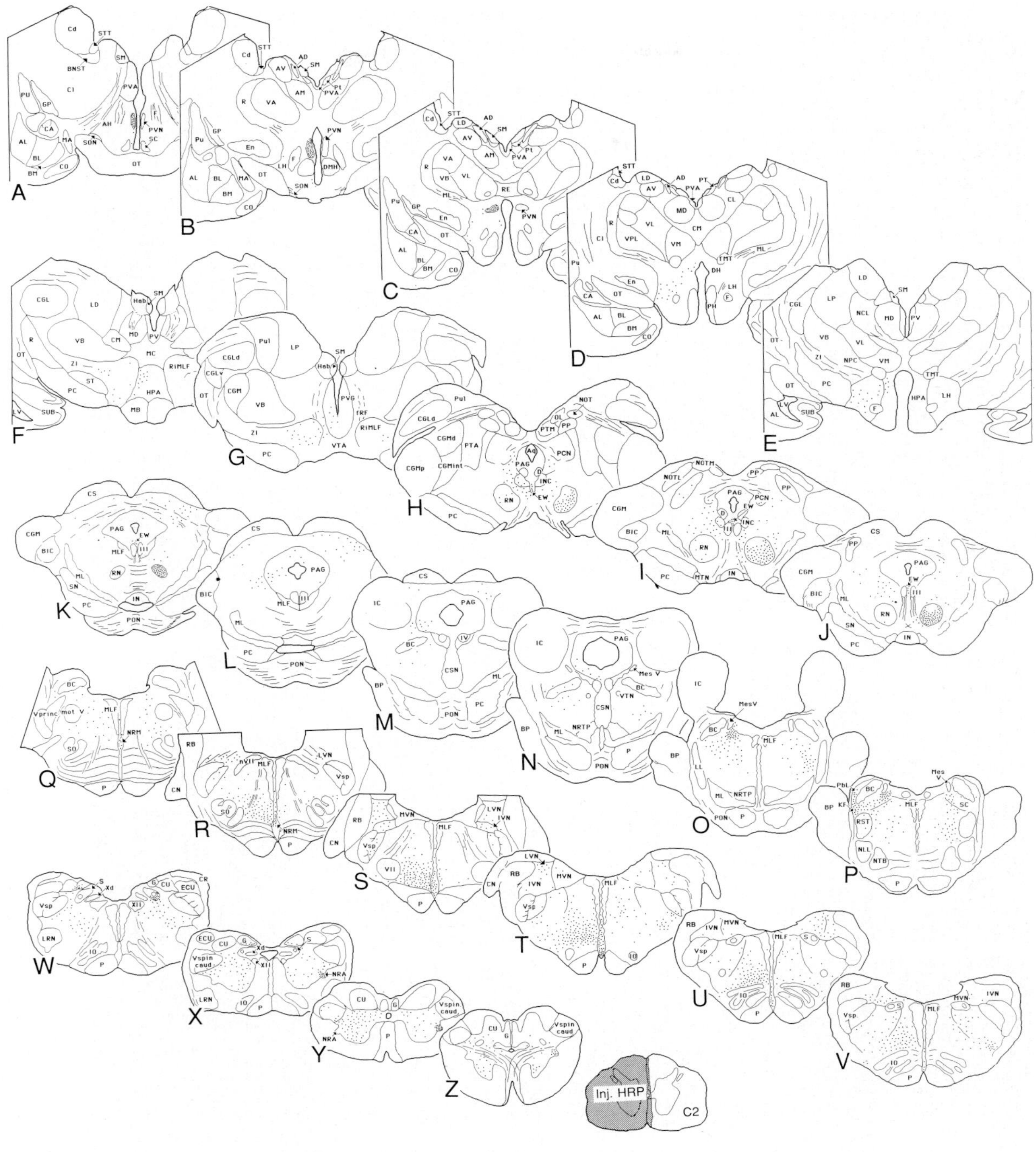

Fig. 32. Schematic representation of the distribution of the HRP labeled neurons in brainstem and diencephalon of the cat after hemi-infiltration of HRP in the C2 spinal cord. (From Holstege, 1988a).

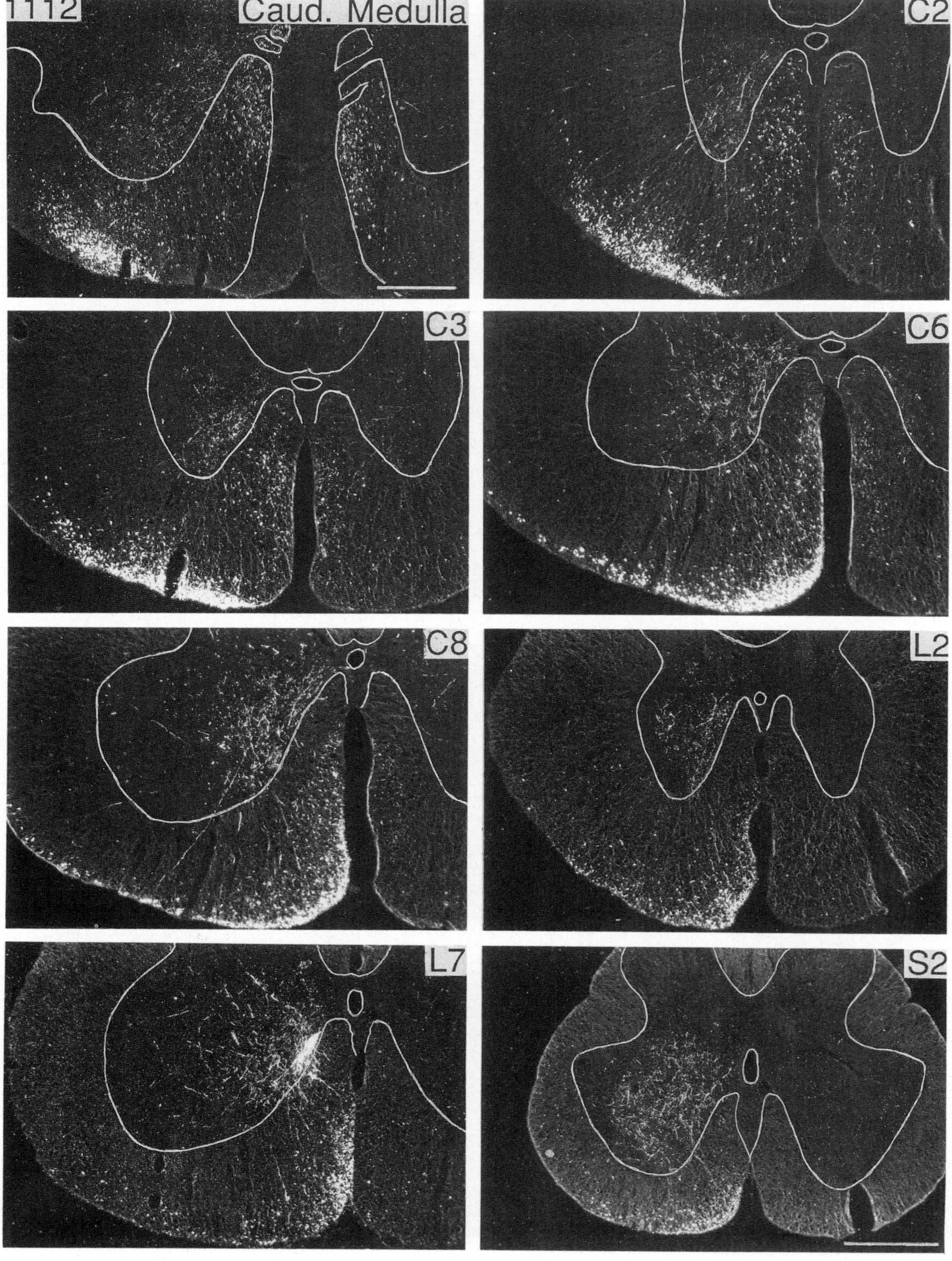
1112
Caud. Medulla
C2
C3
C6
C8
L2
L7
S2

medial tegmentum, a cell group in the contralateral medullary medial tegmental field and the lateral, medial and inferior vestibular nuclei (Fig. 32). They all project (directly or indirectly) to the oculomotor nuclei in the brainstem (see Büttner-Ennever and Büttner, 1988 for review) and to the neck muscle inter- and motoneurons in the first five cervical segments of the spinal cord (Fig. 38) (Holstege, 1988b).

Pathways involved in regulating axial and proximal body movements. Neurons in the pontine and upper medullary medial tegmentum and in the lateral vestibular nucleus (LVN) send a large number of fibers via the ventral funiculus to laminae VIII and the adjoining part of VII throughout the length of the spinal cord (Jones and Yang (1985) in the rat; Martin et al. (1979c) in the opossum; Nyberg-Hansen and Mascitti (1964); Nyberg-Hansen, (1965); Petras, (1967); Holstege, G. and Kuypers, (1982) and Holstege, (1988b) in the cat; Fig. 33). With respect to the neurotransmitters involved in the long reticulo- and vestibulospinal pathways, Kimura et al. (1981), utilizing a polyclonal antibody, reported that the large neurons in the pontine and medullary medial tegmentum and in the LVN were choline acetyl transferase (ChAT) positive, i.e. contained acetylcholine. On the other hand, Jones and Beaudet (1987) utilizing a monoclonal antibody did not find these neurons ChAT positive, but found that some other (smaller) neurons in the inferior and medial vestibular nuclei contained ChAT. Thus, it remains to be determined whether or not the long medially descending systems contain acetylcholine as a neurotransmitter.

The function of the long medially descending systems is nicely illustrated by experiments of Lawrence and Kuypers (1967a,b) in the monkey. They made, after pyramidotomy, (interruption of the corticospinal fibers at the level of the medulla oblongata), a bilateral lesion of the upper medullary medial tegmentum. The lesion not only destroyed the spinal cord projecting neurons in the upper medulla, but also interrupted all the fibers descending medially in the brainstem, e.g. the ponto-, tecto-, interstitio- and vestibulospinal fibers. Such lesions produced monkeys with postural changes of trunk and limbs, inability to right themselves, and a severe deficit in the steering of axial and proximal limb movements. On the other hand picking up pieces of food with the hand was considerably less impaired. Recovery was slow and when the animals were able to walk, they had great difficulty in avoiding obstacles and frequently veered from course. In the examining chair the animals had no problem to pick up pieces of food from a board with their hands and bring them to the mouth. Unlike the animals in which the medial system is intact, they did not orient themselves to the approaching food, but followed the food only with their eyes.

Pathways involved in regulating eye- and head movements. The medial system brainstem structures can be subdivided into cell groups steering vertical eye- and head movements and those steering horizontal eye- and head movements. Examples of the first group are the interstitial nucleus of Cajal and adjacent reticular formation (INC-RF) and Field H of Forel, which includes the rostral interstitital nucleus of the MLF (Büttner-Ennever et al., 1982; Holstege and Cowie, 1989). For the horizontal eye and head movements, the

Fig. 33. Darkfield photomicrographs of the caudal medulla and 7 different levels of the spinal cord in a cat with a ^{3}H-leucine injection in the vestibular complex (lateral vestibular nucleus, rostrodorsal portion of the inferior vestibular nucleus and cell group y). Note the heavily labeled lateral vestibulospinal tract fibers in the ventral part of the ipsilateral ventral funiculus gradually passing medially. Note also the medial vestibulospinal tract fibers on both sides in the dorsal part of the ventral funiculus on the cervical cord. Note further the dense projections to the medial part of the ipsilateral ventral horn throughout the length of the spinal cord and the very strong fiber terminations in a small area at the L7 level. This area contains many neurons projecting to the inferior olive (Armstrong and Schild, 1979). (From Holstege, 1988b).

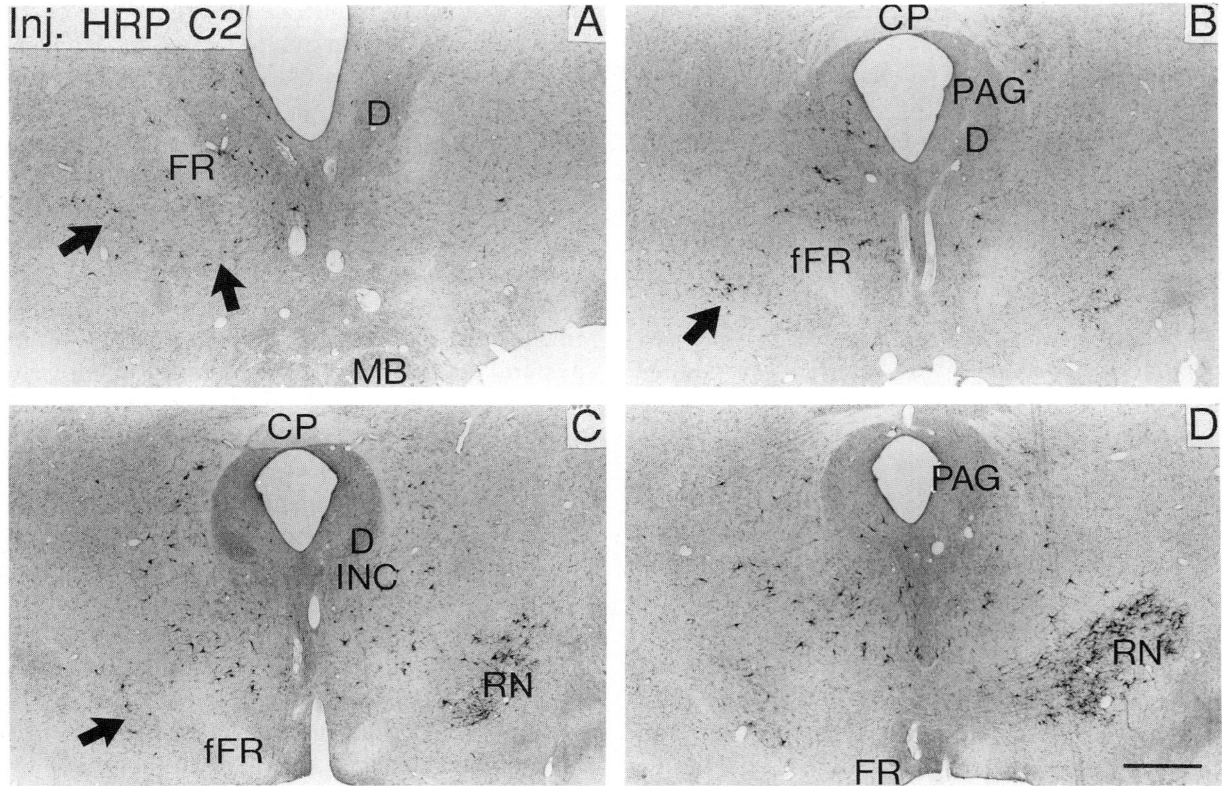

Fig. 34. Brightfield photomicrographs of transverse sections of the ventral part of the rostral mesencephalon in a cat with a left hemi-infiltration of HRP in the C2 spinal cord. Note the scattered HRP labeled neurons in the caudal Field H of Forel (arrows in A, B and C). Note also the many HRP labeled neurons in the reticular areas surrounding the INC in C and D. Many of these neurons are located contralaterally, but some of them may be labeled because the hemi-infiltration extended slightly into the contralateral ventral funiculus of the C2 segment. Note further the many labeled rubrospinal neurons on the contralateral side in B, C and D and one labeled neuron in A. Bar represents 1 mm. (From Holstege and Cowie, 1989).

superior colliculus and the pontine and medullary medial tegmental field are most important (Büttner-Ennever and Holstege, 1986).

Projections of Field H of Forel and interstitial nucleus of Cajal and surrounding areas (INC-RF). Neurons in Field H of Forel and interstitial nucleus of Cajal, projecting to the extra-ocular muscle motoneurons, are mainly located in the so-called rostral interstitial nucleus of the medial longitudinal fasciculus (riMLF), (Graybiel, 1977; Büttner-Ennever and Büttner, 1978), and in the interstitial nucleus of Cajal (INC), (Carpenter et al., 1970; Graybiel and Hartwieg, 1974). The major portion of the spinally projecting neurons are not located in the riMLF of INC proper but in adjacent areas, i.e. the ventral and lateral parts of the caudal third of the Field H of Forel and in the INC-RF (Zuk et al., 1983; Spence and Saint-Cyr, 1988; Holstege, 1988b; Holstege and Cowie, 1989; Figs. 32 and 34).

Neurons in caudal Field H of Forel project to the pontine and upper medullary medial tegmental field (Büttner-Ennever and Holstege, 1986), and via the ventral part of the ventral funiculus, to the lateral part of the upper cervical ventral horn (Holstege, 1988b; Holstege and Cowie, 1989; Fig. 35). This area contains the laterally located motoneuronal cell groups, innervating cleidomastoid, clavotrapezius and splenius muscles (see p. 308 – 309; Fig. 1). At lower cervical levels labeled fibers are distributed to the medial part of the ventral horn. Projections from the caudal Field H of Forel to thoracic or more caudal spinal levels are sparse (Holstege, 1988b; Holstege and Cowie, 1989).

Neurons in the INC-RF, together with a few neurons in the area of the nucleus of the posterior commissure, project bilaterally to the medial part of the upper cervical ventral horn, via the dorsal part of the ventral funiculus (Holstege, 1988b; Holstege and Cowie, 1989). This area includes motoneurons innervating prevertebral flexor muscles and some of the motoneurons of the biventer cervicis and complexus muscles (p. 308 – 309; Fig. 1). Further caudally, labeled fibers are distributed to the medial part of the ventral horn (laminae VIII and adjoining VII) similar to the

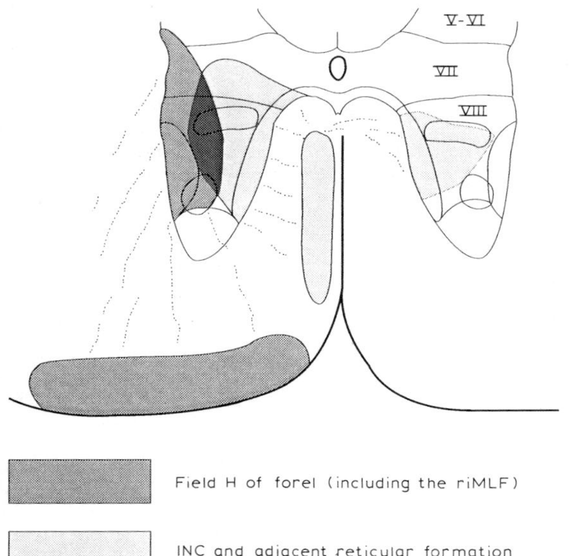

Fig. 35. Schematic drawing showing the pathways as well as the termination zones of the projections originating in caudal Field H of Forel and in the INC-RF. Note that the neurons in the caudal Field H of Forel project to more lateral parts of the ventral horn than the neurons of the INC-RF. Note also that the ventromedial nucleus (see Fig. 1) does not receive direct afferent connections from this part of the brainstem. (From Holstege and Cowie, 1989).

projections of Field H of Forel. A few INC-RF neurons project to low thoracic and lumbosacral levels (Holstege and Cowie, 1989).

Stimulation in the riMLF and adjacent areas produces vertical saccadic eye and fast head movements (Hassler, 1972; Büttner et al., 1977), and lesions in this area, including the H-field of Forel, result in vertical gaze paralysis (Büttner-Ennever et al., 1982; Brandt and Dieterich, 1987). On the other hand, stimulation in the INC-RF was shown to cause ocular torsion, head tilt and head rotation in the frontal plane to the ipsilateral side (Anderson, 1981; Fukushima et al., 1978). Unilateral electrolytic and kainic acid lesions and temporary (procaine) lesions in the INC-RF produce deficits in the vertical vestibulo-ocular and vestibulo-collic reflexes (Anderson, 1981), as well as head tilt to the opposite side (Hyde and Toczek, 1962). Bilateral lesions result in dorsiflexion of the head (Fukushima et al., 1978). These physiological observations suggest that the riMLF is primarily involved in eye and head movement control, while the INC-RF is mainly concerned with eye and head position. The differences in the spinal cord projections from these two areas may form the anatomic framework for the differences in neck muscle control.

Projections from the colliculus superior (CS). Retrograde tracing studies indicate that the neurons in the superior colliculus, projecting to the spinal cord, are mainly located in the lateral portion of its intermediate and deep layers on the contralateral side. Anterograde tracing studies (Nyberg-Hansen, 1964a; Petras, 1967; Coulter et al., 1979; Huerta and Harting, 1982; Holstege, 1988b) show that from the superior colliculus a stream of thick diameter fibers pass lateral and ventral to the PAG and cross the midline via the dorsal tegmental decussation. On the contralateral side the fibers descend in a medial position through the caudal mesencephalon, pons and medulla into the ventromedial funiculus of the spinal cord (Fig. 36), where they continue until the level of C4 and a few until C5 – C6. In the pons and medulla many

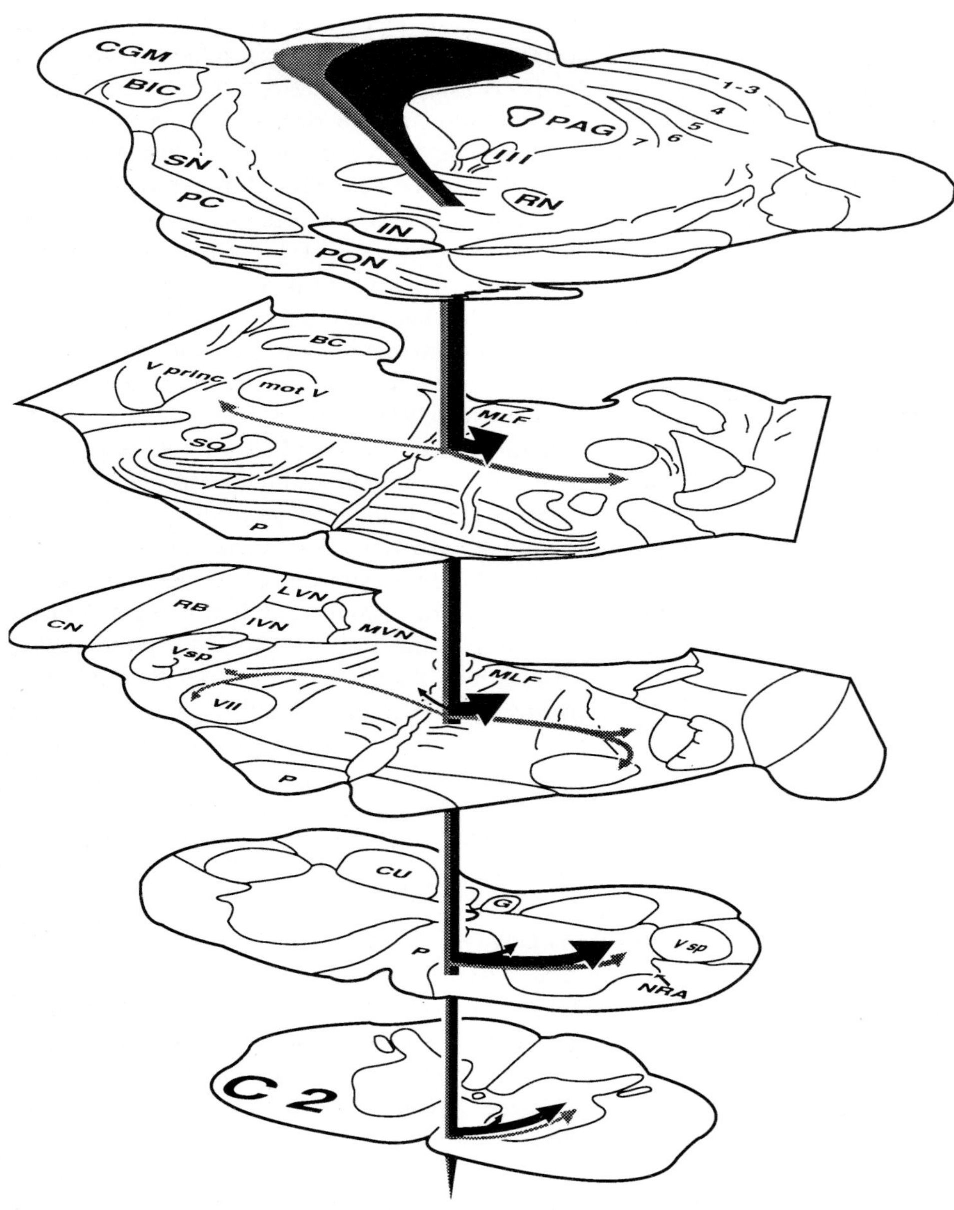

Fig. 36. Schematic drawing of the contralaterally descending pathways of the intermediate deep layers of the superior colliculus to the caudal brainstem. Note the strong projections to the dorsal two thirds of the contralateral pontine and medullary medial tegmental field and the small ipsilateral fiber distribution to this area, mainly at the level of the facial nucleus. Note also that at caudal medullary and upper cervical levels the main contralateral projection is to the lateral part of the intermediate zone, although there exists a small component terminating more medially. Furthermore, originating mainly in the lateral part of the superior colliculus, a specific component is indicated in gray, descending medially with the contralateral tecto-bulbo-spinal tract. The fibers of this component terminate in the lateral tegmental field and lateral facial subnuclei bilaterally, with an ipsilateral preponderance. (From Holstege and Cowie, 1990).

fibers terminate in the medial tegmental field and in the upper cervical cord in the lateral part of the intermediate zone (Fig. 36). The main projection in the spinal cord is on interneurons, which corresponds with the findings of Anderson et al. (1971) who reported disynaptic excitatory tectomotoneuronal projections and only a few monosynaptic ones. Cowie and Holstege (1991) have demonstrated that there exists a lateral component of this medially descending system, which projects to the lateral tegmental field of caudal pons and medulla (see p. 328 – 329) and to the lateral facial subnuclei (Holstege et al., 1984a; Fig. 36). Roucoux et al. (1980) found that stimulation of the anterior part of the CS evokes eye saccades, which were retinotopic and the accompanying head movements were slow and of small amplitude. At intermediate collicular levels CS stimulation produced goal directed eye saccades and synchronous head movements, which were fast and of large amplitude. At posterior collicular levels stimulation evoked goal directed head movements.

Spinal projections from the lateral periaqueductal gray (PAG) and adjacent mesencephalic tegmentum. Retrograde tracing results of Castiglioni et al. (1978) in the monkey, Martin et al. (1979c) in the opossum; Huerta and Harting (1982) and Holstege, (1988a,b) in the cat have demonstrated a spinally projecting group of neurons in the lateral PAG and adjacent mesencephalic tegmentum at levels caudal to the RN (Fig. 32 L, M). According to anterograde tracing studies of Martin et al. (1979c) and Holstege, (1988b), these neurons project to the spinal cord via the central tegmental tract into the ventral and ventrolateral funiculi of the spinal cord. Although some continue until the upper lumbar cord, they are sparse beyond the T3 level. A few descending labeled fibers are observed in the dorsolateral funiculus. At the level of the C1 segment labeled fibers terminate in the lateral part of the intermediate zone and the C2 – C4 levels in more central parts of it (Fig. 37). Further caudally labeled fibers terminate in the medial part of the ventral horn (laminae VIII and adjoining VII). Some labeled fibers, probably derived from the fibers descending in the dorsolateral funiculus, terminate in lamina X and the upper thoracic intermediolateral cell column (Fig. 37). It is not known whether this cell group is involved in eye and head movement control, but exactly this region has been shown to project to an eye movement related area of the central mesencephalic reticular formation (cMRF), (see Büttner-Ennever and Büttner, 1988). Furthermore, stimulation in this area produces horizontal conjugate saccadic eye movements, which are different from eye movements, elicited in the deep layers of the superior colliculus (Robinson, 1972 in the monkey, Collewijn, 1975 in the rabbit). Such an involvement of the PAG and adjacent tegmentum in eye and head movements is interesting, because this area receives its main afferents from limbic structures (Hopkins and Holstege, 1978; Holstege et al., 1985; Holstege, 1987). It implies that these neurons in the lateral PAG and adjacent mesencephalic tegmentum could provide an interaction between the limbic and oculomotor system, which does not occur at "immediate" premotor levels (Büttner-Ennever and Holstege, 1986).

Spinal projections from the pontine and medullary medial tegmentum.

It has been previously indicated (p. 348) that this area maintains long descending projections to the central and medial parts of the intermediate zone (laminae VII and VIII) of the spinal cord. However, at the level of the upper cervical cord, fibers terminate in the lateral and central parts (laminae V – VIII) of the ventral horn. The pontine and upper medullary medial tegmentum plays an important role in the oculomotor control system. The region includes the so-called paramedian pontine reticular formation (PPRF), which is a physiological entity, whose complete anatomic limits are still obscure. It contains many specific cell groups, such as long-lead bursters, short-lead bursters and omnipause neurons, all known to be essential for the generation of saccades (Raphan and Cohen, 1978; Fuchs et al., 1985; Büttner-

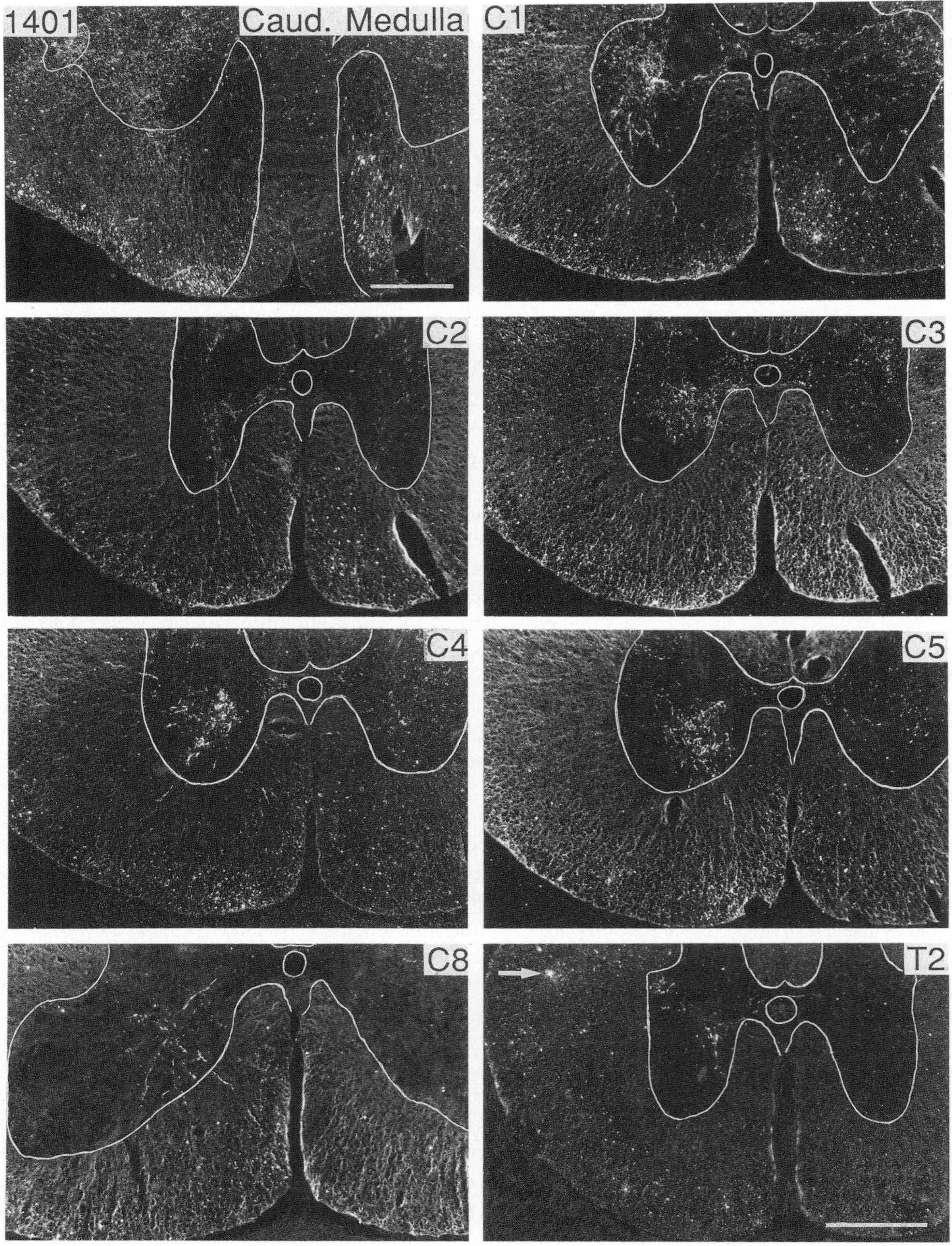
1401
Caud. Medulla
C1
C2
C3
C4
C5
C8
T2

Ennever and Büttner, 1988). The pontine and upper medullary projections to the upper cervical cord are similar to the spinal projections from other saccade related areas, such as the area of the rostral iMLF and the superior colliculus and all 3 regions have strong reciprocal connections (see Büttner-Ennever and Büttner, 1988 for review). Neurons in this region have been reported to receive afferent impulses from the labyrinth (Peterson et al., 1984), cerebellum (Eccles et al., 1975) and superior colliculus (Grantyn et al., 1980). Grantyn et al. (1987) also demonstrated that pontine reticulospinal neurons, on their way to the spinal cord, give off collaterals to the abducens nucleus, facial nucleus, nucleus prepositus hypoglossi and medial vestibular nucleus. This illustrates the close relationship between the oculomotor, neck and axial musculature control systems.

Retrograde tracing results (Holstege, 1988b) have revealed a cell group in the dorsal half of the contralateral medullary medial tegmentum at the level of the inferior olive (Fig. 32 T, U). Anterograde tracing studies of Büttner-Ennever and Holstege, (1986) and Holstege, (1988b) demonstrated that these neurons project through the contralateral ventral funiculus, but only until the level of C5. The fibers, which remain close to the ventral horn, terminate densely in the motoneuronal cell groups of the C1 – C4 segments. The impression was gained that this projection represents one of the strongest direct brainstem projections to neck muscle motoneurons.

The pontine and medullary medial tegmental projections have been extensively investigated physiologically by Peterson et al. (1978, 1979) and Peterson (1979, 1980), who subdivided the pontine and medullary medial tegmentum in 5 different zones. Holstege, (1988b), comparing the anatomic observations with the physiological results of Peterson, concluded that the anatomic tracing studies confirm some of the physiological "tracing" results of Peterson (1979, 1980), but many differences still exist and need to be resolved.

Spinal projections from the vestibular complex. On page 348 it has been indicated that the lateral vestibular nucleus and the pontine and upper medullary medial tegmentum maintain long descending projections to the central and medial parts of the intermediate zone (laminae VII and VIII) of the spinal cord. In the upper cervical cord, the later vestibulospinal tract (LVST) descends through the ventral part of the ipsilateral ventral funiculus. They terminate, unlike the fibers from the medial tegmentum, in the medial and central and not lateral parts of the ventral horn at the level of the upper cervical cord (Fig. 33). Two other bundles of vestibulospinal fibers descended via the ipsi- and contralateral MLF into the medial part of the upper cervical ventral funiculi (Nyberg-Hansen, 1964b; Nyberg-Hansen and Mascitti, 1964; Petras, 1967; Holstege and Kuypers, 1982 and Holstege, 1988b). They belong to the medial vestibulospinal tract, which originates in the lateral, medial and inferior vestibular nuclei. Medial vestibulospinal fibers terminate in the medial part of the ventral horn also. The contralateral medial vestibulospinal tract does not descend beyond cervical levels (Fig. 33). Whether the ipsilateral medial vestibulospinal tract descends beyond cervical levels is difficult to assess, because its fibers join the lateral vestibulospinal tract at low cervical levels. During their descent through the brainstem, the vestibulospinal fibers did not project significantly to the caudal pontine and

Fig. 37. Darkfield photomicrographs of the caudal medulla and 7 different levels of the spinal cord in a cat with an injection of ^{3}H-leucine involving the lateral PAG, the laterally adjoining mesencephalic tegmentum and deep layers of the superior colliculus. Note the ipsilateral fibers derived from the lateral PAG and adjoining tegmentum descending in the ventral and ventrolateral funiculi and terminating in the lateral part of the C1 and the central and/or medial parts of the C2 – T1 ventral horn. Note also the projection to lamina X and the upper thoracic intermediolateral cell column, derived from fibers descending in the dorsolateral funiculus (arrow in T2). Note further the tectospinal fibers in the contralateral ventral funiculus, distributing labeled fibers to the lateral (C1 – C3) or central (C4 – C5) parts of the intermediate zone. Bar represents 1 mm, (from Holstege, 1988b).

medullary medial tegmental field, which suggests that the last two areas have different functions within the medial system.

Stimulation in the lateral vestibular nucleus (LVN) produces mono- and polysynaptic excitatory postsynaptic potentials (EPSPs) in head extensor muscle motoneurons (Wilson and Yoshida, 1969a) and in back muscle motoneurons (Wilson et al., 1970). LVN stimulation also produces some monosynaptic EPSPs in hindlimb extensor muscles, but polysynaptic EPSPs are much more common (Grillner et al., 1970; Wilson and Yoshida, 1969a). Stimulation in the LVN also resulted in disynaptic inhibition of flexor muscles via Ia inhibitory interneurons located in the ventral part of the intermediate zone (Hultborn, 1976). On the other hand, stimulation in the MVN evokes monosynaptic inhibition of neck (Wilson and Yoshida, 1969b) and back motoneurons (Wilson et al., 1970). These inhibitory effects are mediated via the MVST (Akaike et al., 1973). In short, the LVST excites neck, axial and extensor muscle motoneurons and inhibits flexor muscles. The MVST inhibits neck- and axial muscle motoneurons.

Concluding remarks regarding the descending pathways involved in regulating head movements.

Fig. 38 gives an overview of the white matter location of all the descending pathways belonging to the medial descending system in the upper cervical and low thoracic spinal cord. Only the pontine medial tegmental field and the lateral vestibulospinal tract, and to a limited extent the interstitiospinal tract, descend throughout the length of the spinal cord.

At upper cervical levels, the INC-RF and the vestibular nuclei project mainly to the medial portion of the upper cervical intermediate zone, in which area the prevertebral muscle and some biventer cervicis and complexus muscle motoneurons are located (Abrahams and Keane, 1984; Fig. 1). These muscles may be specifically involved in head position, although until now such an involvement has only been described for the biventer cervicis, occipitoscapularis, semispinalis cervicis and rectus capitis (Richmond et al., 1985; Roucoux et al., 1985). In accordance with this concept, both INC-RF and vestibular nuclei are known to be strongly involved in eye position and head posture. On the other hand, the main spinal projection of the caudal Field H of Forel, superior colliculus, lateral PAG and adjacent tegmentum, and pontine medial tegmental field is to the lateral parts of the upper cervical ventral horn, which contains motoneurons innervating cleidomastoid, trapezius and splenius muscles. The latter group of muscles appear best suited to produce rapid or phasic torsional movements of the head such as might occur during orienting movements (Callister et al., 1987). It would correspond with the observation that stimulation in the caudal Field H of Forel, superior colliculus and pontine medial tegmental field produces eye saccades and fast head movements.

In summary, a concept is put forward (Holstege, 1988b) in which the medial somatic system structures are subdivided into two groups; one that controls tonic eye- and head position, and one that produces saccadic eye- and fast head movements.

The lateral descending system

The lateral component of the voluntary motor system produces independent flexion-biased movements of the extremities, in particular of the elbow and hand (Kuypers, 1981). The two most important constituents are the rubro- and corticospinal tracts. Vertebrates without extremities, such as snakes and sharks, do not have a rubro- or corticospinal tract, indicating that the presence of such tracts is related to the presence of limbs or limb like structures (Ten Donkelaar, 1988). Both red nucleus and motor cortex are somatotopically organized, containing regions such as a face area projecting to the face motor- and premotor neurons in caudal pons and medulla, an arm or foreleg area projecting to the cervical cord, and a hindleg portion sending fibers to the lumbosacral cord (Kuypers, 1981; Armand et al., 1985; Holstege, 1987a; Holstege and Tan, 1988). There are differences between the organization of the rubro- and corticospinal tract, which depend for an important part on the species involved.

The rubrobulbar and rubrospinal system. There are two different descending pathways from the red nucleus to the caudal brainstem; 1) a mainly contralateral pathway, which sends fibers to the premotor interneurons in the lateral tegmental field (p. 328–329), the dorsal column nuclei, precerebellar structures other than the inferior olive, and to the spinal cord; 2) an ipsilateral fiber system which terminates on neurons in the inferior olive. Many of the neurons in the red nucleus projecting via the contralateral rubrobulbospinal system are of large diameter and are located in the caudal portions of the red nucleus, while the rubro-olivary neurons are of smaller diameter and are located in the rostral parts of the red nucleus. The caudal part of the red nucleus is usually called magnocellular red nucleus, while the rostral part of the red nucleus is called parvocellular red nucleus. In the cat neurons projecting to both the spinal cord and inferior olive do not exist (Huisman et al., 1982). The subdivision in magno- and parvocellular red nucleus leads to confusion because in the cat the parvocellular (rostral) red nucleus not

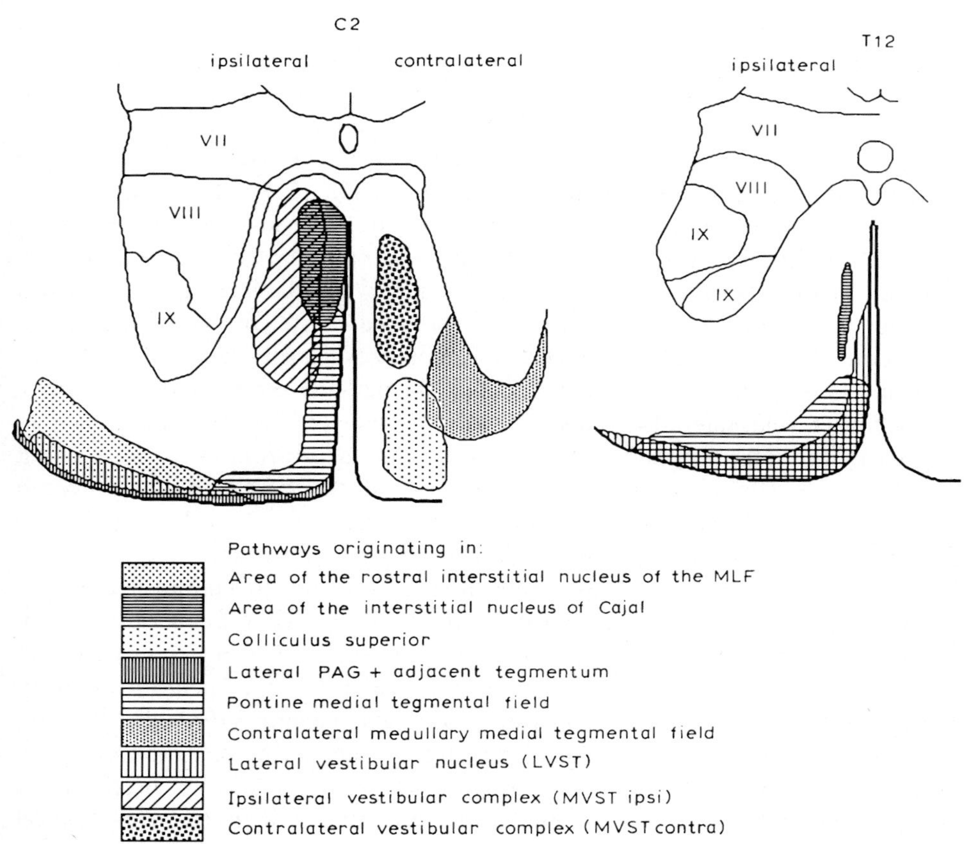

Fig. 38. Schematic representation of the spinal white matter location of the various descending pathways, specifically involved in control of neck and axial muscle inter- and motoneurons. On the left a drawing of the C2 spinal segment and on the right a drawing of the T12 spinal segment. It must be emphasized that this scheme does not give any indication about the number of fibers belonging to the different descending pathways. It must also be noted that many other descending fiber systems pass through the same areas as indicated in the drawing (for example propiospinal, reticulospinal and corticospinal fibers), (from Holstege, 1988b).

only contains neurons projecting to the inferior olive, but also neurons projecting to the spinal cord (Holstege and Tan, 1988). Furthermore there exist important species differences regarding the relation magnocellular-parvocellular red nucleus. Therefore, Holstege and Tan (1988) proposed a new subdivision of the red nucleus based on the projections of the neurons located in it: a rubrobulbospinal red nucleus and a rubro-olivary red nucleus. It must be emphasized that the rubro-olivary neurons form part of a much larger projection system, (see p. 336 – 365).

The rubrobulbospinal projections. The rubrobulbospinal red nucleus is somatotopically organized in such a way that neurons in its dorsal part project to the bulbar lateral tegmental field and facial nucleus (Kuypers et al., 1962; Martin et al., 1974; Holstege and Tan, 1988), neurons in the dorsomedial red nucleus project to the cervical cord and neurons in the ventrolateral red nucleus to the lumbosacral cord (Pompeiano and Brodal, 1957; Murray and Gurule, 1979; Huisman et al., 1982; Holstege and Tan, 1988). In accordance with the somatotopic organization, only very few red nucleus neurons project to both the cervical and lumbar cord (Huisman et al., 1982). All projections are contralateral except for a few ipsilaterally descending fibers, projecting to the intermediate zone of the cervical cord (Holstege, 1987a). The red nucleus also projects to the interpositus nucleus in the cerebellum (Huisman et al., 1982) and to some precerebellar structures in the caudal brainstem, such as the nucleus corporis pontobulbaris, lateral reticular nucleus and external cuneate nucleus (Edwards, 1972; Martin et al., 1974; Holstege and Tan, 1988). Furthermore, neurons in the dorsomedial (foreleg) part of the red nucleus send fibers to the cuneate nucleus, while neurons in the ventrolateral (hindleg) part of the red nucleus project to the gracile nucleus (Edwards, 1972; Martin et al., 1974; Holstege and Tan, 1988). It has been demonstrated that the projections to the interpositus nucleus are collaterals from rubrobulbospinal fibers (Huisman et al., 1982). In all likelihood, this is also true for the red nucleus projections to the precerebellar structures in the brainstem and dorsal column nuclei (see Anderson, 1971), which would correspond with the finding that the latter projections are somatotopically organized (Holstege and Tan, 1988).

In the spinal cord the rubrospinal fibers descend via the dorsolateral funiculus and terminate on interneurons in the lateral part of the intermediate zone (laminae V to VII) and to a limited extent directly to motoneurons. Interneurons receiving rubrospinal fibers receive afferents from other sources also, such as peripheral nerves, propriospinal neurons, and reticulo- and corticospinal tracts. Furthermore, rubrospinal fibers terminate on both first and last order interneurons (Hongo et al., 1969; see also Jankowska, 1988 for review). Apparently the red nucleus uses all the interneurons involved in the reflex pathways in the spinal cord (see p. 322 – 325). Rubrospinal fibers also terminate on interneurons in the upper cervical cord (Holstege et al., 1988b). Upper cervical motoneurons innervate the neckmuscles, which belong to the medial system. Although a red nucleus effect on neck muscles cannot be excluded, it is more likely that the great majority of these projections terminate on interneurons, which in turn project to motoneurons in the lower cervical cord, innervating distal muscles of the forelimb (Holstege, 1988b, see p. 309 – 310). The neurotransmitter utilized by the rubrospinal neurons is not precisely known. According to Kimura et al. (1981) all rubrospinal cells in the red nucleus contain choline acetyl transferase (ChAT), indicating that they use acetylcholine as a neurotransmitter. However, Jones and Beaudet (1987) did not find ChAT positive neurons in the red nucleus.

Although the red nucleus projections to motoneurons are mostly indirect, physiological studies in cat (Shapovalov and Karamyan, 1968) and monkey (Shapovalov et al., 1971; Shapovalov and Kurchavyi, 1974; Cheney, 1980; Cheney et al., 1988) have demonstrated direct red nucleus projections to spinal motoneurons. Anatomically however, there was only evidence for direct red nucleus projections to motoneurons in the facial nucleus (Courville, 1966; Edwards, 1972; Martin et al., 1974; Holstege et al., 1984a; Holstege and Tan, 1988). Only recently, Holstege (1987a; Fig. 39); Robinson et al. (1987) and McCurdy et al. (1987) demonstrated that the red nucleus in the cat projects directly to a specific group of motoneurons in the dorsolateral part of the C8 – T1 ventral horn, innervating forelimb digit muscles (see p. 309 – 310). One year later, Holstege et al. (1988; Figs. 40 and 41) at the light microscopical level and Ralston et al. (1988) at the electron microscopical level revealed rubro-motoneuronal projections in the monkey, which were more extensive than in the cat. These projections involved all distal limb muscle motoneuronal cell groups in the cervical and lumbosacral enlargements. Projections to the axial or proximal muscle motoneurons were never observed. The predominant population of rubromotoneuronal contacts were terminals containing rounded synaptic vesicles, forming asymmetric contacts with motoneuronal somata and primary dendrites. Only occasional terminals with flattened or pleomorphic vesicles were present (Ralston et al., 1988). Gibson et al. (1985) and Cheney et al. (1988) studied the red nucleus projections to flexors and extensor motoneurons of the wrist and fingers in the monkey and observed a strong preference for facilitation of extensor muscles (see also Cheney et al., this volume). Martin and Ghez, (1988) in the cat studied the differential contributions of the motor cortex and red nucleus neurons to the initiation of a targeted limb response and to the control of trajectory. They concluded that both the motor cortex and the red nucleus contributed to the initiation of the motor responses, but that only the motor cortex is involved in the proper scaling of targeted responses.

Direct red nucleus projections to the motoneurons in the intermediate subgroup of the facial nucleus (orbicularis oculi motoneurons) have been described by many authors, and a projection to the dorsal part of the dorsomedial facial subnucleus (pinna muscle motoneurons) by Cour-

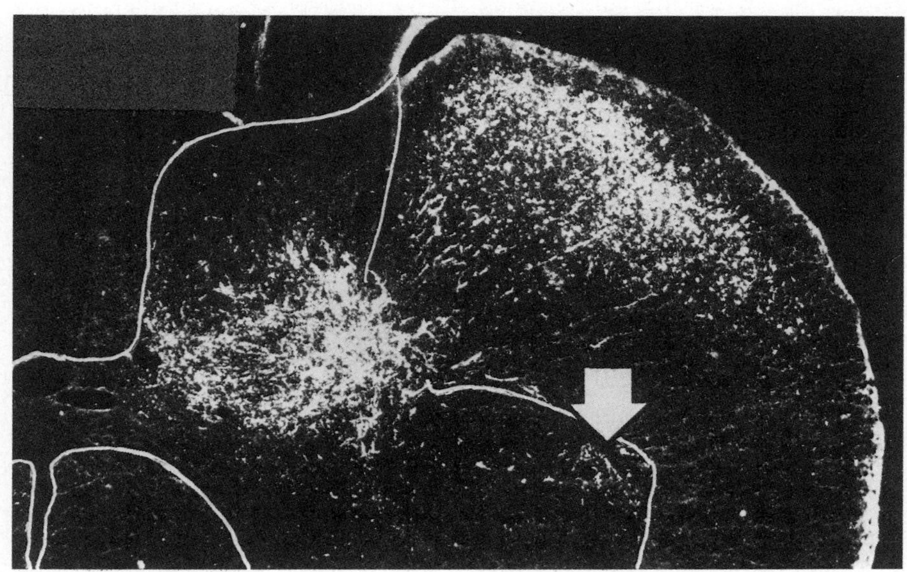

Fig. 39. Darkfield photomicrograph of the contralateral C8 spinal segment of a cat with an injection of ^{3}H-leucine in the dorsomedial (forepaw area) part of the rubrospinal red nucleus. Note the strong projections to the dorsal and lateral intermediate zone and the specific projection to the most dorsolateral portion of the motoneuronal cell group (arrow). (From Holstege, 1987).

C 3

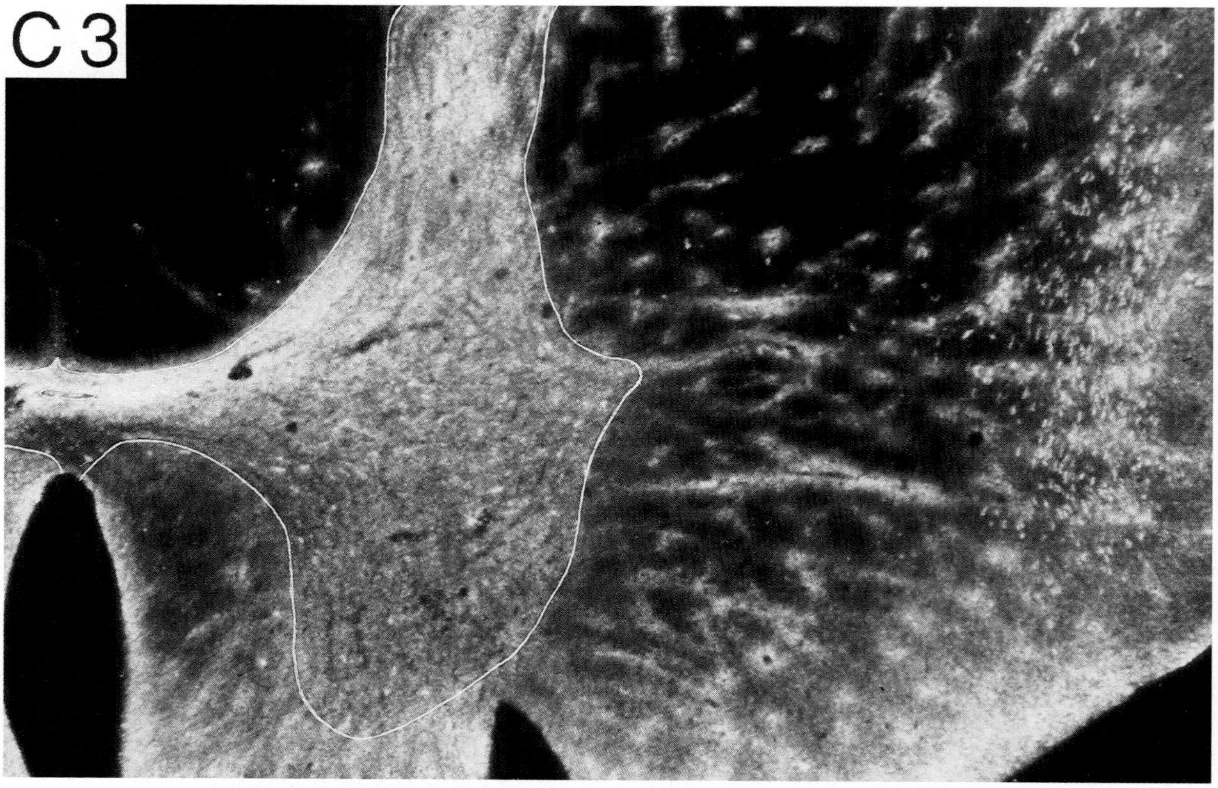

C 7

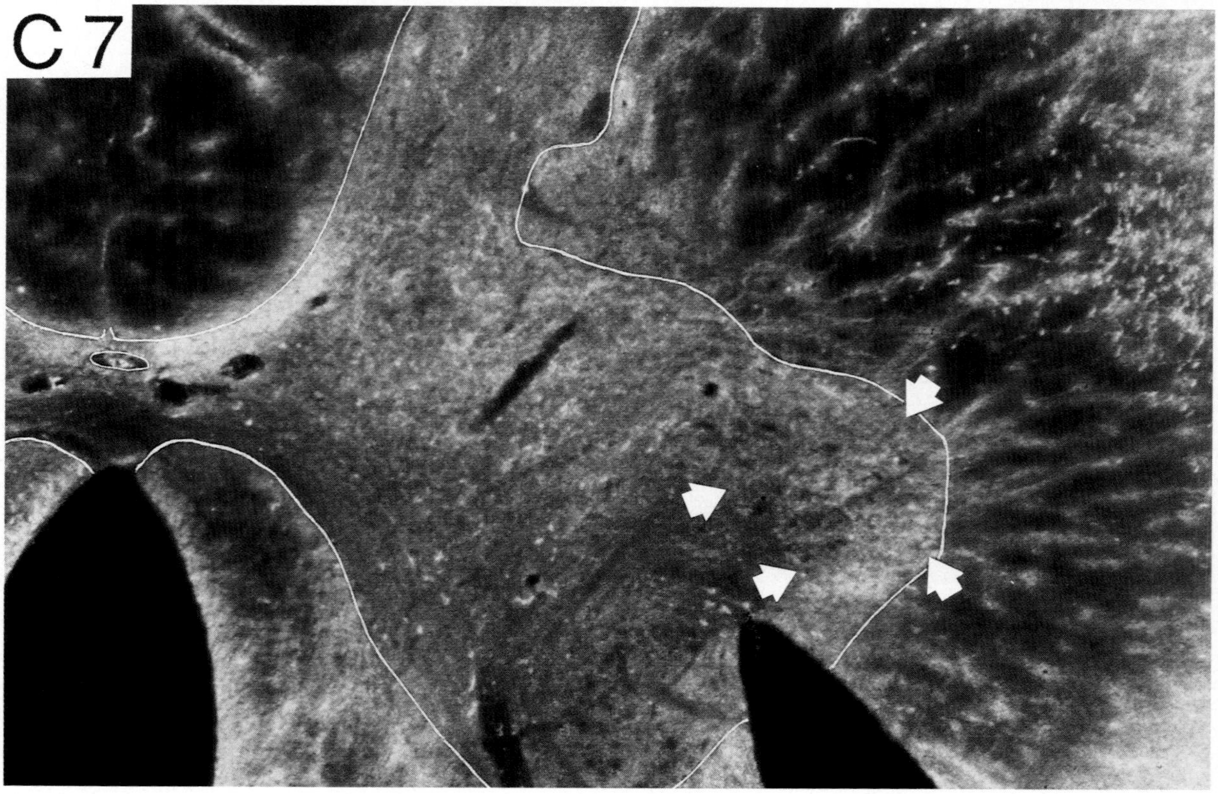

ville, (1966) and Holstege et al., (1984a). However, the literature is not clear about the red nucleus projections to the lateral facial subnuclei (containing peri-oral muscle motoneurons). Martin and Dom (1970) in the opossum, Edwards (1972) and Robinson et al. (1987) in the cat and Miller and Strominger (1973) in the monkey, have reported such projections, but Courville, (1966) and Holstege et al. (1984a) found only fibers of passage and no terminations in this motoneuronal cell group. In a recent study in the cat Holstege and Ralston (1989) at the electron microscopical level observed only occasional terminals in the peri-oral muscle motoneuronal cell group after large injections of WGA-HRP in the red nucleus. On the other hand, abundant terminals (at least 200 times as many as in the lateral and ventrolateral facial subnuclei) were present in the orbicularis oculi and pinna muscle motoneuronal cell groups, indicating that the red nucleus fibers observed among the peri-oral muscle motoneurons were fibers of passage. Fig. 42 gives an overview of the rubrobulbospinal projections.

The red nucleus may have a function in motor learning (Tsukahara, 1981). Schmied et al. (1988), studied the participation of the red nucleus in motor initiation, by training cats to release or not release a lever with its forepaw in response to a certain auditory signal, while other auditory signals were no-go cues. The results led them to propose that the red nucleus responses to a sensory signal depend on its triggering significance, and thus be modifiable by training. In this regard the role of the red nucleus in the conditioned blink reflex is interesting. The conditioned blink reflex or nictitating membrane response (NMR) is a learned response. When a neutral stimulus (visual or auditory) is repeatedly followed by an airpuff to the cornea, the animal will soon develop reflex blinking (i.e. NMR and closure of the eyelids) to the neutral stimulus alone. The reflex pathway goes via the trigeminal nucleus, inferior olive (Yeo et al., 1986), cerebellar cortex (lobule VI), (Yeo et al., 1985b), nucleus interpositus (Yeo et al., 1985a) and red nucleus to the orbicularis oculi and retractor bulbi motoneurons (Holstege et al., 1986a,b). In the latter pathway the pontine blink premotor area may also play a role (Holstege et al., 1986b). It has been demonstrated that lesioning the red nucleus abolishes the conditioned blink reflex (Rosenfield and Moore, 1983) and recently it has been reported that injecting GABA in the red nucleus has also this effect (Haley et al., 1988). The face area of the red nucleus not only receives afferents from the interpositus nucleus, but also directly from the trigeminal nuclei (Holstege et al., 1986b). These projections might be involved in the R2 component of the unconditioned blink reflex, in which the pontine blink premotor area may also be involved (see p. 331 – 333).

As the evolutionary scale is climbed, the rubrospinal red nucleus becomes smaller, and in humans only very few rubrospinal neurons seem to exist, which do not descend further than C3 (see Nathan and Smith, 1982 for review). The most likely reason for such a regression is the development of the corticospinal tract, which is extremely well developed in humans and might render the rubrospinal tract redundant (see Massion, 1988). It remains to be determined whether this is also true for the contralateral rubrobulbar projections.

The rubro-olivary projections. The rubro-olivary projections form part of a large mesencephalo-olivary projection system. In the cat, many neurons in the nucleus of Darkschewitsch, nucleus accessorius medialis of Bechterew, the area of the interstitial nucleus of Cajal, rostral red nucleus and Field H of Forel all contribute to the fiber projections to the inferior olive. Somewhat surprising is

Fig. 40. Darkfield color photographs of the C3 and C7 spinal cord of a monkey after an injection of WGA-HRP in the caudal red nucleus and adjacent areas. The pink labeling in the gray matter represents anterograde labeled rubrospinal fibers. Note that in C3 the rubrospinal fibers terminate in the intermediate zone only, while in C7 they terminate in the intermediate zone and in the dorsolateral motoneuronal cell groups innervating distal forelimb muscles, i.e. muscles involved in movements of wrist and digits.

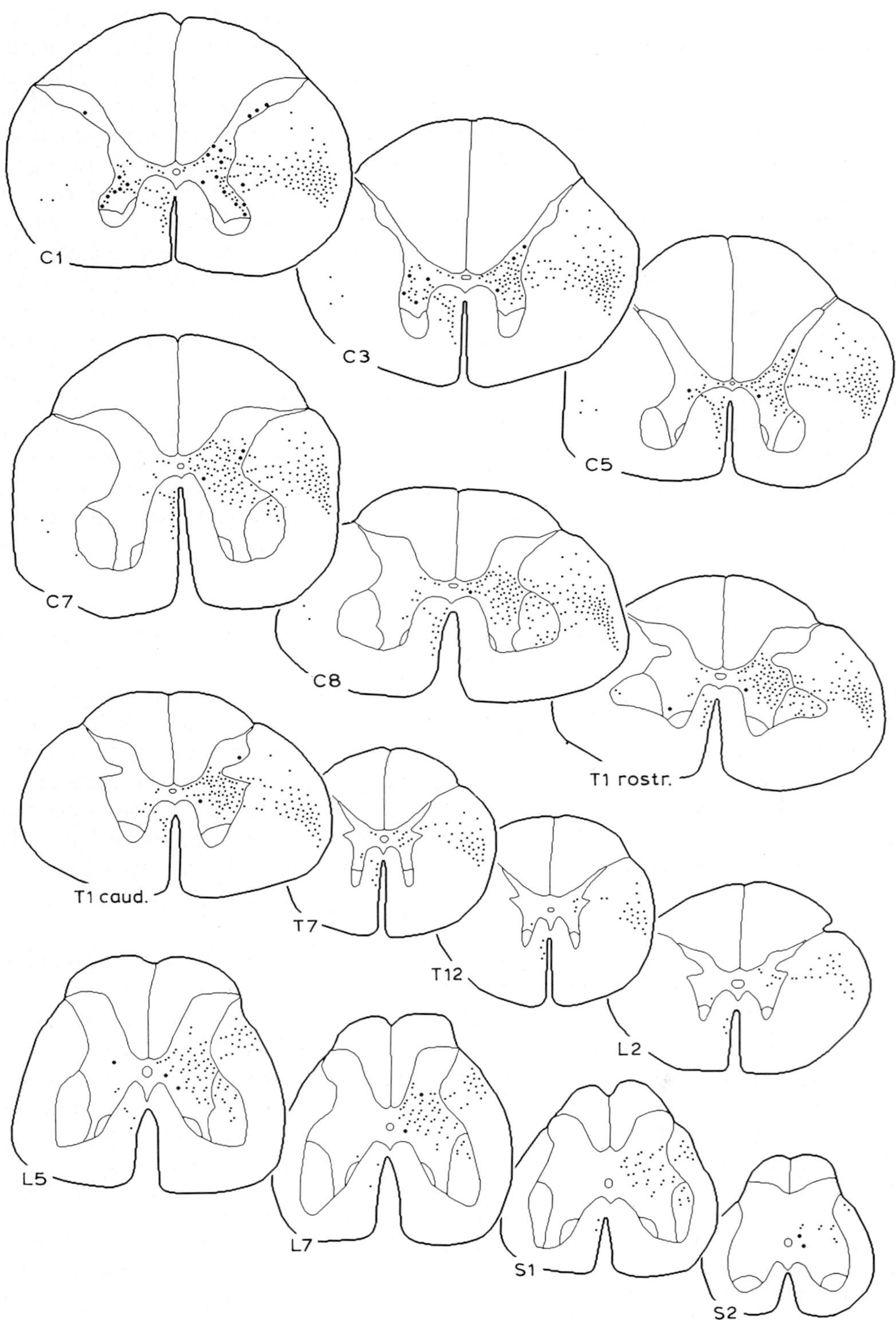
C1
C3
C5
C7
C8
T1 rostr.
T1 caud.
T7
T12
L2
L5
L7
S1
S2

that the termination pattern of all these structures is very similar (Saint-Cyr and Courville, 1982; Oka, 1988; Holstege and Tan, 1988; Fig. 43). Although the upper mesencephalic projections to the inferior olive, including the rubro-olivary ones, are already quite extensive in the cat, climbing the evolutionary scale to humans, the rubro-olivary red nucleus, its projections to the inferior olive via the central tegmental tract as well as the inferior olive itself becomes larger (Nathan and Smith, 1982). In all likelihood, this is due to the enormous growth of the cerebral cortex, because rubro-olivary projections play an important role in the relay cerebral cortex-cerebellum. According to Kuypers and Lawrence (1967) and Humphrey et al. (1984) in the monkey, both the rubrospinal and rubro-olivary neurons receive afferents from the precentral (motor) cortex. However, the cortical projection to the rubro-olivary neurons is much stronger and originates not only in the precentral gyrus, but also in the premotor and supplementary motor areas. It has been demonstrated (Gibson et al., 1985; Cheney et al., 1988) that the discharge of most rubrospinal neurons precedes the onset of movement. Part of this discharge might be elicited by cortical projections to the rubrobulbospinal neurons, which are partly collaterals of corticospinal fibers (Humphrey and Reitz, 1976). Another, (possibly stronger) source of input might be the projections from various motor and premotor cortical areas via the rubro-olivary neurons and the cerebellum, i.e. via the circuit rubro-olivary neurons-inferior olive-cerebellar cortex-deep cerebellar nuclei-rubrobulbospinal red nucleus. A similar pathway exists for the conditioned blink reflex (trigeminal nuclei-inferior olive-cerebellar cortex-deep cerebellar nuclei-face part of the rubrobulbospinal red nucleus). Such a concept, (the cortico-rubrospinal red nucleus projections go via the cerebellum) would provide the anatomic framework for the observation that the rubrospinal red nucleus is so heavily involved in conditioned motor responses (Schmiedt et al., 1988).

The corticobulbar and corticospinal system. The enormous outgrowth of the cerebral cortex in humans, compared to other mammals, is also reflected in the motor cortico-bulbospinal tract, which in primates but especially in humans is the most important descending pathway within the somatic motor system. The motor cortex is somatotopically organized with a foreleg area projecting to the cervical cord, a hindleg area projecting to the lumbosacral cord (Armand et al., 1985) and a face area projecting to the lateral tegmental field of caudal pons and medulla (Kuypers, 1958c; Holstege, unpublished results). In cat, monkey, apes, and humans the motor cortex not only projects mainly contralaterally to the laterally located interneurons in the spinal cord, but, in contrast to the red nucleus, also bilaterally to more medially located interneurons (lamina VIII). These projections are derived from the so-called common zone. In the cat this area is located in the medial part of the motor cortex next to area 6 and extends caudally between the fore- and hindleg areas (Armand and Kuypers, 1980). Stimulation in the area tends to carry the representations of axial movements, i.e. neck, trunk and proximal forelimb movements (Nieoullon and Rispal-Padel, 1976). Strictly speaking, this cortical projection system belongs to the medial descending system, but is presented together with the other corticospinal projections, because it represents a relatively small portion of the descending corticospinal tract. Not surprising-

Fig. 41. Schematic representation of the labeled fibers (small dots) in the spinal cord of a monkey with an injection of WGA-HRP in the rubrospinal red nucleus. The injection-site extended into the area of the interstitial nucleus of Cajal (INC-RF). The retrogradely labeled neurons are indicated with large dots. Note the contralateral projections to the intermediate zone throughout the length of the spinal cord and to the lateral motoneuronal cell groups in the cervical and lumbosacral enlargements. Note also the ipsilateral (interstitiospinal) fibers in the ventral funiculus on the ipsilateral side. Note further the very few ipsilateral rubrospinal fibers, some of which terminate in the lateral motoneuronal cell groups in rostral T1, (from Holstege et al. 1988).

ly, neurons in the common zone, possibly via collaterals of the corticospinal fibers, project to the pontine and upper medullary medial tegmental field, one of the most important parts of the medially descending system (see p. 355 – 357).

In the monkey (Kuypers, 1958b; Ralston and Ralston, 1985), but not in the cat (Armand et al., 1985) there exist direct cortical projections to

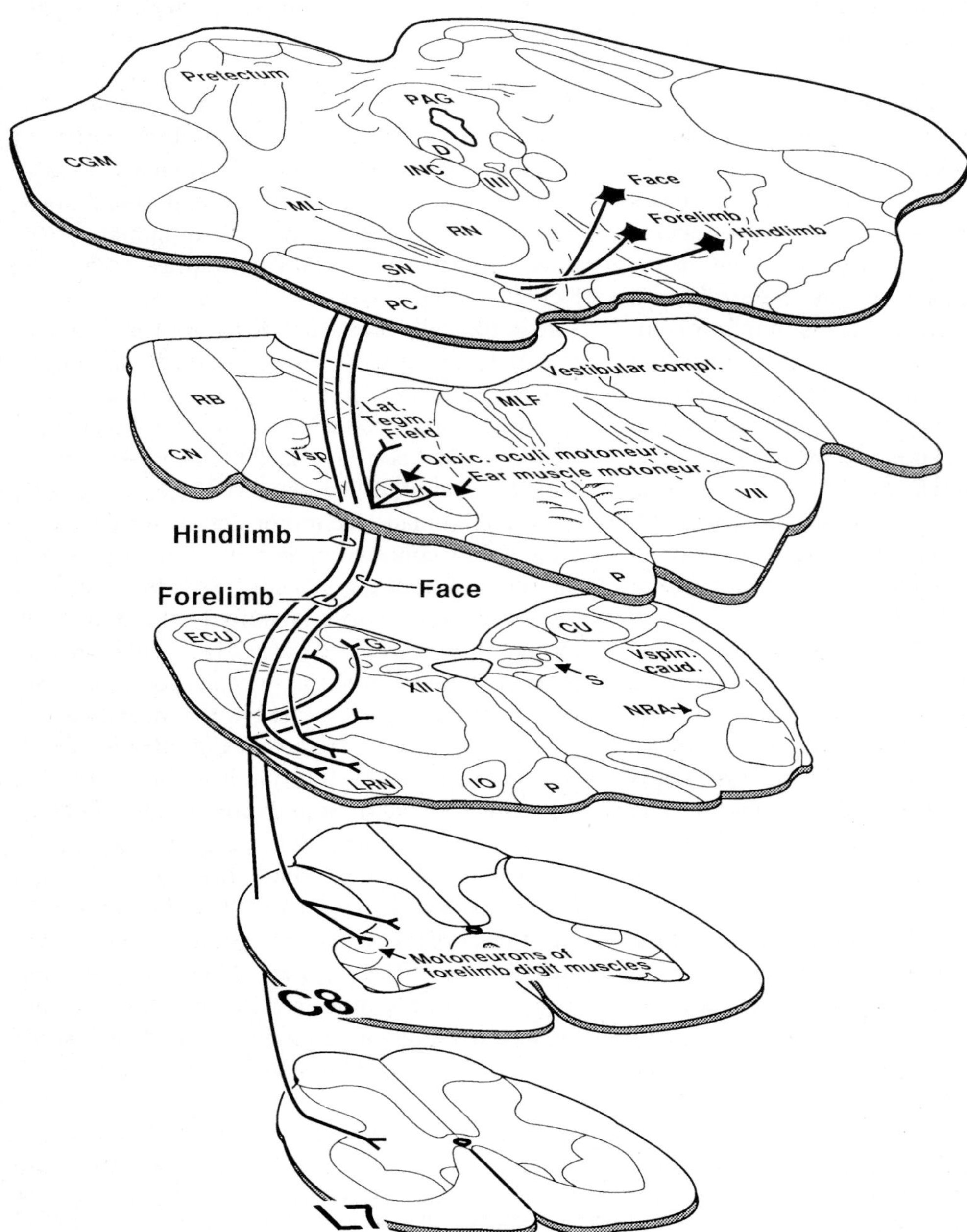

Fig. 42. Schematic overview of the rubrobulbospinal projections in the cat. In the monkey the rubrobulbospinal projections are almost identical, with the exception of more extensive projections to the motoneuronal cell groups.

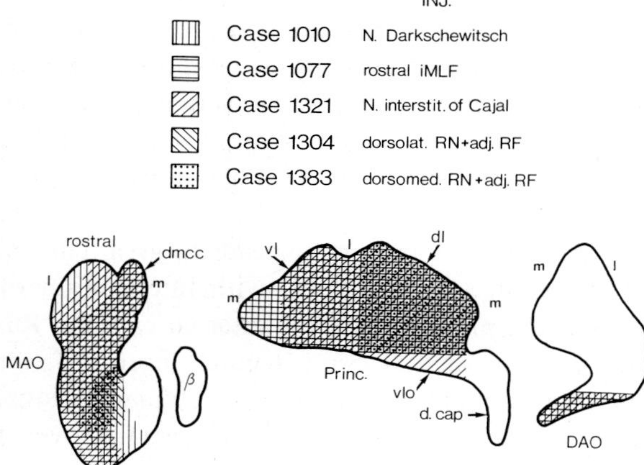

Fig. 43. Schematic diagram of the unfolded inferior olive after Brodal (1940), illustrating the extent of the projections of the rostral mesencephalon. Note the strong overlap of the fiber distributions in the cases with injections of ^{3}H-leucine in the rostral iMLF and Field H of Forel (case 1077), the nucleus of Darkschewitsch and the INC-RF. Note the relatively small contribution of the more caudally located injection sites (cases 1304 and 1383). Injections in the most caudal portion of the red nucleus did not produce labeling in the inferior olive. (From Holstege and Tan, 1988). l = lateral; m = medial; MAO = medial accessory olive; dmcc = dorsomedial cell column; β = nucleus Beta; vl = ventrolateral; dl = dorsolateral; Princ. = principal inferior olive; vlo = ventrolateral outgrowth; d. cap = dorsal cap; DAO = dorsal accessory olive.

motoneurons, innervating the most distal muscles of the extremities. Ralston and Ralston (1985) found electron microscopically that two thirds of the corticomotoneuronal terminals contained round vesicles, suggesting excitatory effects on the motoneuron, and one third pleomorphic or flattened vesicles, suggesting inhibitory effects. It is questionable, however, whether there exist monosynaptic inhibitory corticomotoneuronal connections, but disynaptic connections have been demonstrated (Landgren et al., 1962; see also Cheney et al., this volume, Chapter 11). Jankowska et al., (1975), stimulating the motor cortex in monkeys, observed EPSPs with response latencies of 0.6 – 1.0 ms, indicating monosynaptic contact. The rubro- and corticospinal tract in the monkey are very similar, but there are some differences; 1) the motor cortex projects also to more medial parts of the intermediate zone; 2) corticospinal fibers are at least 100 times more numerous than the rubrospinal ones (Holstege et al., 1988). For the differences between the cortico-motoneuronal and rubro-motoneuronal cells, see Cheney et al. (this volume). In chimpanzees and humans direct cortico-motoneuronal projections are more extensive than in the monkey and terminate also on motoneurons, innervating more proximal muscles of the body (Kuypers, 1958a,b; Schoen, 1964). However, the degeneration findings of Kuypers, 1964 and Schoen, 1964, do not reveal corticospinal projections to the medial motoneuronal cell column in chimpanzee and human. It is possible that more modern tracing techniques in the chimpanzee would reveal direct cortical projections to medial column motoneurons, but such studies have not yet been done. Since the corticospinal and

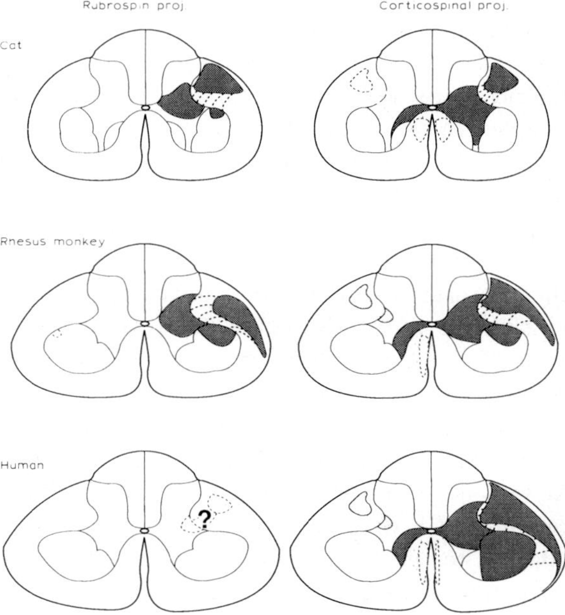

Fig. 44. Schematic representation of the rubrospinal and corticospinal projections in the cat, rhesus monkey and human at the level of C8. The gray areas in the white matter represent the descending pathways, those in the gray matter represent termination zones. Dark gray areas represent strong projections, lighter gray areas represent light projections.

rubrospinal systems are so similar, it is not surprising that collaterals of the corticospinal tract terminate in the magnocellular red nucleus in a somatotopically organized manner (Kuypers, 1981; Holstege, unpublished observations).

Behavioral studies on the lateral system of Lawrence and Kuypers (1967a,b) in the monkey have demonstrated that immediately after pyramidotomy, (interruption of the corticospinal fibers at the level of the medulla oblongata), the animals can sit, walk, run and climb, but cannot pick up pieces of food with their hands. After some recovery they regain this capacity, but individual finger movements such as the thumb and index finger precision grip do not return. In pyramidotomized monkeys, the red nucleus as well as the cortico-rubral fibers are still intact and the recovery of hand movements is probably related to the rubrospinal tract taking over many of the functions of the corticospinal tract. Ablation of the precentral motor cortex in adult monkeys, (thus lesioning the corticospinal as well as the corticorubral fibers) results in a stronger deficit, i.e. a flaccid paresis of the contralateral extremity muscles. In chimpanzee and humans (patients with stroke or tumor interrupting the corticobulbospinal fibers) this flaccid paresis is more severe than in monkeys and much more than in cats. The reason for this difference probably is that the rubrospinal neurons in monkey and cat are much more numerous than in chimpanzee and humans. Correspondingly, if in a monkey a bilateral pyramidotomy is combined with an interruption of the rubrospinal tract on one side, the motor deficit on that side is much more pronounced. The monkey is able to sit up, walk and climb, but in the examining chair the fingers and wrist of the arm ipsilateral to the side of the rubrospinal lesion are noticeably limp. In reaching for food, the hand is brought to the food by turning the arm in the shoulder.

Fig. 44 gives a summary on the rubro- and corticospinal pathways, based on the findings of Kuypers, 1964; Schoen, 1964; Kuypers and Brinkman, 1970; Kuypers, 1973; Kuypers, 1981; Ralston and Ralston, 1985; Armand et al., 1985; Holstege, 1987a; Holstege et al., 1988. The corticospinal fibers become more and more numerous and control larger parts of the spinal gray, going from cat, via monkey to human, which is not true for the rubrospinal tract. The enormous predominance of the corticospinal tract over the rubrospinal tract in humans leads to great clinical problems in stroke patients with interruption of the corticospinal tract in the internal capsule. Recovery from such a lesion is much more difficult than in monkeys or cats with similar lesions, because humans do not have the disposal over a well developed rubrospinal tract.

Descending patways involved in limbic motor control systems

Introduction

It is well known that hemiplegic patients with damage to corticobulbar fibers, resulting in a complete central paresis of the lower face on one side, are able to smile spontaneously, for example when they enjoy a joke. On the other hand, in cases with postencephalitic parkinsonism, patients are able to show their teeth, whistle, frown, i.e. there is no facial palsy, but the patients' emotions are not reflected in their countenance and they have a stiff, masklike facial expression (poker face). Patients with irritative pontine lesions sometimes suffer from non-emotional laughter and crying, and patients with pseudo-bulbar palsy (for example with lesions in the mesencephalon) often suffer from uncontrollable fits of crying or laughter. Such fits are usually devoid of feeling of grief, joy, or amusement; they may even be accompanied by entirely incompatible emotions. Fits of crying and laughter may occur in the same patients, other patients show only one of them (Poeck, 1969; Rinn, 1984). Crying and laughter belong to an expressive behavior, which in animals is called vocalization. It has been shown in many different species that stimulation in the caudal part of the periaqueductal gray (PAG) produces vocalization. Recently Holstege, G. (1989) has demonstrated that vocalization is based on a specific final common pathway, originating from a distinct group of neurons in the PAG that project to the nucleus retroambiguus, which in turn has direct access to all vocalization motoneurons (see p. 382 – 383; see Holstege, G., 1989). In all likelihood, in humans this projection forms the anatomical framework for laughing and crying. The vocalization neurons in the PAG receive their afferents from structures belonging to the limbic system, but not from the voluntary system (see previous section). All this clinical and experimental evidence shows that there exists a complete dissociation between the voluntary and emotional or limbic innervation of motoneurons.

The limbic system is closely involved in the elaboration of emotional experience and expression (MacLean, 1952) and is associated with a wide variety of autonomic, visceral and endocrine functions. The limbic system consists of several cortical and subcortical structures, although there is no agreement on exactly which structures belong to it. Some authors argue that the use of the term limbic system should be abandoned (for example Brodal, 1981). Nevertheless, many scientists still use it and they consider the cingulate, insular, entorhinal, piriform, hippocampal, retrosplenial and orbitofrontal cortex to belong to the limbic system. Subcortical regions usually included in the limbic system are the hypothalamus and the pre-optic region, the amygdala, the bed nucleus of the stria terminalis, the septal nuclei, and the anterior and mediodorsal thalamic nuclei. As early as 1958, Nauta pointed out that the limbic system has extremely strong reciprocal connections with mesencephalic structures such as the periaqueductal gray (PAG) and the laterally and ventrally adjoining tegmentum, (Nauta's limbic system-midbrain circuit). More recent findings strongly support Nauta's concept and has led Holstege, (1990) to consider the mesencephalic periaqueductal gray (PAG) and large parts of the lateral and ventral mesencephalic tegmentum to belong to the limbic system. Nieuwenhuys, (1985; see also Nieuwenhuys et al. 1988), introduces the term "core of the neuraxis" for "a set of neuromediator-rich centers and pathways, which corresponds partly with the limbic system". Nieuwenhuys' core not only involves major parts of the limbic system as defined earlier, but also the ventral parts of the striatum, the thalamic midline nuclei, the parabrachial nuclei, the dorsal vagal complex, the superficial zones of the spinal trigeminal nucleus and of the spinal dorsal horn, and the spinal substantia intermedia centralis. Furthermore Nieuwenhuys (see Nieuwenhuys et al. 1988) introduces the medial and lateral paracore zones. The medial paracore is constituted by the series of raphe nuclei, which extends throughout the brain stem. The lateral paracore consists of the lateral tegmentum of mesencephalon, pons and medulla. It comprizes the substantia nigra, the locus coeruleus and subcoeruleus (A6 group), the nucleus Kölliker-Fuse, and the bulbar lateral tegmental field as defined by Holstege et al. (1977).

Although it is well known that the limbic system exerts a strong influence on somatic and autonomic motoneurons, lesion-degeneration studies did not reveal strong limbic projections to levels caudal to the mesencephalon. This led to the idea that the limbic pathways to caudal brainstem and spinal cord were multisynaptic (Nauta, 1958; Nauta and Domesick, 1981). Since 1975 this view changed dramatically mainly because new tracing techniques became available, such as retrograde tracing using horseradish peroxidase (HRP) (LaVail and LaVail, 1972; Mesulam, 1978), anterograde autoradiographic (Lasek et al., 1968; Cowan et al., 1972) and immuno-histochemical fiber-tracing techniques. Kuypers and Maisky (1975), using the retrograde HRP technique, demonstrated direct hypothalamo-spinal pathways in the cat. Subsequently, the autoradiographic tracing technique has revealed many new limbic system pathways to caudal brainstem and spinal cord. One of the most interesting of these projections are the limbic system projections to the nucleus raphe magnus (NRM) and pallidus (NRP) as well as to the adjacent ventral part of the caudal pontine and medullary reticular formation (the

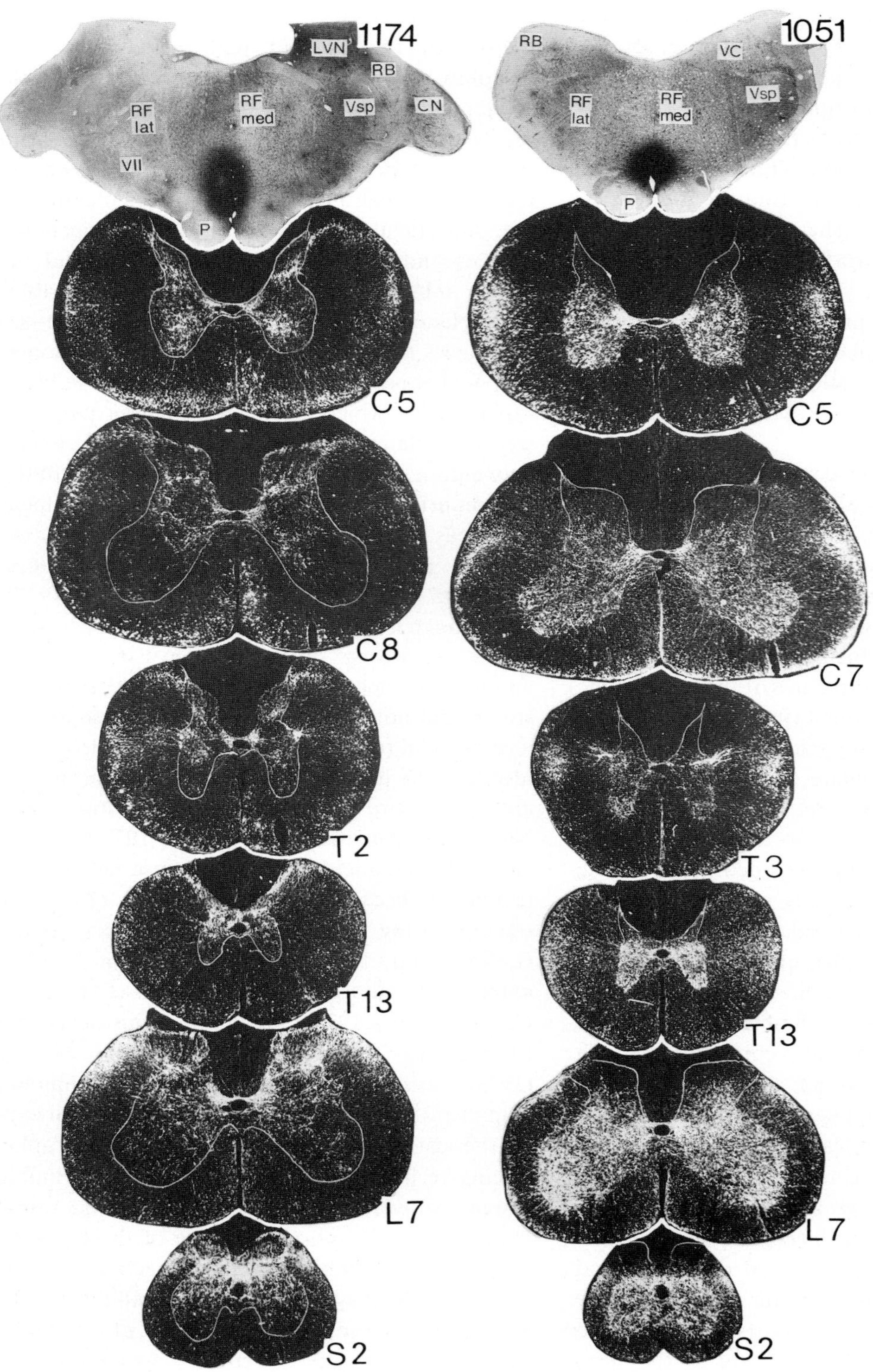
1174
LVN
RB
RF
med
Vsp
CN
RF
lat
VII
P
C5
C8
T2
T13
L7
S2
1051
RB
VC
Vsp
RF
lat
RF
med
P
C5
C7
T3
T13
L7
S2

caudal part of the medial paracore of Nieuwenhuys et al., 1988). These findings are important, because NRM, NRP and adjoining reticular formation in turn project diffusely, but very strongly to all parts of the gray matter throughout the length of the spinal cord. There exist also strong limbic projections to the pontine paralemniscal region and to the area of the locus coeruleus and/or nucleus subcoeruleus, which take part in the lateral paracore of Nieuwenhuys et al. (1988), and also these areas in turn project diffusely to the spinal gray throughout its total length. Therefore, the diffuse brainstem-spinal projections will be discussed in the framework of the descending limbic motor control systems. It should be kept in mind that almost all projections presented in this section have been discovered in the last 15 years.

Pathways projecting diffusely to the spinal gray matter

Projections from the nuclei raphe magnus (NRM), pallidus (NRP) and obscurus (NRO) and the ventral part of the caudal pontine and medullary medial reticular formation. Retrograde HRP results (Kuypers and Maisky, 1975; Tohyama et al., 1979; Holstege, G. and Kuypers, 1982; Holstege, 1988b) indicate that a great number of neurons in the nuclei raphe magnus and pallidus and ventral part of the caudal pontine and medullary medial reticular formation project to the spinal cord (Fig. 32). It was also demonstrated by means of retrograde double labeling tracing techniques that many of these neurons project to cervical as well as lumbar levels of the spinal cord and to the caudal spinal trigeminal nucleus (Martin et al., 1981b; Hayes and Rustioni, 1981; Huisman et al., 1982; Lovick and Robinson, 1983).

Basbaum et al. (1978), using the autoradiographic tracing technique, were the first to demonstrate in the cat that the NRM projects to the marginal layer of the caudal spinal trigeminal nucleus and in the spinal cord to laminae I, II, V, VI and VII, and to the thoracolumbar intermediolateral cell column. Similar projections were observed from the tegmentum located next to the NRM, i.e. the ventral part of the medial tegmental field at the level of the facial nuclei, also called the nucleus reticularis magnocellularis. The results of Basbaum et al. (1978) were confirmed in the opossum and rat (Martin et al., 1981a; 1985) and in the cat (Holstege et al., 1979; Holstege, G. and Kuypers, 1982; Fig. 45 left). Moreover, Holstege, G. and Kuypers (1982) demonstrated that the NRM and adjoining tegmentum project to

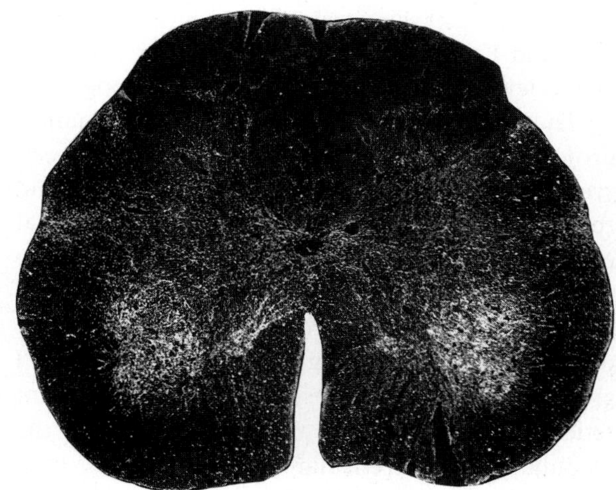

Fig. 46. Darkfield photomicrograph of a section through the lumbar spinal cord in the monkey, after injection of ^{3}H-leucine in the ventral part of the medullary medial tegmental field. Note the diffuse projections to the motoneuronal cell groups.

Fig. 45. Brightfield photomicrographs of autoradiographs showing tritiated leucine injection sites in the raphe nuclei and darkfield photomicrographs showing the distributions of the labeled fibers in the spinal cord. On the left an injection is shown in the caudal NRM and adjoining reticular formation. Note that labeled fibers are distributed mainly to the dorsal horn (laminae I, the upper part of II and V), the intermediate zone and the autonomic motoneuronal cell groups. On the right the injection is placed in the NRP and immediately adjoining tegmentum.Note that the labeled fibers are not distributed to the dorsal horn, but very strongly to the ventral horn (intermediate zone and autonomic and somatic motoneuronal cell groups, (from Holstege, G. and Kuypers, 1982).

the sacral intermedial and intermediolateral cell column. Furthermore they showed that the rostral portion of the NRM and adjoining reticular formation does not project specifically to laminae I and V, but to all laminae of the dorsal horn. Another very important finding was that the NRP and its adjoining reticular formation does not project to the dorsal horn of caudal medulla and spinal cord, but to all other parts of the spinal gray matter, i.e. the intermediate zone and the somatic and autonomic motoneuronal cell groups of the spinal cord (Fig. 45 right) and to the motoneuronal cell groups V, VII, X and XII in the caudal brainstem (Holstege, J.C. and Kuypers, 1982 in the rat; Martin et al., 1979a; 1981a in the opossum; Holstege et al., 1979, Holstege, G. and Kuypers, 1982 in the cat). Such projections have also been shown in the monkey, (Holstege, unpublished observations, Fig. 46). In the rat the projections to the somatic motoneurons have also been demonstrated at the ultrastructural level (Holstege, J.C. and Kuypers, 1982, 1987). Further caudally, at the level of the rostral pole of the hypoglossal nucleus, the medullary medial reticular formation projects mainly to the somatic motoneuronal cell groups, and to a lesser extent to the intermediate zone (Holstege, G. and Kuypers, 1982). Caudal NRM and rostral NRP also project to the thoracolumbar and sacral intermediolateral cell groups (IML), i.e. the autonomic (sympathetic and parasympathetic) preganglionic motoneuronal cell groups (Fig. 45). The rostral NRM and adjacent reticular formation and the ventral part of the medullary medial reticular formation at the level of the rostral pole of the hypoglossal nucleus do not project to the IML.

Summarizing, NRM, NRP and NRO, with their adjoining reticular formation, send fibers throughout the length of the spinal cord, giving off collaterals to all spinal levels. These descending systems are extremely diffuse and are not topographically organized. Furthermore, a strong heterogeneity exists in these projections, in which 1) the rostral NRM and adjoining reticular formation project to all parts of the dorsal horn; 2) the caudal NRM and adjoining reticular formation project mainly to laminae I and V and the autonomic motoneuronal cell groups; 3) the NRP, NRO and ventromedial medulla projects to the intermediate zone and the ventral horn, including the autonomic and somatic motoneuronal cell groups and 4) the ventral part of the medial reticular formation at the level of the rostral pole of the hypoglossal nucleus projects mainly to the somatic motoneuronal cell groups.

Physiological studies are consistent with the anatomy of the descending pathways outlined above. Electrical stimulation in the NRM inhibits neurons in the caudal spinal trigeminal nucleus (Hu and Sessle, 1979; Lovick and Wolstencroft, 1979; Sessle et al., 1981) and spinal dorsal horn (Engberg et al., 1968; Fields et al., 1977, Willis et al., 1977). More recently, stimulation in the NRM was found to produce an inhibitory postsynaptic potential (IPSP) in neurons in laminae I and II of the dorsal horn at a latency consistent with a monosynaptic connection (Light et al., 1986). Not only NRM stimulation, but also stimulation in the adjacent ventral part of the caudal pontine and/or upper part of the medullary medial reticular formation produces inhibition of neurons in the dorsal horn (Fields et al., 1977; Akaike et al., 1978).

The diffuse organization of NRP, NRO and ventromedial medulla projections to the motoneuronal cell groups suggests that they do not steer specific motor activities such as movements of distal (arm, hand or leg) or axial parts of the body, but have a more global effect on the level of activity of the motoneurons. Stimulation of the raphe nuclei has a facilitory effect on motoneurons (Cardona and Rudomin, 1983). There exist many different neurotransmitter substances in this area, of which serotonin is the best known. Serotonin plays a role in the facilitation of motoneurons, probably directly by acting on the Ca^{2+} conductance or indirectly by reduction of K^{+} conductance of the membrane of the motoneuron (McCall and Aghajanian, 1979; White and Neuman, 1980; VanderMaelen and Aghajanian, 1982; Hounsgaard et al., 1986). Thus serotonin enhances the excitability of the motoneurons for inputs from other sources, such as red nucleus or motor cortex (McCall and Aghajanian, 1979). In mammals, there are many serotonergic fibers around the motoneurons (Steinbusch, 1981 and Kojima, 1983b in the rat, Kojima et al., 1982 in the dog, Kojima, 1983a in the monkey). The cell bodies of these serotonergic fibers are mainly located in the NRP, and to a limited extent in the NRO, but not in the NRM (Alstermark et al., 1987).

Not only serotonin, but, at least in the rat, several peptides are also present in the spinally projecting neurons in the ventromedial medulla and NRP and NRO. Many neurons contain substance P, thyrotropin releasing hormone (TRH), somatostatin, methionine (M-ENK) and leucine-enkephalin (L-ENK), while a relatively small number contains vasoactive intestinal peptide (VIP) and cholecystokinin (CCK). It has been demonstrated that most of these peptides coexist to a variable extent with serotonin in the same neuron (Chan Palay et al., 1978; Hökfelt et al., 1978; Hökfelt et al., 1979; Johansson et al., 1981; Hunt and Lovick, 1982; Bowker et al., 1983; Mantyh and Hunt, 1984; Taber-Pierce et al., 1985; Helke et al., 1986; Léger et al., 1986; Bowker et al., 1988). Johansson et al. (1981) have also demonstrated the coexistence of serotonin, substance P and TRH in one and the same neuron. This coexistence of serotonin with different peptides not only occurs in the neuronal cell bodies, but also in their terminals in the ventral horn, (Pelletier et al., 1981; Bowker, 1986; Wessendorf and Elde, 1987). According to Hökfelt et al. (1984), at the ultrastructural level, serotonin, substance P and TRH is stored in the terminal in dense core or granular vesicles, terminals with such vesicles are called G-type terminals (G = granular). Ulfhake, (1987) has recently shown that some of the G-type terminals lack synaptic specialization, suggesting that the content of dense core vesicles may be released at non-synaptic sites of the terminal membrane.

It must be emphasized that a major portion of the diffuse descending pathways to the dorsal horn and the motoneuronal cell groups is not derived from serotonergic neurons (Bowker et al., 1982; Johannessen et al., 1984). At the light microscopical level, Holstege, G. and Kuypers, (1982) showed in the cat that the appearance of the labeling in the motoneuronal cell groups after ^{3}H-leucine injections in the area of the ventral nucleus raphe pallidus, with more than 90% serotonergic neurons, or in the laterally adjacent medullary

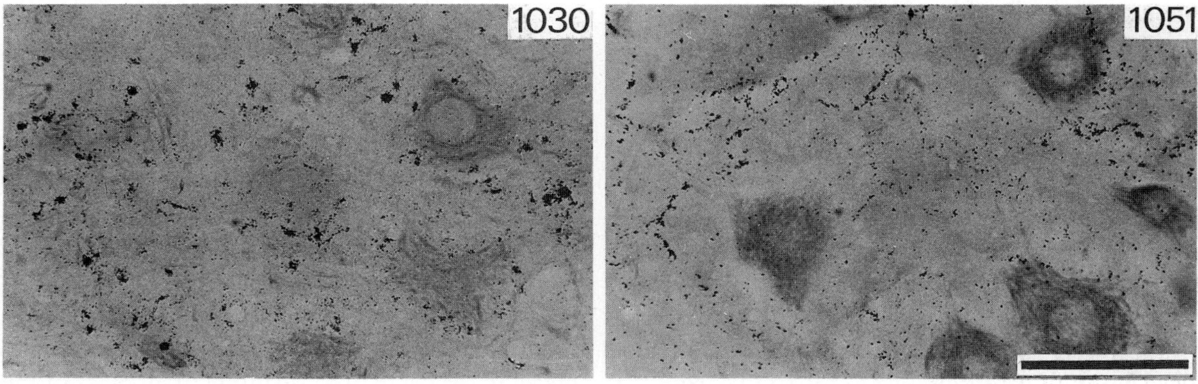

Fig. 47. Brightfield photomicrographs of autoradiographs in the somatic motoneuronal cell groups of the L7 ventral horn in the cat after injections of ^{3}H-leucine in the ventral part of the medullary medial tegmentum. On the left the injection was made at the level just rostral to the hypoglossal nucleus, not involving the raphe nuclei. Note the dominance of clusters of silver grains in the motoneuronal cell groups. On the right the injection was made in the NRP (see Fig. 45 right side). Note that the silver grains are located in strings and not in clusters. These distinct termination patterns probably represent differences in functions and/or neurotransmitter content. Bar represents 0.1 mm. (From Holstege, G. and Kuypers, 1982).

medial tegmentum, with almost no serotonergic neurons (Wiklund et al., 1981), was clearly different (Fig. 47). This suggests that non-serotonergic neurons terminate differently in the motoneuronal cell groups than the fibers of the serotonergic neurons, which may or may not contain other peptides as well. One possible neurotransmitter is acetylcholine, since some of the neurons in the ventromedial medulla are ChAT positive (Jones and Beaudet, 1987). Another candidate is somatostatin, which is present in many of the neurons in especially the more caudal portions of the ventromedial medulla, and in some of the more dorsally located giant cells in the medial tegmentum. Somatostatin containing neurons are not very numerous in the raphe nuclei (Taber-Pierce et al. 1985) and coexists to a small extent with serotonin (Bowker et al. 1988). Electrophoresis of somatostatin in the brain always produces an inhibition of the neurons in the injection-site, which suggests a generalized inhibitory role for somatostatin in the central nervous system. Also GABA may play an important role in these non-serotonergic pathways. Holstege, J.C. (1989) in the rat showed that after injection of WGA-HRP in the ventromedial medulla, 40% of the labeled terminals in the L5 – L6 lateral motoneuronal cell group were also labeled for GABA. Of the double labeled terminals ≈ 80% contained flattened vesicles, indicating an inhibitory function (Krnjévic and Schwarts, 1966). Holstege, J.C. (1989) also found that ≈ 10% of the labeled terminals containing GABA were of the so-called G-type, which probably contain serotonin and/or peptides such as substance P, TRH or enkephalin-like substances (Pelletier et al., 1981; Holstege, J.C. and Kuypers, 1987). This corresponds with the finding of Belin et al. (1983) and Millhorn et al. (1988), who demonstrated co-localization of serotonin and GABA in neurons in the ventral medulla in the rat. Thus, there exist spinally projecting neurons in the ventromedial medulla that contain serotonin as well as GABA. Nicoll (1988) has found that 5HT1A and $GABA_B$ receptors are coupled to the same ion channel. The functional implication of these findings is that some terminals, taking part in this diffuse descending system, may have inhibitory as well as facilitatory effects on the postsynaptic element (i.e. the motoneuron), although the majority is probably either facilitatory or inhibitory. Spinal motoneurons display a bistable behavior, i.e. they can switch back and forth to a higher excitable level (Hounsgaard et al., 1984; 1986; 1988; Crone et al., 1988). Bistable behavior disappears after spinal transection, but reappears after subsequent intravenous injection of the serotonin precursor 5-hydroxy-tryptophan. Thus, intact descending pathways are essential for this bistable behavior of motoneurons and serotonin is one of the neurotransmitters involved in switching to a higher level of excitation. Possibly, GABA may be involved in switching to a lower level of excitation.

In summary, the diffuse descending pathways originating in the ventromedial medulla, including the nucleus raphe pallidus and obscurus, have very general and diffuse facilitatory or inhibitory effects on motoneurons and probably also on interneurons in the intermediate zone. Although most of the terminals have either a facilitatory or an inhibitory function, recent results suggest that there also exist terminals with both facilitatory and inhibitory functions.

Projections from the dorsolateral pontine tegmental field (A7 cell group). Retrograde HRP and anterograde autoradiographic tracing studies (Martin et al., 1979b in the opossum; Holstege, J.C. and Kuypers, 1982, 1987 in the rat; Holstege et al., 1979 and Holstege, G. and Kuypers, 1982 in the cat; Westlund and Coulter, 1980 in the monkey) show that a large number of neurons in the locus coeruleus in the rat or the nucleus subcoeruleus and ventral part of the parabrachial nuclei in the cat project diffusely to all parts of the spinal gray matter. The diffuse dorsolateral pontine projections to the somatic motoneurons have also been demonstrated at the E.M. level (Holstege, J.C. and Kuypers, 1987). In the brainstem some fibers terminate in the NRM and rostral NRP (Holstege, 1988a; Fig. 48). Many neurons in the locus coeruleus, subcoeruleus and the parabrachial nuclei contain noradrenaline (Westlund and Coulter, 1980; Jones and Friedman, 1983; Jones and Beaudet, 1987) or acetylcholine (Kimura et al., 1981; Jones and Beaudet, 1987). Neurons containing both neurotransmitters have not been reported. The diffuse projection from this area to the spinal cord is at least in part noradrenergic, since lesioning the dorsolateral pontine tegmental field, the number of noradrenergic terminals in the spinal gray matter was reduced by 25 – 50% in the dorsal horn and by 95% in the ventral horn (Nygren and Olson, 1977). In addition some serotonergic neurons are present in the dorsolateral pontine tegmental field (Wiklund et al., 1981), and they also project to the spinal cord (Lai and Barnes, 1985).

Electrical stimulation in the area of the locus coeruleus/subcoeruleus in rat (Chan et al., 1986) and cat (Fung and Barnes, 1987) produces a decrease in input resistance and a concurrent nonselective enhancement in motoneuron excitability, indicative of an overall facilitation of motoneurons. Furthermore there is evidence that in the rat noradrenergic fibers derived from the locus coeruleus and descending via the ventrolateral funiculus have an inhibitory effect on nociception (Jones and Gebhart, 1987).

In conclusion, neurons in the area of locus coeruleus/subcoeruleus project diffusely to all parts of the spinal gray throughout the length of

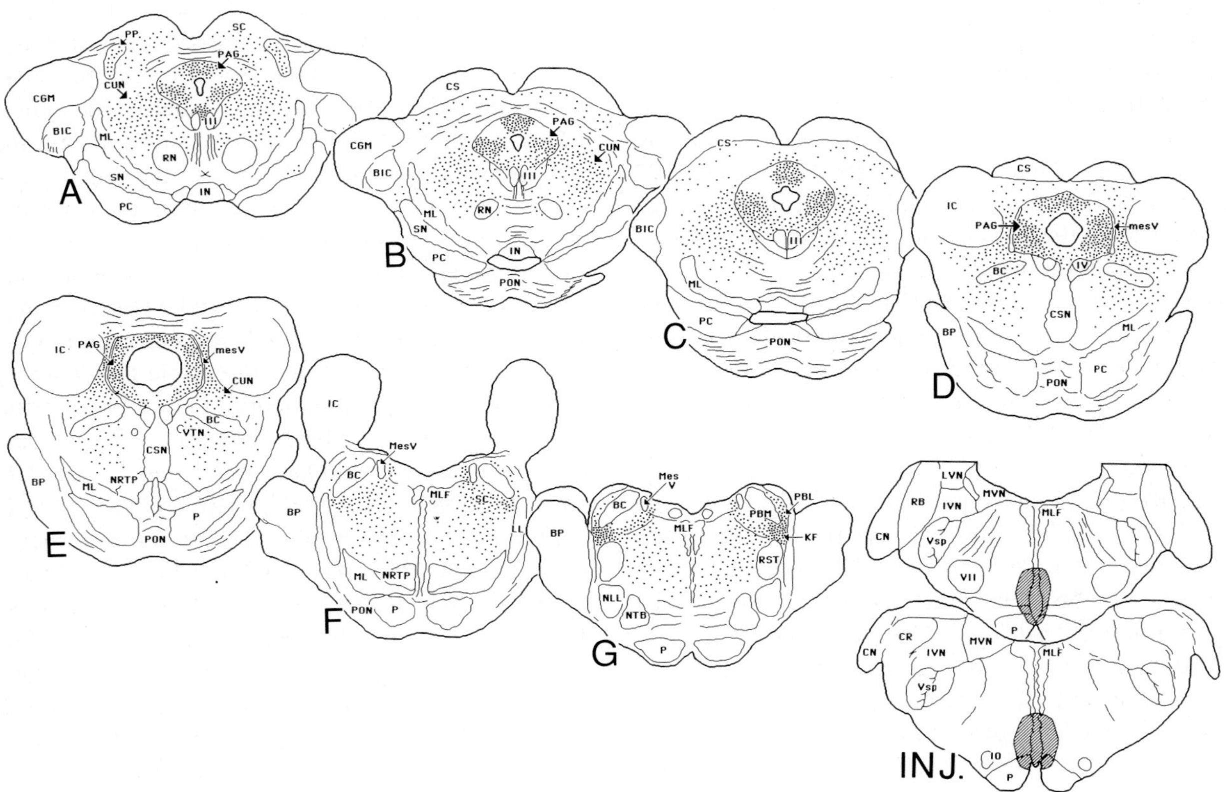

Fig. 48. Schematic drawings of HRP-labeled neurons in mesencephalon and pons after injection of HRP in the NRM/NRP region. Note the dense distribution of labeled neurons in the PAG (except its dorsolateral part) and the tegmentum ventrolateral to it. Note also the distribution of labeled neurons in the area of the ventral parabrachial nuclei and the nucleus Kölliker-Fuse (from Holstege, 1988a).

the spinal cord. They have an inhibitory effect on nociception and a facilitory effect on motoneurons, an influence which is strikingly similar to that obtained after stimulation in NRM and NRP and their adjacent reticular formation.

Projections from the pontine lateral tegmentum (paralemniscal reticular formation). According to retrograde HRP (Fig. 32) and fluorescent tracing studies (Martin et al. 1979b; Holstege and Kuypers, 1982; Huisman et al., 1982) the pontine lateral tegmental field contains a cluster of neurons, which projects contralaterally throughout the length of the spinal cord with a high degree of collateralization. Anterograde autoradiographic tracing studies (Martin et al., 1979b; Holstege et al., 1979; Holstege, G. and Kuypers, 1982; Carlton et al., 1985 and Tan and Holstege, 1986) revealed that fibers originating in this area cross just beneath the floor of the fourth ventricle, and descend through the lateral reticular formation of caudal pons and medulla into the contralateral dorsolateral funiculus of the spinal cord (Fig. 27 right). In the brainstem caudal to the obex, labeled fibers from the pontine lateral tegmental field were distributed to the marginal layer of the caudal spinal trigeminal nucleus and, at the level of C1 – C2, a very strong bilateral projection was observed to the lateral cervical nucleus, a small group of cells lying just lateral to the dorsal horn of the C1 – C2 spinal cord (Westman, 1968). Labeled fibers were distributed throughout the length of the spinal cord to lamina I, the outer part of II, but the strongest projections were to the lateral parts of laminae V and VI. Almost nothing is known about the function of this well defined contralateral pathway. The fact that it is contralateral, that it is located in the dorsolateral funiculus and that it terminates in laminae V and VI suggest a motor function, similar to the rubrospinal tract. On the other hand, the additional projections to laminae I and II and the lateral cervical nucleus and the fact that it is highly collateralized suggest a function in nociception control. In this respect it may be noted that electrical stimulation in the paralemniscal cell group generated a powerful descending inhibition of nociception (Carstens et al., 1980), although it must be kept in mind that many descending fiber systems on their way to the NRM and adjacent tegmentum pass through the paralemniscal area.

Projections from the rostral mesencephalon/caudal hypothalamus (A11 cell group). Skagerberg and Lindvall (1985) in the rat demonstrated that dopamine containing neurons in the A11 cell group projected throughout the length of the spinal cord. The A11 cell group is located in the border region of rostral mesencephalon and dorsal and posterior hypothalamus, extending dorsally along the paraventricular gray of the caudal thalamus. Skagerberg and Lindvall (1985) were not able to determine in which specific parts of the spinal gray matter the A11 dopaminergic fibers terminated. Skagerberg et al. (1982) had demonstrated dopaminergic terminals in the intermediolateral cell column, but Yoshida and Tanaka (1988), using anti-dopamine serum, found dopamine-immunoreactive fibers "throughout the whole gray matter at any level of the spinal cord". Final proof that these dopaminergic fibers originate exclusively in the A11 neurons is still lacking. However, none of the other dopaminergic cell groups (A8 to A10 and A12 to A14) project to the spinal cord (Skagerberg and Lindvall, 1985; see also Albanese et al. 1986), which strongly suggests that the A11 cell group is the only source of the dopaminergic fibers in the spinal cord. The distribution of the dopaminergic fibers in the spinal gray strongly resembles that of the noradrenergic fibers in the spinal cord,

Fig. 49. Darkfield photomicrographs of the brainstem in the cases 1434 and 1338 with injections in respectively the ventrolateral PAG and more rostrally in the lateral PAG. Note the strong projections to the NRM and the ventral part of the medial tegmentum of caudal pons and medulla in both cases. Note that in case 1434, but not in case 1338 labeled fibers were also distributed to the NRP (from Holstege, 1988a).

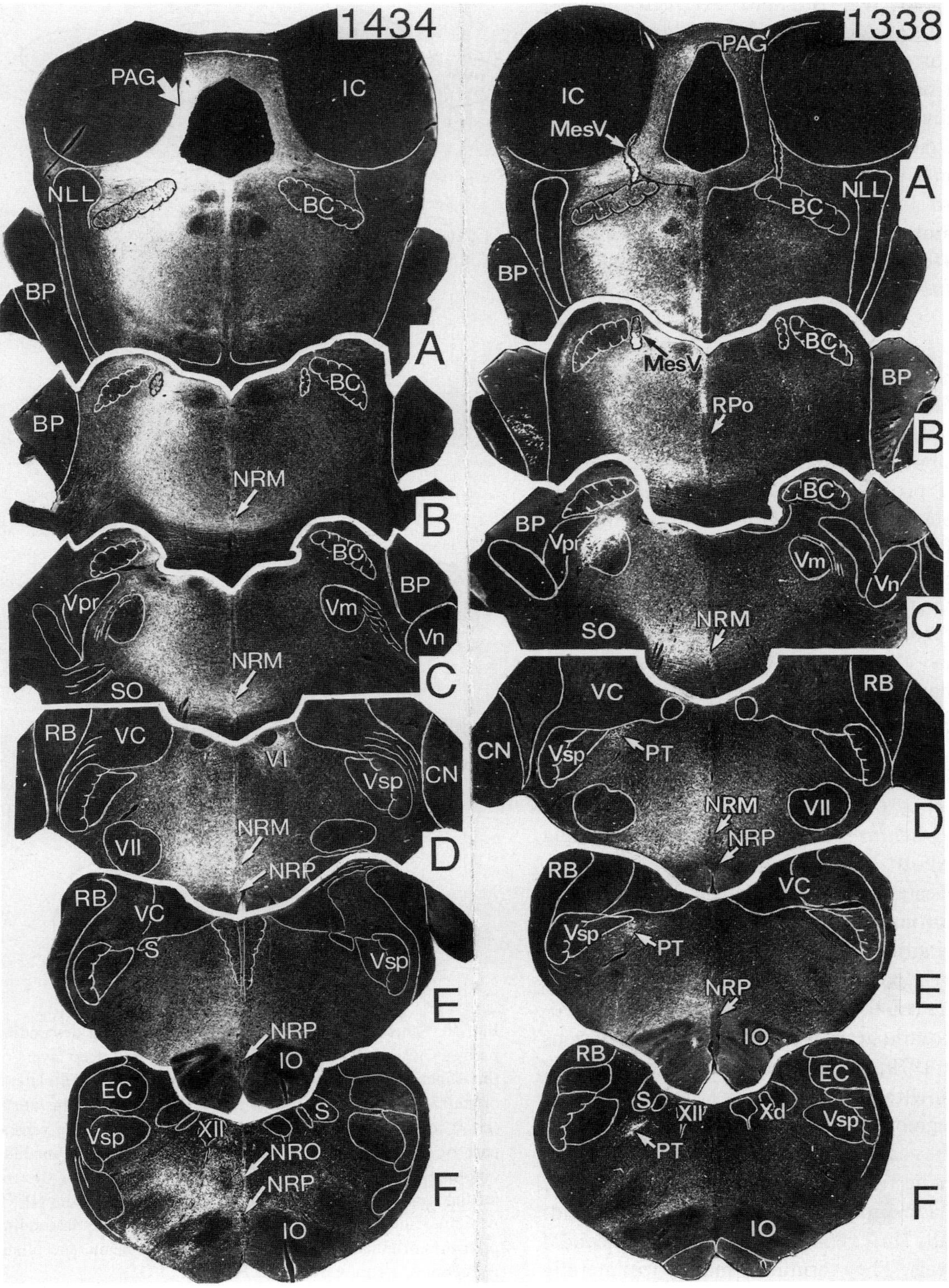
1434
PAG
IC
NLL
BC
BP
A
BP
BC
NRM
B
BC
BP
Vpr
Vm
Vn
NRM
SO
C
RB
VC
VI
CN
Vsp
NRM
VII
NRP
D
RB
VC
S
Vsp
E
NRP
IO
EC
S
Vsp
XII
NRO
NRP
F
IO
1338
PAG
IC
MesV
NLL
A
BC
BP
BC
MesV
BP
RPo
B
BC
BP
Vpr
Vm
Vn
SO
NRM
C
VC
RB
CN
Vsp
PT
NRM
VII
NRP
D
RB
VC
Vsp
PT
NRP
IO
E
RB
EC
S
XII
Xd
Vsp
PT
F
IO

originating in the A5 and A7 cell groups. Therefore the possibility of labeling dopamine as a precursor of noradrenalin must be kept in mind, (for discussion see Yoshida and Tanaka, 1988). Functionally there is also a resemblance between noradrenergic and dopaminergic fiber projections to the spinal cord. Infusion of dopamine in the spinal cord increases (sympathetic) motoneuron activity (Simon and Schramm, 1983) and has an inhibitory effect on noxious input to the spinal cord (Jensen and Smith, 1982; Jensen and Yaksh, 1984).

Projections from the mesencephalon to caudal brainstem and spinal cord

In recent years specific information became available about the anatomy and function of the descending projections of the mesencephalon in relation to emotional behavior. Stimulation in the mesencephalon has been shown to result in pain inhibition, vocalization, aggressive behavior, blood pressure changes, lordosis and locomotion. Many of the neurons involved in these functions are located in the PAG, but neurons in the mesencephalic tegmentum lateral and ventral to the PAG also play a role.

Descending projections to the NRM, NRP and ventral part of the caudal pontine and medullary medial tegmentum. Retrograde HRP tracing studies (Abols and Basbaum, 1981; Holstege, 1988a) indicate that an enormous number of HRP labeled neurons in the PAG and laterally and ventrolaterally adjoining areas project to NRM, NRP and ventral part of the caudal pontine and medullary medial tegmentum (Fig. 48). Anterograde (autoradiographic) tracing studies (Jürgens and Pratt, 1979; Mantyh, 1983; Holstege, 1988a; Fig. 49) show that different parts of the PAG and adjacent tegmentum project in the same basic pattern to the caudal brainstem. The descending mesencephalic fibers pass ipsilaterally through the mesencephalic and pontine lateral tegmental field, but gradually shift ventrally and medially at caudal pontine levels. They terminate mainly ipsilaterally

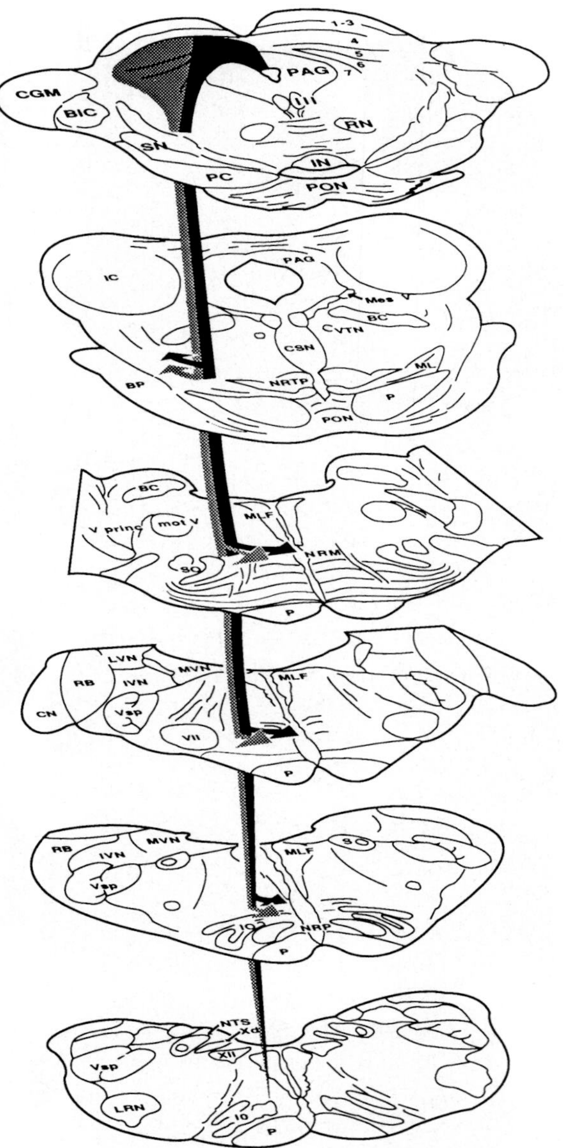

Fig. 50. Schematic representation of the ipsilateral descending pathway, originating from the intermediate and deep layers of the superior colliculus and dorsal PAG. The mediolateral organization of this descending system is illustrated. The lateral (gray) component projects to the lateral aspects of the ventral part of the medial tegmentum of caudal pons and medulla oblongata. The medial (black) component projects to the medial aspects of the medial tegmentum, including the NRM. A similar mediolateral organization exists for the descending pathways originating in more ventral part of the mesencephalic tegmentum, (from Cowie and Holstege, 1991).

in the ventral part of the caudal pontine and medullary medial reticular formation and in the NRM (Fig. 49). On their way to the medulla they give off fibers to the area of the locus coeruleus and nucleus subcoeruleus and the paralemniscal cell group. Neurons in the ventrolateral portion of the caudal PAG and the ventrally adjoining mesencephalic tegmentum send fibers to the NRP (Fig. 49 left). There exists a mediolateral organization within the descending mesencephalic pathways. The main projection of the medially located neurons, i.e. neurons in the medial part of the dorsal PAG, is to the medially located NRM and immediately adjacent tegmentum. On the other hand, neurons in the lateral PAG, the laterally adjacent tegmentum and the intermediate and deep layers of the superior colliculus project mainly laterally to the ventral part of the caudal pontine and upper medullary medial tegmentum with virtually no projections to the NRM (Holstege, 1988a). Fig. 50 from Holstege and Cowie, (1991) is a schematic diagram, showing this mediolateral organization in the descending pathways from the dorsal mesencephalon.

Involvement of the descending mesencephalic projections in control of nociception. In animals (see Besson and Chaouch, 1987 and Willis, 1988 for reviews) as well as in humans (Hosobuchi, 1988; Meyerson, 1988) the PAG is well known for its involvement in the supraspinal control of nociception. The strong impact on nociception is partly mediated via its projections to the NRM and adjacent reticular formation, because in cases with reversible blocks of the NRM and adjacent tegmentum, PAG stimulation results in reduced analgesic effects (Gebhart et al., 1983; Sandkuhler and Gebhart, 1984). However, the analgesic effects do not completely disappear after blocking the NRM and adjacent tegmentum, which suggests that other brainstem regions also play a role. In this respect the PAG projections to the paralemniscal cell group are of interest, since part of the antinociceptive action of the PAG may be exerted through this pathway (see p. 376).

Involvement of the descending mesencephalic projections in the lordosis reflex. Stimulation in the PAG also facilitates the lordosis reflex (Sakuma and Pfaff, 1979a,b). Lordosis, a curvature of the vertebral column with ventral convexity, is an essential element of female copulatory behavior in rodents. The lordosis reflex is facilitated by stimulation of the ventromedial hypothalamic nucleus (Pfaff and Sakuma, 1979a,b) and the PAG (Sakuma and Pfaff, 1979a,b). Stimulation of the L1 through S1 dermatomes is sufficient for eliciting the lordosis reflex, but several studies suggested that it was oestrogen dependent, i.e. would only occur when copulation can result in fertilization. This led to the concept that the lordosis reflex could not be produced in the absence of facilitory forebrain influences. However, it was recently demonstrated that the lordosis reflex can also be elicited in decerebrate rats (Rose and Flynn, 1989). It is also known that descending fibers in the ventrolateral funiculus play a role in the facilitation of the reflex (Kow et al., 1977). It is not possible that these fibers originate from neurons in the ventromedial hypothalamic nucleus or the PAG, because none of the two structures project directly to the lumbosacral spinal cord (Holstege, 1987b; Holstege, 1988a).

Perhaps, the lordosis reflex should be considered as a spinal reflex, in which the L1 – S1 cutaneous input from flank, rump, tailbase and perineum serves as the afferent loop, and the fibers of the back and axial muscle motoneurons form the efferent loop. Both loops are interconnected by spinal interneurons and short and long propriospinal pathways. However, the cutaneous afferents produce lordosis behaviour only when the membrane excitability of the motoneurons is high. This level of excitability is determined by descending pathways, which originate in the NRP and its adjoining ventromedial medullary tegmental field, travel via the ventrolateral funiculus (see Kow et al., 1977) and project diffusely to all inter- and motoneuronal cell groups in the ventral horn throughout the length of the spinal cord (see p. 371 – 374). The NRP and its adjoining ventral part of the medial tegmental field receive their afferents from various structures in the medial limbic system, such as the PAG and anteromedial hypothalamus, but not from the ventromedial hypothalamic nucleus (see Fig. 54). Thus, a concept is put forward in which the ventromedial hypothalamic nucleus controls the lordosis reflex by means of its projections to the ventral part of the medullary medial tegmentum, using the anteromedial hypothalamus (Fuchs et al., 1985) and/or the PAG as relay structures. The medullary ventromedial tegmentum increases the excitability of the motoneurons to such a level that cutaneous L1 – S1 afferent stimulation, which is otherwise ineffective, results in lordosis. Actually, during oestrus the female rat shows several forms of stressful behavior, characterized by frequent locomotion and other stress like phenomena (Pfaff, 1980). It is well known in mammals that various forms of stress, whether it is aggression, fear or sexual arousal, set the motor system at a "high" level. In such circumstances spinal reflexes such as the lordosis reflex can easily be elicited. Pfaff (1980) points to the lateral vestibulospinal tract to play an important role in lordosis behavior, although the lateral vestibular nucleus does not receive afferents from the hypothalamus and PAG. Furthermore, at least in the cat, the majority of the lateral vestibulospinal fibers descend through the ventral funiculus and only to a limited extent through the ventrolateral funiculus (Holstege, 1988b), while the fibers facilitating the lordosis reflex descend exclusively through the ventrolateral funiculus (Kow et al. 1977). On the other hand, lesions in the lateral vestibular nucleus led to decreases in lordosis (Modianos and Pfaff, 1979). In this respect it should be recalled that the lateral vestibulospinal tract has an important influence on all axial movements, thus including the lordosis movements. The question remains whether the lateral vestibular nucleus is specifically involved in lordosis behavior.

Involvement of the descending mesencephalic projections in locomotion. Just lateral to the brachium coniunctivum, just ventral to the cuneiform nucleus and just rostral to the parabrachial nuclei is located the so-called pedunculopontine nucleus. The area contains many ChAT positive neurons (Jones and Beaudet, 1987). Stimulation in the pedunculopontine nucleus induces locomotion in cats (Shik et al., 1966), which is the reason that this area is also termed the mesencephalic locomotor region (MLR). The MLR not only comprises the pedunculopontine nucleus, but extends into the cuneiform nucleus, which is located just dorsal to the pedunculopontine nucleus. Garcia Rill and Skinner, (1988) found that during locomotion neurons in the cuneiform nucleus were related preferentially to rhythmic (bursting) activity, while neurons in the pedunculopontine nucleus are preferentially related to the onset or termination of cyclic episodes (on/off cells).

Anatomical studies (Moon Edley and Graybiel, 1983; Holstege, unpublished results) revealed that the descending projections from this area are organized similar to those from the PAG and adjacent tegmentum. The mainly ipsilateral fiberstream first descends laterally in the mesencephalon and upper pons and then gradually shifts medially to terminate bilaterally, but mainly ipsilaterally in the ventral part of the caudal pontine and medullary medial tegmental field (see also Garcia Rill and Skinner, 1987b). Only sparse projections exist to the nucleus raphe magnus and almost none to the dorsal portions of the caudal pontine and medullary medial tegmentum. By means of low-amplitude ($< 70\ \mu A$), high frequency ($5-60$ Hz) stimulation or via injection of cholinergic agonists in this same area, Garcia Rill and Skinner (1987a) were able to elicit locomotion in the ventral portion of the caudal pontine and medullary medial tegmentum. They also demonstrated that the locomotion in the medioventral medulla could control or override the stepping frequency induced by the mesencephalic locomotor region. Moreover, Garcia Rill and Skinner, (1987b) reported that $\approx 35\%$ of the cells in this area project through the ventrolateral funiculus of the C2 spinal cord and half of these cells received short latency orthodromic input from the mesencephalic locomotor region. Somewhat surprising was that they also found such cells as far rostral as the caudal pontine ventral tegmentum. The latter area, according to the anatomic findings, only projects to the dorsal horn via the dorsolateral funiculus and not to the intermediate zone or ventral horn via the ventrolateral funiculus. Nevertheless, the findings of Garcia Rill and Skinner, (1987a,b) indicate that locomotion, elicited in the mesencephalic locomotor region, is based on the projections from this area to the medial part of the ventral medullary medial tegmentum and on the diffuse projections from the latter area to the rhythm generators in the spinal cord.

The afferent connections of the mesencephalic locomotor area are derived from lateral parts of the limbic system, such as the bed nucleus of the stria terminalis, central nucleus of the amygdala and lateral hypothalamus (Moon Edley and Graybiel, 1983). Strong projections are also derived from the entopeduncular nucleus, subthalamic nucleus and the substantia nigra pars reticulata, but motor cortex projections to the MLR are very scarce (Moon Edley and Graybiel, 1983). These findings indicate that the MLR is influenced by extrapyramidal and lateral limbic structures, and virtually not by somatic motor structures. This corresponds with the fact that the descending projections from the MLR terminate in the ventromedial part of the caudal pontine and medullary tegmental field, which area receives afferents from many other limbic system related areas, but not from the somatic motor structures.

Another area, stimulation of which produces locomotion is the so-called subthalamic locomotor region, which seems to correspond with the caudal hypothalamus (see Armstrong, 1986 and Gelfand et al., 1988 for reviews). After bilateral lesions in the subthalamic locomotor region the cat cannot walk spontaneously for 7 – 10 days, and neither food nor nociceptive stimuli evoke locomotion, although the animal eats food which it can reach without making a step or responds by aggression to pain. Stimulation of the MLR during this period elicits locomotion. The animal walks or runs depending on the strength of stimulation without bumping the walls of the room. Lesioning the MLR, with an intact subthalamic locomotor region does not interfere essentially with motor activity (Sirota and Shik, 1973). In this respect it is important to note that the subthalamic locomotor region (caudal hypothalamus) not only projects to the MLR but also directly to the ventral part of the

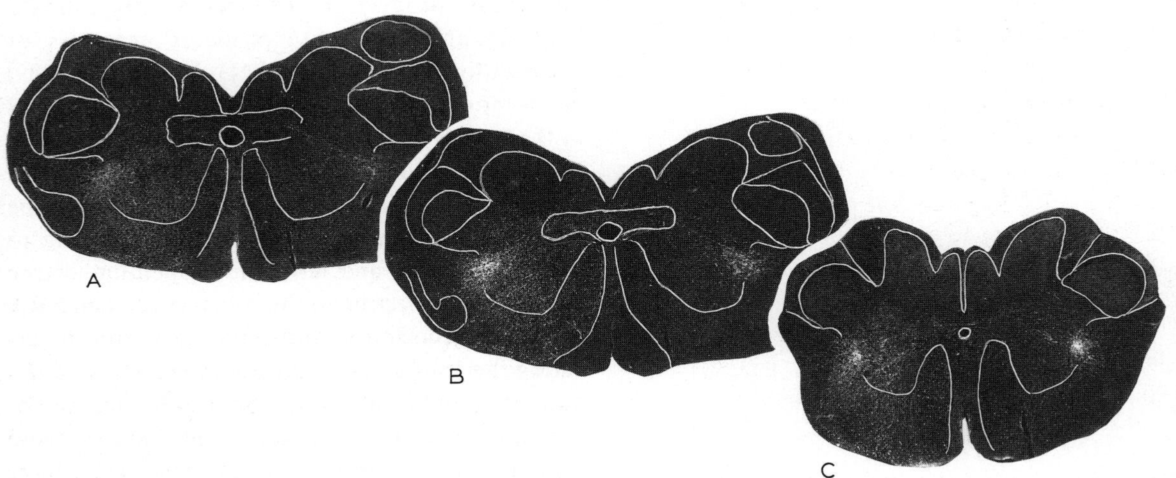

Fig. 51. Darkfield photographs of the caudal medulla in a cat (1434, see also Fig. 48 left) with an injection of ^{3}H-leucine in the ventrolateral part of the caudal PAG. Note the strong bilateral projections to the NRA, (from Holstege, G., 1989).

caudal pontine and medullary medial tegmental field (see p. 389 – 391).

The last region in which locomotion can be elicited is the so called pontomedullary locomotor strip, located in the lateral tegmental field of pons and medulla. This non-continuous tract consists of mainly short propriobulbar axons (Shik, 1983) and probably must be considered as the rostral extent of the spinal interneurons involved in stepping (see p. 328 – 329).

PAG projections to the ventrolateral medulla; involvement in blood pressure control. In an earlier section (p. 346 – 347) it has been shown that neurons in the rostral part of the ventrolateral tegmental field of the medulla (subretrofacial nucleus) are essential for the maintenance of the vasomotor tone and reflex regulation of the systemic arterial blood pressure. Neurons in the rostal part of the subretrofacial nucleus project specifically to the IML neurons, innervating the kidney and adrenal medulla, while neurons in the caudal part of it innervate more caudal parts of the IML, with neurons innervating the hindlimb (Lovick, 1987; Dampney and McAllen, 1988). In a recent study Carrive et al. (1989) have shown that

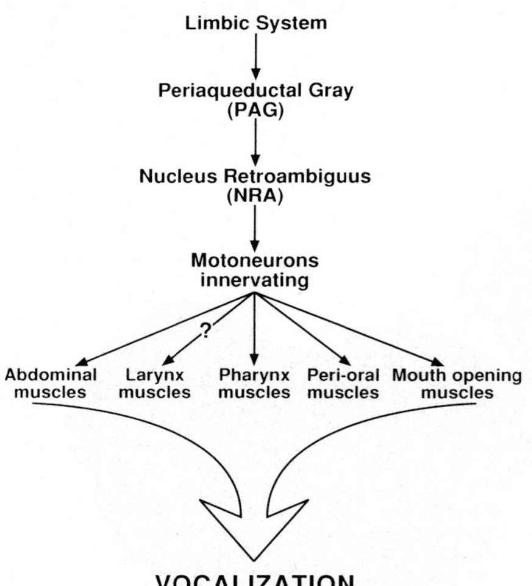

Fig. 52. Schematic representation of the pathways for vocalization from the limbic system to the vocalization muscles, (from Holstege, G., 1989).

neurons in the dorsal portions of the caudal half of the PAG have an excitatory effect on the neurons in the subretrofacial nucleus (increase of blood pressure), while neurons in the ventral part of the PAG have an inhibitory effect (decrease of blood pressure). The same authors also have shown that neurons in the subtentorial portion of the PAG project to the rostral part of the subretrofacial nucleus, which neurons send fibers to the IML motoneurons that innervate the kidney and adrenal medulla. On the other hand, neurons in the caudal part of the pretentorial PAG project to the caudal subretrofacial nucleus, which in turn project to IML motoneurons innervating the hindlimb. In conclusion, there exists a precise organization in the mesencephalic control of blood pressure in different parts of the body. All these projections take part in a descending system involved in the elaboration of emotional motor activities. For an extensive review of this control system, see Richard Bandler, this volume, Chapter 13.

PAG projections to the nucleus retroambiguus; involvement in vocalization. In many different species, from leopard frog to chimpanzee (see Holstege, G., 1989 for review), stimulation in the caudal PAG results in vocalization, i.e. the nonverbal production of sound. In humans laughing and crying are probably examples of vocalization (see section 5a). Holstege, G. (1989) has demonstrated that a specific group of neurons in the lateral and to a limited extent in the dorsal part of the caudal PAG send fibers to the NRA in the caudal medulla (Fig. 51). The cell group in the PAG differs from the smaller cells projecting to the raphe nuclei and adjacent tegmentum or the larger cells projecting to the spinal cord. The NRA in turn projects to the somatic motoneurons innervating the pharynx, soft palate, intercostal and abdominal muscles and probably the larynx (see p. 316; Fig. 52). Direct PAG projections to these somatic motoneurons do not exist (Holstege, 1989). In all likelihood, the projection from the PAG to the NRA forms the final common pathway for vocalization, because DeRossier et al., (1988) found that during vocalization the NRA neurons were more closely related to the vocalization muscle EMG than the PAG. This finding is important, because it shows that a specific expressive motor activity (fixed action pattern) such as vocalization is based on a distinct descending pathway, suggesting that all the other specific motor activities displayed during expressive behavior are based on separate descending pathways.

PAG projections to the spinal cord. Only limited PAG projections to the spinal cord exist (Fig. 32 L – N). Some neurons in the lateral PAG and laterally adjacent tegmentum send fibers through the ipsilateral ventral funiculus of the cervical spinal cord to terminate in laminae VIII and the adjoining part of VII (Martin et al., 1979c; Holstege, 1988a,b; see p. 355). A very few fibers descend ipsilaterally in the lateral funiculus to terminate in the T1 – T2 IML (Holstege, 1988a,b). The projections to the spinal cord may play a role in the defensive behavior observed by Bandler and Carrive (1988), stimulating the PAG. For example, the projection to the medial part of the intermediate zone of the cervical cord may be involved in the contralateral head turning movements as part of defensive behavior, while the projection to the T1 – T2 IML may produce the pupil dilation described by Bandler and Carrive (1988).

Figure 53 gives a schematic overview of the descending projections from the PAG and pedunculopontine and cuneiform nuclei to the caudal brainstem and spinal cord, including the functions in which these projections might be involved.

Projections from the hypothalamus to caudal brainstem and spinal cord

The descending hypothalamic projection systems differ greatly, depending on which part of the hypothalamus is considered. In this section the hypothalamus will be subdivided into the anterior hypothalamus, the paraventricular hypothalamic nucleus, the posterior hypothalamus and the lateral hypothalamus.

Projections from the anterior hypothalamus/preoptic area. According to retrograde HRP studies in the rat, opossum, and cat (Kuypers and Maisky,

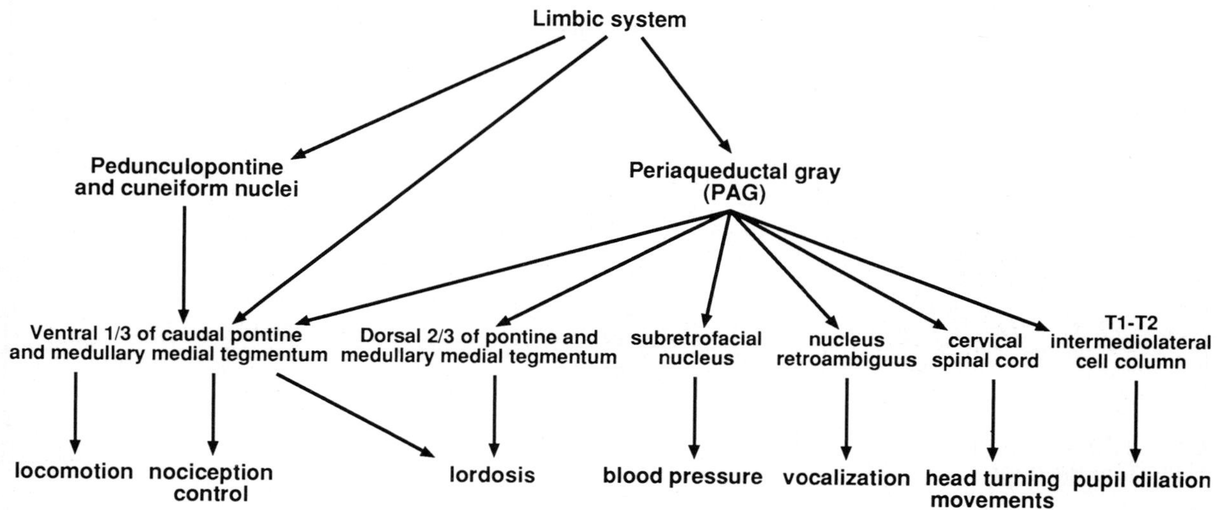

Fig. 53. Schematic overview of the descending projections from the PAG and pedunculopontine and cuneiform nuclei to different regions of the caudal brainstem and spinal cord. The functions in which each of the projections might be involved are also indicated. It should be emphasized that these functional interpretations are only tentative.

1975; Saper et al., 1976; Crutcher et al., 1978; Basbaum et al., 1978 and Holstege, 1987b) neurons in the anterior hypothalamus/preoptic area project strongly to the caudal brainstem, but not to the spinal cord (Fig. 54). Neurons in the medial part of the anterior hypothalamus project (via a medial fiber stream, see large arrows in Fig. 55) to the PAG, the dorsal and superior central raphe nuclei in the pontine tegmentum, and to the ventromedial tegmentum of caudal pons and medulla, including the NRM and NRP (Figs. 55 and 56B).

The anterior hypothalamus receives afferent fiber connections from caudal brainstem structures such as the lateral parabrachial nucleus, the solitary nucleus, and neurons in the ventrolateral

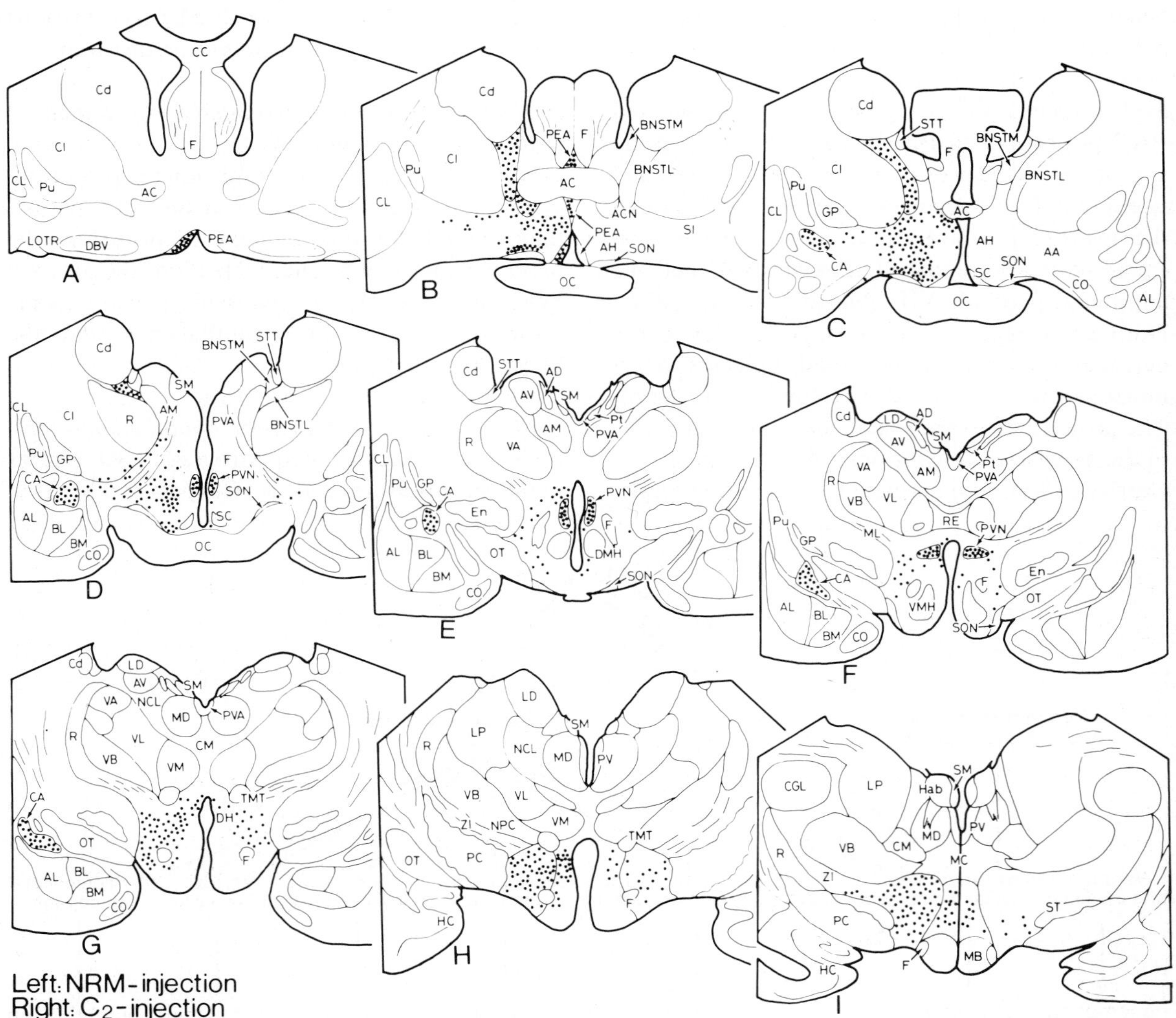

Fig. 54. Schematic drawing of HRP neurons in the hypothalamus, amygdala and bed nucleus of the stria terminalis. On the left of each drawing the pattern of distribution of labeled neurons in after a large injection of HRP in the NRM, rostal NRP and adjoining tegmentum is indicated. On the right of eacht drawing the pattern of distribution of HRP-labeled neurons after hemi-infiltration of HRP in the C2 spinal segment is shown. (From Holstege, 1987).

medulla (Berk and Finkelstein, 1981; Saper and Levisohn, 1983), which suggests that it is involved in cardiovascular regulation. Moreover, application of cholinergic drugs in the anterior hypothalamus results in an emotional aversive response, which includes defense posture and autonomic (e.g., cardiovascular) manifestations (Brudzynski and Eckersdorf, 1984; Tashiro et al., 1985).

Projections from the paraventricular hypothalamic nucleus (PVN). Using the retrograde HRP method in the cat, Kuypers and Maisky (1975) were the first to demonstrate PVN projections to the spinal cord (Fig. 54). Their findings were later confirmed by Hancock (1976) in the rat, Crutcher et al. (1978) in the opossum, Blessing and Chalmers (1979) in the rabbit, Holstege (1987b) in the cat, and Kneisley et al. (1978) in the monkey. The PVN is best known for its projections to the hypophysis, but Hosoya and Matsushita (1979) and Swanson and Kuypers (1980) have shown that the neurons projecting to the hypophysis differ from the ones projecting to the spinal cord. According to Holstege (1987b), the PVN neurons in the cat send their fibers to the caudal brainstem and spinal cord via the medial forebrain bundle and more caudally via a well defined pathway through the lateral part of the mesencephalon and upper pons. At this level they gradually shift medially, filtering through (but not terminating in) the pontine nuclei, to arrive in a very peripheral position lateral to the pyramidal tract (Fig. 58). The PVN fibers descend further into the lateral and dorsolateral funiculus of the spinal cord throughout its total length (Fig. 57). Via this pathway the PVN sends fibers to the NRM, rostral NRP and adjoining reticular formation (Figs. 58 and 56D), and specific parts of the medullary lateral tegmental field (Holstege, 1987b; Fig. 58D – I). In this area lie parasympathetic motoneurons (see p. 317 – 318) and the noradrenergic brainstem nuclei A1 and A2. Specific projections have been demonstrated to the nor-adrenergic A5 area and to the parasympathetic motoneurons in the salivatory nuclei, (Hosoya et al. 1990). Furthermore, PVN fibers terminate in mainly the rostral half of the solitary nucleus (Figs. 58E – G), in all parts of the dorsal vagal nucleus (Swanson and Kuypers, 1980 in the rat; Berk and Finkelstein, 1983 in the pigeon and Holstege, 1987b in the cat; Fig. 58G), and in the area postrema (Hosoya and Matsushita, 1981 in the rat; Holstege, 1987b in the cat; Fig. 58H).

According to the autoradiographic tracing findings of Holstege (1987b; Fig. 57), in the spinal cord the PVN projects bilaterally, but mainly ipsilaterally, to lamina X next to the central canal, the thoracolumbar (T1 – T4) intermediolateral (sympathetic) motoneuronal cell group, and to the sacral intermediomedial and intermediolateral (parasympathetic) motoneuronal cell groups. The projections to the sympathetic intermediolateral cell column at the levels L2, L3 and upper L4 are especially strong and extensive. Finally, the PVN projects to the nucleus of Onuf (Holstege, 1987b; Holstege and Tan, 1987). One might speculate, in view of the strong PVN projections to the L2 – L4 intermediolateral sympathetic motoneurons, the sacral intermediolateral parasympathetic motoneurons and the nucleus of Onuf (Fig. 57 bottom left), that the PVN might play a role in sexual activity and/or control of the uterus contractions in pregnant women (see Holstege and Tan, 1987 for a review). On the other hand, the PVN projects to all preganglionic motoneurons (sympathetic and parasympathetic), which suggests a more general function, for example a similar function as the hormone ACTH. According to Strack et al., 1989, the PVN neurons projecting to the upper thoracic IML are located more medially in the PVN than the neurons projecting to the caudal thoracic and upper lumbar IML, which suggests that there exist some specificity within the PVN spinal pathways (see also Loewy, this volume). The PVN sends its fibers to lamina I of the caudal spinal trigeminal nucleus and throughout the length of the spinal cord (Holstege, 1987b, Fig. 57). This, together with the fact that stimulation in the area of the PVN produces inhibition of spinal dorsal horn neuronal responses to noxious skin heating

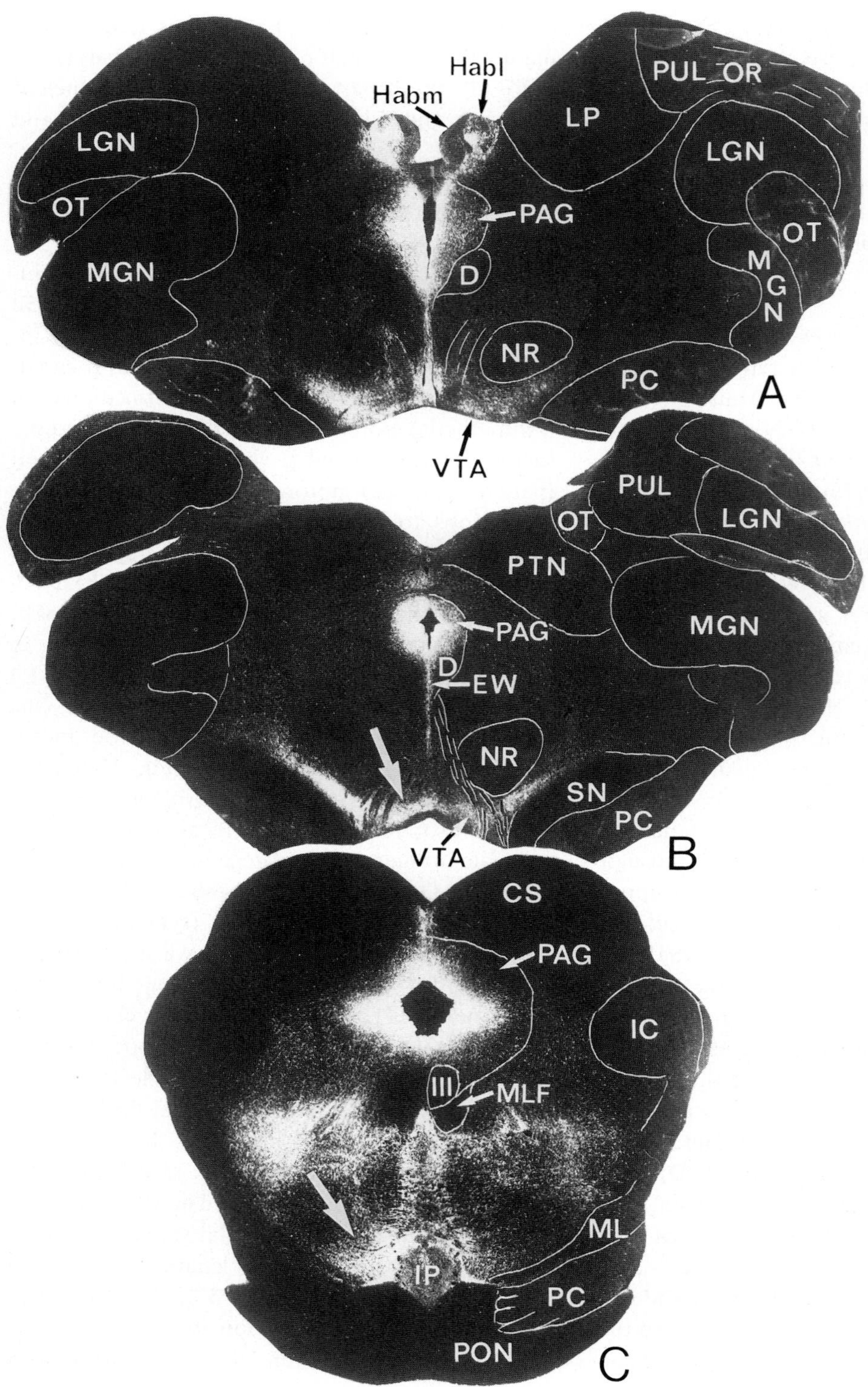

Fig. 55. Darkfield photomicrographs of the brainstem in a case with a ^{3}H-leucine injection in the medial part of the anterior hypothalamic area. Note the strong projections, via a medial fiberstream (see large arrow in B to F) to the medially located

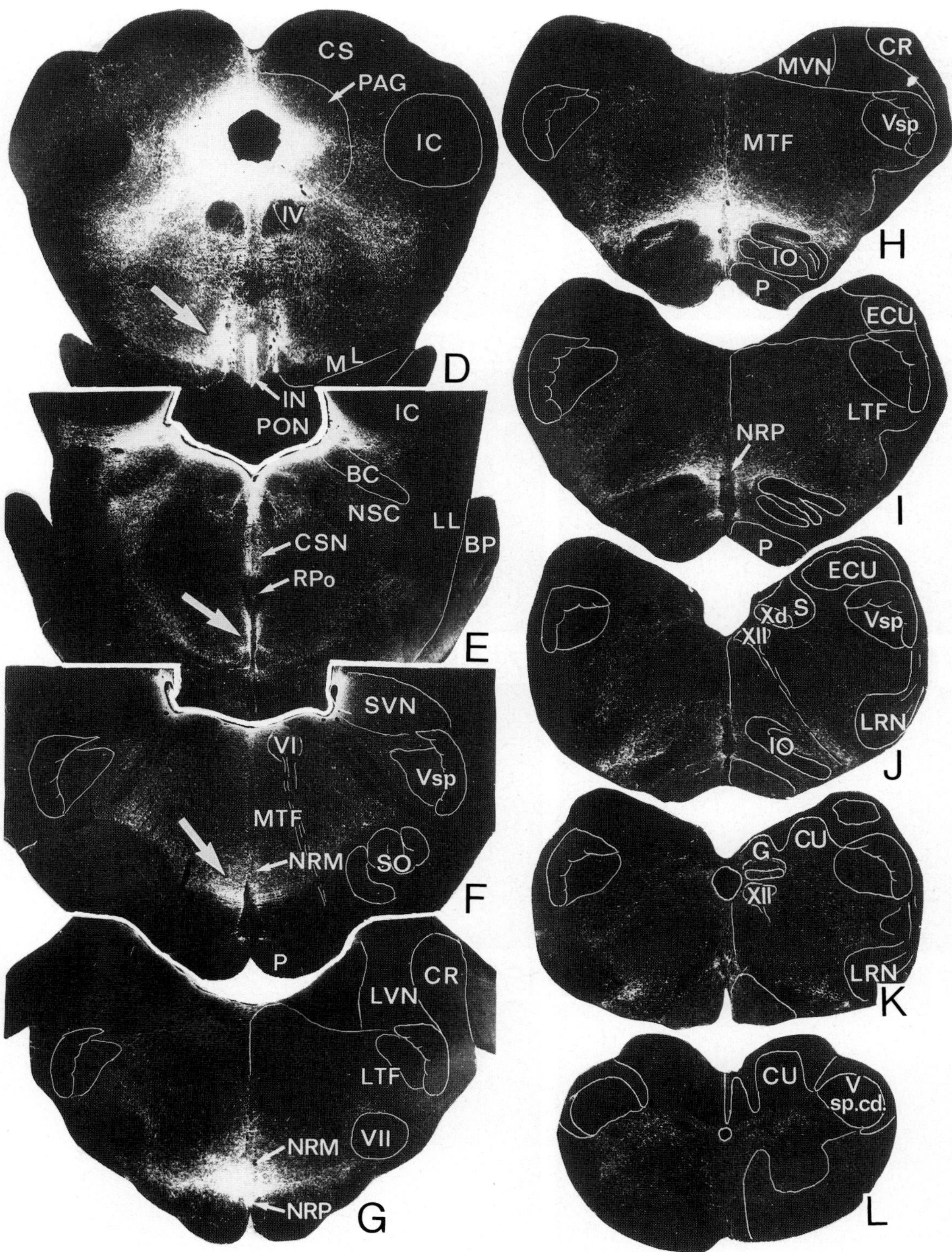

NRM/NRP and to the ventral part of the caudal pontine and upper medullary medial tegmentum. Note also that only the most rostral part of the NRP receives labeled fibers. (From Holstege, 1987).

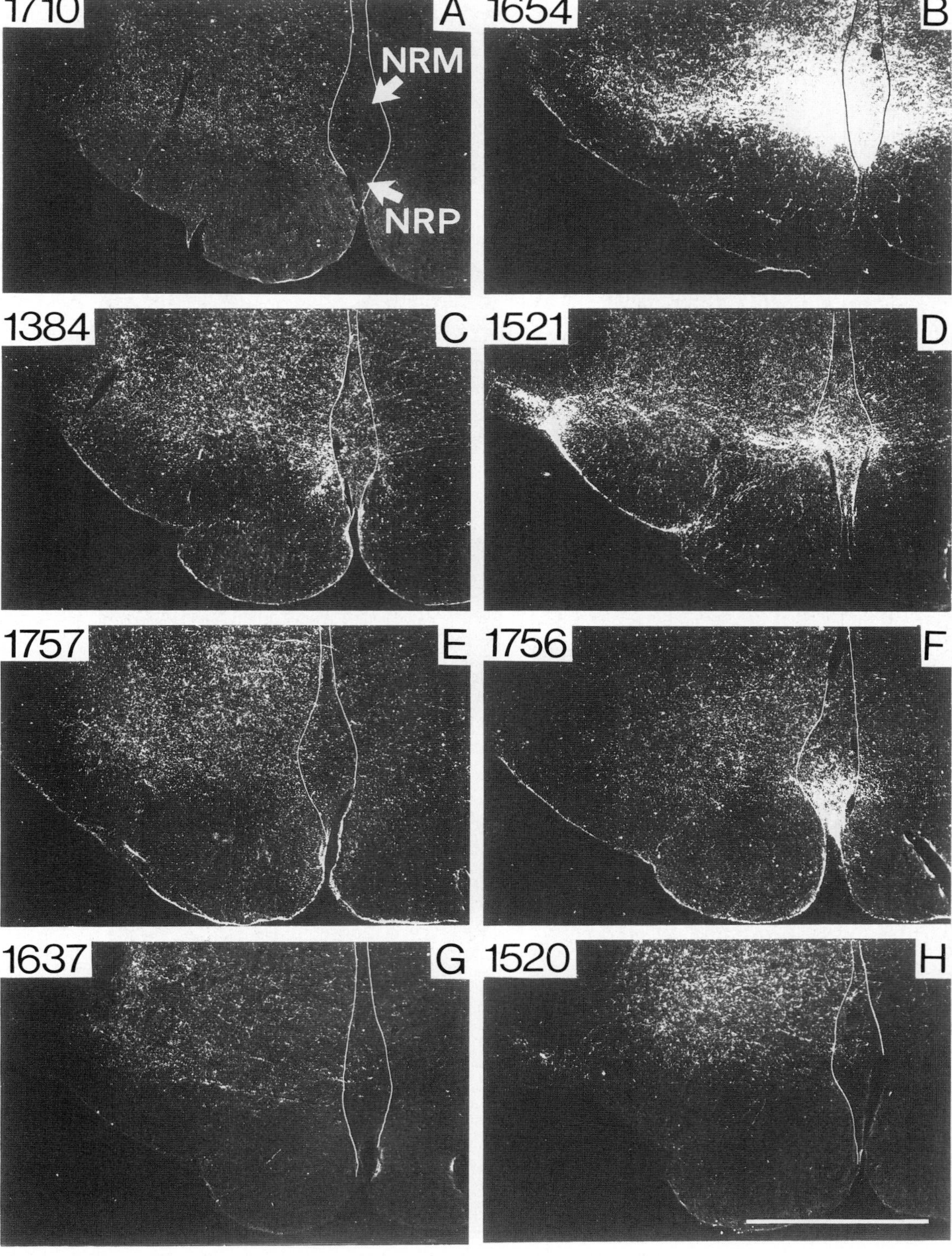
1710
A
NRM
NRP
1654
B
1384
C
1521
D
1757
E
1756
F
1637
G
1520
H

(Carstens, 1982), suggests a role of the PVN in nociception control mechanisms.

The PVN contains a large number of transmitter substances such as oxytocin, vasopressin, somatostatin, dopamine, methionine-enkephalin, leucine-enkephalin, neurotensin, cholecystokinin, dynorphin, substance P, glucogen, renin, and corticotropin releasing factor (see Swanson and Sawchenko, 1983 for a review). Swanson (1977) and Nilaver et al. (1980) traced a pathway containing neurophysin (a carrier protein for oxytocin and vasopressin) from the PVN through the MFB to the caudal brainstem and spinal cord, distributing fibers to the parabrachial nuclei, the nucleus of the solitary tract, the dorsal vagal nucleus and the thoracic intermediolateral cell column and Rexed's laminae I and X. Similar oxytocinergic brainstem projections were found by Hermes et al. (1988) in the garden dormouse, but they also reported oxytocinergic fibers terminating in the nuclei raphe magnus, pallidus and obscurus. Furthermore, Holstege and Van Leeuwen in the cat (unpublished observations) observed oxytocinergic and vasopressinergic fibers in the nucleus of Onuf and the sacral intermediolateral (parasympathetic) cell group. Oxytocin and vasopressin in the spinal cord are only derived from the PVN (Hawthorn et al., 1985), but according to Sawchenko and Swanson (1982) only 20% of the PVN-spinal neurons contain oxytocin or vasopressin and another 5% contain tyrosine hydroxylase (presumably dopamine) and met-enkephalin. Therefore, other neuro-active substances must be involved in this PVN-caudal brainstem/spinal pathway.

The PVN is believed to play an important role in cardiovascular regulation as well as in the feeding mechanism. Feeding behavior in satiated rats can be elicited by injecting clonidine (a noradrenergic agonist) intraperitoneally or in the PVN itself (McCabe et al., 1984). The neural circuitry for this feeding system is believed to start in the noradrenergic neurons of the locus coeruleus (A6 nucleus) that project to the PVN by way of the dorsal pons and dorsal midbrain (Leibowitz and Brown, 1980). The PVN neurons in turn innervate neurons in the dorsal vagal nucleus, which play a crucial role in the noradrenaline-elicited eating response (Sawchenko et al., 1981).

Projections from the medial part of the posterior hypothalamic area. Retrograde tracing studies have demonstrated that the posterior hypothalamus projects to the spinal cord (Kuypers and Maisky, 1975 and Holstege, 1987b in the cat; Fig. 54; Saper et al., 1976; Hancock, 1976 and Hosoya, 1980, in the rat) as well as to the NRM and NRP (Holstege, 1987b). Anterograde autoradiographic tracing studies have revealed that the posterior hypothalamic area sends fibers via a medial pathway to the caudal raphe nuclei and adjoining reticular formation (Hosoya, 1985; Holstege, 1987b). The caudal hypothalamic projections to the NRM are weaker and those to the NRP are much stronger than the PVN projections to this area (compare Figs. 56D (= PVN) and 56F (= caudal hypothalamus). The posterior hypothalamus also projects to the caudal parts of the NRP, which region does not receive afferents from the PVN or other hypothalamic areas (Holstege, 1987b).

The medial part of the posterior hypothalamus sends fibers into the lateral funiculus of the spinal cord, where they terminate in the upper thoracic intermediolateral cell column and in lamina X

Fig. 56. Darkfield photomicrographs of the NRM, rostral NRP and adjoining tegmental field at the level of the facial nucleus in 8 cases with injections in the lateral hypothalamic area (A, C and E), the medial part of the anterior hypothalamic area (B), the PVN of the hypothalamus (D), the medial part of the caudal hypothalamus (F), the central nucleus of the amygdala (G) and bed nucleus of the stria terminalis (H). Note the relative small number of labeled fibers in the NRM/NRP after lateral injections in the limbic system (A, E, G. and H) and the strong projections to the NRM/NRP after medial injections in the limbic system (B, D, and F). The injection in C involved the lateral hypothalamus but extended into the medial hypothalamus, which explains the labeled fibers in NRM/NRP in this case. Bar represents 2 mm. (From Holstege, 1987).

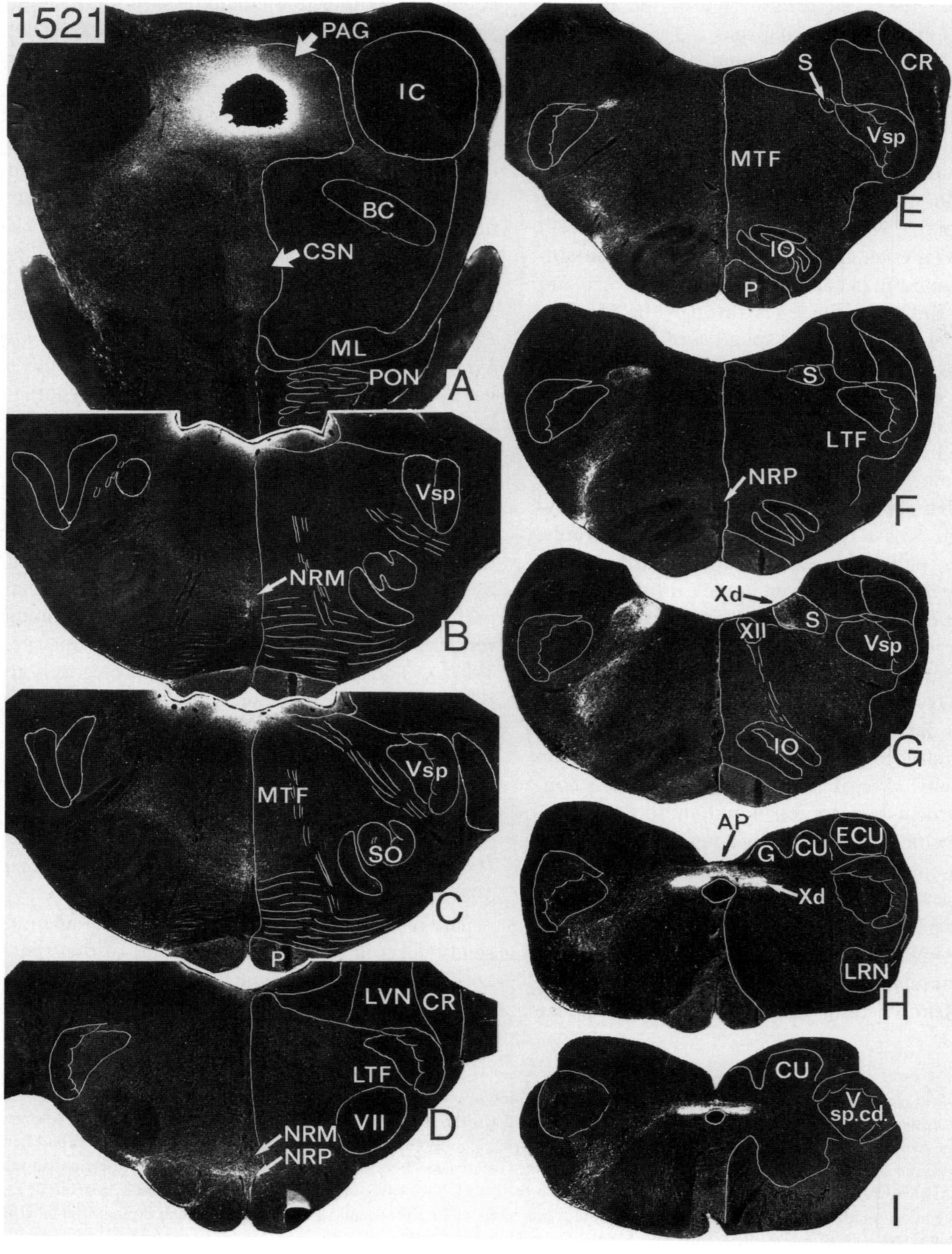
1521
PAG
IC
BC
CSN
ML
PON
A
Vsp
NRM
B
MTF
Vsp
SO
P
C
LVN
CR
LTF
VII
NRM
NRP
D
S
CR
Vsp
MTF
E
IO
P
S
LTF
NRP
F
Xd
S
XII
Vsp
IO
G
AP
G
CU
ECU
Xd
LRN
H
CU
V
sp.cd.
I

throughout the length of the spinal cord (Holstege, 1987b). There seems to exist a rostrocaudal organization in the medial hypothalamic projections to the raphe nuclei and spinal cord, in which the rostral portion of the hypothalamus projects to the rostal parts of the raphe nuclei (i.e. the NRM and the rostal NRP), while the caudal hypothalamus projects to all parts of the NRP and to the spinal cord. Functionally, such differences in projections may be important, because NRM and NRP project to different parts of the spinal gray.

The dorsomedial region of the caudal hypothalamus plays an important role in temperature regulation, and it contains the primary motor center for the production of shivering (Stuart et al. 1961). Shivering is an involuntary response of skeletal muscles which are usually under voluntary control and all skeletal muscle groups can participate (Hemingway, 1963). Shivering does not take place in spinalized animals, indicating that supraspinal mechanisms, i.e. the caudal hypothalamus control this activity. On the other hand, the rhythm of the shiver is probably determined in the spinal cord under the control of the proprioceptive inflow (Birzis and Hemingway, 1957). Possibly the strong caudal hypothalamic projections to the NRP and adjacent tegmentum plays an important role in this "shivering pathway", similar to its role in the descending pathways involved in locomotion, which is also a rhythmical acitivity.

Projections from the lateral hypothalamic area. Functional and anatomical studies on the lateral hypothalamus have always been difficult, because the fibers of the medial forebrain bundle pass through it. This important fiber bundle not only contains fibers originating in the lateral hypothalamus, but also in many other areas, and stimulation or lesions in this area not only affect lateral hypothalamic neurons, but also fibers derived from many other limbic structures (cf. Nieuwenhuys et al., 1982 for a review). Retrograde HRP studies (Saper et al., 1976; Hosoya, 1980 and Holstege, 1987b) reveal that many neurons in the more caudal portions of the lateral hypothalamus project to the spinal cord. Autoradiographic tracing studies (Berk, 1987 in the pigeon; Hosoya and Matsushita, 1981 and Berk and Finkelstein, 1982 in the rat; Holstege, 1987b in the cat), which do not label fibers of passage (Lasek et al., 1968; Cowan et al., 1972), show that the lateral hypothalamus sends fibers to the PAG, the cuneiform nucleus, the parabrachial nuclei and nucleus Kölliker-Fuse, the nucleus subcoeruleus, the locus coeruleus, the caudal pontine and medullary lateral tegmental field, (as defined by Holstege et al., 1977, see p. 328 – 329), and to the ventral part of the caudal pontine and medullary medial tegmentum. Only very few fibers terminate in the area of the NRM and none in the NRP (Fig. 56A and E). Some fibers terminate in the periphery of the dorsal vagal nucleus and in the rostral half of the solitary nucleus. The rostral portion of the lateral hypothalamus also projects strongly to the area just ventral and medial to the mesencephalic trigeminal tract, probably representing Barrington's (1925) nucleus or the M-region of Holstege et al. (1986c). This last area is strongly involved in micturition control (see p. 343 – 346), and an anterior hypothalamic projection to it corresponds with the observation of Grossman and Wang (1956) that stimulation of the preoptic area, which, according to Bleier (1961) is the same as the anterior part of the anterior hypothalamic area, produces micturition-like bladder contractions. Only the caudal portion of the lateral hypothalamus sends fibers throughout the length of the spinal cord via the lateral and dorsolateral funiculi to the intermediate zone, lamina X and the thoracolumbar sympathetic intermediolateral cell column. Köhler et al. (1984) have demonstrated

Fig. 57. Darkfield photomicrographs of 9 brainstem sections of a cat with an injection of ^{3}H-leucine in the area of the PVN of the hypothalamus. Note the distinct descending pathway in the area next to the pyramidal tract and its fiber distribution to the NRM/NRP, dorsal vagal nucleus, area postrema and rostral solitary complex. (From Holstege, 1987).

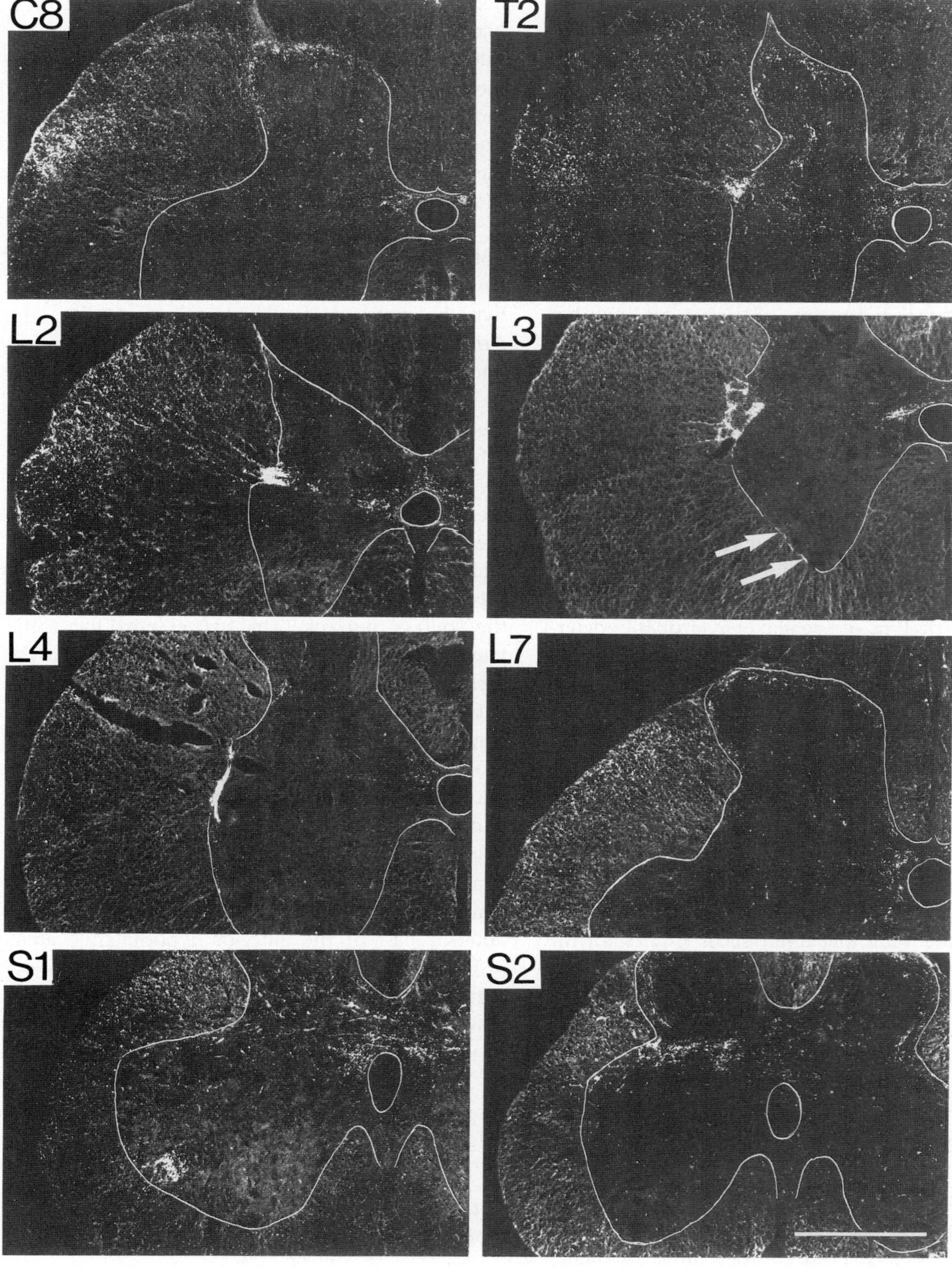
C8
T2
L2
L3
L4
L7
S1
S2

that at least part of the lateral hypothalamo-spinal neurons contain αMSH, and that some of the spinally projecting cells also send fibers to the hippocampus.

The lateral hypothalamic projection to the caudal pontine and medullary lateral tegmental field and to the intermediate zone throughout the length of the spinal cord is interesting, since the caudal brainstem lateral tegmentum can be considered as the rostral continuation of the spinal intermediate zone (see p. 328 – 329). No direct lateral hypothalamic projections exist to the oculomotor, trochlear, trigeminal, abducens, facial and hypoglossal nerve motor nuclei, nor to the retractor bulbi motoneuronal cell group, dorsal group of the nucleus ambiguus or the interneurons of the nucleus retroambiguus. On the other hand, the many parasympathetic motoneurons located in the caudal brainstem lateral tegmentum, such as those innervating the salivatory glands (Hosoya et al., 1983), receive lateral hypothalamic afferents. In summary, the lateral hypothalamus has direct access to autonomic motoneurons in brainstem and spinal cord, and indirect access, via premotor interneurons, to the somatic motoneurons of brainstem and spinal cord.

Many of the brainstem motoneurons are involved in activities such as swallowing, chewing and licking. It is interesting that the lateral hypothalamus is involved in feeding and drinking behavior (Grossman et al., 1978) as well as in salivation (Epstein, 1971). It is probably also involved in cardiovascular control (Stock et al., 1981) and defense behavior (see next section).

Projections from amygdala and bed nucleus of the stria terminalis to caudal brainstem and spinal cord

Hopkins and Holstege (1978), using the autoradiographical tracing method, were the first to describe direct projections from the central nucleus of the amygdala (CA) to the caudal brainstem and first cervical spinal segment. HRP injections in the dorsomedial medulla (Schwaber et al., 1980) and in the NRM and NRP (Holstege et al., 1985) revealed many HRP-labeled neurons in the CA and in the lateral part of the bed nucleus of the stria terminalis (BNSTL). A continuum of HRP labeled neurons was observed in both studies extending from the CA dorsomedially along the medial border of the internal capsule into the BNSTL. Such a distribution pattern is suggestive of a nucleus split into two different parts by the fibers of the internal capsule in the same way as the caudate nucleus and the putamen. As early as 1923 Johnston considered the central and medial amygdaloid nuclei and the BNST as a single anatomic entity, and many others have accepted this concept (see De Olmos et al., 1985, Holstege et al., 1985 and Heimer et al., this volume). In agreement with this concept is that both areas (CA and BNSTL) receive afferents from the same brainstem structures such as the solitary nuclei (Ricardo and Koh, 1978 in the rat, however see Russchen et al., 1982 in the cat and Beckstead et al., 1980 in the monkey) and parabrachial nuclei (Saper and Loewy, 1980). In addition, both areas contain neurons with the same neuropeptides, for example neurotensin, substance P, cholecystokinin, vasoactive intestinal polypeptide, enkephalin, somatostatin and dynorphin. Some of these neurons have also been shown to project to the brainstem (cf. Price et al., 1987, for review). Moreover, the projections from CA and BNST to the caudal brainstem are virtually identical (Hopkins and Holstege, 1978; Holstege et al., 1985). Both structures send many fibers to the lateral hypothalamic area, and via the medial

---

Fig. 58. Darkfield photomicrographs of the spinal cord of the same cat as illustrated in Fig. 57, with a ^{3}H-leucine injection in the area of the PVN of the hypothalamus. Note the projection to lamina I (C8, T2 and L7), the sympathetic intermediolateral cell group (T2, L2, L3 and L4), the nucleus of Onuf (S1) and the parasympathetic intermediomedial and intermediolateral cell group (S2). The arrows in L3 probably indicate projections to distal dendrites of the motoneurons located in the sympathetic intermediolateral cell group. (From Holstege, 1987).

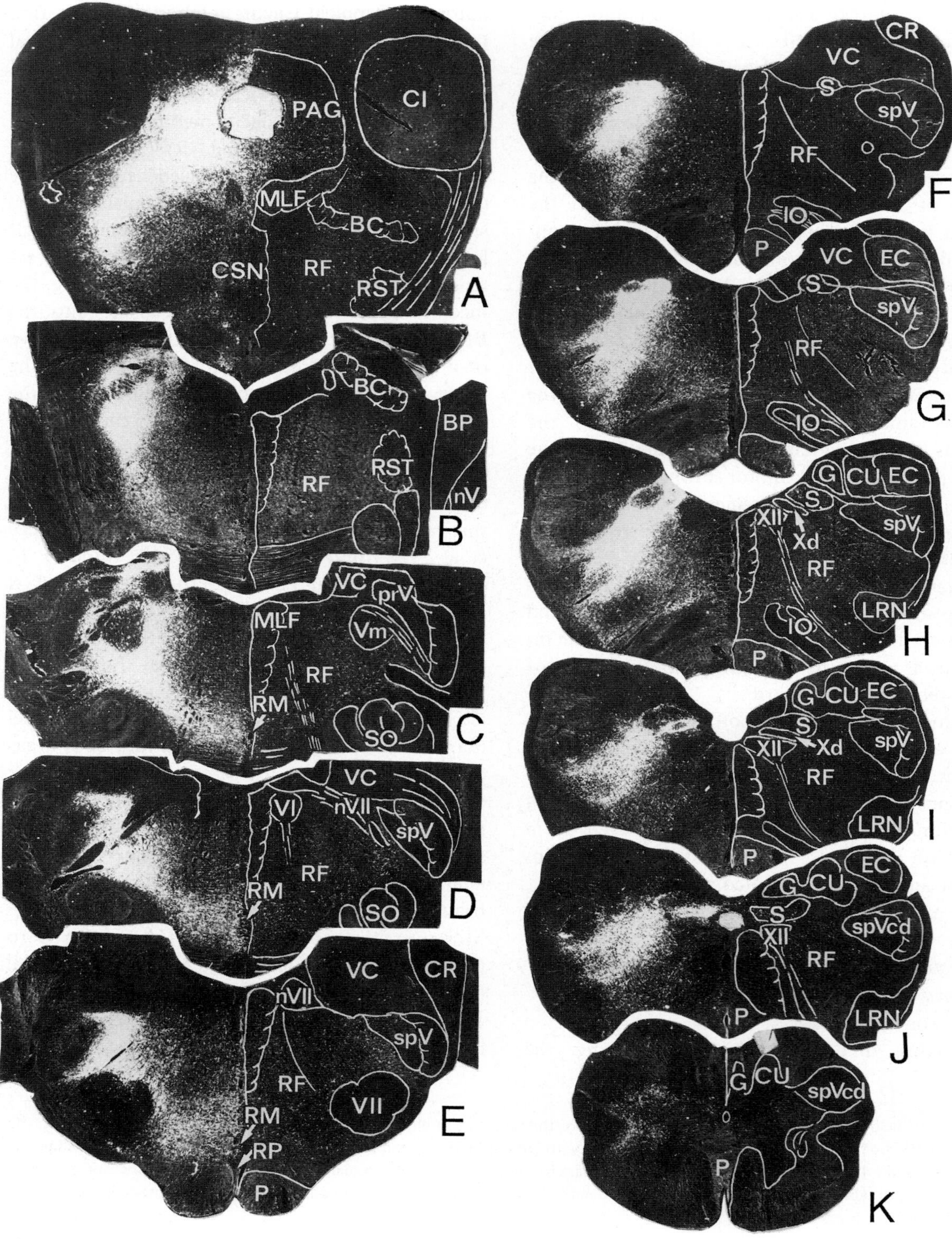
PAG
CI
MLF
BC
CSN
RF
RST
A
BC
BP
RST
RF
nV
B
VC
prV
MLF
Vm
RF
RM
SO
C
VC
VI
nVII
spV
RF
RM
SO
D
VC
CR
nVII
spV
RF
VII
RM
RP
P
E
CR
VC
S
spV
RF
IO
P
F
VC
EC
S
spV
RF
IO
G
G
CU
EC
S
XII
Xd
spV
RF
LRN
IO
P
H
G
CU
EC
S
XII
Xd
spV
RF
LRN
P
I
EC
G
CU
S
XII
spVcd
RF
P
LRN
J
G
CU
spVcd
P
K

forebrain bundle, to the lateral part of the mesencephalon, pons, and medulla oblongata (amygdala: Hopkins and Holstege, 1978 in the cat; Price and Amaral, 1981 in the monkey; BNST: Holstege et al., 1985 in the cat; Fig. 59). At mesencephalic levels fibers were distributed from this fiber bundle to the PAG (except its dorsolateral part), the ventrolaterally adjoining nucleus cuneiformis and pedunculopontine nucleus, and the mesencephalic lateral tegmental field, including the paralemniscal nucleus. Part of these fibers (at least those derived from the BNST) probably contain vasopressin as a neurotransmitter (De Vries and Buys, 1983). In the pons, fibers terminate laterally in the tegmentum, i.e. the medial and lateral parabrachial nuclei, the nucleus Kölliker-Fuse, the nucleus subcoeruleus and the locus coeruleus. With respect to the projections to the locus coeruleus, Price and Amaral (1981) in the monkey did not observe fibers terminating in the nucleus itself, but just lateral to it. At the level of the motor trigeminal nucleus some fibers branch off from the lateral descending fiber bundle, passing ventrally and medially to terminate in the ventral part of the caudal pontine and upper medullary medial tegmentum. A few fibers terminate in the NRM, but none in the NRP (Fig. 56G – H). At medullary levels many fibers terminate in the lateral tegmental field as defined by Holstege et al. (1977) (section 2b) as well as in the rostral and caudal parts of the solitary nucleus and the peripheral parts of the dorsal vagal nucleus. In the same way as the projections from the hypothalamus, no direct projections exist from CA and BNST to the oculomotor, trochlear, trigeminal, abducens, facial and hypoglossal motor nuclei, and also none to the motoneurons in the nucleus retractor bulbi and dorsal group of the

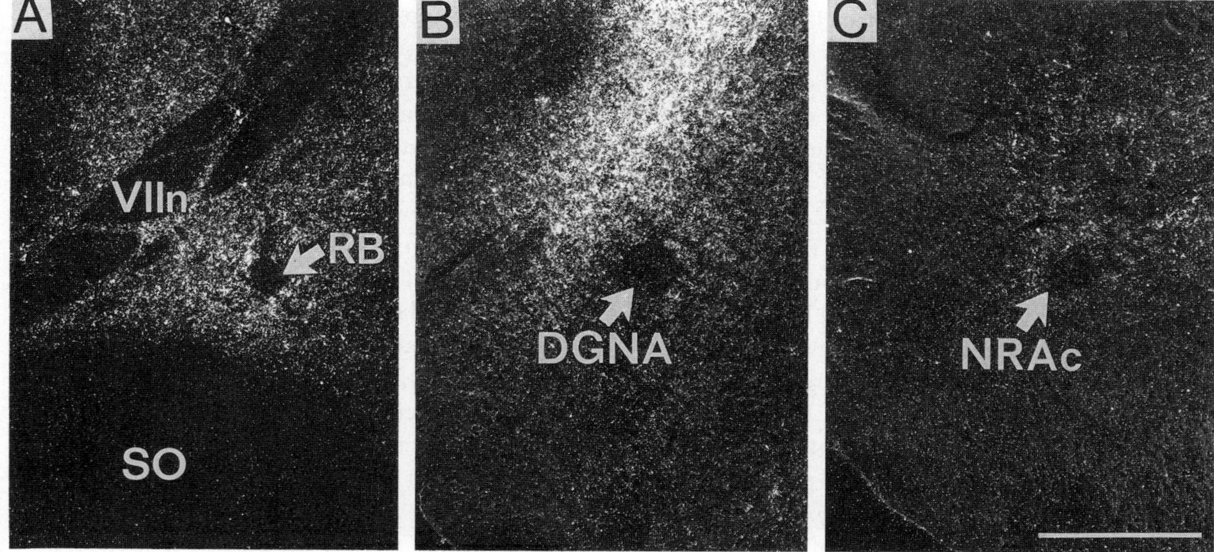

Fig. 60. Darkfield photomicrographs of 3 different rostrocaudal levels of the lateral tegmental field in a cat with an injection centered on the central nucleus of the amygdala. Note the absence of labeled fibers in the motor nucleus of the retractor bulbi motor nucleus (A), the dorsal group of the nucleus ambiguus (B) and the caudal nucleus retroambiguus (C). Bar represents 1 mm.

Fig. 59. Darkfield photomicrographs of 11 brainstem sections of a cat with an injection of ^{3}H-leucine in the bed nucleus of the stria terminalis. Note the strong projection to the PAG, with the exception of its dorsolateral part. Note also the strong projection to the bulbar lateral tegmental field and the projection to the ventral part of the caudal pontine and upper medullary medial tegmentum. (From Holstege et al., 1985).

nucleus ambiguus, nor to the interneurons in the nucleus retroambiguus (Fig. 60). Both CA and BNSTL send a few fibers to the intermediate zone of the C1 spinal cord, but not beyond that level. This corresponds with the finding that a hemi-infiltration of HRP at the level of C2 does not produce HRP labeled neurons in CA or BNSTL, (Holstege et al., 1985; Holstege, 1987b). Thus, there is no evidence for amygdaloid projections to the spinal cord other than to the intermediate zone of the first cervical segment (Mizuno et al., 1985; Sandrew et al., 1986).

A great similarity exists between the caudal brainstem projections originating in the CA and BNSTL on the one hand and the lateral hypothalamic area on the other. All three areas have very strong mutual connections. Neurons in CA and BNSTL receive many afferent fibers from other (basolateral and basomedial) amygdaloid nuclei (Krettek and Price, 1978), but these connections are not reciprocal (see also Price et al., 1987 for review). Apparently, both CA and BNSTL serve as ''output nuclei'' for other parts of the amygdala/bed nucleus of the stria terminalis complex to reach the caudal brainstem. The lateral hypothalamus also may have this function, although its afferent connections are less clearly defined, mainly because of the many fibers of passage in the medial forebrain bundle.

The direct projections from CA, BNSTL and the lateral hypothalamus to the caudal brainstem lateral tegmental field may form the anatomic framework of the final output of the defense response of the animal. Electrical stimulation in the amygdala (especially the basal and central nuclei), bed nucleus of the stria terminalis, lateral hypothalamus, and PAG elicits defensive behavior (Fernandez de Molina and Hunsperger, 1962; Bandler et al., 1990). In fact there exists a column of electrical stimulation sites from CA, BNST, lateral hypothalamus, and PAG through the lateral mesencephalic tegmentum into the lateral tegmentum of the caudal brainstem, which elicits defensive behavior (Abrahams et al., 1960, Coote et al., 1973). Kaada (1972) gives an excellent description of the defense response in cats. The initial phase of such a response is arrest of all spontaneous ongoing activities, and the whole attitude of the animal changes to one of attention. The arousal is followed by orienting or searching movements towards the contralateral side, frequently accompanied by sniffing, swallowing, chewing, and by twitching of the ipsilateral facial musculature. Later in the defense reaction the cat retracts its head and crouches with the ears flattened to a posterior position. The cat growls or hisses, the pupils are dilated and there is piloerection, elevation of blood pressure with bradycardia, increased rate of breathing, alteration of gastric motility and secretion. On stronger stimulation an ''affective'' attack may take place, in which the cat strikes with its paw with claws unsheathed, in a series of swift, accurate blows. If the stimulus continues, the cat will bite savagely. Many of the activities in the beginning of the defense response are coordinated in the caudal brainstem lateral tegmental field. The observation that part of this behavior appears to be ipsilateral corresponds with the predominantly ipsilateral projection of CA, BNSTL and lateral hypothalamus to the caudal brainstem lateral tegmentum. Edwards and Flynn (1971) have shown that during the strike movement in the ''affective'' attack, a pure facilitation of the pyramidal tract neurons of the ipsilateral motor cortex takes place. In addition there are mainly facilitatory influences at the motoneuronal level in the spinal cord, which might be the result of the CA, BNST, lateral hypothalamus, and mesencephalic projections to the ventral part of the medullary medial reticular formation, which in turn projects diffusely to all motoneuronal cell groups in the spinal cord.

Fig. 61 gives a schematic overview of the descending projections to the caudal brainstem from hypothalamus, amygdala and BNST. Similar to the descending projections from the mesencephalon, there is a mediolateral organization within this descending system in which the medial hypothalamus forms the medial, and the lateral hypothalamus, amygdala and BNST the lateral component. The PVN, with its direct projections to all preganglionic (sympathetic and parasympathetic) motoneurons in brainstem and spinal cord, occupies a separate position within this framework.

Projections from the prefrontal cortex to caudal brainstem and spinal cord

In recent years it has been shown that the prefrontal cortex projects directly to the caudal brainstem. Most of these studies are done in the rat, in which the medial frontal cortex sends fibers to the solitary nuclei (NTS), the dorsal parts of the parabrachial nuclei, the PAG and the superior colliculus (Van der Kooy et al., 1984; Neafsy et al., 1986; Terreberry and Neafsy, 1987). The insular cortex projects also to the NTS and PAG (Ruggiero et al., 1987; Neafsy et al., 1986). Ruggiero et al. (1987) also found that electrical stimulation of the rat's insular cortex leads to elevation of arterial pressure and cardioacceleration. Also in the rat projections from the infralimbic cortex to the spinal cord have been reported by Hurley-Gius et al. (1986). After WGA-HRP injections in this part of the cortex, they observed labeled fibers descending contralaterally in the base of the dorsal column and bilaterally in the dorsolateral funiculi. These fibers terminated in laminae I and IV-V throughout the length of the spinal cord and a few in the intermediolateral cell column. Projections from the prefrontal cortex to the NRM, NRP and adjacent tegmentum have not been described. In animals other than the rat studies on the prefrontal cortical projections to the brainstem are extremely

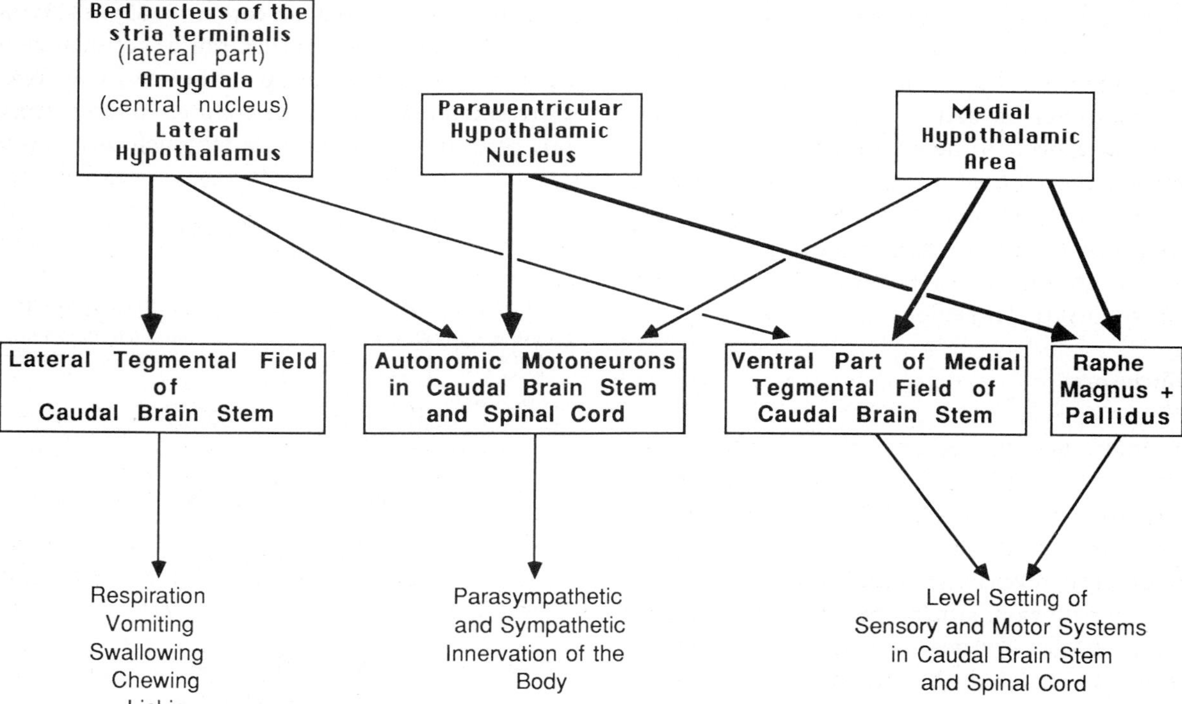

Fig. 61. Schematic overview of the mediolateral organization of the limbic system pathways to brainstem and spinal cord and its possible functional implications. The strongest projections are indicated by thick arrows. (From Holstege, 1988a).

scarce. In the cat, Willett et al. (1986), by means of the WGA-HRP method, found that the orbital gyrus, anterior insular cortex and infralimbic cortex project to the nucleus tractus solitarius. In the monkey, Arnsten and Goldman-Rakic (1984), using the anterograde autoradiographic tracing technique, demonstrated that the dorsolateral and dorsomedial prefrontal cortex projects to the locus coeruleus and nucleus raphe centralis superior. They did not observe labeled fibers beyond the level of the locus coeruleus, and suggested that frontal cortical fibers to more caudal brainstem areas do not exist. It must be emphasized that Arnsten and Goldman-Rakic (1984) in their autoradiographic tracing study used survival times of only 24 – 48 hours. However, much longer survival times are necessary to adequately label the fibers over longer distances (see Holstege 1987b for an extensive review of the use of the autoradiographic tracing technique). Therefore, in the light of the findings in rat and cat, it is extremely unlikely that the frontal cortex in the monkey does not project to the caudal brainstem. In an earlier section (p. 365 – 368) it has been pointed out that there exist major differences between cat, monkey and humans in respect to the projections and the functions of the motor cortex. The motor cortex in primates has taken over many of the ''motor tasks'', performed by brainstem structures in rat and cat. This might also be the case for the fronto-orbital cortical projections in primates.

Conclusions

An enormous number of new studies have been published in the last 10 years on the descending motor pathways to caudal brainstem and spinal cord and about the physiological and pharmacological properties of them. Nevertheless all the new pathways seem to belong to one of three major motor systems in the central nervous system, which determine the activity of the somatic and autonomic motoneurons. In this concept the motoneuronal cell columns themselves are not considered a central motor system, but the beginning of the peripheral motor system (motoneuronal cell body-motor nerve-muscle).

The first motor system

The first system (Fig. 62) is formed by the premotor interneuronal projections to the motoneurons. These neurons receive direct or indirect afferent information from the periphery via peripheral afferent nerves and from the second and/or third motor system. They are of paramount importance for determining the final output of the motoneurons. It is not always true that these interneurons are located close to their target motoneurons. For example those involved in back-musculature control travel over large distances through the spinal cord. Also the interneurons involved in the cutaneus trunci muscle (CTM) reflex send their fibers over large distances, because part the afferent information for the CTM reflex enters the spinal cord far from where the CTM motoneurons are located.

As has been pointed out earlier (p. 328 – 329) the bulbar lateral tegmental field can be considered as the rostral extent of the spinal intermediate zone. Correspondingly this area contains interneurons, not only for the brainstem motoneurons of the

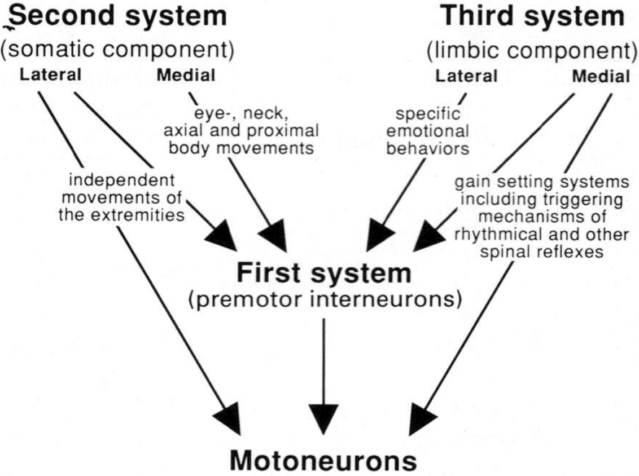

Fig. 62. Schematic overview of the three subdivisions of the motor system.

cranial nerves V, VII, X and XII, but also for some motoneuronal cell groups in the spinal cord. Also these interneurons belong to the first system. Examples are the medullary interneurons projecting to the phrenic and other respiratory related motoneuronal cell groups. Since most of the afferent information from the respiratory organs does not enter the central nervous system via the spinal cord, but via the brainstem (vagal nerve), it is natural that the interneurons involved are located in the region of entrance. The author of this paper reckons the micturition related interneurons in the dorsolateral pons also to this system. They are of enormous importance for micturition,. because via their long descending pathways they determine whether bladder and bladder-sphincter function synergistically. The question arises why these neurons are located so far from their target motoneurons. In that respect it is important to realize that micturition is strongly correlated with the emotional state of the individual. Therefore, the micturition interneurons need to receive afferent information from the limbic system, which is available in the dorsolateral pons, but not in the sacral cord. The interneurons involved in blood-pressure control and projecting to the sympathetic motoneurons in the intermediolateral cell column of the thoracolumbar cord are located in the ventrolateral medulla. Their afferent information enters the central nervous system via the brainstem (vagal nerve), while afferent information from the limbic system, which plays an extremely important role in determining the level of the blood pressure, is also available.

The bulbar lateral tegmental field corresponds with the caudal part of Nieuwenhuys' paracore (Nieuwenhuys et al., 1988), mainly because it receives many afferent connections from the lateral limbic system and because it contains adrenergic (C1 and C2) and nor-adrenergic (A1 – A6) cell groups. However, the great majority of the neurons in the bulbar lateral tegmental field serve as interneurons for motoneurons in caudal brainstem and spinal cord. Although it is true that many of them play a role in the generation of so-called fixed action patterns, such as biting, swallowing and licking, which can be elicited in the limbic system, the same interneurons also receive many afferents from second system structures such as motor cortex and red nucleus. In the present concept the interneurons in the bulbar lateral tegmental field belong to the first and not to the third system.

In summary, the first motor system is formed by the interneuronal projections to the motoneurons. They are present in the caudal brainstem, the spinal cord, and between brainstem and spinal cord.

The second motor system

The second motor system (Fig. 62) is discussed on pp. 348 – 366. The projections of this system have been studied for some time, mainly because they exist of thick fibers, which could be detected with the lesion-degeneration techniques in the nineteen-fifties and sixties. The fibers of this system terminate to only a limited extent directly on motoneurons, but for the most part on the interneurons of the first motor system. Kuypers was the first to point out the mediolateral organization within this system. The medial component originates mainly in the brainstem (dorsal two thirds of the pontine and medullary medial tegmentum, vestibular nuclei, superior colliculus, interstitial nucleus of Cajal and caudal Field H of Forel), descends medially in the ventral funiculus of the spinal cord and terminates on inter- and to a lesser extent motoneurons of the medial motor column in the spinal cord. The medial motor column controls eye- and neck-movements and axial and proximal body movements. The function of the medial system is maintenance of erect posture (antigravity movements), integration of body and limbs, synergy of the whole limb and orientation of body and head (Kuypers, 1981). On the other hand, the lateral component of this second motor system is formed by laterally descending fibersystems, terminating in laterally located inter- and to a more limited extent motoneurons in caudal brainstem and spinal cord (the lateral motor column). These systems are represented by the rubrospinal tract, (of minor importance in humans) and the lateral corticospinal tract, (in humans extremely well developed). The lateral motor column in the spinal cord innervates the distal body musculature, i.e. those of the distal limbs. The lateral component of the voluntary motor system produces independent flexion-biased movements of the extremities, in particular of the elbow and hand (Kuypers, 1981).

The third motor system

The third motor system (Fig. 62) is discovered only recently. Although there was clinical evidence that a separate motor system had to exist, anatomical studies did not find any evidence for such a system. In the last 15 years that has changed drastically. It appeared that modern tracing techniques were able to demonstrate a large number of new pathways. They all consisted of thin fibers, which was the reason that the lesion-degeneration techniques were not able to demonstrate them earlier. The development of the immunohistochemical techniques has revealed a large number of neurotransmitters or neuromodulators within the central nervous system. Interestingly, with the exception of acetylcholine, glutamate and aspertate, all these new monoamines and peptides were found in the third motor system.

The third motor system, which largely corresponds with the core and medial paracore of Nieuwenhuys et al. (1988), is strongly connected with the limbic system and systematically skips the areas belonging to the second one, such as red nucleus, interstitial nucleus of Cajal and other peri-oculomotor areas, the dorsal two thirds of the caudal brainstem medial tegmentum, vestibular nuclei or precerebellar structures as pontine nuclei, inferior olive or lateral reticular nucleus. Reversely, the second motor system does not overlap in its projections with the third motor system. An exception to this rule are the monoaminergic projections originating in the raphe nuclei and locus coeruleus/subcoeruleus complex. These structures, which belong to the third system, send fibers to many structures in the central nervous system, including some belonging to the second system (e.g. the inferior olive and cerebellum).

A mediolateral organization is present within the third motor system. The medial component originates in the medial portions of hypothalamus and in the mesencephalon and terminates in the area of locus coeruleus/subcoeruleus and in the ventral part of the caudal pontine and medullary medial tegmental field. The latter structures determine the final output of this system. The lateral component originates laterally in the limbic system, i.e. in the lateral hypothalamus, central nucleus of the amygdala and bed nucleus of the stria terminalis. These structures project to the lateral tegmental field of caudal pons and medulla, but not to the somatic motoneurons in this area. In how far the prefrontal cortex plays a role within these systems remains to be determined. There are some exceptions on this general subdivision into medial and lateral third motor systems; 1) Within the PAG and lateral adjacent tegmentum, some specific groups of neurons exist, projecting to areas outside the caudal brainstem ventromedial tegmental field, such as the nucleus retroambiguus, cervical spinal cord or subretrofacial nucleus. These neurons are probably related to specific functions, such as vocalization, head movements involved in emotional behavior or blood pressure control. They may serve as final common pathways for especially the lateral component of the third motor system. 2) Some of the fibers of the lateral component of the third descending system terminate in the ventromedial tegmentum at levels around the facial nucleus. Neurons in this area in turn project diffusely to the dorsal horn of the spinal cord. Via these fibers the lateral component structures may have some control over nociception.

The functional implications of the third system motor pathways differ, depending on whether they belong to the medial or lateral system. The medial system, via its projections to the locus coeruleus/ nucleus subcoeruleus and NRM and NRP/NRO and the diffuse coeruleo- and raphe-spinal pathways, has a global effect on the level of activity of the somatosensory and motoneurons in general by changing their membrane excitability. In other words, the emotional brain has a great impact on the sensory as well as on the motor system. In both systems it sets the gain or level of functioning of the neurons. The emotional state of the individual determines this level. For example it is well known that many forms of stress, such as aggression, fear and sexual arousal, induce analgesia, while at the same time the motor system is set at a "high" level and motoneurons can easily be excited by the second motor system. In this concept the brainstem structures, which project diffusely to all parts of the spinal cord, can be considered as tools for the limbic system controlling spinal cord activity. The diffuse descending system is also used to trigger rhythmical (locomotion, shivering) or other (lordosis) in essence spinal reflexes. Whether functions such as locomotion, shivering and lordosis use different or the same diffuse pathways from the caudal brainstem to the spinal cord is not yet clear. If they use the same pathways, the differences lie in the function of the spinal generators for each of these functions. The lateral component of the third motor system project to the caudal brainstem lateral tegmental field, which contains first motor system interneurons involved in specific functions such as respiration, vomiting, swallowing, chewing, and licking. These activities are displayed in the beginning of flight or defense response and can be easily elicited by stimulation of the lateral parts of the limbic system. Therefore it seems that the lateral component of the third motor systems is involved in more specific activities, related to emotional behavior.

It is intriguing that both the medial and lateral components of the second and third motor systems are involved in similar activities. The medial components are involved in general activities such as in integration of body and limbs and orientation of body and head for the second system and level setting of neurons for the third system. On the other hand, the lateral components are involved in specific activities such as independent movements of the extremities for the second motor system and blood pressure and respiration control, vocalization, vomiting, swallowing, chewing, and licking for the third motor system.

Acknowledgements

This work was supported by NASA Grant NCC 2 – 491 to Gert Holstege. The author thanks Drs. Han Collewijn, R. Nieuwenhuys and J. Voogd for reading the manuscript and their comments. Furthermore he thanks his brother Joan Holstege for the helpful discussions and suggestions about the text on the diffuse descending pathways.

Abbreviations

AA	anterior amygdaloid nucleus
AC	anterior commissure
ACN	nucleus of the anterior commissure
AD	anterodorsal nucleus of the thalamus
AH	anterior hypothalamic area
AL	lateral amygdaloid nucleus
AM	anteromedial nucleus of the thalamus
AP	area postrema
Aq	aqueduct of Sylvius
AV	anteroventral nucleus of the thalamus
BC	brachium conjunctivum
BIC	brachium of the inferior colliculus
BL	basolateral amygdaloid nucleus
BM	basomedial amygdaloid nucleus
BNST	bed nucleus of the stria terminalis
BNSTL	lateral part of the bed nucleus of stria terminalis
BNSTM	medial part of the bed nucleus of the stria terminalis
BP	brachium pontis
CA	central amygdaloid nucleus
CC	corpus callosum
Cd	caudate nucleus
CGL	lateral geniculate body
CGLd	lateral geniculate body (dorsal part)
CGLv	lateral geniculate body (ventral part)
CGM	medial geniculate body
CGMd	medial geniculate body, dorsal part
CGMint	medial geniculate body, interior division

CGMp medial geniculate body, principal part
CI capsula interna
CL claustrum
CL nucleus centralis lateralis of the thalamus
CM centromedian thalamic nucleus
CN cochlear nuclei
CO cortical amygdaloid nucleus
CP posterior commissure
CR corpus restiforme
cru cruciate sulcus
CS superior colliculus
CSN nucleus raphe centralis superior
CU nucleus cuneatus
CUN cuneiform nucleus
D nucleus of Darkschewitsch
DBV nucleus of the diagonal band of Broca
DGNA dorsal group of the nucleus ambiguus
DH dorsal hypothalamic area
DMH dorsomedial hypothalamic nucleus
DTN dorsal tegmental nucleus
EC external cuneate nucleus
ECU external cuneate nucleus
En entopeduncular nucleus
EW nucleus Edinger-Westphal
F fornix
fRF fasciculus retroflexus
G nucleus gracilis
GP globus pallidus
Hab habenular nucleus
Habl lateral habenular nucleus
Habm medial habenular nucleus
HC hippocampus
HPA posterior hypothalamus area
IC inferior colliculus
IN interpeduncular nucleus
INC interstitial nucleus of Cajal
IO inferior olive
IP interpeduncular nucleus
IVN inferior vestibular nucleus
KF nucleus Kölliker-Fuse
Latiss latissimus dorsi muscle
LD nucleus lateralis dorsalis of the thalamus
LGN lateral geniculate nucleus
LH lateral hypothalamic area
LL lateral lemniscus
LONGISS longissimus dorsi muscle
LOTR lateral olfactory tract
LP lateral posterior nucleus of the thalamus
LRN lateral reticular nucleus
LTF lateral tegmental field
LV lateral ventricle
LVN lateral vestibular nucleus
MA medial amygdaloid nucleus
MB mammillary body
MC nucleus medialis centralis of the thalamus
MD nucleus medialis dorsalis of the thalamus
MesV mesencephalic trigeminal tract
ML medial lemniscus
MLF medial longitudinal fasciculus
motV motor trigeminal nucleus
MTF medial tegmental field
mV motor trigeminal nucleus
MVN medial vestibular nucleus
MTN medial terminal nucleus
NCL nucleus centralis lateralis
NLL nucleus of the lateral lemniscus
NOT nucleus of the optic tract
NOTL lateral nucleus of the optic tract
NOTM medial nucleus of the optic tract
NPC nucleus paracentralis of the thalamus
NTB nucleus of the trapezoid body
NR red nucleus
NRA nucleus retroambiguus
NRAc caudal nucleus retroambiguus
NRM nucleus raphe magnus
NRP nucleus raphe pallidus
NRTP nucleus reticularis tegmenti pontis
NSC nucleus subcoeruleus
NTB nucleus of the trapezoid body
nVI abducens nerve
nVII facial nerve
nVIII vestibulocochlear nerve
OBL. EXT. external oblique abdominal muscle
OBL. INT. internal oblique abdominal muscle
OC optic chiasm
OL olivary pretectal nucleus
OR optic radiation
OT optic tract
P pyramidal tract
PAG periaqueductal gray
PbL lateral parabrachial nucleus
PBM medial parabrachial nucleus
TMT mammillothalamic tract

PC	pedunculus cerebri
PCN	nucleus of the posterior commissure
PEA	anterior part of periventricular hypothalamic nucleus
PH	periventricular hypothalamic nucleus
PON	pontine nuclei
PONT Med RF	pontine medial reticular formation
PP	posterior pretectal nucleus
Pt	parataenial nucleus of the thalamus
PT	Probst tract
PTA	anterior pretectal nucleus
PTM	medial pretectal nucleus
Pu	putamen
Pul	pulvinar nucleus of the thalamus
PV	posterior paraventricular nucleus of the thalamus
PVA	paraventricular nucleus of the thalamus (anterior part)
PVG	periventricular gray
PVN	paraventricular hypothalamic nucleus
R	reticular nucleus of the thalamus
RB	restiform body
RB	retractor bulbi motor nucleus
RE	nucleus reuniens of the thalamus
RECTUS	rectus abdominis muscle
RF	reticular formation
RFmed	medial reticular formation
RFlat	lateral reticular formation
RiMLF	rostral interstitial nucleus of the MLF
RM	nucleus raphe magnus
RN	red nucleus
Rpo	nucleus raphe pontis
RST	rubrospinal tract
S	solitary complex
SC	suprachiasmatic nucleus
SC	nucleus subcoeruleus
SI	substantia innominata
SM	stria medullaris
SN	substantia nigra
SO	superior olivary complex
SON	supraoptic nucleus
spin V	spinal trigeminal complex
ST	subthalamic nucleus
STT	stria terminalis
SUB	subiculum
SVN	superior vestibular nucleus
Transv.	transversus abdominis muscle
TMT	mammillothalamic tract
TS	tract of the solitary nucleus
VA	ventroanterior nucleus of the thalamus
VB	ventrobasal complex of the thalamus
VC	vestibular complex
VL	ventrolateral nucleus of the thalamus
VM	ventromedial nucleus of the thalamus
VMH	ventromedial nucleus of the hypothalamus
VPL	nucleus ventralis posterolateralis of the thalamus
VTA	ventral tegmental area of Tsai
VTN	ventral tegmental nucleus
ZI	zona incerta
III	oculomotor nucleus
IV	trochlear nucleus
Vm	motor trigeminal nucleus
Vn	trigeminal nerve
Vpr.	principal trigeminal nucleus
Vprinc.	principal trigeminal nucleus
Vsp.	spinal trigeminal complex
V sp. cd.	spinal trigeminal complex pars caudalis
V spin.caud.	spinal trigeminal complex pars caudalis
VI	abducens nucleus
VII	facial nucleus
VIIn	facial nerve
XII	hypoglossal nucleus

References

Abols, I.A. and Basbaum, A.I. (1981) Afferent connections of the rostral medulla of the cat: a neural substrate for midbrain-medullary interactions in the modulation of pain. *J. Comp. Neurol.,* 201: 285 – 297.

Abrahams, V.C., Hilton, S.M. and Zbrozyna, A. (1960) Active muscle vasodilatation produced by stimulation of the brain stem: its significance in the defence reaction. *J. Physiol.,* 154: 491 – 513.

Abrahams, V.C. and Keane, J. (1984) Contralateral, midline and commissural motoneurons of neck muscles: a retrograde HRP study in the cat. *J. Comp. Neurol.,* 223: 448 – 456.

Akaike, T., Fanardjian, V.V., Ito, M. and Ohno, T. (1973) Electrophysiological analysis of the vestibulospinal reflex pathway in the rabbit. II. Synaptic actions upon spinal neurons. *Exp. Brain Res.,* 17: 497 – 515.

Akaike, A., Shibata, T., Satoh, M. and Takagi, H. (1978) Analgesia induced by microinjection of morphine into, and electrical stimulation of, the nucleus reticularis paragigantocellularis of rat medulla oblongata. *Neuropharmacol.,* 17:

775 – 778.

Albanese, A., Altavista, M.C. and Rossi, P. (1986) Organization of central nervous system dopaminergic pathways. *J. Neural. Transm.*, 22 (Suppl.): 3 – 17.

Alstermark, B., Kimmel, H. and Tantisira, B. (1987) Monosynaptic raphespinal and reticulospinal projection to forelimb motoneurons in cats. *Neurosci. Lett.*, 74: 286 – 290.

Alstermark, B., Kummel, H., Pinter, M.J. and Tantisira, B. (1987) Branching and termination of C3 – C4 propriospinal neurones in the cervical spinal cord of the cat. *Neurosci. Lett.*, 74: 291 – 296.

Alstermark, B., Lundberg, A., Norsell, U. and Sybirska, E. (1981) Integration in descending motor pathways controlling the forelimb in the cat. 9. Differential behavioral defects after spinal cord lesions interrupting defined pathways from higher centers to motoneurones. *Exp. Brain Res.*, 42: 299 – 318.

Anderson, J.H. (1981) Ocular torsion in the cat after lesions of the interstitial nucleus of Cajal. *Ann. NY Acad. Sci.*, 374: 865 – 871.

Anderson, M.E. (1971) Cerebellar and cerebral inputs to physiologically identified efferent cell groups in the red nucleus of the cat. *Brain Res.*, 30: 49 – 66.

Anderson, M.E., Yoshida, M. and Wilson, V.J. (1971) Influence of superior colliculus on cat neck motoneurons. *J. Neurophysiol.*, 34: 898 – 907.

Appenteng, K., O'Donovan, M.J., Somjen, G. and Stephens, J.A. (1978) The projection of jaw elevator muscle spindle afferents to fifth nerve motoneurons in the cat. *J. Physiol. (Lond.)*, 279: 409 – 424.

Armand, J. and Kuypers, H.G.J.M. (1980) Cells of origin of crossed and uncrossed corticospinal fibers. A quantitative horseradish peroxidase study. *Exp. Brain Res.*, 42: 299 – 318.

Armand, J., Holstege, G. and Kuijpers, H.G.J.M. (1985) Differential corticospinal projections in the cat. An autoradiographical tracing study. *Brain Res.*, 343: 351 – 355.

Armstrong, D.M. (1986) Supraspinal contributions to the initiation and control of locomotion in the cat. *Prog. Neurobiol.*, 26: 273 – 361.

Armstrong, D.M. and Schild, R.F. (1979) Spino-olivary neurones in the lumbo-sacral cord of the cat demonstrated by retrograde transport of horseradish peroxidase. *Brain Res.*, 168: 176 – 179.

Arnsten, A.F.T. and Goldman-Rakic, P.S. (1984) Selective prefrontal cortical projections to the region of the locus coeruleus and raphe nuclei in the rhesus monkey. *Brain Res.*, 306: 9 – 18.

Averill, D.B., Cameron, W.E. and Berger, A.J. (1984) Monosynaptic excitation of dorsal medullary respiratory neurons by slowly adapting pulmonary stretch receptors. *J. Neurophysiol.*, 52: 771 – 785.

Bach-y-Rita, P. (1971) Neurophysiology of eye movements. In: P. Bach-y-Rita and C.C. Collins (Eds.), *The control of eye movements.* Academic Press, New York pp. 7 – 45.

Baldissera, F., Hultborn, H. and Illert, M. (1981) Integration in spinal neuronal systems. In: R.E. Burke (Ed.), *Handbook of Physiology, Section I, The Nervous System, Vol. II, Motor Systems.* Washington American Physiological Society. 509 – 595.

Bandler, R. and Carrive, P. (1988) Integrated defence reaction elicited by excitatory amino acid microinjection in the midbrain periaqueductal grey region of the unrestrained cat. *Brain Res.*, 439: 95 – 106.

Bandler, R., Carrive, P. and Zhang, S.P. (1991) Integration of somatic and autonomic reactions within the midbrain periaqueaductal grey: Viscerotopic, somatotopic and functional organization. In: G. Holstege (Ed.), *Role of the forebrain in sensation and behavior,* Chapter 13. Elsevier, Amsterdam, Progr. Brain Res. Vol. 87, pp. 269 – 305.

Barbas-Henry, H. and Wouterlood, F.G. (1988) Synaptic connections between primary trigeminal afferents and accessory abducens motoneurons in the monitor lizard varanus-exanthematicus. *J. Comp. Neurol.*, 267: 387 – 397.

Barrington, F.J.F. (1925) The effect of lesions of the hind- and mid-brain on micturition in the cat. *Quart. J. Exp. Physiol. Cogn. Med.*, 15: 81 – 102.

Basbaum, A.I., Clanton, C.H. and Fields, H.L. (1978) Three bulbospinal pathways from the rostral medulla of the cat: an autoradiographic study of pain modulating system. *J. Comp. Neurol.*, 178: 209 – 224.

Batini, C., Buisseret-Delmas, C. and Corvisier, J. (1976) Horseradish peroxidase localization of masticatory muscle motoneurons in cat. *J. Physiol.*, 72: 301 – 309.

Baulac, M. and Meininger, V. (1981) Organisation des motoneurones des muscles pectoraux chez le chat. Contribution à l'étude de l'arc axillaire (Achselbogen). *Acta Anat.*, 109: 209 – 217.

Baumgarten, R.von, Baumgarten, C.von, and Schäfer, K.P. (1957) Beitrag zur Lokalisationsfrage bulboreticularer respiratorischer Neurone der Katze. *Pflügers Archiv.*, 264: 217 – 227.

Beckstead, R.M., Morse, J.R. and Norgren, R. (1980) The nucleus of the solitary tract in the monkey: projections to the thalamus and brain stem nuclei. *J. Comp. Neurol.*, 190: 259 – 282.

Belin, M.F., Nanopoulos, D., Didier, M., Aguera, M., Steinbusch, H., Verhofstad, A., Maitre, M. and Pujol, J.-F. (1983) Immunohistochemical evidence for the presence of gamma-aminobutyric acid and serotonin in one nerve cell. A study on the raphe nuclei of rat using antibodies to glutamate decarboxylase and serotonin. *Brain Res.*, 275: 329 – 339.

Berger, A.J. (1977) Dorsal respiratory group neurons in the medulla of cat: spinal projections, responses to lung inflation and superior laryngeal nerve stimulation. *Brain Res.*, 135: 231 – 254.

Berger, A.J. (1980) The distribution of the cat's carotid sinus nerve afferent and efferent cell bodies using the horseradish peroxidase technique. *Brain Res.*, 190: 309 – 320.

Berger, A.J. and Averill, D.B. (1983) Projection of single pulmonary stretch receptors to solitary tract region. *J. Neurophysiol.,* 49: 819 – 830.

Berk, M.L. (1987) Projections of the lateral hypothalamus and bed nucleus of the stria terminalis to the dorsal vagal complex in the region. *J. Comp. Neurol.,* 260: 140 – 156.

Berk, M.L. and Finkelstein, J.A. (1981) Afferent projections to the preoptic area and hypothalamic regions in the rat brain. *Neuroscience,* 6 no. 8: 601 – 624.

Berk, M.L. and Finkelstein, J.A. (1982) Efferent connections of the lateral hypothalamic area of the rat: an autoradiographic investigation. *Brain Res. Bull.,* 8: 511 – 526.

Berthier, N.E. and Moore, J.W. (1983) The nictitating membrane response: an electrophysiological study of the abducens nerve and nucleus and the accessory abducens in rabbit. *Brain Res.,* 258: 201 – 211.

Bertrand, F. and Hugelin, A. (1971) Respiratory synchronizing funtion of nucleus parabrachialis medialis: pneumotaxic mechanisms. *J. Neurophysiol.,* 34: 189 – 207.

Bertrand, F., Hugelin, A. and Vibert, J.F. (1974) A stereologic model of pneumotaxic oscillator based on spatial and temporal distributions of neuronal bursts. *J. Neurophysiol.,* 37: 91 – 107.

Besson, J-M. and Chaouch, A. (1987) Peripheral and spinal mechanisms of nociception. *Physiological Rev.,* 67: 67 – 186.

Bieger, D. and Hopkins, D.A. (1987) Viscerotopic representation of the upper alimentary tract in the medulla oblongata in the rat: the nucleus ambiguus. *J. Comp. Neurol.,* 262: 546 – 562.

Birzis, L. and Hemingway, A. (1957) Shivering as a result of brain stimulation. *J. Neurophysiol.,* 20: 91 – 99.

Blaivas, J.G. (1982) The neurophysiology of micturition: a clinical study of 550 patients. *J. Urol.,* 127: 958 – 963.

Bleier, R. (1961) The hypothalamus of the cat: a cytoarchitectonic atlas in the Horsley-Clarke coordinate system. J. Hopkins Press, Baltimore.

Blessing, W.W. and Chalmers, J.P. (1979) Direct projection of catecholamine (presumably dopamine) containing neurons from hypothalamus to spinal cord. *Neurosci. Lett.,* 11: 35 – 41.

Bolk, L., Groppert, E., Kallius, E. and Lubosch, W. (1938) Handbuch der vergleichende Anatomie der Wirbeltiere. Urban and Schwarzenberg, Berlin.

Bongianni, F., Fontana, G. and Pantaleo, T. (1988) Effects of electrical and chemical stimulation of the Bötzinger complex on respiratory activity in the cat. *Brain Res.,* 445: 254 – 261.

Bowker, R.M. (1986) Serotonergic and peptidergic inputs to the primate ventral spinal cord as visualized with multiple chromagens on the same tissue section. *Brain Res.,* 375: 345 – 350.

Bowker, R.M., Westlund, K.N., Sullivan, M.C. and Coulter, J.D. (1982) Organization of serotonergic projections to the spinal cord. *Progr. Brain Res.,* 57: 239 – 265.

Bowker, R.M., Westlund, K.N., Sullivan, M.C., Wilber, J.F. and Coulter, J.D. (1983) Descending serotonergic, peptidergic and cholinergic pathways from the raphe nuclei: A multiple transmitter complex. *Brain Res.,* 288: 33 – 48.

Bowker, R.M., Abbott, L.C. and Dilts, R.P. (1988) Peptidergic neurons in the nucleus raphe magnus and the nucleus gigantocellularis: their distributions, interrelationships, and projections to the spinal cord. In: H.L. Fields and J.M. Besson (Eds.), *Pain Modulation.* Elsevier, Amsterdam *Progr. Brain Res.,* 77: 95 – 127.

Brandt, T. and Dieterich, M. (1987) Pathological eye-head coordination in roll: tonic occular tilt reaction in mesencephalic and medullary lesions. *Brain,* 110: 649 – 666.

Brink, E.E., Morrell, J.I. and Pfaff, D.W. (1979) Localization of lumbar epaxial motoneurons in the rat. *Brain Res.,* 170: 23 – 43.

Brodal, A. (1940) Experimentelle Untersuchungen über die olivocerebellare Lokalisation. *Z. Gesamte Neurol. Psychiatr.,* 169: 1 – 153.

Brodal, A. (1981) *Neurological Anatomy in Relation to Clinical Medicine.* Third Edition, Oxford University Press, Inc.

Brown, A.G. and Fyffe, R.E.W. (1978) The morphology of group Ia afferent fibre collaterals in the spinal cord of the cat. *J. Physiol.* 274: 111 – 128.

Burde, R.M. and Loewy, A.D. (1980) Central origin of oculomotor parasympathetic neurons in the monkey. *Brain Res.,* 198: 434 – 440.

Burke, R.E., Strick, P.L., Kanda, K., Kim, C.C. and Walmsley, B. (1977) Anatomy of medial gastrocnemius and soleus motor nuclei in cat spinal cord. *J. Neurophysiol.,* 40: 667 – 680.

Büttner-Ennever, J.A. and Büttner, U. (1978) A cell group associated with vertical eye movements in the rostral mesencephalic reticular formation of the monkey. *Brain Res.,* 151: 31 – 48.

Büttner-Ennever, J.A. and Büttner, U. (1988) The reticular formation. In: J.A. Büttner-Ennever (Ed.), *Neuroanatomy of the oculomotor system.* Elsevier Science Publishers BV, Amsterdam, New York, Oxford, 119 – 176.

Büttner-Ennever, J.A., Büttner, U., Cohen, B. and Baumgarter, G. (1982) Vertical gaze paralysis and the rostral interstitial nucleus of the medial longitudinal fasciculus. *Brain,* 105: 125 – 149.

Büttner-Ennever, J. and Holstege, G. (1986) Anatomy of premotor centers in the reticular formation controlling oculomotor, skeletomotor and autonomic motor systems. *Progr. Brain Res.,* 64: 89 – 98.

Büttner, U., Büttner-Ennever, J.A. and Henn, V. (1977) Vertical eye movement related unit activity in the rostral mesencephalic reticular formation of the alert monkey. *Brain Res.,* 130: 239 – 253.

Callister, R.J., Brichta, A.M. and Peterson, E.H. (1987) Quantitative analysis of cervical musculature in rats: histochemical composition and motor pool organization. II. deep dorsal muscles. *J. Comp. Neurol.,* 255: 369 – 385.

Cameron, W.E., Averill, D.B. and Berger, A.J. (1983) Morphology of cat phrenic motoneurons as revealed by intracellular injection of horseradish peroxidase. *J. Comp. Neurol.,* 219: 70 – 80.

Cardona, A. and Rudomin, P. (1983) Activation of brainstem serotonergic pathways decreases homosynaptic depression of monosynaptic responses of frog spinal motoneurons. *Brain Res.,* 280: 373 – 378.

Carlton, S.M., Chung, J.M., Leonard, R.B. and Willis, W.D. (1985) Funicular trajectories of brainstem neurons projecting to the lumbar spinal cord in the monkey (Macaca fascicularis): A retrograde labeling study. *J. Comp. Neurol.,* 241: 382 – 404.

Carpenter, M.B., Harbison, J.W. and Peter, P. (1970) Accessory oculomotor nuclei in the monkey: projections and effects of discrete lesions. *J. Comp. Neurol.,* 140: 131 – 154.

Carrive, P., Bandler, R. and Dampney, R.A.L. (1989) Viscerotopic control of regional vascular beds by discrete groups of neurons within the midbrain periaqueductal gray. *Brain Res.,* 493: 385 – 390.

Carstens, E. (1982) Inhibition of spinal dorsal horn neuronal responses to noxious skin heating by medial hypothalamic stimulation in the cat. *J. Neurophysiol.,* 48: 808 – 822.

Carstens, E., Klumpp, D. and Zimmermann, M. (1980) Differential inhibitory effects of medial and lateral midbrain stimulation on spinal neuronal discharges to noxious skin heating in the cat. *J. Neurophysiol.,* 43: 332 – 342.

Castiglioni, A.J., Gallaway, M.C. and Coulter, J.D. (1978) Spinal projections from the midbrain in monkey. *J. Comp. Neurol.,* 178: 329 – 346.

Chan, J.Y.H., Fung, S.J., Chan, S.H.H. and Barnes, C.D. (1986) Facilitation of lumbar monosynaptic reflexes by locus coeruleus in the rat. *Brain Res.,* 369: 103 – 109.

Chan Palay, V., Jonsson, G. and Palay, S.L. (1978) Serotonin and substance P coexist in neurons of the rat's central nervous system. *Proc. Natl. Acad. Sci.,* 75: 1582 – 1586.

Cheney, P.D., Mewes, K. and Fetz, E.E. (1988) Encoding of motor parameters by corticomotoneuronal (CM) and rubromotoneuronal (RM) cells producing postspike facilitation of forelimb muscles in the behaving monkey. *Beh. Brain Res.,* 28: 181 – 191.

Ciriello, J., Caverson, M.M. and Polosa, C. (1986) Function of the ventrolateral medulla in the control of the circulation. *Brain Res. Rev.,* 11: 359 – 391.

Cleaton-Jones, P. (1972) Anatomical observations on the soft palate of the albino rat. *Anat. Anz.,* 131: 419 – 424.

Cohen, M.I. (1971) Switching of the respiratory phases and evoked phrenic responses produced by rostral pontine electrical stimulation. *J. Physiol.,* 217: 133 – 258.

Cohen, M.I., Piercey, M.F. Gootman, P.M. and Wolotsky, P. (1974) Synaptic connections between medullary inspiratory neurons and phrenic motoneurons as revealed by cross-correlation. *Brain Res.,* 81: 319 – 324.

Collewijn, H. (1975) Oculomotor areas in the rabbit's midbrain and pretectum. *J. Neurobiol.,* 6: 3 – 22.

Collewijn, H. and Holstege, G. (1984) Effects of neonatal and late unilateral enucleation on optokinetic responses and optic nerve projections in the rabbit. *Exp. Brain Res.,* 57: 138 – 150.

Connelly, C.A. and Wurster, R.D. (1985) Sympathetic rhythms during hyperventilation-induced apnea. *Am. J. Physiol.,* 249: R424 – 431.

Contreras, R.J., Gomez, M.M. and Norgren, R. (1980) Central origins of cranial nerve parasympathetic neurons in the rat. *J. Comp. Neurol.,* 190: 373 – 395.

Coote, J.H., Hilton, S.M. and Zbrozyna, A.W. (1973) The ponto-medullary area integrating the defence reaction in the cat and its influence on muscle blood flow. *J. Physiol.,* 229: 257 – 274.

Coulter, J.D., Bowker, R.M., Wise, S.P., Murray, E.A., Castiglioni, A.J. and Westlund, K.N. (1979) Cortical, tectal and medullary descending pathways to the cervical spinal cord. *Progr. Brain Res.,* 50: 263 – 279.

Courville, J. (1966) The nucleus of the facial nerve; the relation between cellular groups and peripheral branches of the nerve. *Brain Res.,* 1: 338 – 354.

Courville, J. (1966) Rubrobulbar fibres to the facial nucleus and the lateral reticular nucleus (nucleus of the lateral funiculus). An experimental study in the cat with silver impregnation methods. *Brain Res.,* 1: 317 – 337.

Cowan, W.M., Gottlieb, D.I., Hendrickson, A.E., Price, J.L. and Woolsey, T.A. (1972) The autoradiographic demonstration of axonal connections in the central nervous system. *Brain Res.,* 37: 21 – 51.

Cowie, R.J. and Holstege, G. (1991) Dorsal mesencephalic projections to pons, medulla oblongata and spinal cord in the cat. Limbic and non-limbic components. *Neuroscience,* (submitted).

Crone, C., Hultborn, H., Kiehn, O., Mazieres, L. and Wigstrom, H. (1988) Maintained changes in motoneuronal excitability by short-lasting synaptic inputs in the decerebrate cat. *J. Physiol.,* 405: 321 – 343.

Crouch, J.E. (1969) *Text-Atlas of Cat Anatomy.* Lea and Febiger, Philadelphia.

Crutcher, K.A., Humbertson, A.O. jr. and Martin, G.F. (1978) The origin of brainstem spinal pathways in the North American Opossum (Didelphis virginiana). Studies using the horseradish peroxidase. *J. Comp. Neurol.,* 179: 169 – 194.

Cullheim, S. and Kellerth, J.-O (1978) A morphological study of the axons and recurrent axon collaterals of cat α-motoneurones supplying different funtional types of muscle unit. *J. Physiol.,* 281: 301 – 314.

Czarkowska, J., Jankowska, E. and Sybirska, E. (1976) Axonal projections of spinal interneurones excited by group I afferents in the cat, revealed by intracellular staining with horseradish peroxidase. *Brain Res.,* 118: 115 – 118.

Dampney, R.A.L. and McAllen, R.M. (1988) Differential control of sympathetic fibres supplying hindlimb skin and muscle by retrofacial neurones in the cat. *J. Physiol. (Lond.)* 395: 41 – 56.

Davies, J.G. McF., Kirkwood, P.A. and Sears, T.A. (1985) The detection of monosynaptic connexions from inspiratory bulbospinal neurones to inspiratory motoneurones in the cat. *J. Physiol. (Lond.)* 368: 33 – 62.

Davies, J.G. McF., Kirkwood, P.A. and Sears, T.A. (1985) The distribution of monosynaptic connexions from inspiratory bulbospinal neurones to inspiratory motoneurones in the cat. *J. Physiol.* 368: 63 – 87.

Davis, P.J. and Nail, B.S. (1984) On the location and size of laryngeal motoneurons in the cat and rabbit. *J. Comp. Neurol.,* 230: 13 – 32.

Decima, E.E., Von Euler, C. and Thoden, U. (1969) Intercostal-to-phrenic reflexes in the spinal cat. *Acta Physiol. Scand.* 75: 568 – 579.

Dekker, J.J., Lawrence, D.G. and Kuypers, H.G.J.M. (1973) The location of longitudinally running dendrites in the ventral horn of the cat spinal cord. *Brain. Res.,* 51: 319 – 325.

De Olmos, J.S., Alheid, G.F. and Beltramino, C.A. (1985) Amygdala. In: G. Paxinos, (Ed.), *The Rat Nervous System.* Academic Press, Sydney, pp. 223 – 334.

DeRosier, E.A., West, R.A. and Larson, C.R. (1988) Comparison of single unit discharge properties in the periaqueductal gray and nucleus retroambiguus during vocalization in monkeys. *Soc. Neurosci. Abstr.,* 14: 1237.

Dom, R., Falls, W. and Martin, G.F. (1973) The motor nucleus of the facial nerve in the opossum (Didelphis marsupialis virginiana). Its organization and connections. *J. Comp. Neurol.,* 152: 373 – 402.

ten Donkelaar, H.J. (1988) Evolution of the red nucleus and rubrospinal tract. *Behav. Brain Res.,* 28: 9 – 20.

Donoghue, S., Garcia, M., Jordan, D. and Spyer, K.M. (1982) The brain-stem projections of pulmonary stretch afferent neurons in cats and rabbits. *J. Physiol. (Lond.)* 322: 352 – 364.

Doty, R.W. and Bosma, J.F. (1956) An electromyographic analysis of reflex deglutition. *J. Neurophysiol.,* 19: 44 – 60.

Duffin, J. and Lipski, J. (1987) Monosynaptic excitation of thoracic motoneurones by inspiratory neurones of the nucleus tractus solitarius in the cat. *J. Physiol.,* 390: 415 – 431.

Duron, B., Jung-Caillol, M.C. and Marlot, D. (1978) Myelinated nerve fiber supply and muscle spindles in the respiratory muscles of cat: a quantitative study. *Anat. Embryol.,* 152: 171 – 192.

Duron, B., Marlot, D., Larnicol, N., Jung-Caillol, M.C. and Macron, J.M. (1979) Somatotopy in the phrenic motor nucleus of the cat as revealed by retrograde transport of horseradish peroxidase (HRP). *Neurosci. Lett.,* 14: 159 – 163.

Eccles, J.C., Nicoll, R.A., Schwartz, W.F., Táboríková, H. and Willey, T.J. (1975) Reticulospinal neurons with and without monosynaptic inputs from cerebellar nuclei. *J. Neurophysiol.,* 38: 103.

Edwards, S.B. (1972) Descending projections of the midbrain reticular formation of the cat: an experimental study using a "protein transport", tracing method. *Anat. Rec.,* 172: 305.

Edwards, S.B. and Flynn, J.P. (1972) Corticospinal control of striking in centrally elicited attack behavior. *Brain Res.,* 41: 51 – 65.

Ellenberger, H.H. and Feldman, J.L. (1988) Monosynaptic transmission of respiratory drive to phrenic motoneurons from brainstem bulbospinal neurons in rats. *J. Comp. Neurol.,* 269: 47 – 57.

Engberg, I., Lundberg, A. and Ryall, R.W. (1968) Reticulospinal inhibition of interneurones. *J. Physiol.,* 194: 225 – 236.

Epstein, A.N. (1971) The lateral hypothalamic syndrome: its implications for the physiological psychology of hunger and thirst. In E. Stellar and J.M. Sprague (Eds.), *Progress in Physiological Psychology, Vol. 4.* Academic Press, New York. pp. 263 – 317.

Erzurumlu, R.S., Bates, C.A. and Killackey, H.P. (1980) Differential organization of thalamic projection cells in the brain stem trigeminal complex of the rat. *Brain Res.,* 198: 427 – 434.

Euler, C.von, Martilla, I. Remmers, J.E. and Trippenbach, T. (1976) Effects of lesions in the parabrachial nucleus on the mechanisms for central and reflex termination of inspiration in the cat. *Acta Physiol. Scand.,* 96: 324 – 337.

Evinger, C. (1988) Extraocular motor nuclei: location, morphology and afferents. In J.A. Büttner-Ennever (Ed.), *Neuro-anatomy of the oculomotor system.* Elsevier, Amsterdam, New York, Oxford. pp. 81 – 117.

Fedorko, L. and Merrill, E.G. (1984) Axonal projections from the rostral expiratory neurones of the Bötzinger complex to medulla and spinal cord in the cat. *J. Physiol.,* 350: 487 – 496.

Fedorko, L., Merrill, E.G. and Lipski, J. (1983) Two descending medullary inspiratory pathways to phrenic motoneurons. *Neurosci. Lett.,* 43: 285 – 291.

Feldman, J.L. (1986) Neurophysiology of breathing in mammals. In F.E. Bloom (Ed.), *Handbook of Physiology, Sect. 1: The Nervous System,* vol. IV. Intrinsic Regulatory Systems of the Brain. American Physiological Soc., Bethesda, MD. pp. 463 – 524.

Feldman, J.L., Loewy, A.D. and Speck, D.F. (1985) Projections from the ventral respiratory group to phrenic and intercostal motoneurons in cat: An autoradiographic study. *J. Neurosci.,* 5: 1993 – 2000.

Fernandez de Molina, A. and Hunsperger, R.W. (1959) Central representation of affective reactions in forebrain and brain stem: electrical stimulation of amygdala, stria terminalis, and adjacent structures. *J. Physiol.,* 145: 251 – 265.

Fernandez de Molina, A. and Hunsperger, R.W. (1962) Organization of the subcortical system governing defense and flight reactions in the cat. *J. Physiol. (Lond.)* 160: 200 – 213.

Fetcho, J.R. (1987) A review of the organization and evolution of motoneurons innervating the axial musculature of vertebrates. *Brain Res. Rev.,* 12: 243 – 280.

Fetz, E.E., Jankowska, E., Johannisson, T. and Lipski, J. (1979) Autogenetic inhibition of motoneurones by impulses in group Ia muscle spindle afferents. *J. Physiol.,* 293: 173 – 197.

Fields, H.L., Basbaum, A.I., Clanton, C.H. and Anderson, S.D. (1977) Nucleus raphe magnus inhibition of spinal cord dorsal horn neurons. *Brain Res.,* 126: 441 – 453.

Friauf, E. and Baker, R. (1985) An intracellular HRP-study of cat tensor tympani motoneurons. *Exp. Brain Res.,* 57: 499 – 511.

Friauf, E. and Herbert, H. (1985) Topographic organization of facial motoneurons to individual pinna muscles in rat and bat. *J. Comp. Neurol.,* 240: 161 – 170.

Fritz, N., Illert, M. and Reeh, P. (1986) Location of motoneurones projecting to the cat distal forelimb. II. Median and ulnar motornuclei. *J. Comp. Neurol.,* 244: 302 – 312.

Fritz, N., Illert, M. and Saggau, P. (1986) Location of motoneurones projecting to the cat distal forelimb. I. Deep radial motornuclei. *J. Comp. Neurol.,* 244: 286 – 301.

Fritz, N., Illert, M. and Saggau, P. (1978) Monosynaptic convergence of group I muscle afferents from the forelimb onto interosseus motoneurones. *Neurosci. Lett. Suppl. I:* S 95.

Fritz, N., Illert, M., de la Motte, S. and Reeh, P. (1984) Pattern of monosynaptic Ia connections from forelimb nerves onto median and ulnar motoneurones. *Neurosci. Lett.,* 18: S264.

Fuchs, A.F., Kaneko, C.R.S. and Scudder, C.A. (1985) Brainstem control of saccadic eye movements. *Ann. Rev. Neurosci.,* 8: 307 – 337.

Fuchs, S.A., Edinger, H.M. and Siegel, A. (1985) The organization of the hypothalamic pathways mediating affective defence behavior in the cat. *Brain Res.,* 330: 77 – 92.

Fukushima, K., Pitts, N.G. and Peterson, B.W. (1978) Direct excitation of neck motoneurons by interstitiospinal fibers. *Exp. Brain Res.,* 33: 565 – 583.

Fung, S.J. and Barnes, C.D. (1987) Membrane excitability changes in hindlimb motoneurons induced by stimulation of the locus coeruleus in cats. *Brain Res.,* 402: 230 – 242.

Garcia-Rill, E. and Skinner, R.D. (1987) The mesencephalic locomotor region. I. Activation of a medullary projection site. *Brain Res.,* 411: 1 – 12.

Garcia-Rill, E. and Skinner, R.D. (1987) The mesencephalic locomotor region. II. Projections to reticulospinal neurons. *Brain Res.,* 411: 13 – 20.

Garcia-Rill, E. and Skinner, R.D. (1988) Modulation of rhythmic function in the posterior midbrain. *Neuroscience,* 27: 639 – 654.

Gebhart, G.F., Sandkühler, J., Thalhammer, J.G. and Zimmermann, M. (1983) Quantitative comparision of inhibition in spinal cord of nociceptive information by stimulation in periaqueductal gray or nucleus raphe magnus of the cat. *J. Neurophysiol.,* 50: 1433 – 1445.

Gelfand, I.M., Orlovsky, G.N. and Shik, M.L. (1988) Locomotion and scratching in tetrapods. In A.H. Cohen, S. Rossignol and S. Grilner (Eds.), Neural control of rhythmic movements in verebrates. John Wiley and Sons Inc., New York. pp. 167 – 199.

Gibson, A.R., Houk, J.C. and Kohlerman, N.J. (1985) Magnocellular red nucleus activity during different types of limb movement in the macaque monkey. *J. Physiol.,* 358: 527 – 549.

Giovanelli Barilari, M.S. and Kuypers, H.G.J.M. (1969) Propriospinal fibers interconnecting the spinal enlargements in the cat. *Brain Res.,* 14: 321 – 330.

Gormezano, I., Schneiderman, N., Deaux, E. and Fuentes, I. (1962) Nictitating membrane: classical conditioning and extinction in the albino rabbit. *Science,* 138: 33 – 34.

Grafstein, B. and Laureno, R. (1973) Transport of radioactivity from eye to visual cortex in the mouse. *Exp. Neurol.,* 39: 44 – 57.

Grant, K., Guéritaud, J.P., Horcholle-Bossavit, G. and Tyc-Dumont, S. (1979) Anatomical and electrophysiological identification of motoneurones supplying the cat retractor bulbi muscle. *Exp. Brain Res.,* 34: 541 – 550.

Grant, K., Guegan, M. and Horcholle-Bossavit, G. (1981) The anatomical relationship of the retractor bulbi and posterior digastric motoneurones to the abducens and facial nuclei in the cat. *Arch. Ital. Biol.,* 119: 195 – 207.

Grantyn, A., Ong-Meang Jacques, V. and Berthoz, A. (1987) Reticulo-spinal neurons participating in the control of synergic eye and head movements during orienting in the cat. *Exp. Brain Res.,* 66: 355 – 377.

Grantyn, R., Baker, R. and Grantyn, A. (1980) Morphological and physiological identification of excitatory pontine reticular neurons projecting to the cat abducens nucleus and spinal cord. *Brain Res.,* 198: 221 – 229.

Graybiel, A.M. (1977) Direct and indirect preoculomotor pathways of the brain stem: an autoradiographic study of the pontine reticular formation in the cat. *J. Comp. Neurol.,* 175: 37 – 78.

Graybiel, A.M. and Hartwieg, E.A. (1974) Some afferent connections of the oculomotor complex in the cat: an experimental study with tracer techniques. *Brain Res.,* 81: 543 – 551.

Griffiths, D., Holstege, G., Dalm E. and de Wall, H. (1990) Control and coordination of bladder and urethral function in the brain stem of the cat. *Neurourol. Urodynam.,* pp. 9: 360 – 382.

Grillner, S. (1981) Control of locomotion in bipeds, tetrapods, and fish. In: R.E. Burke (Ed.), *Handbook of Physiology, Section I, The Nervous System, Vol. II, Motor Systems.* Washington, American Physiological Society 2, part 2: 1179 – 1236.

Grillner, S., Hongo, T. and Lund, S. (1970) The vestibulospinal tract. Effects on alpha motoneurons in the lumbosacral spinal cord in the cat. *Exp. Brain Res.,* 10: 94 – 120.

Grossman, R.G. and Wang, S.C. (1956) Diencephalic mechanism of control of the urinary bladder of the cat. *Yale J. Biol. Med.,* 28: 285 – 297.

Grossman, S.P., Dacey, D., Halaris, A.E., Collier, T. and Routtenberg, A. (1978) Aphagia and adipsia after preferential destruction of nerve cell bodies in hypothalamus. *Science,* 202: 537 – 539.

Guégan, M. and Horcholle-Bossavit, G. (1981) Reflex control of the retractor bulbi muscle in the cat. *Pflügers Arch.,* 389: 143 – 148.

Guinan Jr., J.J., Joseph, M.P. and Norris, B.E. (1989) Brainstem facial-motor pathways from two distinct groups of stapedius motoneurons in the cat. *J. Comp. Neurol.,* 287: 134 – 144.

Haase, P. and Hrycyshyn, A.W. (1985) Labelling of motoneurons supplying the cutaneous maximus in the rat, following injection of the triceps brachii muscle with horseradish peroxidase. *Neurosci. Lett.,* 60: 313 – 318.

Hagg, S. and Ha, H. (1970) Cervicothalamic Tract in the Dog. *J. Comp. Neurol.,* 139: 357 – 374.

Hahne, M., Illert, M. and Wietelmann, D. (1988) Recurrent inhibition in the cat distal forelimb. *Brain Res.,* 456: 188 – 192.

Haley, D.A., Thompson, R.F. and Madden, J. IV (1988) Pharmacological analysis of the magnocellular red nucleus during classical conditioning of the rabbit nictitating membrane response. *Brain Res.,* 454: 131 – 139.

Hancock, M.B. (1976) Cells of origin of hypothalamo-spinal projections in the rat. *Neurosci. Lett.,* 3: 179 – 184.

Harvey, J.A., Land, T. and McMaster, S.E. (1984) Anatomical study of the rabbit's corneal-VIth nerve reflex: connections between cornea, trigeminal sensory complex, and the abducens and accessory abducens nuclei. *Brain Res.,* 301: 307 – 321.

Hassler, R. (1972) Supranuclear structures regulating binocular eye and head movements. *Bibl. Ophthal.,* 82: 207 – 219.

Hawthorn, J., Ang, V.T.Y. and Jenkins, J.S. (1985) Effects of lesions in the hypothalamic paraventricular, supraoptic and suprachiasmatic nuclei on vasopressin and oxytocin in the rat brain and spinal cord. *Brain Res.,* 346: 51 – 57.

Hayes, N.L. and Rustioni, A. (1981) Descending projections from brainstem and sensorimotor cortex to spinal enlargements in the cat. *Exp. Brain Res.,* 41: 89 – 107.

Heimer, L., de Olmos, J., Alheid, G.F. and Zaborsky, L. (1991) "Peristroika" in the basal forebrain; Opening the border between neurology and psychiatry. In G. Holstege (Ed.), *Role of the forebrain in senszation and behavior* Elsevier Amsterdam, Progr. Brain Res., Vol. 87, pp. 109 – 165.

Helke, C.J., Sayson, S.C., Keeler, J.R. and Charlton, C.G. (1986) Thyrotropin-releasing hormoneimmunoreactive neurons project from the ventral medulla to the intermediolateral cell column: partial coexistence with serotonin. *Brain Res.,* 381: 1 – 7.

Hemingway, A. (1963) Shivering. *Phys. Rev.,* 43: 397 – 422.

Henneman, E. and Mendell, L.M. (1981) Functional organization of motoneuron pool and its inputs. In R.E. Burke (Ed.), *Handbook of Physiology, Section I, The Nervous System, Vol. II, Motor Systems* Washington American Physiology Society. pp. 423 – 507.

Henry, J.L. and Calaresu, F.R. (1972) Topography and numerical distribution of neurons of the thoraco-lumbar intermediolateral nucleus in the cat. *J. Comp. Neurol.,* 144: 205 – 214.

Hermes, M.L., Buijs, R.M., Masson-Pevet, M. and Pevet, P. (1988) Oxytocinergic innervation of the brain of the garden dormouse *(Eliomys quercinus* L.). *J. Comp. Neurol.,* 273: 252 – 262.

Hilaire, G. and Monteau, R. (1976) Connexions entre les neurones inspiratoire bulbaires et les motoneurones phrénique et intercosteaux. *J. Physiol. (Paris),* 72: 987 – 1000.

Hinrichsen, C.F.L. and Watson, C.D. (1984) The facial nucleus of the rat: Representation of facial muscles revealed by retrograde transport of HRP. *Anat. Rec.,* 209: 407 – 415.

Hiraoka, M. and Shimamura, M. (1977) Neural mechanisms of the corneal blinking reflex in cats. *Brain Res.,* 125: 265 – 275.

Hökfelt, T., Ljungdahl, A., Steinbusch, H., Verhofstad, A., Nilsson, G., Brodin, E., Pernow, B. and Goldstein, M. (1978) Immunohistochemical evidence of substance P-like immunoreactivity in some 5-hydroxtryptamine-containing neurons in the rat central nervous system. *Neuroscience,* 3: 517 – 538.

Hökfelt, T., Terenius, T., Kuypers, H.G.J.M. and Dann, O. (1979) Evidence for enkephalin immunoreactivity neurons in the medulla oblongata projecting to the spinal cord. *Neurosci. Lett.,* 14: 55 – 61.

Hökfelt, T., Skirboll, L., Rehfeld, J.F., Goldstein, M., Markey, K. and Dann, O. (1980) A subpopulation of mesencephalic dopamine neurons projecting to limbic areas contains a cholecystokinin-like peptide: evidence from immunohistochemistry combined with retrograde tracing. *Neuroscience,* 5: 2093 – 2124.

Hökfelt, T., Johansson, O. and Goldstein, M. (1984) Chemical neuroanatomy of the brain. *Science,* 225: 1326 – 1334.

Holstege, G. (1987a) Anatomical evidence for an ipsilateral rubrospinal pathway and for direct rubrospinal projections to motoneurons in the cat. *Neurosci. Lett.,* 74: 269 – 274.

Holstege, G. (1987b) Some anatomical observations on the projections from the hypothalamus to brainstem and spinal cord: and HRP and autoradiographic tracing study in the cat. *J. Comp. Neurol.,* 260: 98 – 126.

Holstege, G. (1988a) Direct and indirect pathways to lamina I in the medulla oblongata and spinal cord of the cat. In H.L. Fields and J.M. Besson (Eds.), *Descending brainstem controls of nociceptive transmission.*Progr. Brain Res. vol. 77 Elsevier, Amsterdam. pp. 47 – 94.

Holstege, G. (1988b) Brainstem-spinal cord projections in the cat, related to control of head and axial movements. In J.A. Büttner-Ennever (Ed.), Neuroanatomy of the oculomotor system Elsevier, Amsterdam chapter 11: 429 – 468.

Holstege, G. (1988c) Anatomical evidence for a strong ventral parabrachial projection to nucleus raphe magnus and adjacent tegmental field. *Brain Res.,* 447: 154 – 158.

Holstege, G. (1989a) An anatomical study on the final common pathway for vocalization in the cat. *J. Comp. Neurol.,* 284: 242 – 252.

Holstege, G. (1990) Subcortical limbic system projections to caudal brainstem and spinal cord. In G. Paxinos (Ed.), *The human nervous system.* Acad. Press Sydney, Tokyo. pp. 261 – 286.

Holstege, G. and Blok, B. (1986) The afferent projections of the motor trigeminal nucleus in the cat. An autoradiographical tracing study. *Neurosci. Lett.,* 26: S. 435.

Holstege, G. and Blok, B. (1989) Descending pathways to the cutaneus trunci muscle motoneuronal cell group in the cat. *J. Neurophysiol.,* 62: 1260 – 1269.

Holstege, G. and Collewijn, H. (1982) The efferent connections of the nucleus of the optic tract and the superior colliculus in the rabbit. *J. Comp. Neurol.,* 209: 139 – 175.

Holstege, G. and Cowie, R.J. (1989) Projections from the rostral mesencephalic reticular formation to the spinal cord. *Exp. Brain Res.,* 75: 265 – 279.

Holstege, G. and Griffiths, D. (1990) Neuronal organization of micturition In G. Paxinos (Ed.), *The human nervous system.* Acad. Press Sydney, Tokyo, pp. 297 – 306.

Holstege, G. and Kuypers, H.G.J.M. (1977) Propriobulbar fibre connections to the trigeminal, facial and hypoglossal motor nuclei I. An anterograde degeneration study in the cat. *Brain,* 100: 239 – 264.

Holstege, G. and Kuypers, H.G.J.M. (1982) The anatomy of brain stem pathways to the spinal cord in the cat. A labeled amino acid tracing study. *Progr. Brain Res.,* 57: 145 – 175.

Holstege, G. and Ralston, D.D. (1989) Rubrofacial projections in the cat. An anterograde L.M. and E.M. study utilizing WGA-HRP as a tracer. *Soc. Neurosci. Abstr.,* 15: p. 389.

Holstege, G. and Tan, J. (1987) Supraspinal control of motoneurons innervating the striated muscles of the pelvic floor including urethral and anal sphincters in the cat. *Brain,* 110: 1323 – 1344.

Holstege, G. and Tan, J. (1988) Projections from the red nucleus and surrounding areas to the brainstem and spinal cord in the cat. An HRP and autoradiographical tracing study. *Beh. Brain Res.,* 28: 33 – 57.

Holstege, G. and Van Krimpen, L. (1986) Afferent connections to the pharynx and soft palate motoneuronal cell group. An autoradiographical study in the cat. *Neurosci. Lett. Suppl.* 26: S437.

Holstege, G., Blok, B.F. and Ralston, D.D. (1988) Anatomical evidence fot red nucleus projections to motoneuronal cell groups in the spinal cord of the monkey. *Neurosci. Lett.,* 95: 97 – 101.

Holstege, G., Kuypers, H.G.J.M. and Boer, R.C. (1979) Anatomical evidence for direct brain stem projections to the somatic motoneuronal cell groups and autonomic preganglionic cell groups in cat spinal cord. *Brain Res.,* 171: 329 – 333.

Holstege, G., Kuypers, H.G.J.M. and Dekker, J.J. (1977) The organization of the bulbar fibre connections to the trigeminal, facial and hypoglossal motor nuclei. II. an autoradiographic tracing study in cat. *Brain,* 100: 265 – 286.

Holstege, G., Meiners, L. and Tan, K. (1985) Projections of the bed nucleus of the stria terminalis to the mesencephalon, pons, and medulla oblongata in the cat. *Exp. Brain Res.,* 58: 379 – 391.

Holstege, G., van Ham, J.J. and Tan, J. (1986a) Afferent projections to the orbicularis oculi motoneuronal cell group. An autoradiographical tracing study in the cat. *Brain Res.,* 374: 306 – 320.

Holstege, G., Van Neerven, J. and Evertse, F. (1984b) Some anatomical observations on axonal connections from brain stem areas physiologically identified as related to respiration. *Neurosci. Lett., Suppl. 18:* S83.

Holstege, G., Van Neerven, J. and Evertse, F. (1987) Spinal cord location of the motoneurons innervating the abdominal, cutaneous maximus, latissimus dorsi and longissimus dorsi muscles in the cat. *Exp. Brain Res.,* 67: 179 – 194.

Holstege, G., Graveland, G., Bijker-Biemond, C. and Schuddeboom, I. (1983) Location of motoneurons innervating soft palate, pharynx and upper esophagus. Anatomical evidence for a possible swallowing center in the pontine reticular formation. An HRP and autoradiographical tracing study. *Brain Behav. Evol.,* 23: 47 – 62.

Holstege, G., Griffiths, D., De Wall, H. and Dalm, E. (1986c) Anatomical and physiological observations on supraspinal control of bladder and urethral sphincter muscles in the cat. *J. Comp. Neurol.,* 250: 449 – 461.

Holstege, G., Tan, J., van Ham, J. and Bos, A. (1984a) Mesencephalic projection to the facial nucleus in the cat. An autoradiographic tracing study. *Brain Res.,* 311: 7 – 22.

Holstege, G., Tan, J., van Ham, J.J. and Graveland, G.A. (1986b) Anatomical observations on the afferent projections to the retractor bulbi motoneuronal cell group and other pathways possibly related to the blink reflex in the cat. *Brain Res.,* 374: 321 – 334.

Holstege, J.C. (1989) Ultrastructural evidence for GABA-ergic brainstem projections to spinal motoneurons. *Soc. Neurosci. Abstr.,* 15 part 1: p. 308.

Holstege, J.C. and Kuypers, H.G.J.M. (1982) Brain stem projections to spinal motoneuronal cell groups in rat studied by means of electron microscopy autoradiography. *Progr. Brain Res.,* 57: 177 – 183.

Holstege, J.C. and Kuypers, H.G.J.M. (1987) Brainstem projections to lumbar motoneurons in rat-I. An ultrastructural study using autoradiography and the combination of autoradiography and horseradish peroxidase histochemistry. *Neuroscience,* 21: 345 – 367.

Hongo, T., Jankowska, E. and Lundberg, A. (1969) The

rubrospinal tract. I. Effects on alphamotoneurons innervating hindlimb muscles in cats. *Exp. Brain Res.,* 7: 344 – 364.

Hopkins, D.A. and Armour, J.A. (1982) Medullary cells of origin of physiologically identified cardiac nerves in the dog. *Brain Res. Bull.,* 8: 359 – 365.

Hopkins, D.A. and Holstege, G. (1978) Amygdaloid projections to the mesencephalon, pons, and medulla oblongata in the cat. *Exp. Brain Res.,* 32: 529 – 547.

Horcholle-Bossavit, G., Jami, L., Thiesson, D. and Zytnicki, D. (1988) Motor nuclei of peroneal muscles in the cat spinal cord. *J. Comp. Neurol.,* 277: 430 – 440.

ter Horst, G.J., Luiten, P.G.M. and Kuipers, F. (1984) Descending pathways from hypothalamus to dorsal motor vagus and ambiguus nuclei in the rat. *J. Auton. Nerv. Syst.,* 11: 59 – 75.

Hosobuchi, Y. (1988) Current issues regarding subcortical electrical stimulation for pain control in humans. In H.L. Fields and J.M. Besson (Eds.), *Nociception control.* Elsevier Amsterdam *Progr. Brain Res.,* 77: 189 – 192.

Hosoya, Y. (1980) The distribution of spinal projection neurons in the hypothalamus of the rat, studied with the HRP method. *Exp. Brain Res.,* 40: 79 – 87.

Hosoya, Y. (1985) Hypothalamic projections to the ventral medulla oblongata in the rat, with special reference to the nucleus raphe pallidus: a study using autoradiographic and HRP techniques. *Brain Res.,* 344: 338 – 350.

Hosoya, Y. and Matsushita, M. (1979) Identification and distribution of the spinal and hypophyseal projection neurones in the paraventricular nucleus of the rat. A light and electron microscopic study with the HRP method. *Exp. Brain Res.,* 35: 315 – 331.

Hosoya, Y. and Matsushita, M. (1981) Brainstem projections from the lateral hypothalamic area in the rat, as studied with autoradiography. *Neurosci. Lett.,* 24: 111 – 116.

Hosoya, Y., Matsushita, M. and Sugiura, Y. (1983) A direct hypothalamic projection to the superior salivatory nucleus neurons in the rat. A study using anterograde autoradiographic and retrograde HRP methods. *Brain Res.,* 266: 329 – 334.

Hosoya, Y., Sugiura, Y., Ito, R. and Kohno, K. (1990) Descending projections from the hypothalamic paraventricular nucleus to the A5 area, including the superior salivatory nucleus in the rat, using anterograde and retrograde transport techniques. *Exp. Brain Res.,* (in press).

Hounsgaard, J., Hultborn, H., Jespersen, B. and Kiehn, O. (1984) Intrinsic membrane properties causing a bistable behavior of α-motoneurons. *Exp. Brain Res.,* 55: 391 – 394.

Hounsgaard, J., Hultborn, H. and Kiehn, O. (1986) Transmitter-controlled properties of α-motoneurones causing long-lasting motor discharge to brief excitatory inputs. *Progr. Brain Res.,* 64: 39 – 49.

Hounsgaard, J., Hultborn, H., Jespersen, B. and Kiehn, O. (1988) Bistability of alpha-motoneurones in the decebrate cat and in the acute spinal cat after intravenous 5-hydroxytryptophan. *J. Physiol.,* 405: 345 – 367.

Hu, J.W. and Sessle, B.J. (1979) Trigeminal nociceptive and non-nociceptive neurones: brain stem intranuclear projections and modulation of orofacial, periaqueductal gray and nucleus raphe magnus stimuli. *Brain Res.,* 170: 547 – 553.

Huerta, M.F. and Harting, J.K. (1982) Tectal control of spinal cord activity: neuroanatomical demonstration of pathways connecting the superior colliculus with the cervical spinal cord. *Progr. Brain Res.,* 57: 293 – 328.

Huisman, A.M., Kuypers, H.G.J.M. and Verburgh, C.A. (1982) Differences in collateralization of the descending spinal pathways from red nucleus and other brain stem cell groups in cat and monkey. *Progr. Brain Res.,* 57: 185 – 217.

Hultborn, H. (1976) Transmission in the pathway of reciprocal 1a inhibition to motoneurons and its control during the tonic stretch reflex. In: S. Homma (Ed.). Understanding the Stretch Reflex. *Progr. Brain Res.,* 44: 235 – 255.

Humphrey, D.R. and Reitz, R.R. (1976) Cells of origin of corticorubral projections from the arm area of primate cortex and their presynaptic actions in the red nucleus. *Brain Res.,* 110: 219.

Humphrey, D.R., Gold, R. and Reed, D.J. (1984) Sizes, laminar and topographic origins of cortical projections to the major divisions of the red nucleus in the monkey. *J. Comp. Neurol.,* 225: 75 – 94.

Hunt, S.P. and Lovick, T.A. (1982) The distribution of serotonin, met-enkephalin and β-lipotropin-like immunoreactivity in neuronal perikarya of the cat brainstem. *Neurosci. Lett.,* 30: 139 – 145.

Hurley-Gius, K.M., Cechetto, D.F. and Saper, C.B. (1986) Spinal connections of the infralimbic autonomic cortex. *Soc. Neurosc. Abstr.,* 12: pp. 538.

Hyde, J.E. and Toczek, S. (1962) Functional relation of interstitial nucleus to rotatory movements evoked from zona incerta stimulation. *J. Neurophysiol.,* 25: 455 – 466.

Illert, M., Lundberg, A., Padel, Y. and Tanaka, R. (1978) Integration in descending motor pathways controlling the forelimb in the cat. 5. Properties of and monosynaptic excitatory convergence on C3-C4 propriospinal neurones. *Exp. Brain Res.,* 33: 101 – 130.

Ishizuka, N., Mannen, H., Hongo, T. and Sasaki, S. (1979) Trajectory of group Ia afferent fibers stained with horseradish peroxidase in the lumbosacral spinal cord of the cat: three dimensional reconstructions from serial sections. *J. Comp. Neurol.,* 186: 189 – 213.

Jänig, W. and McLachlan, E.M. (1986) Identification of distinct topographical distributions of lumbar sympathetic and sensory neurons projecting to end organs with different functions in the cat. *J. Comp. Neurol.,* 246: 104 – 112.

Jankowska, E. (1988) Target cells of rubrospinal tract fibres within the lumbar spinal cord. *Behav. Brain Res.,* 28: 91 – 96.

Jankowska, E. and Lindström, S. (1971) Morphological identification of Renshaw cells. *Acta Physiol. Scand.*, 81: 428 – 430.

Jankowska, E. and Lindström, S. (1972) Morphology of interneurones mediating Ia reciprocal inhibition of motoneurones in the spinal cord of the cat. *J. Physiol.*, 226: 805 – 823.

Jankowska, E., McCrea, D. and Mackel, R. (1981) Oligosynaptic excitation of motoneurones by impulses in group Ia muscle spindle afferents in the cat. *J. Physiol.*, 316: 411 – 425.

Jankowska, E. and McCrea, D.A. (1983) Shared reflex from Ib tendon organ afferents and Ia muscle spindle afferents in the rat. *J. Physiol.*, 338: 99 – 111.

Jankowska, E., Padel, Y. and Tanaka, R. (1975) Projections of pyramidal tract cells to alpha motoneurons innervating hindlimb muscles in the monkey. *J. Physiol. (Lond.)*, 249: 637 – 667.

Jankowska, E. and Roberts, W.J. (1972) An electrophysiological demonstration of the axonal projections of single spinal interneurones in the cat. *J. Physiol.*, 222: 597 – 622.

Jensen, T.S. and Smith, D.F. (1982) Dopaminergic effects on tail-flick response in spinal rats. *Europ. J. Pharmacol.*, 79: 129 – 133.

Jensen, T.S. and Yaksh, T.L. (1984) Effects of an intrathecal dopamine agonist, apomorphine, on thermal and chemical evoked noxious responses in rats. *Brain Res.*, 296: 285 – 293.

Johannessen, J.N., Watkins, L.R. and Mayer, D.J. (1984) Non-serotonergic origins of the dorsolateral funiculus in the rat ventral medulla. *J. Neurosci.*, 4: 757 – 766.

Johansson, O., Hökfelt, T., Pernow, B., Jeffcoate, S.L., White, N., Steinbusch, H.W.M., Verhofstad, A.A.J., Emson, P.C. and Spindel, E. (1981) Immunohistochemical support for three putative transmitters in one neuron: coexistence of 5-hydroxytryptamine, substance P- and thyrotropin releasing hormone-like immunoreactivity in medullary neurons projecting to the spinal cord. *Neuroscience*, 6: 1857 – 1881.

Johnston, J.B. (1923) Further contributions to the study of the evolution of the forebrain. *J. Comp. Neurol.*, 35: 337 – 481.

Jones, B.E. and Beaudet, A. (1987) Distribution of acetylcholine and catecholamine neurons in the cat brainstem: A choline acetyltransferase and tyrosine hydroxylase immunohistochemical study. *J. Comp. Neurol.*, 261: 15 – 32.

Jones, B.E. and Friedman, L. (1983) Atlas of catecholamine perikarya, varicosities and pathways in the brainstem of the cat. *J. Comp. Neurol.*, 215: 382 – 396.

Jones, B.E. and Yang, T.-Z (1985) The efferent projections from the reticular formation and the locus coeruleus studied by anterograde and retrograde axonal transport in the rat. *J. Comp. Neurol.*, 242: 56 – 92.

Jones, S.L. and Gebhart, G.F. (1987) Spinal pathways mediating tonic, coeruleospinal, and raphe-spinal descending inhibition in the rat. *J. Neurophysiol.*, 58: 138 – 159.

Joseph, M.P., Guinan, J.J. jr., Fullerton, B.C., Norris, B.E. and Kiang, N.Y.S. (1985) Number and distribution of stapedius motoneurons in cats. *J. Comp. Neurol.*, 232: 43 – 54.

Jürgens, U. and Pratt, R. (1979) The singular vocalization pathway in the squirrel monkey. *Exp. Brain Res.*, 34: 499 – 510.

Kaada, B. (1972) Stimulation and regional ablation of the amygdaloid complex with reference to functional representation. In: B.E. Eleftheriou (Ed.), *The Neurobiology of the Amygdala.* Plenum Press, New York. pp. 145 – 204.

Kalia, M. (1981) Brain stem localization of vagal preganglionic neurons. *J. Autonomic Nerv. Syst.*, 3: 451 – 481.

Kalia, M. and Mesulam, M.M. (1980) Brain stem projections of sensory and motor components of the vagus complex in the cat: II. laryngeal, tracheobronchial, pulmonary, cardiac and gastrointestinal branches. *J. Comp. Neurol.*, 193: 467 – 508.

Kalia, M. and Mesulam, M.M. (1980) Brain stem projections of sensory and motor components of the vagus complex in the cat: I. The cervical vagus and nodose ganglion. *J. Comp. Neurol.*, 193: 435 – 465.

Keller, J.T., Saunders, M.C., Ongkiko, C.M., Johnson, J., Frank, E., Van Loveren, H. and Tew, J.M. jr. (1983) Identification of motoneurons innervating the tensor tympani and tensor veli palatini muscles in the cat. *Brain Res.*, 270: 209 – 215.

van Keulen, L.C.M. (1979) Axon trajectories of Renshaw cells in the lumbar spinal cord of the cat as reconstructed after intracellular staining with horseradish peroxidase. *Brain Res.*, 167: 157 – 163.

Kidokoro, Y., Kubota, K., Shuto, S. and Sumino, R. (1968) Possible interneurons responsible for reflex inhibition of motoneurons of jaw-closing muscles from the inferior dental nerve. *J. Neurophysiol.*, 31: 709 – 716.

Kimura, H., McGeer, P.L., Peng, J.H. and McGeer, E.G. (1981) The central cholinergic system studied by choline acetyltransferase immunohistochemistry in the cat. *J. Comp. Neurol.*, 200: 151 – 201.

Klein, B.G. and Rhoades, R.W. (1985) Representation of Whisker follicle intrinsic musculature in the facial motor nucleus of the rat. *J. Comp. Neurol.*, 232: 55 – 69.

Kneisley, L.W., Biber, M.P. and LaVail, J.H. (1978) A study of the origin of brain stem projections to monkey spinal cord using retrograde transport method. *Exp. Neurol.*, 60: 116 – 139.

Köhler, C., Haglund, L. and Swanson, L.W. (1984) A diffuse αMSH-immunoreactive projection to the hippocampus and spinal cord from individual neurons in the lateral hypothalamic area and zona incerta. *J. Comp. Neurol.*, 223: 501 – 514.

Kojima, M., Takeuchi, Y., Goto, M. and Sano, Y. (1982) Immunohistochemical study on the distribution of serotonin fibers in the spinal cord of the dog. *Cell Tissue Res.*, 226: 477 – 491.

Kojima, M., Takeuchi, Y., Goto, M. and Sano, Y. (1983) Immunohistochemical study on the localization of serotonin fibers and terminals in the spinal cord of the monkey. *(Macaca fuscata). Cell Tissue Res.*, 229: 23 – 36.

Kojima, M., Takeuchi, Y., Kawata, M. and Sano, Y. (1983) Motoneurons innervating the cremaster muscle of the rat are characteristically densely innervated by serotonergic fibers as revealed by combined immunohistochemistry and retrograde fluorescence DAPI-labeling. *Anat. Embryol.*, 168: 41 – 49.

Komiyama, M., Shibata, H. and Suzuki, T. (1984) Somatotopic representation of facial muscles within the facial nucleus of the mouse. *Brain Behav. Evol.*, 24: 144 – 151.

Kow, L.-M, Montgomery, M.O. and Pfaff, D.W. (1977) Effects of spinal cord transections on lordosis reflex in female rats. *Brain Res.*, 123: 75 – 88.

Krettek, J.E. and Price, J.L. (1978) A description of the amygdaloid complex in the rat and cat with observations on intra-amygdaloid axonal connections. *J. Comp. Neurol.*, 178: 225 – 280.

Krnjévic, K. and Schwartz, S. (1966) Is gamma-aminobutyric acid an inhibitory transmitter? *Nature*, 211: 1372 – 1374.

Krogh, J.E. and Denslow, J.S. (1979) The cutaneus trunci muscle in spinal reflexes. *Electromyogr. Clin. Neurophysiol.*, 19: 157 – 164.

Krogh, J.E. and Towns, L.C. (1984) Location of the cutaneus trunci motor nucleus in the dog. *Brain Res.*, 295: 217 – 225.

Kugelberg, E. (1952) Facial reflexes. *Brain*, 75: 385 – 396.

Kume, M., Uemura, M., Matsuda, K., Matsushima, K. and Mizuno, N. (1978) Topographical representation of peripheral branches of the facial nerve within the facial nucleus: An HRP study in the cat. *Neurosci. Lett.*, 8: 5 – 8.

Kuo, D.S., Yamasaki, D.S. and Krauthamer, G.M. (1980) Segmental organization of sympathetic preganglionic neurons of the splanchinc nerve as revealed by retrograde transport of horseradish peroxidase. *Neurosci. Lett.*, 17: 11 – 17.

Kuypers, H.G.J.M. (1958) An anatomical analysis of corticobulbar connections to the pons and lower brain stem in the cat. *J. Anat. (Lond.)*, 92: 198 – 218.

Kuypers, H.G.J.M. (1958) Corticobulbar connections to the pons and lower brain stem in man. An anatomical study. *Brain*, 81: 364 – 388.

Kuypers, H.G.J.M. (1958) Some projections from the pericentral cortex to the pons and lower brain stem in monkey and chimpanzee. *J. Comp. Neurol.* 110: 221 – 255.

Kuypers, H.G.J.M. (1964) The descending pathways to the spinal cord, their anatomy and function. In J.C. Eccles and J.P. Schadé (Eds.), *Organization of the Spinal Cord* Elsevier Amsterdam, Progr. Brain Res. 11: 178 – 200.

Kuypers, H.G.J.M. (1973) The anatomical organization of the descending pathways and their contributions to motor control especially in primates. N. Develop. *EMG Clin. Neurophysiol.* 3: 38 – 68.

Kuypers, H.G.J.M. (1981) Anatomy of the descending pathways. In: R.E. Burke (Ed.), *Handbook of Physiology, Section I, The Nervous System*, Vol. II, Motor Systems Washington American Physiological Society 597 – 666.

Kuypers, H.G.J.M. and Brinkman J. (1970) Precentral projections to different parts of the spinal intermediate zone in the rhesus monkey. *Brain Res.*, 24: 29 – 48.

Kuypers, H.G.J.M. and Lawrence, D.G. (1967) Cortical projections to the red nucleus and the brain stem in the rhesus monkey. *Brain Res.*, 4: 151 – 188.

Kuypers, H.G.J.M. and Maisky, V.A. (1975) Retrograde axonal transport of horseradish peroxidase from spinal cord to brain stem cell groups in the cat. *Neurosci. Lett.*, 1: 9 – 14.

Kuypers, H.G.J.M., Fleming, W.R. and Farinholt, J.W. (1962) Subcorticospinal projections in the rhesus monkey. *J. Comp. Neurol.*, 118: 107 – 137.

Kuzuhara, S., Kanazawa, I. and Nakanishi, T. (1980) Topographical localization of the Onuf's nuclear neurons innervating the rectal and vesical striated sphincter muscles: a retrograde fluorescent double labeling in cat and dog. *Neurosci. Lett.*, 16: 125 – 130.

Lai, Y.-Y, and Barnes, C.D. (1985) A spinal projection of serotonergic neurons of the locus coeruleus in the cat. *Neurosci. Lett.*, 58: 159 – 164.

Landgren, S., Phillips, C.G. and Porter, R. (1962) Minimal synaptic actions of pyramidal impulses on some alpha motoneurons of the baboon's hand and forearm. *J. Physiol. (Lond.)*, 161: 91 – 111.

Lasek, R., Joseph, B.S. and Whitlock, D.G. (1968) Evaluation of a radioautographic neuroanatomical tracing method. *Brain Res.*, 8: 319 – 336.

Lavail, J.H. and Lavail, M.M. (1972) Retrograde axonal transport in the central nervous system. *Science*, 176: 1416 – 1417.

Lawn, A.M. (1966) The nucleus ambiguus of the rabbit. *J. Comp. Neurol.*, 127: 307 – 320.

Lawrence, D.G. and Kuypers, H.G.J.M. (1968) The functional organization of the motor system in the monkey. I. The effects of bilateral pyramidal lesions. *Brain*, 91: 1 – 14.

Lawrence, D.G. and Kuypers, H.G.J.M. (1968) The functional organization of the motor system in the monkey II. The effects of lesions of the descending brainstem pathways. *Brain*, 91: 15 – 36.

Léger, L., Charnay, Y., Dubois, P.M. and Jouvet, M. (1986) Distribution of enkephalin-immunoreactive cell bodies in relation to serotonin-containing neurons in the raphe nuclei of the cat: immunohistochemical evidence for the coexistence of enkephalins and serotonin in certain cells. *Brain Res.*, 362: 63 – 73.

Leibowitz, S.F. and Brown, L.L. (1980) Histochemical and pharmacological analysis of noradrenergic projections to the paraventricular hypothalamus in relation to feeding stimulation. *Brain Res.*, 201: 289 – 314.

Light, A.R., Casale, E.J. and Menetrey, D.M. (1986) The effects of local stimulation in nucleus raphe magnus and periaqueductal gray on intracellularly recorded neurons in spinal laminae I and II. *J. Neurophysiol.,* 56 no. 3: 555 – 571.

Lindquist, C. and Martensson, A. (1970) Mechanisms involved in the cat's blink reflex. *Acta Physiol. Scand.,* 80: 149 – 159.

Lipski, J. and Duffin, J. (1986) An electrophysiological investigation of propriospinal inspiratory neurons in the upper cervical cord of the cat. *Exp. Brain Res.,* 61: 625 – 637.

Lipski, J. and Martin-Body, R.L. (1987) Morphological properties of respiratory intercostal motoneurons in cats as revealed by intracellular injection of horseradish peroxidase. *J. Comp. Neurol.,* 260: 423 – 434.

Loewy, A.D. and Burton, H. (1978) Nuclei of the solitary tract: efferent projections to the lower brain stem and spinal cord of the cat. *J. Comp. Neurol.,* 181: 421 – 450.

Loewy, A.D., Saper, C.B. and Baker, R.P. (1979) Descending projections from the pontine micturition center. *Brain Res.,* 172: 533 – 539.

Loewy, A.D., Saper, C.B. and Yamodis, N.D. (1978) Re-evaluation of the efferent projections of the Edinger-Westphal nucleus in the cat. *Brain Res.,* 141: 153 – 159.

Loewy, A.D., Wallach, J.H. and McKellar, S. (1981) Efferent connections of the ventral medulla oblongata in the rat. *Brain Res. Rev.,* 3: 63 – 80.

Long, S. and Duffin, J. (1986) The neural determinants of respiratory rhythm. *Progr. Neurobiol.,* 27: 101 – 182.

Lorenz, R.G., Saper, C.B., Wong, D.L., Ciaranello, R.D. and Loewy, A.D. (1985) Co-localization of substance P and phenylethanolamine-n-methyltransferase-like immunoreactivity in neurons of ventrolateral medulla that project to the spinal cord: potential role in control of vasomotor tone. *Neurosci. Lett.,* 55: 255 – 260.

Lovick, T.A. (1987) Differential control of cardiac and vasomotor activity by neurones in nucleus paragigantocellularis lateralis in the cat. *J. Physiol. (Lond.),* 389: 23 – 35.

Lovick, T.A. and Robinson, J.P. (1983) Bulbar raphe neurones with projections to the trigeminal nucleus caudalis and the lumbar cord in the rat: A fluorescence double-labelling study. *Exp. Brain Res.,* 50: 299 – 309.

Lovick, T.A. and Wolstencroft, J.H. (1979) Inhibitory effects of nucleus raphe magnus on neuronal responses in the spinal trigeminal nucleus to nociceptive compared to non-nociceptive inputs. *Pain,* 7: 135 – 145.

Lumsden, T. (1923) Observations on the respiratory centres in the cat. *J. Physiol. (Lond.),* 57: 153 – 160.

Lundberg, A. (1975) Control of spinal mechanisms from the brain. In D.B. Tower (Ed.), *The Nervous System.* The Basic Neurosciences. New York Raven. vol.I: 253 – 265.

Luschei, E.S. (1987) Central projections of the mesencephalic nucleus of the fifth nerve: An autoradiographic study. *J. Comp. Neurol.,* 263: 137 – 145.

Lyon, M.J. (1975) Localization of the efferent neurons of the tensor tympani muscle of the newborn kitten using horseradish peroxidase. *Exp. Neurol.,* 49: 439 – 455.

Lyon, M.J. (1978) The central location of the motor neurons to the stapedius muscle in the cat. *Brain Res.,* 143: 437 – 444.

Mackel, R. (1979) Segmental and descending control of the external urethral and anal sphincters in the cat. *J. Physiol.,* 294: 105 – 123.

MacLean, P.D. (1952) Some psychiatric implications of physiological studies on frontotemporal portion of limbic system. *EEG Clin. Neurophysiol.,* 4: 407 – 418.

Mannen, T., Iwata, M., Toyokura, Y. and Nagashima, K. (1982) The Onuf's nucleus and the external anal sphincter muscles in amyotrophic lateral sclerosis and Shy-Drager Syndrome. *Acta Neuropathol.,* 58: 255 – 260.

Mantyh, P.W. (1983) Connections of midbrain periaqueductal gray in the monkey. II. Descending efferent projections. *J. Neurophysiol.,* 49: 582 – 595.

Mantyh, P.W. and Hunt, S.P. (1984) Evidence for cholecystokinin-like immunoreactive neurons in the rat medulla oblongata which project to the spinal cord. *Brain Res.,* 291: 49 – 54.

Martin, G.F., Cabana, T. and Humbertson, A.O. Jr. (1981) Evidence for collateral innervation of the cervical and lumbar enlargements of the spinal cord by single reticular and raphe neurons. Studies using fluorescent markers in double-labelling experiments on the North American opossum. *Neurosci. Lett.,* 24: 1 – 6.

Martin, G.F., Cabana, T., Humbertson, A.O. Jr., Laxson, L.C. and Panneton, W.M. (1981) Spinal projections from the medullary reticular formation of the North American Opossum: Evidence for connectional heterogeneity. *J. Comp. Neurol.,* 196: 663 – 682.

Martin, G.F. and Dom, R. (1970) Rubrobulbar projections of the opossum *(Didelphis virginiana). J. Comp. Neurol.,* 139: 199 – 214.

Martin, G.F., Dom, R., Katz, S. and King, J.S. (1974) The organization of projection neurons in the opossum red nucleus. *Brain Res.,* 78: 17 – 34.

Martin, G.F., Holstege, G. and Mehler, W.R. (1990) The reticular formation of the pons and medulla. In G. Paxinos (Ed.), *The Human Nervous System.* Academic Press pp. 203 – 220.

Martin, G.F., Humbertson, A.O. Jr., Laxson, C. and Panneton, W.M. (1979a) Evidence for direct bulbospinal projections to laminae IX, X and the intermediolateral cell column. Studies using axonal transport techniques in the North American opossum. *Brain Res.,* 170: 165 – 171.

Martin, G.F., Humbertson, A.O. Jr., Laxson, C. and Panneton, W.M. (1979b) Dorsolateral pontospinal systems. Possible routes for catecholamine modulation of nociception. *Brain Res.,* 163: 333 – 339.

Martin, G.F., Humbertson, A.O. Jr., Laxson, L.C., Panneton, W.M. and Tschismadia, I. (1979c) Spinal projections from the mesencephalic and pontine reticular formation in the North American opossum: A study using axonal transport techniques. *J. Comp. Neurol.,* 187: 373 – 401.

Martin, G.F., Vertes, R.P. and Waltzer, R. (1985) Spinal projections of the gigantocellular reticular formation in the rat. Evidence for projections from different areas to laminae I and II and lamina IX. *Exp. Brain Res.,* 58: 154 – 162.

Martin, J.H. and Ghez, C. (1988) Red nucleus and motor cortex: parallel motor systems for the initiation and control of skilled movement. *Behav. Brain Res.,* 28: 217 – 223.

Massion, J. (1988) Red nucleus: past and future. *Behav. Brain Res.,* 28: 1 – 8.

Matsushita, M. and Ueyama, T. (1973) Ventral motor nucleus of the cervical enlargement in some mammals; its specific afferents from the lower cord levels and cytoarchitecture. *J. Comp. Neurol.,* 150: 33 – 52.

McGabe, J.T., deBellis, M. and Leibowitz, S.F. (1984) Clonidine-induced feeding: Analysis of central sites of action and fiber projections mediating this response. *Brain Res.,* 309: 85 – 104.

McCall, R.B. and Aghajanian, G.K. (1979) Serotonergic facilitation of facial motoneuron excitation. *Brain Res.,* 169: 11 – 29.

McCormick, D.A., Lavond, D.G. and Thompson, R.F. (1982) Concomitant classical conditioning of the rabbit nictitating membrane and eyelid responses: correlations and implications. *Physiol. Behav.,* 28: 769 – 775.

McCue, M.P. and Guinan, Jr., J.J. (1988) Anatomical and functional segregation in the stapedius motoneuron pool of the cat. *J. Neurophysiol.,* 60: 1160 – 1180.

McCurdy, M.L., Hansma, D.I., Houk, J.C. and Gibson, A.R. (1987) Selective projections from the cat red nucleus to digit motor neurons. *J. Comp. Neurol.,* 265: 367 – 379.

McKenna, K.E. and Nadelhaft, I. (1986) The organization of the pudendal nerve in the male and female rat. *J. Comp. Neurol.,* 248: 532 – 549.

Meessen, H. and Olszewski, J. (1949) A Cytoarchitectonic Atlas of the Rhombencephalon of the Rabbit. S. Karger, Basel, New York.

Mehler, W. (1969) Some neurological species differences - A posteriori. *Ann. N.Y. Acad. Sci.* 167: 424 – 468.

Meyerson, B.A. (1988) Problems and controversies in PVG and sensory thalamic stimulation as treatment for pain. In: H.L. Fields and J.M. Besson (Eds.), *Nociception control* Progr. Brain Res. Elsevier, Amsterdam 77: 175 – 188.

Mendell, L.M. and Henneman, E. (1971) Terminals of single 1a fibers: location, density, and distribution withing a pool of 300 homonymous motoneurons. *J. Neurophysiol.,* 34: 171 – 187.

Merrill, E.G. (1974) Finding a respiratory function for the medullary respiratory neurons. In R. Bellairs and E.G. Gray (Ed.), *Essays on the Nervous System.* Clarendon, Oxford. pp. 451 – 486.

Merrill, E.G. (1970) The lateral respiratory neurones of the medulla: their associations with nucleus ambiguus, nucleus retroambigualis, the spinal accessory nucleus and the spinal cord. *Brain Res.,* 24: 11 – 28.

Merrill, E.G. and Fedorko, L. (1984) Monosynaptic inhibition of phrenic motoneurons: A long descending projection from Bötzinger neurons. *Neuroscience,* 4 no. 9: 2350 – 2353.

Merrill, E.G. and Lipski, J. (1987) Inputs to intercostal motoneurons from ventrolateral medullary respiratory neurons in the cat. *J. Neurophysiol.,* 57 no. 4: 1837 – 1853.

Merrill, E.G., Lipski, J., Kubin, L. and Fedorko, L. (1983) Origin of expiratory inhibition of nucleus tractus solitarius inspiratory neurones. *Brain Res.,* 263: 43 – 51.

Mesulam, M. (1978) Tetramethyl benzidine for horseradish peroxidase neurohistochemistry: a noncarcinogenic blue reaction-product with superior sensitivity for visualizing neural afferents and efferents. *J. Histochem. Cytochem.,* 26: 106 – 117.

Miller, A.J. (1972) Characteristics of the swallowing reflex induced by peripheral nerve and brain stem stimulation. *Exp. Neurol.,* 34: 210 – 222.

Miller, A.D. (1987) Localization of motoneurons innervating individual abdominal muscles of the cat. *J. Comp. Neurol.,* 256: 600 – 606.

Miller, A.D., Tan, L.K. and Suzuki, I. (1987) Control of abdominal and expiratory intercostal muscle activity during vomiting: role of ventral respiratory group expiratory neurons. *J. Neurophysiol.,* 57: 1854 – 1866.

Miller, R.A. and Strominger, N.L. (1973) Efferent connections of the red nucleus in the brainstem and spinal cord of the rhesus monkey. *J. Comp. Neurol.,* 152: 327 – 346.

Millhorn, D.E., Hökfelt, T., Seroogy, K. and Verhofstad, A.A.J. (1988) Extent of colocalization of serotonin and GABA in neurons of the ventral medulla oblongata in rat. *Brain Res.,* 461: 169 – 174.

Miyazaki, T., Yoshida, Y., Hirano, M., Shin, T. and Kanaseki, T. (1981) Central location of the motoneurons supplying the thyrohyoid and the geniohyoid muscles as demonstrated by horseradish peroxidase method. *Brain Res.,* 219: 423 – 427.

Mizuno, N., Konishi, A. and Sato, M. (1975) Localization of masticatory motoneurons in the cat and rat by means of retrograde axonal transport of horseradish peroxidase. *J. Comp. Neurol.,* 164: 105 – 116.

Mizuno, N., Nomura, S., Konishi, A., Uemura-Sumi, M., Takahashi, O., Yasui, Y., Takada, M. and Matsushima, R. (1982) Localization of motoneurons innervating the tensor tympani muscles: an horseradish peroxidase study in the guinea pig and cat. *Neurosci. Lett.,* 31: 205 – 208.

Mizuno, N., Yasui, Y., Nomura, S., Itoh, K., Konishi, A., Takada, M. and Kudo, M. (1983) A light and electron microscopic study of premotor neurons for the trigeminal motor nucleus. *J. Comp. Neurol.,* 215: 290 – 299.

Mizuno, N., Takahashi, O., Satoda, T. and Matsushima, R. (1985) Amygdalospinal projections in the macaque monkey. *Neurosci. Lett.,* 53: 327 – 330.

Modianos, D. and Pfaff, D.W. (1979) Medullary reticular formation lesions and lordosis reflex in female rats. *Brain Res.,* 171: 334 – 338.

Molenaar, I. (1978) The distribution of propriospinal neurons projecting to different motoneuronal cell groups in the cat's brachial cord. *Brain Res.,* 158: 203 – 206.

Molenaar, I. and Kuypers, H.G.J.M. (1978) Cells of origin of propriospinal, ascending supraspinal and medullospinal fibers. A HRP study in cat and Rhesus monkey. *Brain Res.,* 152: 429 – 450.

Molenaar, I., Rustioni, A. and Kuypers, H.G.J.M. (1974) The location of cells of origin of the fibers in the ventral and the lateral funiculus of the cat's lumbosacral cord. *Brain Res.,* 78: 239 – 254.

Moon Edley, S. and Graybiel, A.M. (1983) The afferent and efferent connections of the feline nucleus tegmenti pedunculopontine, pars compacta. *J. Comp. Neurol.,* 217: 187 – 216.

Morgan, C., De Groat, W.C. and Nadelhaft, I. (1986) The spinal distribution of sympathetic preganglionic and visceral primary afferent neurons that send axons into the hypogastric nerves of the cat. *J. Comp. Neurol.,* 243: 23 – 40.

Morgan, C., Nadelhaft, I. and De Groat, W.C. (1979) Location of bladder preganglionic neurons within the sacral parasympathetic nucleus of the cat. *Neurosci. Lett.,* 14: 189 – 195.

Mraovitch, S., Kumada, M. and Reis, D.J. (1982) Role of the nucleus parabrachialis in cardiovascular regulation in cat. *Brain Res.,* 232: 57 – 75.

Murray, H.M. and Gurule, M.E. (1979) Origin of the rubrospinal tract of the rat. *Neurosci. Lett.,* 14: 19 – 25.

Nadelhaft, I., De Groat, W.C. and Morgan, C. (1980) Location and morphology of parasympathetic preganglionic neurons in the sacral spinal cord of the cat revealed by retrograde axonal transport of horseradish peroxidase. *J. Comp. Neurol.,* 193: 265 – 281.

Nakano, K., Tokushige, A., Hasegawa, Y. and Kohno, M. (1986) An autoradiographic study of the spinofacial projection in the monkey. *Brain Res.,* 372: 338 – 344.

Nathan, P.W. and Smith, M.C. (1958) The centrifugal pathway for micturition within the spinal cord. *J. Neurol. Neurosurg. Psychiat.,* 21: 177 – 189.

Nathan, P.W. and Smith, M.C. (1982) The rubrospinal and central tegmental tracts in man. *Brain,* 105: 223 – 269.

Nauta, W.J.H. (1958) Hippocampal projections and related neural pathways to the mid-brain in the cat. *Brain,* 80: 319 – 341.

Nauta, W.J.H. and Domesick, V.B. (1981) Ramifications of the limbic system. In S. Matthysse (Ed.), *Psychiatry and the Biology of the Human Brain:* A Symposium Dedicated to Seymour S. Kety. Elsevier North Holland, Amsterdam. pp. 165 – 188.

Neafsy, E.J., Hurley-Gius, K.M. and Arvanitis, D. (1986) The topographical organization of neurons in the rat medial frontal, insular and olfactory cortex projecting to the solitary nucleus, olfactory bulb, periaqueductal gray and superior colliculus. *Brain Res.,* 377: 261 – 270.

Newsom Davis, J. (1970) An experimental study of hiccup. *Brain,* 93: 851 – 872.

Newsom Davis, J. and Plum, F. (1972) Separation of descending spinal pathways to respiratory motoneurons. *Exp. Neurol.,* 34: 78 – 94.

Nicoll, R.A. (1988) The coupling of neurotransmitter receptors to ion channels in the brain. *Science,* 241: 545 – 551.

Nieoullon, A. and Rispal-Padel, L. (1976) Somatotopic localization in cat motor cortex. *Brain Res.,* 105: 405 – 422.

Nieuwenhuys, R. (1985) Chemoarchitecture of the brain. Springer, Berlin, Heidelberg, New York, Tokyo, p. 246.

Nieuwenhuys, R., Geeraedts, L.M.G. and Veening, J. (1982) The medial forebrain bundle of the rat. I. General introduction. *J. Comp. Neurol.,* 206: 49 – 81.

Nieuwenhuys, R., Voogd, J. and Van Huijzen, C. (1988) *The Human Central Nervous System.* 3rd. revised edition, Springer, Berlin, Heidelberg, New York, Tokyo. p. 437.

Nilaver, G., Zimmerman, E.A., Wilkins, J., Michaels, J., Hoffman, D. and Silverman, A. (1980) Magnocellular hypothalamic projections to the lower brain stem and spinal cord of the rat. *Neuroendocrinology,* 30: 150 – 158.

Ninane, V., Gilmartin, J.J. and De Troyer, A. (1988) Changes in abdominal muscle length during breathing in supine dogs. *Respir. Physiol.,* 73: 31 – 41.

Nomura, S. and Mizuno, N. (1982) Central distribution of afferent and efferent components of the glossopharyngeal nerve: An HRP study in the cat. *Brain Res.,* 236: 1 – 13.

Nomura, S. and Mizuno, N. (1981) Central distribution of afferent and efferent components of the chorda tympani in the cat as revealed by horseradish peroxidase. *Brain Res.,* 214: 229 – 237.

Nosaka, S., Yamamoto, T. and Yasunaga, K. (1979) Localization of vagal cardioinhibitory preganglionic neurons within rat brain stem. *J. Comp. Neurol.,* 186: 79 – 93.

Nyberg-Hansen, R. (1965) Sites and mode of termination of reticulo-spinal fibers in the cat. An experimental study with silver impregnation methods. *J. Comp. Neurol.,* 124: 71 – 100.

Nyberg-Hansen, R. (1964) The location and termination of tectospinal fibers in the cat. *Exp. Neurol.,* 9: 212 – 227.

Nyberg-Hansen, R. (1964) Origin and termination of fibers from the vestibular nuclei and descending in the Medial Longitudinal Fasciculus. An experimental study with silver impregnation methods in the cat. *J. Comp. Neurol.,* 122: 355 – 367.

Nyberg-Hansen, R. and Brodal, A. (1964) Sites and mode of termination of rubrospinal fibres in the cat. *J. Anat. Lond.,* 98: 235 – 253.

Nyberg-Hansen, R. and Mascitti, T.A. (1964) Sites and mode of termination of fibres of the vestibulospinal tract in the cat. An experimental study with silver impregnation methods. *J. Comp. Neurol.,* 122: 369 – 387.

Nygren, L.G. and Olson, L. (1977) A new major projection from locus coeruleus: the main source of noradrenergic nerve terminals in the ventral and dorsal columns of the spinal cord. *Brain Res.,* 132: 85 – 93.

Oka, H. (1988) Functional organization of the parvocellular red nucleus in the cat. *Behav. Brain Res.,* 28: 233 – 240.

Olszewski, J. and Baxter, D. (1954) *Cytoarchitecture of the Human Brain Stem.* J.B. Lippincott Company, Switzerland.

Onai, T. and Miura, M. (1986) Projections of supraspinal structures to the phrenic motor nucleus in cats studied by a horseradish peroxidase microinjection method. *J. Auton. Nerv. Syst.,* 16: 61 – 77.

Ongerboer de Visser, B.W. and Kuypers, H.G.J.M. (1978) Late blink reflex changes in lateral medullary lesions. *Brain,* 101: 285 – 295.

Onufrowicz, B. (1899) Notes on the arrangement and function of the cell groups in the sacral region of the spinal cord. *J. Nerv. Mental Dis.,* 26: 498 – 504.

Otake, K., Sasaki, H., Ezure, K. and Manabe, M. (1988) Axonal projections from Bötzinger expiratory neurons to contralateral ventral and dorsal respiratory groups in the cat. *Exp. Brain Res.,* 72: 167 – 177.

Panneton, W.M. and Burton, H. (1981) Corneal and periocular representation within the trigeminal sensory complex in the cat studied with transganglionic transport of horseradish peroxidase. *J. Comp. Neurol.,* 199: 327 – 344.

Panneton, W.M. and Martin, G.F. (1983) Brainstem projections to the facial nucleus of the opossum. *Brain Res.,* 267: 19 – 33.

Papez, J.W. (1927) Subdivisions of the facial nucleus. *J. Comp. Neurol.,* 43: 159 – 191.

Paxinos, G. and Watson, C. (1986) *The Rat Brain in Stereotaxic Coordinates* (Second Edition) Academic Press, San Diego.

Pelletier, G., Steinbusch, H.W.M. and Verhofstad, A.A.J. (1981) Immunoreactive substance P and serotonin present in the same dense core vesicles. *Nature,* 293: 71 – 72.

Peterson, B.W. (1979) Reticulospinal projections to spinal motor nuclei. *Ann. Rev. Physiol.,* 41: 127 – 140.

Peterson, B.W. (1980) Participation of pontomedullary reticular neurons in specific motor activity. In J.A. Hobson and M.A.B. Brazier (Eds.), *The Reticular Formation Revisited.* Raven Press, New York, pp. 171 – 192.

Peterson, B.W., Fukushima, K., Hirai, N., Schor, R.H. and Wilson, V.J. (1984) Responses of vestibulospinal and reticulospinal neurons to sinusoidal vestibular stimulation. *J. Neurophysiol.,* 43: 1236 – 1251.

Peterson, B.W., Pitts, N.G., Fukushima, K. and Mackel, R. (1978) Reticulospinal excitation and inhibition of neck motoneurons. *Exp. Brain Res.,* 32: 471 – 489.

Peterson, B.W., Pitts, N.G. and Fukushima, K. (1979) Reticulospinal connections with limb and axial motoneurons. *Exp. Brain Res.,* 36: 1 – 20.

Petras, J.M. (1967) Cortical, tectal and tegmental fiber connections in the spinal cord of the cat. *Brain Res.,* 6: 275 – 324.

Pfaff, D.W. (1980) *Estrogens and brain function.* Neuronal analysis of a hormone-controlled mammalian reproductive behavior. Springer-Verlag, New York, Heidelberg, Berlin. pp. 281.

Pfaff, D.W. and Sakuma, Y. (1979) Deficit in the lordosis reflex of female rats caused by lesions in the ventromedial nucleus of the hypothalamus. *J. Physiol.,* 288: 203 – 211.

Pfaff, D.W. and Sakuma, Y. (1979) Facilitation of the lordosis reflex of female rats from the ventromedial nucleus of the hypothalamus. *J. Physiol.,* 288: 189 – 203.

Pfaller, K. and Arvidsson, J. (1988) Central distribution of trigeminal and upper cervical primary afferents in the rat studied by anterograde transport of horseradish peroxidase conjugated to wheat germ agglutinin. *J. Comp. Neurol.,* 268: 91 – 108.

Plecha, D.M., Randall, W.C., Geis, G.S. and Wurtser, R.D. (1988) Localization of vagal preganglionic somata controlling sinoatrial and atrioventricular nodes. *Am. J. Physiol.,* 255: R703 – 708.

Poeck, K. (1969) Pathophysiology of emotional disorders associated with brain damage. In P.J. Vinken and G.W. Bruyn (Eds.), *Handbook of clinical neurology (Vol. 3)* North-Holland, Amsterdam. pp. 343 – 367.

Pompeiano, O. and Brodal, A. (1957) Experimental demonstration of a somatotopical origin of rubrospinal fibers in the cat. *J. Comp. Neurol.,* 108: 225 – 252.

Price, J.L. and Amaral, D.G. (1981) An autoradiographic study of the projections of the central nucleus of the monkey amygdala. *J. Neurosci.,* 1 no. 11: 1242 – 1259.

Price, J.L., Russchen, F.T. and Amaral, D.G. (1987) The limbic region. II. The amygdaloid complex. In A., Björklund, T., Hökfelt, L.W. Swanson (Eds.), *Handbook of Chemical Neuroanatomy.* Vol. 5. Integrated Systems of the CNS. Part I Hypothalamus, Hippocampus, Amygdala, Retina. Elsevier Science Publishers, Amsterdam. pp. 279 – 388.

Provis, J. (1977) The organization of the facial nucleus of the brush-tailed possum (Trichosurus vulpecula). *J. Comp. Neurol.,* 172: 177 – 188.

Pullen, A.H. (1988) Quantitative synaptology of feline motoneurones to external anal sphincter muscle. *J. Comp. Neurol.,* 269: 414 – 424.

Ralston, D.D. and Ralston, H.J. III (1985) The terminations of corticospinal tract axons in the macaque monkey. *J. Comp. Neurol.,* 242: 325 – 337.

Ralston, D.D., Milroy, A.M. and Holstege, G. (1988) Ultrastructural evidence for direct monosynaptic rubrospinal connections to motoneurons in *Macaca mulatta. Neurosci. Lett.,* 95: 102 – 106.

Raphan, T. and Cohen, B. (1978) Brain stem mechanisms for rapid and slow eye movements. *Annu. Rev. Physiol.,* 40: 527 – 552.

Rexed, B. (1952) The cytoarchitectonic organization of the spinal cord in the cat. *J. Comp. Neurol.,* 96: 415 – 496.

Rexed, B. (1954) A cytoarchitectonic atlas of the spinal cord in the cat. *J. Comp. Neurol.,* 100: 297 – 380.

Ricardo, J.A. and Koh, E.T. (1978) Anatomical evidence of

direct projections from the nucleus of the solitary tract to the hypothalamus, amygdala, and other forebrain structures in the rat. *Brain Res.,* 153: 1 – 26.

Richmond, F.J.R. and Abrahams, V.C. (1975) Morphology and enzyme histochemistry of dorsal muscles of the cat neck. 1312 – 1321.

Richmond, F.J.R., Loeb, G.E. and Reesor, D. (1985) Electromyographic activity in neck muscles during head movements in the alert, unrestrained cat. *Soc. Neurosci. Abstr.,* 11: 83.

Richmond F.J.R., MacGillis, D.R.R. and Scott, D.A. (1985) Muscle-fiber compartmentalization in cat splenius muscles. *J. Neurophysiol.,* 53: 868 – 885.

Rikard-Bell, G.C., Bystrzycka, E.K. and Nail, B.S. (1984) Brainstem projections to the phrenic nucleus: a HRP study in the cat. *Brain Res. Bull.,* 12: 469 – 477.

Rinn, W.E. (1984) The neurophysiology of facial expression: a review of the neurological and psychological mechanisms for producing facial expressions. *Psychol. Bull.,* 95: 52 – 77.

Robinson, D.A. (1972) Eye movements evoked by collicular stimulation in the alert monkey. *Vision Res.,* 12: 1795 – 1808.

Robinson, F.R., Houk, J.C. and Gibson, A.R. (1987) Limb specific connections of the cat magnocellular red nucleus. *J. Comp. Neurol.,* 257: 553 – 577.

Romanes, G.J. (1951) The motor cell columns of the lumbosacral spinal cord of the cat. *J. Comp. Neurol.,* 94: 313 – 363.

Roppolo, J.R., Nadelhaft, I. and de Groat, W.C. (1985) The organization of pudendal motoneurons and primary afferent projections in the spinal cord of the rhesus monkey revealed by horseradish peroxidase. *J. Comp. Neurol.,* 234: 475 – 488.

Rose, J.D. and Flynn, F.W. (1989) Lordosis can be elicited in chronically-decerebrate rats by combined lumbosacral and vagino-cervical stimulation. *Soc. Neurosci. Abstr.,* 15: p. 1100.

Rosenfield, M.E. and Moore, J.W. (1983) Red nucleus lesions disrupt the classically conditioned nictitating membrane response in rabbits. *Behav. Brain Res.,* 10: 393 – 398.

Ross, C.A., Ruggiero, D.A., Park, D.H., Joh, T.H., Sved, A.F., Fernandez-Pardal, J., Saavedra, J.M. and Reis, D.J. (1984) Tonic vasomotor control by the rostral ventrolateral medulla: effect of electrical or chemical stimulation of the area containing C1 adrenaline neurons on arterial pressure, heart rate and plasma catecholamines and vasopressin. *J. Neurosci.,* 4: 474 – 494.

Røste, G.K. (1989) Non-motoneurons in the facial and motor trigeminal nuclei projecting to the cerebellar flocculus in the cat. A fluorescent double-labelling and WGA-HRP study. *Exp. Brain Res.,* 75: 295 – 305.

Roucoux, A., Guitton, D. and Crommelinck, M. (1980) Stimulation of the superior colliculus in the alert cat II. Eye and head movements evoked when the head is unrestrained. *Exp. Brain Res.,* 39: 75 – 85.

Roucoux, A., Crommelinck, M., Decostre, M.F. and Crémieux, J. (1985) Gaze shift related neck muscle activity in trained cats. *Soc. Neurosci. Abstr.,* 11: 83.

Rubin, E. and Purves, D. (1980) Segmental organization of sympathetic preganglionic neurons in the mammalian spinal cord. *J. Comp. Neurol.,* 192: 163 – 175.

Ruggiero, D.A., Mraovitch, S., Granata, A.R., Anwar, M. and Reis, D.J. (1987) A role of insular cortex in cardiovascular function. *J. Comp. Neurol.,* 257: 189 – 207.

Russchen, F.T. (1982) Amygdalopetal projections in the cat: II. Subcortical afferent connections. A study with retrograde tracing techniques. *J. Comp. Neurol.,* 207: 157 – 176.

Rustioni, A., Kuypers, H.G.J.M. and Holstege, G. (1971) Propriospinal projections from the ventral and lateral funiculi to the motoneurons in the lumbosacral cord of the cat. *Brain Res.,* 34: 255 – 275.

Saint-Cyr, J.A. and Courville, J. (1982) Descending projections to the inferior olive from the mesencephalon and superior colliculus in the cat. *Exp. Brain Res.,* 45: 333 – 348.

Sakuma, Y. and Pfaff, D.W. (1979) Mesencephalic mechanisms for integration of female reproductive behavior in the rat. *Am. J. Physiol.,* 237: R285 – R290.

Sakuma, Y. and Pfaff, D.W. (1979) Facilitation of female reproductive behavior from mesencephalic central gray in the rat. *Am. J. Physiol.,* 237: R278 – R284.

Sandkuhler, J. and Gebhart, G.F. (1984) Characterization of inhibition of a spinal nociceptive reflex by stimulation medially and laterally in the midbrain and medulla in the pentobarbital-anesthetized rat. *Brain Res.,* 305: 67 – 76.

Sandrew, B.B., Edwards, D.L., Poletti, C.E. and Foote, W.E. (1986) Amygdalospinal Projections in the Cat. *Brain Res.,* 373: 235 – 239.

Saper, C.B. and Levisohn, D. (1983) Afferent connections of the median preoptic nucleus in the rat: Anatomical evidence for a cardiovascular integrative mechanism in the anteroventral third ventricular (AV3V) region. *Brain Res.,* 288: 21 – 31.

Saper, C.B., Loewy, A.D., Swanson, L.W. and Cowan, W.M. (1976) Direct hypothalamo-autonomic connections. *Brain Res.,* 117: 305 – 312.

Saper, C.B. and Loewy, A.D. (1980) Efferent connections of the parabrachial nucleus in the rat. *Brain Res.,* 197: 291 – 317.

Sato, M., Mizuno, N. and Konishi, A. (1978) Localization of motoneurons innervating perineal muscles: a HRP study in cat. *Brain Res.,* 140: 149 – 154.

Satoda, T., Takahashi, O., Tashiro, T., Matsushima, R., Uemura-Sumi, M. and Mizuno, N. (1987) Representation of the main branches of the facial nerve within the facial nucleus of the Japanese monkey (Macaca fuscata). *Neurosci. Lett.,* 78: 283 – 287.

Sawchenko, P.E., Gold, R.M. and Leibowitz, S.F. (1981) Evidence for vagal involvement in the eating elicited by adrenergic stimulation of the paraventricular nucleus. *Brain Res.,* 225: 249 – 269.

Sawchenko, P.E. and Swanson, L.W. (1982) Immunohistochemical identification of neurons in the paraventricular nucleus of the hypothalamus that project to the medulla or to the spinal cord in the rat. *J. Comp. Neurol.,* 205: 260 – 272.

Schmied, A., Amalric, M., Dormont, J.F., Conde, H. and Farin, D. (1988) Participation of the red nucleus in motor initiation: unit recording and cooling in cats. *Behav. Brain Res.,* 28: 207 – 216.

Schoen, J.H.R. (1964) Comparative aspects of the descending fibre systems in the spinal cord. In J.C. Eccles and J.P. Schadé, (Eds.), *Organization of the Spinal Cord, Progr. Brain Res.,* 11: 203 – 222.

Schomburg, E.D., Meinck, H.-M, and Haustein, J. (1975) A fast propriospinal inhibitory pathway from forelimb afferents to motoneurones of hindlimb flexor digitorum longus. *Neurosci. Lett.,* 1: 311 – 314.

Schrϕder, H.D. (1981) Onuf's nucleus X: A morphological study of a human spinal nucleus. *Anat. Embrol.,* 162: 443 – 453.

Schrϕder, H.D. (1980) Organization of the motoneurons innervating the pelvic muscles of the rat. *J. Comp. Neurol.,* 192: 567 – 587.

Schwaber, J.S., Knapp, B.S. and Higgins, G. (1980) The origin and extent of direct amygdala projections to the region of the dorsal motor nucleus of the vagus and the nucleus of the solitary tract. *Neurosci. Lett.,* 20: 15 – 21.

Sears, T.A., Kirkwood, P.A. and Davies, J.G. McF. (1985) Cross-correlation analysis of connections between bulbospinal neurones and respiratory motoneurones. In A.L. Bianchi and M. Denavit-Saubie (Eds.), Neurogenesis of Central Respiratory Rhytm. MTP Press Limited Lancaster. 216 – 222.

Sessle, B.J., Hu, J.W., Dubner, R. and Lucier, G.E. (1981) Functional properties of neurons in cat trigeminal subnucleus caudalis (medullary dorsal horn) II: Modulation of responses to noxious and nonnoxious stimuli by periaqueductal gray, nucleus raphe manus, cerebral cortex and afferent influences and effect of naloxone. *J. Neurophysiol.,* 45: 193 – 207.

Shahani, B.T. and Young, R.R. (1972) Human orbicularis oculi reflexes. *Neurology (Minneap.),* 22: 149 – 154.

Shapovalov, A.I. and Karamyan, O.A. (1968) Short-latency interstitiospinal and rubrospinal synaptic influences on alpha-motoneurons. *Bull. Eksp. Biol. Med.,* 66: 1297 – 1300.

Shapovalov, A.I., Karamyan, O.A., Kurchavyi, G.G. and Repina, Z.A. (1971) Synaptic actions evoked from the red nucleus on the spinal alpha-motoneurons in the rhesus monkey. *Brain Res.,* 32: 325 – 348.

Shapovalov, A.I. and Kurchavyi, G.G. (1974) Effects of transmembrane polarization and TEA injection on monosynaptic actions from motor cortex, red nucleus and group Ia afferents on lumbar motoneurons in the monkey. *Brain Res.,* 82: 49 – 67.

Shaw, M.D. and Baker, R. (1983) The locations of stapedius and tensor tympani motoneurons in the cat. *J. Comp. Neurol.,* 216: 10 – 19.

Sherrey, J.H. and Megirian, D. (1975) Analysis of the respiratory role of pharyngeal constrictor motoneurons in the cat. *Exp. Neurol.,* 49: 839 – 851.

Shigenaga, Y., Chen, I.C., Suemune, S., Nishimori, T., Nasution, I.D., Yoshida, A., Sato, H., Okamoto, T., Sera, M. and Hosoi, M. (1986) Oral and facial representation within the medullary and upper cervical dorsal horns in the cat. *J. Comp. Neurol.,* 243: 388 – 408.

Shigenaga, Y., Yoshida, A., Mitsuhiro, Y., Doe, K. and Suemune, S. (1988) Morphology of single mesencephalic trigeminal neurons innervating periodontal ligament of the cat. *Brain Res.,* 448: 331 – 8.

Shik, M.L. (1983) Action of the brain stem locomotor region on spinal stepping generators via propriospinal pathways. In C.C. Kao, R.P. Bunge and P.J. Reier. (Eds.), *Spinal Cord Reconstruction.* Raven Press, New York. pp. 421 – 434.

Shik, M.L., Severin, F.V. and Orlovski, G.N. (1966) Control of walking and running by means of electrical stimulation of the mid-brain. *Biophysics,* 11: 756 – 765.

Shohara, E. and Sakai, A. (1983) Localization of motoneurons innervating deep and superficial facial muscles in the rat: A horseradish peroxidase and electrophysiologic study. *Exp. Neurol.,* 81: 14 – 33.

Sica, A.L., Cohen, M.I., Connelly, D.F. and Zhang, H. (1984) Hypoglossal motoneuron responses to pulmonary and superior laryngeal afferent inputs. *Respir. Physiol.,* 56: 339 – 357.

Simon, O.R. and Schramm, L.P. (1983) Spinal superfusion of dopamine excites renal sympathetic nerve activity. *Neuropharmacology,* 22: 287 – 293.

Sirkin, D.W. and Feng, A.S. (1987) Autoradiographic study of descending pathways from the pontine reticular formation and the mesencephalic trigeminal nucleus in the rat. *J. Comp. Neurol.,* 256: 483 – 493.

Sirota, M.G. and Shik, M.L. (1973) The cat locomotion elicited through the electrode implanted in the midbrain. *Sechenov Physiol. J. (Leningrad),* 59: 1314 – 1321.

Skagerberg, G., Bjϕrklund, A., Lindvall, O. and Schmidt, R.H. (1982) Origin and termination of the diencephalo-spinal dopamine system in the rat. *Brain Res. Bull.,* 9: 237 – 244.

Skagerberg, G. and Lindvall, O. (1985) Organization of diencephalic dopamine neurones projecting to the spinal cord in the rat. *Brain Res.,* 342: 340 – 351.

Smith, C.L. and Hollyday, M. (1983) The development and postnatal organization of motor nuclei in the rat thoracic spinal cord. *J. Comp. Neurol.,* 220: 16 – 28.

Spence, S.J. and Saint-Cyr, J.A. (1988) Comparative topography of projections from the mesodiencephalic junctions to the inferior olive, vestibular nuclei, and upper cervical cord in the cat. *J. Comp. Neurol.,* 268: 357 – 374.

Spencer, R.F., Baker, R. and McCrea, R.A. (1980) Localization and morphology of cat retractor bulbi motoneurons. *J. Neurophysiol.,* 43: 754 – 771.

Sprague, J.M. (1948) A study of motor cell localization in the spinal cord of the rhesus monkey. *Am. J. Anat.,* 82: 1 – 26.

Steinbusch, H.W.M. (1981) Distribution of serotonin-immunoreactivity in the central nervous system of the rat: cell-bodies and terminals. *Neuroscience,* 6 no. 4: 557 – 618.

Sterling, P. and Kuypers, H.G.J.M. (1967) Anatomical organization of the brachial spinal cord of the cat. II. The motoneuron plexus. *Brain Res.,* 4: 16 – 32.

Sterling, P. and Kuypers, H.G.J.M. (1968) Anatomical organization of the brachial spinal cord of the cat. III. The propriospinal connections. *Brain Res.,* 7: 419 – 443.

Stock, G., Rupprecht, U., Stumpf, H. and Schlör, K.H. (1981) Cardiovascular changes during arousal elicited by stimulation of amygdala, hypothalamus and locus coeruleus. *J. Auton. Nerv. Syst.,* 3: 503 – 510.

Strack, A.M., Sawyer, W.B., Marubio, L.M. and Loewy, A.D. (1988) Spinal origin of sympathetic preganglionic neurons in the rat. *Brain Res.,* 455: 187 – 191.

Strack, A.M., Sawyer, W.B., Hughes, J.H., Platt, K.B. and Loewy, A.D. (1989) A general pattern of CNS innervation of the sympathetic outflow demonstrated by transneuronal pseudorabies viral infections. *Brain Res.,* 491: 156 – 162f.

Strassman, A., Mason, P., Eckenstein, F., Baughman, R.W. and Maciewicz, R. (1987) Choline acetyltransferase immunocytochemistry of Edinger-Westphal and ciliary ganglion afferent neurons in the cat. *Brain Res.,* 423: 293 – 304.

Stuart, D.G., Kawamura, Y. and Hemingway, A. (1961) Activation and suppression of shivering during septal and hypothalamic stimulation. *Exp. Neurol.,* 4: 485 – 506.

Swanson, L.W. (1977) Immunohistochemical evidence for a neurophysin-containing autonomic pathway arising in the paraventricular nucleus of the hypothalamus. *Brain Res.,* 128: 346 – 353.

Swanson, L.W. and Kuypers, H.G.J.M. (1980) The paraventricular nucleus of the hypothalamus: cytoarchitectonic subdivisions and organization of projections to the pituitary, dorsal vagal complex, and spinal cord as demonstrated by retrograde fluorescence double labeling methods. *J. Comp. Neurol.,* 194: 555 – 570.

Swanson, L.W. and Sawchenko, P.E. (1983) Hypothalamic integration. Organization of the paraventricular and supraoptic nuclei. *Ann. Rev. Neurosci.,* 6: 269 – 324.

Taber-Pierce, E., Lichtenstein, E. and Feldman, S.C. (1985) The somatostatin systems of the guinea-pig brainstem. *Neuroscience,* 15: 215 – 235.

Takeuchi, Y., Nakano, K., Uemura, M., Matsuda, K., Matsushima, R. and Mizuno, N. (1979) Mesencephalic and pontine afferent fiber system to the facial nucleus in the cat: a study using the horseradish peroxidase and silver impregnation techniques. *Exp. Neurol.,* 66: 330 – 343.

Tan, J. and Holstege, G. (1986) Anatomical evidence that the pontine lateral tegmental field projects to lamina I of the caudal spinal trigeminal nucleus and spinal cord and to the Edinger-Westphal nucleus in the cat. *Neurosci. Lett.,* 64: 317 – 322.

Tashiro, N., Tanaka, T., Fukumoto, T., Hirata, K. and Nakao, H. (1985) Emotional behavior and arrhytmias induced in cats by hypothalamic stimulation. *Life Science,* 36: 1087 – 1094.

Terreberry, R.R. and Neafsey, E.J. (1987) The rat medial frontal cortex projects directly to autonomic regions of the brainstem. *Brain Res. Bull.,* 19: 639 – 649.

Theriault, E. and Diamond, J. (1988) Intrinsic organization of the rat cutaneus trunci motor nucleus. *J. Neurophysiol.,* 60: 463 – 477.

Thompson, G.C., Igarashi, M. and Stach, B.A. (1985) Identification of stapedius muscle motoneurons in squirrel monkey and bush baby. *J. Comp. Neurol.,* 231: 270 – 279.

Tohyama, M., Sakai, K., Salvert, D., Touret, M. and Jouvet, M. (1979) Spinal projections from the lower brain stem in the cat as demonstrated by the horseradish peroxidase technique. I. Origins of the reticulospinal tracts and their funicular trajectories. *Brain Res.,* 173: 383 – 405.

Toyoshima, K., Kawana, E. and Sakai, H. (1980) On the neuronal origin of the afferents to the ciliary ganglion in cat. *Brain Res.,* 185: 67 – 76.

Tramonte, R. and Bauer, J. (1986) The location of the preganglionic neurons that innervate the submandibular gland of the cat. A horseradish peroxidase study. *Brain Res.,* 375: 381 – 384.

Travers, J.B. and Norgren, R. (1983) Afferent projections to the oral motor nuclei in the rat. *J. Comp. Neurol.,* 220: 280 – 298.

Tsukahara, N. (1981) Classical conditioning mediated by the red nucleus in the cat. *J. Neurosci.,* 1: 72 – 79.

Uemura, M., Matsuda, K., Kume, M., Takeuchi, Y., Matsushima, R. and Mizuno, N. (1979) Topographical arrangement of hypoglossal motoneurons: An HRP study in the cat. *Neurosci. Lett.,* 13: 99 – 104.

Ueyama, T., Mizuno, N., Nomura, S., Konishi, A., Itoh, K. and Arakawa, H. (1984) Central distribution of afferent and efferent components of the pudendal nerve in cat. *J. Comp. Neurol.,* 222: 38 – 46.

Ulfhake, B., Arvidsson, U., Cullheim, S., Hokfelt, T., Brodin, E., Verhofstad, A. and Visser, T. (1987) An ultrastructural study of 5-hydroxytryptamine-, thyrotropin-releasing hormone- and substance P- immunoreactive axonal boutons in the motor nucleus of spinal cord segments L7-S1 in the adult cat. *Neuroscience,* 23: 917 – 929.

Van der Kooy, D., Koda, L.Y., McGinty, J.F., Gerfen, C.R. and Bloom, F.E. (1984) The organization of projections from the cortex, amygdala, and hypothalamus to the nucleus of the solitary tract in rat. *J. Comp. Neurol.,* 224: 1 – 24.

VanderMaelen, C.P. and Aghajanian, G.K. (1982) Serotonin-induced depolarization of rat facial motoneurons in vivo: comparison with amino acid transmitters. *Brain Res.*, 239: 139 – 152.

de Vries, G.J. and Buijs, R.M. (1983) The origin of the vasopressinergic and oxytocinergic innervation of the rat with special reference to the lateral septum. *Brain Res.*, 273: 307 – 317.

Weaver, Fr C. (1980) Localization of parasympathetic preganglionic cell bodies innervating the pancreas within the vagal nucleus and nucleus ambiguus of the rat brain stem: evidence of dual innervation based on the retrograde axonal transport of horseradish peroxidase. *J. Auton. Nerv. Syst.*, 2: 61 – 71.

Wessendorf, M.W. and Elde, R. (1987) The coexistence of serotonin- and substance P-like immunoreactivity in the spinal cord of the rat as shown by immunofluorescent double labeling. *J. Neuroscience,* 7: 2352 – 2363.

Westlund, K.N. and Coulter, J.D. (1980) Descending projections of the locus coerculeus and subcoeruleus/medial parabrachial nuclei in monkey: axonal transport studies and dopamine-β-hydroxylase immunocytochemistry. *Brain Res. Rev.*, 2: 235 – 264.

Westman, J. (1968) The lateral cervical nucleus in the cat. I. A Golgi study. *Brain Res.*, 10: 352 – 368.

White, S.R. and Neuman, R.S. (1980) Facilitation of spinal motoneurone excitability by 5-hydroxytryptamine and noradrenaline. *Brain Res.*, 188: 119 – 127.

Wiklund, L., Léger, L. and Persson, M. (1981) Monoamine cell distribution in the cat brain stem. A fluorescence histoschemical study with quantification of indolaminergic and locus coeruleus cell groups. *J. Comp. Neurol.*, 203: 613 – 647.

Willett, C.J., Gwyn, D.G., Rutherford, J.G. and Leslie, R.A. (1986) Cortical projections to the nucleus of the tractus solitarius: An HRP study in the cat. *Brain Res. Bull.*, 16: 497 – 505.

Willis, W.D. (1988) Anatomy and physiology of descending control of nociceptive responses of dorsal horn neurons: comprehensive review. In H.L. Fields and J.M. Besson (Eds.), *Pain Modulation* Progr. Brain Res., Elsevier Amsterdam 77: 1 – 29.

Willis, W.D., Haber, L.H. and Martin, R.F. (1977) Inhibition of spinothalamic tract cells and interneurons by brain stem stimulation in the monkey. *J. Neurophysiol.*, 40: 968 – 982.

Wilson, V.J. and Yoshida, M. (1969) Comparison of effects of stimulation of Deiters' nucleus and medial longitudinal fasciculus on neck, forelimb, and hindlimb motoneurons. *J. Neurophysiol.*, 32: 743 – 758.

Wilson, V.J. and Yoshida, M. (1969) Monosynaptic inhibition of neck motoneurons by the medial vestibular nucleus. *Exp. Brain Res.*, 9: 365 – 380.

Wilson, V.J., Yoshida, M. and Schor, R.H. (1970) Supraspinal monosynaptic excitation and inhibition of thoracic back motoneurons. *Exp. Brain Res.*, 11: 282 – 295.

Yamada, H., Ezure, K. and Manabe, M. (1988) Efferent projections of inspiratory neurons of the ventral respiratory group. A dual labeling study in the rat. *Brain Res.*, 455: 283 – 294.

Yeo, C.H., Hardiman, M.J. and Glickstein, M. (1985) Classical conditioning of the nictitating membrane response of the rabbit: I. Lesions of the cerebellar nuclei. *Exp. Brain Res.*, 60: 87 – 98.

Yeo, C.H., Hardiman, M.J. and Glickstein, M. (1985) Classical conditioning of the nictitating membrane response of the rabbit: III. Connections of cerebellar lobule HVI. *Exp. Brain Res.*, 60: 114 – 126.

Yeo, C.H., Hardiman, M.J. and Glickstein, M. (1986) Classical conditioning of the nictitating membrane response of the rabbit: IV. Lesions of the inferior olive. *Exp. Brain Res.*, 63: 81 – 92.

Yoshida, M. and Tanaka, M. (1988) Existence of new dopaminergic terminal plexus in the rat spinal cord: assessment by immunohistochemistry using anti-dopamine serum. *Neurosci. Lett.*, 94: 5 – 9.

Yoshida, Y., Miyazaki, O., Hirano, M., Shin, T., Totoki, T, and Kanaseki, T. (1981) Localization of efferent neurons innervating the pharyngeal constrictor muscles and the cervical esophagus muscle in the cat by means of the horseradish peroxidase method. *Neurosci. Lett.*, 22: 91 – 95.

Zuk, A., Rutherford, J.G. and Gwyn, D.G. (1983) Projections from the interstitial nucleus of Cajal to the inferior olive and to the spinal cord in cat: a retrograde fluorescent double-labeling study. *Neurosci. Lett.*, 38: 95 – 103.

Subject Index